Introduction to Health Care Delivery

A Primer for Pharmacists

FOURTH EDITION

Robert L. McCarthy, PhD
Dean and Professor
School of Pharmacy
University of Connecticut
Storrs, Connecticut

Kenneth W. Schafermeyer, PhD
Professor and Director of Graduate Studies
St. Louis College of Pharmacy
St. Louis, Missouri

JONES AND BARTLETT PUBLISHERS
Sudbury, Massachusetts
BOSTON   TORONTO   LONDON   SINGAPORE

World Headquarters

Jones and Bartlett Publishers
40 Tall Pine Drive
Sudbury, MA 01776
978-443-5000
info@jbpub.com
www.jbpub.com

Jones and Bartlett Publishers
Canada
6339 Ormindale Way
Mississauga, Ontario L5V 1J2
Canada

Jones and Bartlett Publishers
International
Barb House, Barb Mews
London W6 7PA
United Kingdom

Jones and Bartlett's books and products are available through most bookstores and online booksellers. To contact Jones and Bartlett Publishers directly, call 800-832-0034, fax 978-443-8000, or visit our website www.jbpub.com.

This publication is designed to provide accurate and authoritative information in regard to the Subject Matter covered. It is sold with the understanding that the publisher is not engaged in rendering legal, accounting, or other professional service. If legal advice or other expert assistance is required, the service of a competent professional person should be sought.

Production Credits
Executive Editor: David Cella
Production Director: Amy Rose
Editorial Assistant: Lisa Gordon
Associate Production Editor: Jamie Chase
Marketing Manager: Jennifer Bengston
Manufacturing and Inventory Coordinator: Amy Bacus
Composition: Shawn Girsberger
Cover Design: Kate Ternullo
Cover Image: © Image100/Alamy Image
Cover Image © Obvious/ShutterStock, Inc
Cover Image © Bluestocking/ShutterStock, Inc.
Cover Image © Agb/ShutterStock, Inc.
Printing and Binding: Malloy, Inc.
Cover Printing: Malloy, Inc.

Library of Congress Cataloging-in-Publication Data
Introduction to health care delivery : a primer for pharmacists / [edited by] Robert L. McCarthy, Kenneth W. Schafermeyer. -- 4th ed.
    p. ; cm.
   Includes index.
   Includes bibliographical references and index.
   ISBN-13: 978-0-7637-4353-6
   ISBN-10: 0-7637-4353-4
  1. Medical care--United States. 2. Pharmaceutical services--United States. I. McCarthy, Robert L. II. Schafermeyer, Kenneth W.
  [DNLM: 1. Delivery of Health Care--United States. 2. Drug Industry--United States. 3. Economics, Pharmaceutical--United States. 4. Pharmaceutical Services--United States. W 84 AA1 I88 2007]
   RA395.A3I567 2007
   362.1'0973--dc22
                        2006035596

6048
Printed in the United States of America
11 10 09 08   10 9 8 7 6 5 4 3

To over two decades of extraordinary students
whom I have been privileged to teach
at three colleges of pharmacy.

Robert L. McCarthy

To Wowie and all of my students
from the St. Louis College of Pharmacy.

Kenneth W. Schafermeyer

Contents

Chapter 18—Pharmacoeconomics
Emily R. Cox and Kenneth W. Schafermeyer

Chapter 19—International Health Care Services
Ana C. Quiñones and Linda E. Barry Dunn

Contributors

Emily R. Cox, RPh, PhD
Senior Director, Research
Express Scripts, Inc.
Maryland Heights, MO

Shane P. Desselle, PhD, FAPhA
Professor
Pharmacy Administration
Duquesne University
Mylan School of Pharmacy
Bayer Learning Center
Pittsburgh, PA

Ernest J. Dole, PharmD
Coordinator, Clinical Pharmacy
  Services
Lovelace Sandia Health System
Clinical Associate Professor
College of Pharmacy
University of New Mexico Health
  Sciences Center
Albuquerque, NM

Linda E. Barry Dunn, MPP
Associate Professor
Social, Behavioral, and Adminis-
  trative Sciences
Touro University
College of Pharmacy
Vallejo, CA

Dana P. Hammer, PhD, MS
Director, Bracken Pharmaceutical
  Care Learning Center and Teach-
  ing Certificate
Programs in Pharmacy Education
University of Washington
School of Pharmacy
Seattle, WA

Ardis Hanson, MLS
Library Director
Louis de la Parte Florida Mental
  Health Institute
University of South Florida
Tampa, FL

Edward Krupat, PhD
Associate Professor of Psychology
Director of Evaluation
Harvard Medical School
Center for Evaluation
Boston, MA

**Bruce Lubotsky Levin, DrPH,
  MPH**
Associate Professor and Head
Graduate Studies in Behavioral
  Health
Editor-in-Chief
Journal of Behavioral Health Ser-
  vices and Research
De la Parte Institute and College of
  Public Health
University of South Florida
Tampa, FL

Earlene E. Lipowski, PhD
Associate Professor
College of Pharmacy
Pharmacy Health Care Administra-
  tion
University of Florida
Gainesville, FL

William W. McCloskey, PharmD
Associate Professor
Pharmacy Practice
Massachusetts College of Pharmacy
and Health Sciences
Boston, MA

Helen Meldrum, EdD, MEd
Associate Professor
Psychology
Bentley College
Waltham, MA

Kristin B. Meyer, PharmD, CGP
Assistant Professor
Pharmacy Practice
Drake University
Des Moines, IA

Michael Montagne, PhD
Professor of Social Pharmacy
Acting Associate Dean of Graduate
Studies
Interim Chair, Department of
Pharmaceutical Sciences
School of Pharmacy
Massachusetts College of Pharmacy
and Health Sciences
Boston, MA

Catherine N. Otto, PhD, MBA
Associate Professor and Clinical
Coordinator
Clinical Laboratory Science
Oregon Health and Science University
Oregon Institute of Technology
Portland, OR

Craig A. Pedersen, PhD
Associate Professor
Director of Graduate Studies
Division of Pharmacy Practice and
Administration
College of Pharmacy
Ohio State University
Columbus, OH

Kimberly S. Plake, PhD, RPh
Assistant Professor of Pharmacy
Practice
School of Pharmacy and Pharma-
ceutical Sciences
Purdue University
West Lafayette, IN

Ana C. Quiñones, PhD, MS
Assistant Professor
Pharmacy Administration
Midwestern University
Chicago College of Pharmacy
Downers Grove, IL

Alice M. Sapienza, MS, MBA, DBA
Professor of Healthcare Adminis-
tration
School for Health Studies
Simmons College
Boston, MA

David M. Scott, PhD, MPH
Associate Professor
College of Pharmacy
North Dakota State University
Fargo, ND

Peter L. Steere, MBA
Associate Director
University Health Services
Yale University
New Haven, CT

Jennifer L. Tebbe-Grossman, PhD, MA
Professor of Political Science and
    American Studies
School of Arts and Sciences
Massachusetts College of Pharmacy
    and Health Sciences
Boston, MA

Alan P. Wolfgang, MS, PhD
Associate Professor
University of Georgia
College of Pharmacy
Athens, GA

Preface

Before embarking on the Fourth Edition, we surveyed instructors who use this book in courses at pharmacy schools throughout the country and incorporated their suggestions to make this text more useful for pharmacy students and their instructors. Based on the suggestions received, we have made several significant changes to the fourth edition including:

1. The revised edition has been shortened by consolidating some chapters and deleting others (a chapter on ethics and a chapter on public health). Deleting these chapters was not an easy decision, but necessary to keep the book a reasonable length. These two chapters were chosen partly because there are textbooks available on both of these topics, including a new book from Jones and Bartlett, *Introduction to Public Health for Pharmacists* by Levin, Hurd, and Hanson. We recommend these books for students and instructors who want to cover these topics in-depth. For those instructors who are looking for single chapters on public health or health care ethics, the chapters on these topics from the Third Edition are available on the book's Web site at www.jbpub.com. These chapters may be reproduced for students who are using this textbook.
2. A comprehensive new glossary.
3. We also reorganized the chapters to more closely reflect how instructors are using the book in their courses. The chapters are still grouped into three parts: Part 1, The Social Aspects of Health Care Delivery (Chapters 1–5), Part 2, Organizational Aspects of Health Care Delivery (Chapters 6–11), and Part 3, The Economic Aspects of Health Care Delivery (Chapters 12–20).

OVERVIEW OF CHAPTERS:

- **Chapter 1**—Health Care Delivery in America: Historical and Policy Perspectives includes new information about factors that make our health care system unique. Additional material discusses why the U.S. health care system can simultaneously be praised by some as superior, yet criticized by others as too costly, ineffective, of insufficient quality, and inaccessible to many of our citizens.

- **Chapter 2**—Health Care Professionals and Interdisciplinary Care, includes updated data on the various health care professions, as well as a brief description of the concept of pay for performance.

- **Chapter 3**—The Pharmacist and the Pharmacy Profession, provides new information about the Medicare Modernization Act of 2003 and supplements new material regarding Web-based pharmacy and e-technology as it relates to health and pharmacy care.

- **Chapter 4**—The Patient, includes updated information on patients, their environment, their expectations, and their access to health care information.

- **Chapter 5**—Drug Use, Access, the Pharmaceutical Industry, and Supply Chain in the United States, has been significantly revised, reflected by the new chapter title. In addition to updated data, the chapter includes new information about drug distribution, both licit and illicit.

- **Chapter 6**—Hospitals, contains up-to-date data on the state of American hospitals, as well as the continued impact of technology on hospital pharmacy practice.

- **Chapter 7**—Ambulatory Care, provides updated data on ambulatory care practice, including information about collaborations between schools and colleges of pharmacy, as well as community health centers and the establishment of mini-clinics in community pharmacies.

- **Chapter 8**—Long-Term Care, includes the latest information about the growing delivery segment of extended care, including the impact of Medicare Part D and the growing interest in LTC insurance.

- **Chapter 9**—Mental Health Services Delivery, contains an update of legislative and regulatory action related to mental health and trends in diagnosis and treatment.

- **Chapter 10**—Home Care, provides the latest information about available services, financing, and delivery options related to health services in the home.

- **Chapter 11**—Informatics in Health Care, reviews current technology trends that facilitate and enhance the delivery of contemporary health care services.

- **Chapter 12**—Basic Economic Principles Affecting Health Care, provides background on important economic concepts that are vital to understanding our health care system.

- **Chapter 13**—Unique Aspects of Health Economics, describes the challenges associated with allocating health care services and controlling costs.

- **Chapter 14**—Private Health Insurance, covers the basic principals of health insurance and provides new information on the uninsured and much more detail about insurance programs' reimbursement for prescription drugs.

- **Chapter 15**—Government Involvement in Health Care, updates information explaining the influence that federal, state, and local governments have with regard to the financing, delivery, and regulation of health care services.

- **Chapter 16**—Managed Health Care, provides updated information of managed health care in general and prescription drugs in particular.

- **Chapter 17**—Medicare and Medicaid, is an updated consolidation of two separate chapters from the Third Edition and includes a new section on Medicare Part D.

- **Chapter 18**—Pharmacoeconomics, contains updated information about the rationale and methods for determining the cost-effectiveness, cost benefit, and cost utility of health care services and provides more details about pharmacoeconomic modeling. The chapter also demonstrates how this information is used in health care decision making.

- **Chapter 19**—International Health Care Services, has been extensively revised once again with updated information and a new emphasis on illustrating lessons from other health systems that could be applied to the U.S. health care system.

- **Chapter 20**—Health Care Reform, describes the changes that have occurred in the delivery, financing, and regulation of health care since publication of the third edition, including medical savings accounts, health savings accounts, and various state initiatives to increase patients' access to health care.

With changes in health care occurring at an ever increasing pace, a health care systems textbook must be revised frequently. Since the First Edition, we have tried to ensure that this book has the latest and most accurate information possible and are pleased that our publisher shares this goal. We are also appreciative of the feedback we receive from users. Your comments and our aggressive revision schedule helps to ensure the utility of this book for both you and your students. Please continue to offer your comments and suggestions as we continue to meet our goal of offering a book that provides a comprehensive overview of the American health care delivery system from a pharmacist's unique perspective.

Robert L. McCarthy
Storrs, Connecticut

Kenneth W. Schafermeyer
St. Louis, Missouri

Acknowledgments

It is hard for us to believe that this is the Fourth Edition of our book. A text does not reach a Fourth Edition without the commitment and dedication of many people. Beyond our students—who have inspired us for a combined nearly fifty years and to whom this edition is dedicated—we are most grateful to our contributors, many of whom have been with us from the start. Their commitment to quality is largely responsible for any success this book has enjoyed. They are indeed special colleagues and friends.

We are equally grateful to the many instructors who have adopted our book and provided us with thoughtful and important feedback. Their suggestions have enhanced its value as we developed this fourth iteration.

We have also enjoyed strong support from the staff at Jones & Bartlett, especially David Cella, Lisa Gordon, and Jamie Chase. We are deeply grateful for their advice, encouragement, and, most of all, patience.

Robert L. McCarthy

Kenneth W. Schafermeyer

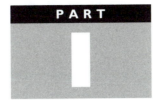

SOCIAL ASPECTS OF HEALTH CARE DELIVERY

CHAPTER

1

Health Care Delivery in America: Historical and Policy Perspectives

Jennifer L. Tebbe-Grossman

Case Scenario

The Palmers, a large extended family, emigrated to New England in the early 1700s. In the 18th and early 19th centuries, the family and their descendants lived on farms in New England. They prospered through farming and some occasional work in small factories in nearby towns. Around 1860, family members moved to the growing cities. A number took jobs in factories; others were fortunate enough to go to high school and even college and found positions in the new professions of teaching, business, and health care. In the 20th century, some family members thrived, especially in the period of rapid economic growth after World War II. Others were barely able to make ends meet, relying at times on government programs and private charity help to get by.

One constant in the extended Palmer family is that from the time of their arrival in New England in 1740, various family members kept diaries, recording information about their extended family members' daily lives. In the 21st century, in the attic of your grandmother, you have found these diaries spanning several centuries. As a future health professional, you learn from these diaries about the health and disease history of your family members: how they thought about what caused disease and what their philosophies of health and disease were when they made their choices to seek health services; what kinds of diseases family members confronted; the differences public health improvements and technological changes made in their lives; how their health services were paid for; from whom and where they got or didn't get their health services and why; and what they thought about different health care policies presented by politicians and branches of government as these policies changed over time in the United States. In other words, the diaries cover much of what appears in this first chapter of the text.

Based on the material in this chapter, what might you find out about the health experiences and beliefs of the Palmer family members, given their differing economic backgrounds over time? What might you think about how much or how little health care services and their delivery have improved over time for all Americans?

LEARNING OBJECTIVES

Upon completion of this chapter, the student shall be able to:

- explain paradoxes of the U.S. health care system
- explain health conditions in 18th- and 19th-century America in relation to disease patterns and causation theories
- explain types of health practices and practitioners and factors explaining access to health care in 19th-century America
- explain the various roles of government in health care delivery in 18th- and 19th-century America
- explain the differences between orthodox and sectarian practitioners and their patients in relation to their perspectives on therapeutics and the delivery of health care
- explain changes in the character, organization, and purposes of hospitals as health delivery sites from the early 19th century through the 20th century
- describe reforms in medical education at the turn of the 20th century and the consequences of the Flexner Report of 1910
- identify the "golden age of medicine" and describe what replaced it in the late 20th century
- explain the ways in which medicine and pharmacy pursued "professionalization" in the late 19th and 20th centuries and how these professions define themselves in the 21st century
- explain how the factors of public health, lifestyle (diet, housing, personal hygiene), and medical practice influenced the decline of infectious diseases and increase in life expectancy at the turn of the 20th century
- discuss the occurrences of infectious and chronic diseases in the 21st century
- discuss the types of government policy that affected health care delivery in the 20th century, particularly in relation to the implementation of public and private health insurance
- discuss the implementation of Medicare and Medicaid in the 1960s, the 1973 Health Maintenance Organization Act, the 1996 Health Insurance Portability and Accountability Act, and the 1997 Children's Health Insurance Program
- explain the benefits and costs of the Medicare Part D Drug Plan
- explain problems associated with incremental and comprehensive health care reform

CHAPTER QUESTIONS

1. What kinds of health beliefs did Americans hold in the 18th and 19th centuries?
2. What factors account for the decline in mortality rates and increases in life expectancy at the turn of the 20th century?
3. Describe the reforms in education that pharmacists and physicians implemented in the early 20th century as part of the "professionalization" process.
4. Who provided healthcare services for Americans and in what kinds of settings during the 18th, 19th, and 20th centuries?
5. What kinds of changes in private and public health insurance plans were considered by Americans in the past?
6. What are the differences between incremental and comprehensive healthcare reform in the contexts of finance, organization, and delivery? What are the chances of achieving comprehensive health care reform in the near future? Does the United States need comprehensive health care reform?

INTRODUCTION

This chapter examines the evolution of health care and health services in the United States by taking a historical perspective. Of particular concern in the context of changes in attitudes and practice toward individual and social responsibility in the delivery of health care services is the transformation in the use of social spaces where health care services have been distributed: the home, office, dispensary, drugstore, hospital, and health maintenance organization (HMO). Patterns of health and illness in the United States are examined in the context of mortality and life expectancy and the occurrence of infectious and chronic diseases. The changing social meanings of health and disease, the roles of health professionals such as pharmacists and physicians, and the expectations of citizens as patients and consumers in an increasingly complex health care delivery environment are explored.

PARADOXES OF THE U.S. HEALTH CARE SYSTEM

The U.S. health care system is characterized by many paradoxes. The United States has the best, most advanced technology available—yet we have a very high rate of medical errors. There are gaps in who has access to health care, with almost one of every six Americans lacking health insurance (Fuchs and Emmanuel, 2005, pp. 1399–1400). Compared to other industrialized nations, the level of spending in the United States means that the country has one of the most expensive health systems, especially in terms of administrative costs. The U.S. health system is also fragmented in terms of how it is financed and how health care services are organized and delivered. The following brief listing of problems connected to the paradoxes of health in America highlights some key components of the continuing crisis.

Technology

Magnetic resonance imaging systems, new diagnostics, transplant surgeries, biotechnology-based products, genetic engineering, health care informatics, telemedicine, and new reproductive technologies are just a few of the rapid technological advances that have emerged in recent years in the United States. These developments offer hopes for improved quality of life, quicker diagnoses and better treatments, and increased life expectancy. Reliance on technological innovation also creates problems, however. Most Americans expect to receive only the best technical care available, which often leads to overuse of technological advances. New technologies tend to be updated quickly, often without sufficient examination of cost and effectiveness issues, once they have initially been implemented within the health care system. Health professionals are educated to primarily focus on the "scientific problem to be solved," deemphasizing the personal aspect of delivering care to the patient. And finally, technology is not equally distributed among patient populations—significant disparities exist based on poverty and race (Weiss and Lonnquist, 2006, pp. 332–333; Torrens, 1989, pp. 10–12).

Health Expenditures

The United States easily surpassed all other countries in spending, yet millions of its citizens lack adequate access to health care. Almost 16% of the U.S. gross domestic product (GDP) was spent on health care in 2004, representing annual growth of almost 8% since 2003 and putting total spending at nearly $1.6 trillion. In 2004, national health spending continued to rise faster than both wages and overall economic growth, with "workers paying much more in health premiums than just a few years ago" (Smith, Cowan, Heffler, Catlin, National Health Accounts Team, 2006, p. 195; Kaufman and Stein, 2006, p. A01).

Despite this high level of spending, the United States saw only a 2.8% improvement in quality improvement on the 44 core measures included among health care objectives for *Healthy People 2010,* according to data available for 2005 (The 2005 National Health Quality report, 2006, p. 3). According to a study comparing the United States with such industrialized nations as Canada, Switzerland, and the United Kingdom, the United States pays higher prices for aspects of care such as physician visits, pharmaceuticals, and hospital stays. Unfortunately, in comparing "demonstrably better technical quality of care or better patient satisfaction with care," the United States does not do as well as other industrialized nations (Anderson, Hussey, Frogner, and Waters, 2005, p. 912). It does not reach the median set by the Organization for Economic Cooperation and Development (OECD; the United States is one of 30 industrialized member-countries) in three major categories of health resources: magnetic resonance imaging (MRI) and computed tomography (CT) scanners per capita, hospital beds per capita, and physicians and nurses per capita (Anderson, Hussey, Frogner, and Waters, 2005, p. 906).

In 2004 (the most recent year in which statistics are available), 45.8 million Americans—15.7% of the population—had no public or private health insurance coverage. In addition, many more Americans have insurance policies but are underinsured. Their policies often don't cover important aspects of care, and they usually require significant out-of-pocket payments for services (DeNavas-Walt, Proctor, and Lee, 2005).

HEALTH STANDARDS

While health care standards in the United States are considered the highest in the world, inadequate, improper, and even dangerous care is all too prevalent in this country. On a worldwide basis, the United States has the highest standards in such areas as licensure of health care personnel, certification of providers and facilities, and approval and regulation of drugs and devices by the Food and Drug Administration with regard to safety and effectiveness (White House Domestic Policy Council, 1993). Nevertheless, as noted earlier, the United States does not compare favorably to other countries in relation to access to important health care resources. Also, other countries have better ratios of population to nurses and population to physicians (Reinhardt, Hussey, and Anderson, 2004, p. 13).

Quackery and medical errors in the United States are also major problems. Consider the proliferation of anti-aging quackery and hucksterism. It is illegal to distribute or administer human growth hormones for "age-related problems" according to federal law, yet treatments are widely advertised on the Internet and in clinics and generate millions of dollars for the industry while "exacting great monetary, health and social costs" (Perls, 2004, p. B682.)

Medical errors are one of the leading causes of death and injury in the United States, with 44,000 to 98,000 people dying in U.S. hospitals each year as a consequence of these mistakes. In 1999, the Institute of Medicine issued a major report outlining ways to reduce medical errors and urging that Congress create a national patient safety center. The focus on medical errors has resulted in some recent successes. Through a "100,000 Lives Campaign," in which 3,100 hospitals representing about 75% of the nation's acute care beds participated, U.S. hospitals have saved an estimated 122,300 lives since early 2005 by focusing on patient safety (*Wall Street Journal*, 2006).

Health Outcomes

A recent study comparing health outcomes in the United States and the United Kingdom concluded that "based on self-reported illnesses and biological markers of disease, U.S. residents are much less healthy than their English counterparts" (Banks, Marmot, Oldfield, and Smith, 2006, p. 2037). The study found that differences exist at all levels of socioeconomic status, although health disparities are largest for those who have the least education and income. The health states whose outcomes were compared in the two populations were diabetes, hypertension, heart disease, myocardial infarction, strokes, lung disease, and cancer. The paradox: The United States spends far more on medical care than the United Kingdom does on a per capita basis (Banks, Marmot, Oldfield, and Smith, 2006, p. 2037).

An oft-cited statistic is that the United States ranks lower than many other nations—especially industrialized nations including Germany, Sweden, and Canada—in terms of infant mortality rates while spending more to prevent this problem. In the early years of the 21st century, 42 out of the 226 countries that reported infant mortality statistics outranked the United States on this statistic (*The World Factbook*, 2006). A number of reasons account for the United States' relatively low standing among other nations, despite the fact that there has been a significant decline in infant mortality rates among all groups in the United States during the 20th century. For instance, the United States still has significant disparities in infant mortality rates based on race. In a study of standardized mortality rates between 1960 and 2000, the overall infant mortality rate showed a drop from 26.0 deaths per 1,000 infants to 6.9 deaths per 1,000 infants. For African American infants, however, this drop was far less impressive: from 44.3 deaths per 1,000 infants in 1960 to 14.1 deaths per 1,000 infants in 2000 (Satcher, Fryer, McCann, Troutman, Woolf, and Rust, 2005, p. 460). Overall, the U.S. infant mortality rate has leveled off at a relatively high rate compared to other countries.

Such programs as the "Every Child Succeeds" effort in Cincinnati, Ohio, have achieved better success in lowering these rates. In seven counties in the Cincinnati area, 8.3 of every 1,000 infants die before the age of 1 year. In the "Every Child Succeeds" project, which enrolled 1,800 mothers, the infant mortality rate was "2.8—much lower than in virtually every industrialized country." Yet the program's funding is so low that it can be extended to only one-fifth of the needy women in the Cincinnati area (Naik, 2006).

Comparisons of life expectancy show similar race-based disparities. Life expectancy increased for all racial groups in the United States from the late 19th century to the early 21st century, with life expectancies for women increasing from 51 to 80 years over this period and life expectancies for men increasing from 48 to 77.5 years. Life expectancy for African American males is 68.3 years, however, versus 74.8 years for white males. For black females, life expectancy is 75 years versus 80 years for white females. Many factors account for these racial disparities, especially differences in quality of neighborhood living environments and access to prevention care services (Epstein, 2003; Maciosek, Coffield, Edwards, Flottemesch, Goodman, and Solberg, 2006).

All of these existing paradoxes in the U.S. health care system are important to think about when reviewing the evolution of health care and the delivery of health care services over time in America.

HEALTH, DISEASE, AND HEALTH PRACTITIONERS IN COLONIAL AMERICA

As different groups of European settlers arrived in the Americas in the 16th and 17th centuries, they found a variety of societies and cultures. Some of the indigenous inhabitants of North America only hunted and gathered. Other groups occupied more permanent settlements and subsisted through both agricultural production and hunting and gathering. Contrary to the belief of many Europeans that the Americas promised a new Eden of good health, Native Americans endured significantly high mortality rates. Malnutrition, violence, accidents, fungal infections, anthrax, tapeworms, tuberculosis, yaws, and syphilis were common causes of death. European settlers brought influenza—which may not have been seen previously in the Americas—and new illnesses—including yellow fever, malaria, smallpox, and measles—against which Native Americans had no immunity. Thus, as Gerald Grob notes, the result of early contact between Europeans and Native Americans "was a catastrophe of monumental proportions that resulted in the destruction of a large majority of the indigenous population and facilitated European domination of the Americas" (2002, p. 27).

Arriving debilitated from sea travel, settlers of England's North American colonies did not encounter an edenic utopian environment. Rather, in the early years, many fell victim to malnutrition and dysentery—the consequences of a poor food and water supply. The colonists suffered from a wide range of endemic and epidemic infectious diseases such as yellow fever, measles, smallpox, and malaria. The British government did not implement broad public policies to address problems of health and illness or encourage the establishment of health practitioners or institutions (Cassedy, 1991). Colonial officials addressed such public health problems as garbage disposal, street maintenance, and the regulation of water supply and sanitation occasionally and with little success in enforcement. Partially because of health emergencies (especially epidemic outbreaks), towns and cities did become accustomed to the idea and practice of health legislation enacted by local government authorities but, as James Cassedy argues, the public health benefit "must have been negligible" (1991, p. 14).

When colonists became sick, they depended on various members of the community for access to the healing arts, looking as much for simple human and religious comforts as for therapeutic services. Physicians, apothecaries, midwives, clergy, public officials, and family members or neighbors—often the females in the household who diagnosed, made medicines, and physically supported the sick—responded to individual or community health needs. Until at least 1825, women commonly depended on their female friends and relatives, and midwives when they were available, to attend to them in childbirth in their homes (Bogdan, 1992). European physicians did not look to the colonies, which had small and widely scattered populations, as locations that offered great professional or economic opportunity. Few physicians emigrated, and since medical education in the North American colonies was not considered a priority of government or private agencies, only a minority of physicians or apothecaries completed formal training. Physicians often compounded and dispensed medicines in shops next door to their medical practices. Apothecaries appeared only in small numbers as compounders, dispensers, or sometimes manufacturers and wholesalers of medicines.

In the growing colonies, all of these practitioners of the "healing arts" improvised based on what they found in their environments and shared health beliefs that relied on a combination of folklore; mineral, plant, and vegetable herbal remedies; and magic. The colonists used health practices and medications that were common in Europe and England, such as mercury and opium preparations. They also adopted such Native American health remedies as cinchona bark, which contained quinine (Christianson, 1987; Duffy, 1993; Tannenbaum, 2002).

AMERICA IN THE NINETEENTH CENTURY: THE HEALTH CARE ENVIRONMENT

As the nation expanded westward and its population grew in the early 19th century, Americans exhibited a local outlook on health care that was similar to their attitudes toward economic and political life. A person's health experience as a resident of a town or city on the Eastern Seaboard was different from the health experience of a farmer in the rural southern or midwestern areas or of an immigrant traveling west into the new territories.

Rural and Urban Health

Self-reliance was a necessity for farmers and travelers. Poverty, loneliness, exhaustion, accidents, exposure to the elements, and dangerous plant and animal life took their toll. Family members and midwives who also functioned as "social healers" within communities played the most important roles in caring for ordinary people in times of illness. During the era of the American Revolution, in rural areas and small towns the number of physicians who practiced medicine in their own homes and traveled to make "house calls" in the homes of their patients increased significantly. Both midwives, or "social healers," and physicians treated entire families—men, women, and children—and juggled the responsibilities of their health practices with their domestic and community responsibilities. Payment for services was in cash and often "in kind," what families produced by their labor. Many patients could not pay, however, so midwives and physicians needed to rely on other sources of income. Rural and small-town residents could request compounded and proprietary medicines through both physicians and pharmacists. They could also purchase proprietary medicines in the general store and from "itinerant healers" or "medicine men" who regularly traveled from town to town (Cassedy, 1991; Leavitt, 1995, p. 4; Ulrich, 1990; Young, 1992).

In urban areas, social class largely affected a person's quality of life and access to health care. The wealthy and growing upper middle class, including those members of the family (introduced in the case scenario at the beginning of the chapter) who were well off, lived in neighborhoods that provided clean air and water, gardens and parks, servants, and health practitioners of their choice. The lower middle classes—including skilled workers, clerks, tradesmen, and widows—could afford food and housing and occasional visits to public parks. They tried to keep their domestic spaces clean despite the unsanitary living conditions offered by tenement landlords. They could pay minimal amounts for self-dosing remedies, medicines, or doctor bills. When such health care as surgery or vaccinations was required, most major towns and cities provided dispensaries for workers who could pay little or nothing at all.

As the 19th century progressed, the working classes shared problems with the poor, including lack of such basic municipal services as garbage and sewage removal. As part of the Industrial Revolution, members of the working classes breathed air polluted by coal dust from the factories and railroads that were next to their residences. Congestion, noise, the frenetic pace of commercial life, and the accelerated influx of new waves of immigrants led to a rapid accumulation of new and old health problems, especially rising mortality rates due to infectious diseases. In addition, African Americans confronted even higher degrees of difficulty in relation to quality of life indicators because of slavery and discrimination. They experienced lack of access to health education, health facilities, and basic public health services (Byrd and Clayton, 2000; Cassedy, 1991; Hoy, 1995; Rosenberg, 1985a).

Health Values, Therapeutics, and Practitioners

Health practitioners and the general public have long disagreed about theories regarding the causes of disease and the public policies needed to address them. Some believed that supernatural forces inflicted disease because of human sin. Some believed in contagion or environmental (miasmic) theories of disease. Still others believed that the individual who did not take precautions to lead a healthful life was responsible for disease (Tesh, 1988).

Regardless of their beliefs about disease causation, most Americans generally shared the same values when it came to health, disease, and the body—that is, they looked to Galen's 2nd-century concept of humoralism. The body was an "interconnected whole" with a natural balance (Warner, 1997, p. 87). As Charles Rosenberg (1985b) noted, "every part of the body was related inevitably and inextricably with every other. In health, the body's system was in balance; in disease, the body lost its balance and suffered disequilibrium. If health practitioners were to treat effectively, they needed knowledge of individual patients and the body's system of 'intake and outgo'" (p. 40). What could be observed empirically happening to the patient's body was therapeutically important.

Orthodox physicians (also referred to as allopathic, regular, or mainstream physicians), who could usually show evidence of some didactic medical education or at least apprenticeship under a practicing physician, offered their mostly middle- and upper-class patients "heroic" medicine. They adopted mostly depletive measures, whereas members of the lay public—drawing upon popular domestic medical texts and almanacs—more often employed both depletive and strengthening measures (tonics and astringents) (Horrocks, 2003). Orthodox physicians assumed an active, aggressive role whereby the patient and the family could see very visible changes in secretions and excretions in the body as a result of the physician's interventions. Using leeches, medical instruments, and a variety of drug therapies, orthodox physicians bled, purged, puked, and sweated their patients. Because cures were not often the result of a physician's care during serious illnesses, patients and families could at least share in the knowledge that they had observed the physician's efforts to do something. Rosenberg has noted the ways in which depletive drugs were used in this system:

> Drugs had to be seen as adjusting the body's internal equilibrium; in addition, the drug's action had, if possible, to alter these visible products of the body's otherwise inscrutable internal state. Logically enough, drugs were not ordinarily viewed as specifics for particular disease entities; material medics texts were generally arranged not by drug or disease, but in categories reflecting the drug's physiological effects: diuretics, cathartics, narcotics, emetics, diaphoretics. (1985b, p. 41)

Orthodox physicians competed with sectarians (also called irregulars), who offered a variety of alternative practices, cures, and remedies that were less heroic, including folk medicines, strengthening tonics, and astringents sold by both itinerant quacks and druggists. Sectarians advocated temperance from alcohol; homeopathy, the "infinitesimal dose" therapeutic that differed significantly from the usually higher levels of medicines required by heroic dosing (Kaufman, 1971); and regimens of fresh air, exercise, and water cures (hydropathy) taken in what Susan E. Cayleff has referred to as comfortable "cure establishments," situated in "natural surroundings" in "country settings" (1987, p. 77). In his popular *Thomson's Almanac*, Samuel Thomson vigorously attacked the orthodox physician primary reliance on what he deemed excessive depletive measures and advocated his own medical philosophy primarily emphasizing self-treatment through the use of his regimen of herbal medicines, "sweating" baths, emetics, and purgatives (Haller, 2000; Horrocks, 2003, p. 120). Sylvester Graham worried about the sexual passions and advocated a vegetarian and high-fiber diet and exercise regime that forbade spices, alcohol, tea, and coffee, in an effort to control those passions (Nissenbaum, 1980).

Even in the 20th and 21st centuries, these so-called alternative health practices continue to flourish. Folk medicine traditions vary by region and ethnicity, ranging from Chinese acupuncture to Japanese shiatsu to Pennsylvania German (or "Dutch") "powpow." New Age practitioners, appealing primarily to white middle- and upper-middle-class adherents, advocate such therapies as "crystal healing" and meditational systems (Fuller, 1993).

The commercial manufacture of proprietary medicines developed rapidly during the first half of the 19th century, replacing the functions of the domestic practitioner who formulated the family's home remedies over the hearth fire. Physicians dispensed drugs in their offices and on home visits while "pharmacists began to open stores in towns and cities to fill prescriptions for patients of physicians and to compound drugs requested by their customers" (Cowen and Kent, 1997, p. 98; Rothstein, 1996a, p. 376). Gregory Higby has observed that pharmacists, as part of a shift of "allegiance from physicians to their customers," also began "counter prescribing"—that is, "refilling prescriptions without physician authorization, and diagnosing and treating customers" (1992, p. 5). By 1860, many Americans could buy relatively cheap commodities called "patent medicines," which were manufactured in small factories, advertised in newspapers, and delivered to any town or city through improved transportation systems. As the 19th century progressed, pharmacists "sold bottles of their own or physicians' concoctions" and became "retailers" of the "prepared drugs" (Rothstein, 1996a, p. 376).

At the same time, social reformers and public officials sought to label the production and distribution of patent medicines as "quackery" and warned the consuming public that patent medicine products were dangerous and fraudulent in their claims. Reformers were unsuccessful in their efforts to pass national legislation regulating the industry until the enactment of the Pure Food and Drug Act (1906), which addressed accurate labeling. Nevertheless, such patent medicines as Lydia Pinkham's Vegetable Compound remained popular among middle-class women as a treatment for "female complaints" because it was seen as an "alternative to orthodox treatments they believed to be unsafe" (Cayleff, 1992, p. 317).

Americans sought out a variety of alternative therapies because they often viewed orthodox (regular) physicians as elitist practitioners who sought to monopolize health care. Many Americans accepted the egalitarian view that a variety of philosophies of health care practice should be available to all people. Thus health care services were most commonly delivered in the home, the physician's office, the drugstore, and the "cure establishment" for the middle and upper classes. The working classes and the poor did not participate in the world of these health care services on a regular basis because of the necessity to pay out-of-pocket at the moment of receiving services. Instead, when most ordinary Americans became sick, they first sought treatment from someone in their own household because health care payment was "fee-for-service"—that is, patients paid a health practitioner directly at the time of service. They often dosed themselves with self-help remedies that they could afford in an attempt to avoid the cost of treatment from an orthodox physician or one of the many sectarian physicians (Stage, 1979).

The Rise and Transformation of the Hospital

The early 19th-century hospital had its origins in the almshouse or pest-house, identifying it as an institution with charitable and welfare functions. Most Americans saw the hospital as a place that protected the community from those hospitalized and as a place where patients usually died. Aseptic practices were not commonplace. Admittance for care could be gained if a prominent member of the community was willing to vouch for the prospective patient's moral character. Patients entering the hospital throughout most of the 19th century were those with the least resources—the "deserving" poor, with so few ties to family or community that no one could care for them. Often they were recent immigrants; however, charitable hospitals sometimes refused certain immigrant populations, particularly the Irish in Eastern Seaboard cities, and categorically denied admission to African Americans.

Male and female custodial caretakers of the sick were former patients who worked for room and board or local wage-earning residents from the community who had no formal training. Distinguished members of the community served as trustees who financed the institutions, and physicians from upper-class families provided free care to patients, developing new knowledge from the treatment of the very sick (Rosenberg, 1987; Vogel, 1979).

Charitable dispensaries were used by the poor and lower classes, including the poorer members of the Palmer family mentioned in this chapter's case scenario, far more than hospitals from the late 18th century until around 1920. These autonomous, freestanding institutions were located primarily in urban, often new immigrant, neighborhoods and provided such outpatient services as prescribing, dental work, and minor surgery. There were few employees: a steward, a "house physician," and sometimes a druggist, although the house physician might also act as druggist as well. Later in the nineteenth century, established consulting physicians volunteered from the local community (Rosenberg, 1985b; Starr, 1991).

Over a 50-year period after the Civil War, the number of U.S. hospitals grew from fewer than 100 to more than 6,000 general and specialty institutions (such as mental facilities, children's hospitals, and tuberculosis sanitariums). The new hospitals were sponsored and financed by such disparate groups as religious organizations, ethnic associations, women's groups, physician groups (including African American physician associations), and homeopathists and other sects.

As the 19th century drew to a close, the chiefly welfare or charitable nature of the hospital declined. Orthodox physicians and trustees sought private, paying patients from the middle and upper classes. Physicians grew to reject Galen's system of therapeutics with its "heroic" remedies, replacing it with an increasing acceptance of the germ theory of disease (whereby specific microorganisms were believed to be responsible for the spread of disease). Hospitals introduced new elements, including the enforcement of new aseptic and antiseptic techniques; new technological methods, including regular anesthetization in surgery and the initial medical application of X rays; and applied nursing methods patterned on the model developed by Florence Nightingale in England (Kevles, 1997; Pernick, 1985; Reverby, 1987). Architectural designs were planned to provide personal service in a pleasant, clean decor with comfortable furnishings.

General practitioners, as well as elite physicians, sought to admit patients to these hospitals to enhance the growth of their private medical practices. Hospitals continued to take "charity patients," but the numbers decreased and these individuals received a lesser level of care. By the end of the 19th century, hospitals were well on their way in a journey from "charitable guest houses to biomedical showcases," with the wealthier members of the Palmer family having the greatest access to the new technological miracles (Risse, 1999, p. 4; Ludmerer, 1999; Rosenberg, 1987, p. 47; Rosner, 1979, p. 127).

The growth of the modern hospital as "an indispensable element in American health care" was ensured by the 1946 National Hospital Survey and Construction Act (Hill-Burton Act) and subsequent amendments, which provided federal funding for planning and assisting in the construction of new hospital and public health centers (Rosenberg, 1987, p. 343). While the Hill-Burton Act led to an overabundance of hospital beds and "funds went disproportionately to middle-income communities," Rosenberg says that technological innovation, increasing application of business management policies, and establishment of "the principles of local initiative, state review, and federal support sharing" provided for some degree of planning on a state level. Hospitals in the post–World War II era organized the financing and delivery of care around an acute disease model.

While the operation of hospitals and conducting of medical education and research became more dependent on federal government funding, hospitals found increasingly in the 1970s through much of the 1990s that government had become more interested in pursuing service programs. This was particularly connected to the federal funding of Medicare and Medicaid programs beginning in the 1960s. A new emphasis was also placed on encouraging preventive health and pursuing cost-cutting and efficiency measures. At the same time, continued idealistic commitment of hospitals as "exemplary social institutions" to the local community defined the development of the hospital until the 1990s (Litman, 1997, p. 3; Fox, 1993, p. 17; Starr, 1982; Stevens, 1989, p. 364).

In the 1990s, some community hospital mergers and nonprofit–to–for-profit hospital conversions resulted in the maintenance of clear social missions to local communities, while others led to the closing of many community hospitals that had previously treated the poor and less well-off (Bell, 1996; Blumenthal and Weissman, 2000; Cahill, 1997; Lukas and Young, 2000; Opdycke, 1999; Young, Dasai, and Lukas, 1997). In the context of thinking of the patient as a consumer, the hospital as an "industry" sought to attract the sufficiently insured through "a patient-centered care scheme designed to achieve customer satisfaction by striving to make hospitals more pleasant, comfortable, and user friendly" (Essoyan, 2000, p. A19; La Ferla, 2000, p. 4; Risse, 1999, p. 681). Hospitals were redesigned to "streamline health care delivery," enhancing efficiency and cost savings by using such strategies as placing patients in "focused settings" with satellite pharmacy, laboratory, and radiological facilities and employing "cross-trained multidisciplinary caregiving teams" (e.g., a nurse, practical aide, and technician) (Risse, 1999, pp. 682–683). However, given the managed care focus on financial incentives and customer orientation, scholars, the public, health professionals, and public officials have raised ethical issues and expressed concerns about whether health professionals have indeed become more efficient but lost autonomy to the extent of becoming mere "providers of health services" (Aroskar, 1999, p. 518; Gordon, 1997; Risse, 1999, p. 682). To what extent the hospital remains an environment where the human being is the center of care remains an important question (see Chapter 8).

CONTINUITY AND CHANGE IN HEALTH INSTITUTIONS AND PROFESSIONS

As part of a continuing process during the early years of the 20th century, medicine and pharmacy instituted important changes in their pursuit of modern, credential-based professionalization. As self-defined members of individual professions, physicians and pharmacists sought to strengthen their positions in society by employing a variety of strategies. These professions placed new emphasis on their special expertise within their own field of study and practice, the pursuit of rigorous educational reform, professional autonomy, a pronounced idealistic commitment to altruism that placed their clientele above any commercial concern for profit, increased authority and purview of professional organizations, and strengthened licensing and self-regulation standards.

Medicine

Beginning in 1908, at the urging of the American Medical Association (AMA), Abraham Flexner conducted a study of medical schools sponsored by the Carnegie Foundation. He published *Medical Education in the United States and Canada* in 1910, recommending numerous changes in the focus, education, and practice of medicine in the 20th century (Flexner, 1910). The Flexner Report paved the way for effectively making allopathic medicine the legally sanctioned form of practice and abandoning the apprenticeship model of medical education and the primarily commercial financing of medical schools by physician-entrepreneurs. In the early 1900s, medical educators and leaders had already reached some consensus on the direction of change as proposed in the Flexner Report, and by 1930 many reforms were in place. Chiefly, these reforms included most states' acceptance that medical schools would be accredited under the control of the American Medical Association; the graduation of fewer students; and the closing of weaker medical schools with the remaining stronger institutions obtaining funding from such sources as state governments and philanthropists to pursue further discoveries in bacteriology and other biomedical sciences and to produce trained clinicians and specialists in such areas as obstetrics, cardiology, and surgery. These reforms also resulted in the reduction of the number of students admitted from the lower classes, ethnic minorities, and women. Their numbers did not reappear in any strength until the 1970s and 1980s when the number of African Americans and women admitted to medical schools began to increase (Ludmerer, 1985; Markowitz and Rosner, 1979; Morantz-Sanchez, 1992; More, 1999; Starr, 1982).

Nonetheless, the "medical reform" of the early 20th century ushered in what John C. Burnham has termed a "golden age" in which "American physicians enjoyed social esteem and prestige along with an admiration for their work that was unprecedented in any age" (Burnham, 1982, p. 284). In post–World War II America, the biomedical model predominated in research and in areas of clinical care. An emphasis was placed on the "subcellular and molecular level, and life processes were increasingly understood in physical and chemical terms" (Ludmerer, 1999, p. 148). This golden age did not begin to be seriously challenged until the 1960s, when questions were raised both from within the profession and by the public about the physician's "priestly pretension" and "technical performance" (Burnham, 1982, p. 291).

From the 1970s through the 1990s, medical education and academic health centers came under increasing duress. Some social inequities were addressed as increasing numbers of women and minorities were admitted to medical schools and such new pedagogies as problem-based learning were widely introduced in medical school curricula to improve clinical skills. At the same time, the new managed care practice made inroads against the pursuit of academic research and the provision of "the importance to the physician's work of having sufficient time with patients" (Ludmerer, 1999, p. 383).

At the beginning of the 21st century, physicians continue to express concern about their roles in managed care systems. They have shown a willingness to treat patients in new ways, including group visits where chronically ill patients with such diseases as diabetes, hypertension, and arthritis attend seminars led by physicians (Martinez, 2000). Physicians have also raised concerns about whether the quality of patient care and their decision-making autonomy are unduly threatened by managed care's increased emphasis on linking the number of patients whom physicians treat to their fees and salaries (Kowalczyk, 2000). Deborah A. Stone argues that the "doctor has been reconceived as an entrepreneur who is now in the business of insuring patients as well as caring for them" (1997, p. 534).

Pharmacy

As the 20th century began, pharmacists pursued several approaches in an effort to change their practice to modern credential-based professionalization. Challenges to the apprenticeship model of training pharmacists had already occurred in the 1860s and 1870s, when state universities established the first pharmacy curricula, based primarily on study in the basic sciences and laboratory instruction. By 1900, there were 53 colleges and departments of pharmacy in the United States. Most had minimal standards for admission and length of study. Colleges organized their own association (renamed the American Association of Colleges of

Pharmacy [AACP] in 1925) and struggled to reach their goals of establishing more rigorous standards of education and practice. The AACP instituted the requirement of high school graduation for admission, and by 1932, it mandated 4 years of study for graduation (Deno, Rowe, and Brodie, 1959; Sonnedecker, 1976).

In 1900, more than 38,000 U.S. drugstores served a population of 76 million, translating to one store per 2,000 people (Deno et al., 1959). Known as both druggists and pharmacists, few practitioners operated in individual establishments devoted exclusively to professional services. Instead, most worked in independent, druggist-owned stores or shops that provided a variety of services and products, including soda fountain service, perfumes, telephone booths, magazines, and popular books. Chain drugstores, with the same ownership and the same product lines, began to appear in the early years of the 20th century and expanded regionally and nationally across the United States.

In their effort to professionalize, pharmacists confronted a difficult problem: Most Americans used pharmacists' services in the neighborhood drugstore, a commercial enterprise identified with the profit motive. The 1922 code of ethics established by the American Pharmaceutical Association, however, stated that the pharmacy's "primary object" was "the service it can render to the public in safeguarding the handling, sale, compounding and dispensing of medicinal substances" (APA, 1922, p. 728). In a variety of contexts throughout the 20th century, including the ongoing economic struggle between independent, chain, and superstore pharmacies; HMO pharmacies; and Internet and mail-order pharmacies, pharmacists as entrepreneurs have promoted the image that members of the public are customers who should be sold good products. At the same time, pharmacists have asked the public to seek out their services because they possess the "specialized knowledge and professional training" and the moral character necessary for the exercise of civic responsibility in their communities (Apple, 1996).

The practice of hospital pharmacy has been of great significance in enabling pharmacists to implement their professionalization goals. While independent and chain-store pharmacists grappled with image problems, hospital pharmacy thrived as a "bastion of high pharmaceutical technology, art, and science" during the 1920s (Higby with Gallagher, 1992, p. 507). Between 1930 and the present, many pharmacy educators and practitioners moved toward the incorporation of a clinical component in pharmacy practice and the acceptance of a doctor of pharmacy (PharmD) curriculum in pharmacy schools throughout the United States. A culminating point in the expression of educational reform was presented in 1975 in *Pharmacists for the Future: The Report of the Study Commission on Pharmacy* (Millis, 1975). The underpinning for the new program of study and practice was the concept of pharmaceutical care, to be implemented in community and institutional settings such as hospitals and long-term care facilities. Some educators believed that this reform would allow pharmacists to become equal members of the health care team with physicians, nurses, and other allied health professionals. According to Charles D. Hepler, pharmaceutical care is "defined as a relationship between a patient and a pharmacist in which the pharmacist accepts responsibility for drug-use functions and provides those services governed by awareness of, and commitment to, the patient's interests" (1988, p. 26). In implementing the goals of pharmaceutical care, the pharmacy accrediting association, the American Council on Pharmaceutical Education, mandated the doctor of pharmacy, a 6-year degree program, as the entry-level requirement.

Pharmacists are confronting difficult dilemmas in the managed care era as they seek to implement pharmaceutical care (Navarro, 1999). Recent studies of pharmacists' work environments show that most community pharmacists are increasingly busy and, despite the presence of more pharmacy technicians, still spend most of their time in dispensing roles. Some inroads have been made in moving toward more pharmacist involvement in patient care and drug therapy, but pharmacists continue to report dissatisfaction with their general lack of opportunities to more effectively fulfill this role. Some community pharmacists have become more deeply involved in providing expanded pharmaceutical-care services by, for example, helping patients better monitor such chronic diseases as diabetes, asthma, and hypertension. These pharmacists generally document their care for patients using charts and computer technology; this documentation, in turn, serves to improve patient quality of care and to provide evidence of outcomes so that the pharmacists can seek compensation for the pharmaceutical-care services (Kreling, Doucette, Mott, Gaither, Pedersen, and Schommer, 2006; Brock, Casper, Green, and Pedersen, 2006). (For further reading, see Chapter 3.)

HEALTH AND SICKNESS PATTERNS IN HISTORICAL PERSPECTIVE

Definitions of Health and Disease

Elliot Mishler notes that broader definitions of health "are neither obsolete, nor of historical and esoteric interest only," when he refers to the World Health Organization's definition of health as a "state of complete physical, mental, and social well-being and not merely the absence of disease or infirmity" (1981, p. 3). In addition, Charles Rosenberg argues for not thinking in narrow constructs:

> Disease is at once a biological event, a generation-specific repertoire of verbal constructs reflecting medicine's intellectual and institutional history, an occasion of and potential legitimization for public

policy, an aspect of social role and individual—intrapsychic—identity, a sanction for cultural values, and a structuring element in doctor and patient interactions. In some ways disease does not exist until we have agreed that it does, by perceiving, naming, and responding to it. (1992, p. xiii)

In studying health care delivery in the United States, how we perceive, name, and respond to health and disease and what we make the primary focus of the health care system are major concerns. What is the best balance among biomedical treatments; health prevention, maintenance, promotion, and education; and changes in how we deal with environmental carcinogens or industrial pollution? Depending on the focus adopted, how should the health care system provide for better access to health care services for the public (Brandt, 1997; Tesh, 1988)?

Each year the mass media headline statistics reported by government and research institutions about health and disease levels, mortality and life expectancy, and causes of death both worldwide and within the United States. Historians have also sought, within biomedical, cultural, social, economic, and political contexts, to account for increases in life expectancy, declines in mortality rates, and changes in causes of death from acute and infectious diseases and, more recently, from chronic illnesses.

Health Demographics and Causes of Death

Settlers in colonial America confronted malnutrition daily, making them susceptible to endemic and epidemic infectious illnesses. During the 18th century, Americans were most often affected by such endemic illnesses as dysentery, malaria, and respiratory infections, with occasional epidemics, including smallpox and yellow fever. As the 19th century progressed, Americans became more concerned with illnesses related to the increasing population that lived in cities, experiencing rapid urbanization and industrialization. Deaths continued to result from dysentery and respiratory infections, but also increasingly from smallpox, cholera, scarlet fever, whooping cough, measles, diphtheria, and—above all—tuberculosis (Leavitt and Numbers, 1997). Improvements in public health could be noted as the 19th century ended. In particular, death rates declined—especially infant mortality rates—and life expectancy increased, as noted earlier in this chapter.

Causes of Death and Disease

In 1900, the leading causes of death were infectious diseases, including both epidemic and endemic diseases, influenza and pneumonia, tuberculosis, gastritis and enteritis, diphtheria, measles, scarlet fever, and whooping cough. Some chronic diseases, such as heart and cerebrovascular disease, and cancer were also among the top 10 causes of death in the United States (Lerner, M. & Anderson, O.W., 1963, p. 16). At the end of the 20th century, the 10 leading causes of death reported in the United States were heart disease, cancer, cerebrovascular disease, chronic lower respiratory diseases, accidents, diabetes mellitus, influenza and pneumonia, Alzheimer's disease, kidney disease, and septicemia (U.S. Census Bureau, 2002). Obviously, causes of death were increasingly attributed to chronic illnesses in the late 20th century, both in the United States and worldwide.

The 10-volume *Global Burden of Disease* project, edited by Christopher J. L. Murray of Harvard University and Alan D. Lopez of the World Health Organization, estimates that between 1990 and 2020, infectious, nutritional, and childbirth–associated deaths will decrease in absolute numbers from 17.2 million to 10.3 million and will decrease as a proportion of all deaths from 34% to 15% (Murray and Lopez, 1996). Noncommunicable diseases, including unipolar major depression, ischemic heart disease, cerebrovascular and chronic obstructive pulmonary diseases, however, will increase by 77%, with the number of related deaths increasing from 28 million to nearly 50 million annually (Knox, 1996a). However, critics point out that developing countries continue to struggle with health problems and diseases linked to poverty, such as malnutrition, dysentery, malaria, and tuberculosis. And, with the increase in global travel and the lack of funding for the public health infrastructure, these diseases (as well as the recently emerged threats of West Nile virus, AIDS, and avian flu) have caused the United States to take note of the changes in patterns of increase in infectious diseases outside its national borders and to ponder the capability of public health agencies to deliver appropriate services (Garrett, 2000; Steinhauer, 2000a). In the aftermath of the terrorist attacks on September 11, 2001, the United States has also become concerned about bioterrorist threats to health, including the possibility that smallpox could be used as a bioterrorist weapon.

Factors Explaining Health Demographic Change

To understand the meaning of statistics that report declines in infant mortality rates, increases in life expectancy, declines in communicable diseases, and increases in chronic, degenerative illnesses, historians have analyzed the possible factors that account for the changing numbers and have explored public authorities' explanations for these changes. Three factors are generally cited as explanations: (1) changes in standard of living or lifestyle, including improvements in personal hygiene, diet, nutrition, and housing; (2) advances in public health measures; and (3) progress in medical practice, including therapeutic interventions in the treatment of patients.

In examining the documentary evidence, health care historians have found that changes in public health measures and lifestyle contributed more to health improvements than therapeutic interventions by physicians in the 19th and early 20th centuries (Leavitt and Numbers, 1997; Rothstein, 1996b). In the latter half of the 19th century, such cities as New York began to recognize the importance of connecting the new knowledge linked to the germ theory of disease with the city's environment and its people's health, including improved sanitation, water supply and delivery, and refuse collection and waste removal (Melosi, 2000). In 1865, New York commissioned a report on public health and later formed a board of health with responsibilities to include enforcing sanitary regulations and controlling epidemics. By 1912, as David Rosner has noted, "garbage collection, meat and milk inspections, pure water, and sewerage systems had been installed throughout the city. Dead animals were now regularly picked up off the streets, and fire safety codes augmented stricter enforcement of housing laws" (1995, p. 15). The department of health, in its annual report, attributed "over the course of just forty-five years . . . a decrease of over 50 percent" in the death rate to public sanitation measures (1995, p. 15).

William Rothstein emphasizes the importance of educating the public about specific behaviors related to standards of living and public health:

> Until well into the 20th century, millions of Americans drank from metal drinking cups kept next to fountains for all to use, did not sterilize bottles or take other measures necessary for hygienic feeding of infants, let their children sleep in the same bed and play with siblings with contagious diseases like diphtheria and scarlet fever, purchased unrefrigerated and bacteria-laden milk and meat, used polluted wells and water supplies without boiling the water, and took baths in bathtubs after others had used the same water. These and many other similar behaviors have disappeared because the public has been educated about personal hygiene. (1996b, pp. 77–78)

At the same time, public health campaigns in the late 19th and early 20th centuries against specific diseases must be seen within the context of how health professionals, public officials, and the general public felt that disease and "outsiders" threatened the civic order. They often linked epidemics of infectious diseases—including smallpox, tuberculosis, bubonic plague, typhoid, and polio—to new immigrant populations. Some public health efforts focused on isolation, quarantine, and destruction of housing, often using violence to implement these policies. The founding of ethnic and religious hospitals; the establishment of visiting and public health nursing, neighborhood clinics, and settlement houses; health advocacy programs to foster individual efforts to improve domestic hygiene; and struggles for effective public health legislation and enforcement were all examples of efforts to assist immigrants in preventive health measures, in improving the living conditions in urban housing, and in occupational safety and health on the job (Kraut, 1994; Leavitt, 1996; Ott, 1996; Tomes, 1998).

Health care historians have also rightly documented the significance of the role of clinical medicine and therapeutic intervention in contributing to the decline of mortality rates in infectious diseases, with arguably the most striking example occurring in the middle of the 20th century. In citing the role of antibiotics, John Parascandola points out that "within a decade after penicillin was first made freely available for civilian use in the United States in 1945, the antibiotics had become the most important class of drugs in the treatment of infectious disease. In 1948, antibiotics prescriptions accounted for only 1.5% of the total number written in the United States; by 1952, that figure had risen to 13.7%" (1997, pp. 108–109). Parascandola also cites a Federal Trade Commission report from 1958, which indicates a decrease of 56.4% in the total number of deaths from 1945 to 1955 for eight major diseases responsive to antibiotic therapy, versus a decline of only 8.1% for all other causes of death.

In 1997, the power of antibiotic treatment, coupled with public health measures, was documented in the announcement from the Centers for Disease Control and Prevention (CDC) that during the previous year new cases of syphilis in the United States—"curable with penicillin since 1947"—fell "to their lowest rate in 40 years" (Okie, 1997, p. A3). Officials voiced their belief that it was possible to eliminate the transmission of this sexually transmitted disease through a plan that would continue to involve treatment efforts by public health officials. The CDC started a National Plan to Eliminate Syphilis in 1999 and in 2000, the Center requested $15 million from the U.S. Congress "to wipe out syphilis from the United States by 2005" through programs that include laboratory services, free diagnosis and treatment, and epidemiological tracking for carriers and those at risk in local communities. In 2007, the American Society for Microbiology in testimony before Congress reported that the 2005 goals listed above were not reached in that the CDC Plan requires further support with syphilis rates among U.S. men unfortunately increasing in the United States ("Comment: Cheap and Easy," 2000; Goldberg, 2000; American Society for Microbiology, 2007). In the 21st century, major public health efforts will continue to focus on when and how to implement programs such as the targeting of syphilis and on how to educate the public about the "misuse and overuse of antibiotics," stressing the limitations of "wonder drugs" (Parascandola, 1997, pp. 109, 110).

Successful public health measures are often cited to help explain the declines in infant death rates in U.S. cities during the 1990s. These measures have included better access to stable housing, prenatal care for pregnant women who qualify for such government programs as Healthy Start or Medicaid, better education provided to new mothers from pediatricians about sudden infant death syndrome, and medical and technological advances in neonatal intensive care (Knox, 1997; Kong, 1997; Neergaard, 1995). Conversely, when funding has decreased in a community for various programs aimed at healthy mothers and babies, the infant mortality rate has risen (Steinhauer, 2000b). As such reports as *For a Healthy Nation: Returns on Investment in Public Health* point out, increases in life expectancy in the 20th century have been more directly linked to improved public health measures than to any innovations in medical interventions (U.S. Department of Health and Human Services [DHHS], 1994).

Chronic Illness

Government agencies, biomedical health researchers, and health professionals have recognized since the 1920s that chronic disease must be a health policy priority in the United States (Fox, 1988). In discussing how the United States should address the fact that chronic illnesses afflict close to half the population, costing nearly $470 billion in 1990, a number of issues related to public health measures, environmental factors, standard of living, lifestyle, and therapeutic interventions are raised. Medical researchers cite such "diseases of affluence" as sedentary lifestyle, poor diet, smoking, and alcohol abuse as major causes of chronic illness (Knox, 1996b, p. A11). Other researchers document concerns about the lack of good management of chronic disease and people's inability to receive the help they need to live on an everyday basis with chronic health conditions. Dr. Halstad R. Holman, director of an arthritis center at Stanford University, notes, "Our health care system—its structure, practices, education, and even research agendas—was developed for acute disease. We have a profound mismatch between our entire health care system and what it's structured to do and what we need it to do" (Knox, 1996b, p. A11).

HEALTH POLICY OVERVIEW: 1900–1950

New Legislation in the Early 20th Century

The major hallmark of 20th-century health care was the increased role of government policy making at the local, state, and especially the federal level. During the first two decades of the 20th century, the federal government assumed a more vigorous role in public health, symbolized by its renaming of the Marine Hospital Service as the U.S. Public Health Service in 1912. Partially as a consequence of "muckraking" journalists' exposure of dangerous practices in the food and drug industries, the U.S. Congress enacted the Pure Food and Drug Act in 1906, then significantly strengthened its oversight of this industry with more comprehensive legislation under the 1938 Federal Food, Drug and Cosmetic Act (Temin, 1980). In addressing the plight of America's poor children, many of whom lacked good nutrition and housing and were forced to work in dangerous conditions, Congress established the Children's Bureau in 1912. This legislation was followed in 1921 by the Sheppard-Towner Maternity and Infancy Act, which provided federal funding to support children's health clinics until 1929 (King, 1993). In addition, Congress approved important legislation establishing the National Institutes of Health in 1930 and passed the National Cancer Act in 1937 to further biomedical research (Patterson, 1987).

Public and Private Health Insurance

Twentieth-century changes in health insurance can be traced back to at least 1798, when government hospitals were established in some coastal cities to provide care for merchant seamen. In the 19th century, small numbers of Americans obtained some form of "insurance against sickness" primarily by gaining "income protection" through such groups as trade unions and fraternal organizations or through their employers (Numbers, 1997, p. 277). Some purchased protection against sickness from commercial insurers. Generally, only mining and lumber companies provided actual medical benefits.

In the early 20th century, progressive reformers and labor unions began to talk about some form of government-sponsored health insurance. In 1914, workers' compensation or compulsory sickness insurance programs appeared. Operating on a state level, they generally provided cash payments for injuries or disease related to the workplace. In later decades, payments were made for medical expenses and death benefits. Employers usually purchased these programs from commercial insurers. As early as 1917, several states considered health insurance bills (Numbers, 1997; Starr, 1982; Stevens, 1971).

As various state-supported health proposals appeared, opposition to government intervention was voiced by individual health practitioners, including physicians and pharmacists, the pharmaceutical industry, and employers. Following the significant drops in physician and hospital income that occurred in the wake of the Great Depression, hospitals eventually reconsidered insurance plans. In 1929, the "Father" of the Blue Cross movement, Baylor University Hospital, enrolled public school teachers in a plan covering hospital costs (Numbers, 1997). In the same year, Blue Cross was established to cover hospital costs; in 1939, Blue Shield was created to cover physician fees. These insurance programs, which served as a third-party payment system, presented an attractive alternative to the tradition of patients' paying health practitioners directly for health services, and the AMA expressed its support for their implementation (see Chapter 18).

During the Franklin D. Roosevelt administration, Congress considered the Murray-Wagner-Dingall bill, which proposed to provide health care for the poor primarily through federal grants given to the states. Ultimately, this national health effort was defeated (Numbers, 1997).

POST-WORLD WAR II HEALTH CARE CHANGES

In the second half of the 20th century, President Harry Truman spoke forcefully in favor of a national health insurance proposal that offered protection to all Americans (Poen, 1979). At the time, these proposals failed largely because they evoked strong opposition from the AMA. As part of its effort to defeat the Truman proposal, the AMA undertook a $4.5 million "national education campaign," warning that "national health insurance would lead to federal control of health care" (Johnson and Broder, 1996, p. 66). In the Cold War era, which was characterized by a virulent anticommunism movement, the AMA's public relations campaign equated national health insurance with socialized medicine.

In the 1950s, with support from the federal government through tax-deductibility rulings, employers and labor unions increasingly offered U.S. workers health care plans as part of their benefits programs. In addition, in 1965, the federal government increased the health care system's dependence on third-party payments by establishing Medicare, a program that covers hospital insurance and doctor visits for Americans older than age 65, and Medicaid, a joint federal and state program that provides health care for the poor and disabled (Patel and Rushefsky, 1995; see Chapters 19 and 20). While a push for these programs began under the John F. Kennedy administration, President Lyndon Johnson was successful in achieving their passage with his landslide victory in the 1964 presidential election and his leadership in directing his Great Society legislation through Congress.

Despite these incremental reforms, health care costs continued to rise in the 1960s and 1970s, and problems of access to services for the uninsured increased. Once again raising the possibility of a comprehensive national health policy, Senator Edward Kennedy and President Jimmy Carter launched unsuccessful attempts in the 1970s to pass such legislation as Kennedy's Health Security Act, which was designed to "assure every American quality health care at a price he can afford" (Kennedy, 1972). By 1980, the "mostly private" model of a health care system best described how most Americans were covered—that is, by private insurance programs purchased through plans offered by their employers. Coverage of the health care costs of only a few needy groups (e.g., veterans and the elderly) was provided through government-sponsored "public insurance programs" (Patel and Rushefsky, 1995, p. 25).

Prepaid Health Care and Health Maintenance Organizations

While Congress did not adopt broad health insurance coverage, in 1973 it passed the Health Maintenance Organization Act. This legislation required every employer with more than 25 employees that offered a health plan to include at least one HMO plan providing comprehensive medical care for a fixed fee to its enrollees. A companion bill "requiring employers to provide a basic minimum package of benefits to all their employees" failed, with the AMA and the health insurance industry leading lobbying against the bill (Johnson and Broder, 1996, p. 67).

Prepaid health programs were first introduced in the 1920s. The highly successful Kaiser Permanente Medical Care Program initially offered health care services to the workers employed by Henry F. Kaiser in the building of the Grand Coulee Dam in 1938. The prepaid program expanded its provision of comprehensive care to workers in his steel mills and shipyards, and eventually to the general public on the West Coast and to a lesser extent in the Midwest.

Despite the passage of the 1973 law, rapid growth of HMOs did not become pronounced until the 1990s. In 1995, HMOs covered nearly 60 million individuals, and the less structured preferred provider organizations (PPOs) covered an additional 91 million people (Anders, 1996; Peterson, 1997; see Chapter 21). By 1998, 77 million Americans—or 29% of the total U.S. population—had enrolled in an HMO (U.S. DHHS, 1999).

Renewed Efforts for National Health Insurance

As the 20th century ended, the American public experienced significant social, economic, and political changes that affected both the U.S. health care system and the delivery of health care services. In 1991, national health care insurance again emerged as a major congressional and presidential campaign issue. Harris Wofford, a Pennsylvania Democrat running for a seat in the Senate, chose to emphasize health care as a voter concern in his race against a Republican candidate who was a popular former governor of the state and was strongly favored to win the race. In his first political ad, Wofford looked into the camera and told Pennsylvania residents, "If criminals have a right to a lawyer, I think working Americans should have the right to a doctor." He won the Senate seat by a 55% to 45% margin (Johnson and Broder, 1996, p. 60). In the same year, Bill Clinton made health care a major issue in his presidential campaign, offering a step-by-step plan to achieve universal health care coverage for all Americans through his Health Security Plan.

Incremental Policy Proposals

Despite the AMA dropping its opposition to national health insurance, in 1994 Congress once again defeated proposals for implementing national health insurance, including President Clinton's Health Security Plan, largely because of strong lobbying campaigns waged by the pharmaceutical, hospital, and health insurance industries. In 1996, incremental legislation to decrease the number of uninsured persons was passed in the form of the Health Insurance Portability and Accountability Act. This law specified that employers or insurers of new employees could impose a waiting period of no more than 12 months before covering them under the employer's health plan. In addition, for workers who had health benefits prior to losing their job, the law provided that they could purchase individual insurance policies for at least 18 months. Congress also passed the Children's Health Insurance Program in 1997 with the intent that it would provide health insurance for at least half of the 11 million children who lack such coverage (Atchinson and Fox, 1997; Castellblanch, 1996; Goldstein, 1999; Pear, 1997).

Citizens, scholars, and public officials continue to call for incremental improvements in managed care services and for incremental increases in access to health benefits that will work over the long term. While many states used the 1997 federal legislation to significantly extend their health insurance coverage to children in low-income families, other states have forfeited the funds they received from the legislative program because of their failure to move quickly in using their allotments to provide health care to more children (Pear, 2000; Steinhauer, 2000c). Clearly, critics argue, government at all levels needs to address problems of partisan politics and legislative and bureaucratic roadblocks when dealing with national health problems.

In the 2000 election, a single-payer national health insurance plan, more health coverage for uninsured working adults, better access to health services for children, more prescription drug benefits for the elderly, and a Patients' Bill of Rights were all topics of debate (Enthoven and Vorhaus, 1997; Hacker, 1997; Halfon, Inkelas, DuPlessis, and Newacheck, 1999; Hellander, Himmelstein, Wolfe, and Woolhandler, 1994; Kronick and Gilmer, 1999; Skocpol, 1997). The Patients' Bill of Rights called for limiting the power of HMOs and other types of managed care plans in deciding on the degree of care patients receive, and permitting patients and employers to sue their HMOs. However, the highly partisan Democrats and Republicans in the U.S. Congress could not reach a compromise on such issues in 2003, and the Patients' Bill of Rights was not enacted into law (Lewis, 2000; Goldstein, 2003).

Since 2000, Congress has also considered several bills to reduce drug prices and to expand Medicare coverage by including prescription medications. Democrats and Republicans ultimately passed the Medicare Prescription Drug, Improvement, and Modernization Act of 2003, which budgeted nearly $400 billion to provide such benefits as a drug discount card (which became available in 2004–2005) and a guaranteed new drug benefit (beginning in 2006). Medicare beneficiaries could pay a new premium for the drug benefit if they chose to participate in this program. In an experimental plan to begin in 2010 in some regions of the United States, beneficiaries will be able to join a private health plan that offers drug coverage.

Almost immediately after passage of the Medicare reforms, concerns on several fronts emerged. Critics wondered whether low-income elderly persons would be worse off in some states as a result of the new federal

law because state pharmaceutical assistance programs offered better programs; whether private employers would be encouraged to drop more
generous drug benefit packages that they currently provide to retirees;
and whether the bill weakened Medicare in general by emphasizing an
increasing role for the private sector in administration of the drug benefit
and in direct competition with traditional Medicare (McClellan, Spatz,
and Carney, 2000; Pear and Bogdanich, 2003; Pear, 2003; Harris, 2003;
Hernandez and Pear, 2004).

The initial enrollment period for the new Medicare drug benefit ended
in May 2006. The enrollment process was not without problems: Beneficiaries faced enormous difficulties in determining the best combination
of benefits versus costs as they negotiated the maze of too many choices
offered by the plans. Doctors and pharmacists encountered problems in
trying to answer patients' many questions about plans' drug coverage.
Independent community pharmacists especially faced problems of lower
reimbursement rates and slow payment by the Medicare bureaucracy.
Some community pharmacies, including those in rural areas where their
services were most needed, closed their doors. Chain pharmacies had
better success in coping with the Medicare changes, as the lower rein-
bursement rates they received were offset by an increase in the volume
of prescriptions they filled. Patients who enrolled paid a $250 deductible
and then often reported delight at incurring lower prescription expenses.
However, their delight was often tempered when they reached the $2,000
limit on coverage and had to pay out-of-pocket for each medicine's full
cost until they spent $2,850; coverage of medications at 95% of their
cost then went into effect at that point. While some of the initial administrative and bureaucratic confusion reported by health professionals
and beneficiaries abated, new problems also arose, including errors on
monthly Medicare statements.

Concerns continued to be expressed about who most benefits from the
new plan: patients or pharmaceutical and insurance companies. Surveys and studies are under way to determine whether drug prices have
become lower as a result of the plans or if health outcomes for the
elderly beneficiaries have improved (Pear, 2006; Cardinale, 2006; Bach
and McClellan, 2006; Slaughter, 2006; Merrick, 2006; Zhang, 2006;
Freudenheim, 2006).

HEALTH CARE REFORM: A CONTINUING PARADOX

Despite its outstanding achievements, Americans repeatedly report
significant dissatisfaction with the U.S. health care system. In a recent
examination of the potential for comprehensive health care change,
economist Victor R. Fuchs and ethicist Ezekiel J. Emanuel (2005) note
that many ideas have been put forward about reforming the system from

both incremental and comprehensive policy approaches. Critics argue for financial, organizational, and delivery reforms. Incremental reform suggestions have included mandates that all employers offer some kind of health insurance for all employees; changes in Medicaid and Medicare that would extend eligibility to greater numbers of uninsured persons; health savings accounts; and mandatory managed competition plans offered by employers. Comprehensive reform suggestions have included providing universal coverage for all Americans through a single-payer plan (e.g., a Canada-style plan) or health care vouchers (public insurance that provides for choice and competition).

To date, the United States has consistently relied on incremental reform, as in the Children's Health Insurance Program or Medicare Part D. However, as Fuchs and Emmanuel point out, many obstacles confront comprehensive reform, including single-issue lobbying constituencies and checks and balances in the U.S. constitutional system that resist radical change. Fuchs and Emanuel observe that such events as war, depression, major civil unrest, or a pandemic might be needed to "set in motion a change in the political climate" that would lead to comprehensive health reform (2005, p. 1412).

As this historical overview shows, the U.S. health care system has undergone many changes over time. Some of these changes have benefited most Americans; others have resulted in denial of services for significant portions of the population. Health care expenditures will increase significantly as the 21st century advances, especially as life expectancy increases and the public's expectations for improved health outcomes and quality of life grow. Americans have very hard economic and social choices to make in a rapidly changing global environment.

QUESTIONS FOR FURTHER DISCUSSION

1. How will the conflict between the entrepreneurial role of health delivery organizations and the health professional's responsibility to serve the community be resolved in the future?
2. Lifestyle improvements, public health measures, and therapeutic interventions all affect health and disease patterns. How much money and effort should be devoted to these areas to address the health problems of Americans? What should the priorities be among the three areas? What roles should private and public institutions play? What roles should health professionals play?
3. To what degree is the health care system "in crisis" in the 21st century?

KEY TOPICS AND TERMS

Self-dosing
Social healers
Humoralism
Orthodox physicians
Heroic medical therapy
Sectarians
Patent medicines
Quackery
Dispensary
Charitable hospitals
Hospitals at the turn of the 20th century
Asepsis
Flexner Report (1910)
Infectious versus chronic disease
Factors explaining changes in mortality rates and life expectancy
Hill-Burton legislation (Hospital Survey and Construction Act of 1946)
Blue Cross and Blue Shield
Medicare
Medicaid
Pharmaceutical care
1973 Health Maintenance Organization Act
1996 Health Insurance Portability and Accountability Act
1997 Children's Health Insurance Program
Medicare Part D
Incremental health care reform
Comprehensive health care
Single-payer plan
Employer mandate

REFERENCES

The American Health Quality Association. (2006). *The 2005 National Healthcare Quality Report.* Retrieved June 19, 2006 from www.quality tools.ahrq.gov.

American Pharmaceutical Association. (1922). Code of ethics of the American Pharmaceutical Association. *Journal of the American Pharmaceutical Association, 11*(9), 728–729.

American Society for Microbiology. (2007). Statement submitted to Congress in support of increased funding for the Centers of Disease Control and Prevention. Retrieved November 1, 2006 from http://www.asm.org/Policy/index.asp?bid=41962

Anders, G. (1996). *Health against wealth: HMOs and the breakdown of medical trust.* Boston: Houghton Mifflin.

Anderson, G. F., Hussey, P. S., Frogner, B. K., & Waters, H. R. (2005, July/August). Health spending in the United States and the rest of the industrialized world. *Health Affairs, 24*(4), 903–914.

Apple, R. D. (1996). *Vitamania: Vitamins in American culture.* New Brunswick, NJ: Rutgers University Press.

Aroskar, M. A. (1999). Ethical aspects of pharmacy practice in managed care. In Robert P. Navarro (Ed.), *Managed care pharmacy practice* (pp. 507–524). Gaithersburg, MD: Aspen Publications.

Atchinson, B. K., & Fox, D. M. (1997). From the field: The politics of the Health Insurance Portability and Accountability Act. *Health Affairs, 16*(3), 146–150.

Bach, P. B., & McClellan, M. B. (2006, June 1). The first months of the prescription-drug benefit—ACMS update. *New England Journal of Medicine, 354*(22), 2313–2314.

Banks, J., Marmot, M., Oldfield, Z., & Smith, J. P. (2006, May 3). Disease and disadvantage in the United States and in England. *Journal of the American Medical Association. 295*(17), 2037–2045.

Bell, J. E. (1996, May/June). Saving their assets: How to stop plunder at Blue Cross and other nonprofits. *The American Prospect,* (26), 60–66.

Blumenthal, D., & Weissman, J. (2000). Trends: Selling teaching hospitals to investor-owned hospital chains: Three case studies. *Health Affairs, 19,* 158–166.

Bogdan, J. C. (1992). Childbirth in America, 1650–1990. In R. D. Apple (Ed.), *Women, health, and medicine in America: A historical handbook* (pp. 101–120). New Brunswick, NJ: Rutgers University Press.

Brandt, A. M. (1997). The cigarette, risk, and American culture. In W. G. Rothstein (Ed.), *Readings in American health care: Current issues in socio-historical perspective* (pp. 138–150). Madison, WI: University of Wisconsin Press.

Brock, K. A., Casper, K. A., Green, T. R., & Pedersen, C. A. (2006). Documentation of patient care services in a community pharmacy setting. *Journal of the American Pharmaceutical Association, 46*(3), 378–384.

Burnham, J. C., (1982, March 19). American medicine's golden age: What happened to it? *Science, 245,* pp. 1474-1479.

Byrd, W. M., & Clayton, L. A. (2000). *An American health dilemma: A medical history of African Americans and the problem of race, beginning to 1900* (Vol. 1). New York: Routledge.

Cahill, S. (1997). The Wal-Mart of hospitals. *In These Times, 21*(8), 14–16.

Cardinale, V. (2006, April 17). Bewitched, bothered, and bewildered: Consumers view the new drug benefit with caution, concern, and some optimism. *Drug Topics,* (150), 30, 32, 35–37.

Cassedy, J. H. (1991). *Medicine in America: A short history.* Baltimore: Johns Hopkins University Press.

Castellblanch, R. (1996). Legislation for sale. *In These Times, 20,* 14–16.

Cayleff, S. E. (1987). *Wash and be healed: The water-cure movement and women's health.* Philadelphia: Temple University Press.

Cayleff, S. E. (1992). Self-help and the patent medicine business. In R. D. Apple (Ed.), *Women, health, and medicine in America: A historical handbook* (pp. 303–328). New Brunswick, NJ: Rutgers University Press.

Central Intelligence Agency. (2006). *The World Factbook.* Washington, DC. Retrieved November 1, 2006 from http://www.odci.gov/cia/publications/factbook/docs/randorderguide.html

Christianson, E. H. (1987). Medicine in New England. In R. L. Numbers (Ed.), *Medicine in the New World: New Spain, New France, and New England* (pp. 101–153). Knoxville, TN: University of Tennessee Press.

Comment: Cheap and easy. (2000, July 10). *The New Yorker,* p. 21.

Cowen, D. L., & Kent, D. F. (1997). Medical and pharmaceutical practice in 1854. *Pharmacy in History, 39,* 91–100.

DeNavas-Walt, C., Proctor, B., & Lee. C. H. (2005). *Income, poverty, and health insurance coverage in the United States: 2004.* Washington, DC: U. S. Census Bureau, Government Printing Office.

Deno, R. A., Rowe, T. D., & Brodie, D. C. (1959). *The profession of pharmacy: An introductory textbook.* Philadelphia: J. B. Lippincott.

Duffy, J. (1993). *From humors to medical science: A history of American medicine* (2nd ed.). Urbana and Chicago: University of Illinois Press.

Enthoven, A. C., & Vorhaus, C. B. (1997). A vision of quality in health care delivery. *Health Affairs, 16*(3), 44–57.

Epstein, H. (2003, October 12). Enough to make you sick? *New York Times Sunday Magazine,* pp. 75ff.

Essoyan, S. (2000, August 13). Hospital mixes high-tech, human touch. *Boston Globe,* p. A19.

Flexner, A. (1910). *Medical education in the United States and Canada* (Bulletin No. 4). New York: Carnegie Foundation for the Advancement of Teaching.

Fox, D. M. (1988). An historical perspective: Health policy and changing epidemiology in the United States—Chronic disease in the twentieth century. In R. C. Maulitz (Ed.), *Unnatural causes: The three leading killer diseases in America* (pp. 11–31). New Brunswick, NJ: Rutgers University Press.

Fox, D. M. (1993). *Power and illness: The failure and future of American health.* Berkeley, CA: University of California Press.

Freudenheim, M. (2006, June 21). Drug prices up sharply this year. *New York Times,* pp. 1C, C9.

Fuchs, V. R., & Emanuel, E. J. (2005). Health care reform: Why? What? When? *Health Affairs, 24*(6), 1399–1414.

Fuller, R. C. (1993). Alternative medicine. In *Macmillan compendium: Everyday life: American social history.* New York: Simon and Schuster Macmillan.

Garrett, L. (2000). *Betrayal of trust: The collapse of global public health.* New York: Hyperion.

Goldberg, C. (2000, July 4). Fight on syphilis is timely, officials say, and in danger. *New York Times,* p. A8.

Goldstein, A. (1999, October 11). Who lacks health insurance? *Washington Post Weekly Edition,* p. 18.

Goldstein, A. (2003, September 12). For Patients Rights, a quiet fadeaway. *Washington Post,* p. A4.

Gordon, S. (1997). *Life support: Three nurses on the front lines.* Boston: Little, Brown.

Grob, G. N. (2002). *The deadly truth: A history of disease in America.* Cambridge, MA: Harvard University Press.

Hacker, J. S. (1997). *The road to nowhere: The genesis of President Clinton's plan for health security.* Princeton, NJ: Princeton University Press.

Halfon, N., Inkelas, M., DuPlessis, H., & Newacheck, P. W. (1999). Challenges in securing access to care for children. *Health Affairs, 18*(2), 48–63.

Haller, J. S., Jr. (2000). *The people's doctors: Samuel Thomson and the American botanical movement, 1790–1860.* Carbondale, IL: Southern Illinois University Press.

Harris, G. (2003, November 26). Some experts foresee revolt by elderly over drug benefits. *New York Times,* p. A18.

Hellander, I., Himmelstein, D. U., Wolfe, S., & Woolhandler, S. (1994). Health care paper chase, 1993: The cost to the nation, the states, and the District of Columbia. *International Journal of Health Services, 24*(1), 1–9.

Hepler, C. D. (1988). Unresolved issues in the future of pharmacy. *American Journal of Hospital Pharmacy, 45,* 1071–1081.

Hernandez, R., & Pear, R. (2004, January 4). State officials are cautious on Medicare drug benefits. *New York Times,* p. A15.

Higby, G. J. (1992). *In service to American pharmacy: The professional life of William Procter, Jr.* Tuscaloosa, AL: University of Alabama Press.

Higby, G. J. (with Gallagher, T. C.). (1992). Pharmacists. In R. D. Apple (Ed.), *Women, health, and medicine in America: A historical handbook* (pp. 489–508). New Brunswick, NJ: Rutgers University Press.

Horrocks, T. A. (2003). Rules, remedies, and regimens: Health advice in early American almanacs. In C. E. Rosenberg (Ed.), *Right living: An Anglo-American tradition of self-help medicine and hygiene* (pp. 112–146). Baltimore: Johns Hopkins University Press.

Hoy, S. (1995). *Chasing dirt: The American pursuit of cleanliness.* New York: Oxford University Press.

Johnson, H., & Broder, D. (1996). *The system: The American way of politics at the breaking point.* Boston: Little, Brown.

Kaufman, M. (1971). *Homeopathy in America: The rise and fall of a medical heresy.* Baltimore: Johns Hopkins University Press.

Kennedy, E. M. (1972). *In critical condition: The crisis in America's health care.* New York: Simon and Schuster.

Kevles, B. H. (1997). *Medical imaging in the twentieth century.* New Brunswick, NJ: Rutgers University Press.

King, C. R. (1993). *Children's health in America: A history.* New York: Twayne.

Knox, R. A. (1996a, September 16). Changing world, changing ailments. *Boston Globe,* pp. C1–C3.

Knox, R. A. (1996b, November 13). Widespread chronic illness cited. *Boston Globe,* p. A11.

Knox, R. A. (1997, April 10). Health care inflation likely to accelerate, report predicts. *Boston Globe,* p. A28.

Kaufmann, M. & Stein, R. (2006, January 10). Record share of economy spent on health care. *Washington Post,* p. A01.

Kong, D. (1997, June 10). Infant deaths down, but city worries. *Boston Globe,* p. A1.

Kowalczyk, L. (2000). A stretched-thin doctor draws a line. *Boston Globe,* pp. A1, C6.

Kraut, A. M. (1994). *Silent travelers: Germs, genes, and the "immigrant menace."* New York: Basic Books.

Kreling, D. H., Doucette, W. R., Mott, D. A., Gaither, A., Pedersen, C. A., & Schommer, J. C. (2006). Community pharmacists' work environments: Evidence from the 2004 national pharmacist workforce study. *Journal of the American Pharmaceutical Association, 46*(3), 331–339.

Kronick, R., & Gilmer, T. (1999, March/April). Explaining the decline in health insurance coverage, 1979–1995. *Health Affairs, 18*(2), 30–47.

La Ferla, R. (2000, August 13). Hospitals are discovering their inner spa. *New York Times,* sect. 9, pp. 1, 4.

Leavitt, J. W. (1995). A worrying profession: The domestic environment of medical practice in mid-19th century America. *Bulletin of the History of Medicine, 69,* 1–29.

Leavitt, J. W. (1996). *Typhoid mary: Captive to the public's health.* New York: Beacon Press.

Leavitt, J. W., & Numbers, R. L. (1997). Sickness and health: An overview. In J. W. Leavitt & R. L. Numbers (Eds.), *Sickness and health in America: Readings in the history of medicine and public health* (3rd ed.) (pp. 3–10). Madison, WI: University of Wisconsin Press.

Lerner, M., & Anderson, O. W. (1963). *Health progress in the United States: 1900-1960.* Chicago: University of Chicago Press.

Lewis, N. A. (2000, July 7). Patient's bill set to become an issue for campaign. *New York Times,* p. A10.

Litman, T. J. (1997). The relationship of government and politics to health and health care—a sociopolitical overview. In T. J. Litman & L. S. Robins (Eds.), *Health politics and policy* (3rd ed.) (pp. 3–45). New York: Delmar.

Ludmerer, K. M. (1985). *Learning to heal: The development of American medical education.* New York: Basic Books.

Ludmerer, K. M. (1999). *Time to heal: American education from the turn of the century to the era of managed care.* New York: Oxford University Press.

Lukas, C. V. &Young, G. J. (2000, March-April). Trends: Public hospitals, privatization and uncompensated care. *Health Affairs.* p. 1-6.

Maciosek, M. V., Coffield, A. B., Edwards, N. M., Flottemesch, T. J., Goodman, M. J., & Solberg, L. I. (2006). Priorities among effective clinical preventive services: Results of a systematic review and analysis. *American Journal of Preventive Medicine, 20*(10), 1–10.

Markowitz, G. E., & Rosner, D. (1979). Doctors in crisis: Medical education and medical reform during the progressive era, 1895–1915. In S. Reverby & D. Rosner (Eds.), *Health care in America: Essays in social history* (pp. 185–205). Philadelphia: Temple University Press.

Martinez, B. (2000, August 21). Now it's mass medicine. *Wall Street Journal,* pp. B1, B4.

McClellan, M., Spatz, I. D., & Carney, S. (2000, March/April). Designing a Medicare prescription drug benefit: Issues, obstacles, and opportunities. *Health Affairs,* 26–41.

Melosi, M. V. (2000). *The sanitary city: Urban infrastructure in America from colonial times to the present.* Baltimore: Johns Hopkins University Press.

Merrick, A. (2006, June 21). Getting an "A" in Part D: While others complained Walgreen found way to profit from drug plan for seniors. *Wall Street Journal,* pp. 1–2.

Millis, J. S. (1975). *Pharmacists for the future: The report of the Study Commission on Pharmacy.* Ann Arbor, MI: Health Administration Press.

Mishler, E. G. (1981). Viewpoint: Critical perspectives on the biomedical model. In E. G. Mishler (Ed.), *Social contexts of health, illness, and patient care* (pp. 1–13). New York: Cambridge University Press.

Morantz-Sanchez, R. (1992). Physicians. In R. D. Apple (Ed.), *Women, health, and medicine in America: A historical handbook* (pp. 469–487). New Brunswick, NJ: Rutgers University Press.

More, E. S. (1999). *Restoring the balance: Women physicians and the profession of medicine, 1850–1995.* Cambridge, MA: Harvard University Press.

Murray, C. J. L., & Lopez, A. D. (Eds.). (1996). *The global burden of disease: A comprehensive assessment of mortality and disability from diseases, injuries, and risk factors in 1990 and projected to 2020.* Cambridge, MA: Harvard University Press.

Naik, G. (2006, June 20). Cincinnati applies a corporate model to saving infants. *Wall Street Journal,* pp. A01, A14.

Navarro, R. P. (1999). *Managed care pharmacy practice.* Gaithersburg, MD: Aspen Publications.

Neergaard, L. (1995, July 10). Infant deaths at record low, but gap exists. *Boston Globe,* p. A3.

Nissenbaum, S. (1980). *Sex, diet, and debility in Jacksonian America: Sylvester Graham and health reform.* Westport, CT: Greenwood Press.

Numbers, R. L. (1997). The third party: Health insurance in America. In J. W. Leavitt & R. L. Numbers (Eds.), *Sickness and health in America: Readings in the history of medicine and public health* (3rd ed.) (pp. 269–283). Madison, WI: University of Wisconsin Press.

Okie, S. (1997, May 26). Syphilis drop sparks hope of eradication in U. S. *Boston Globe,* p. A3.

Opdycke, S. (1999). *No one was turned away: The role of public hospitals in New York City since 1900.* New York: Oxford University Press.

Ott, K. (1996). *Fevered lives: Tuberculosis in American culture since 1870.* Cambridge, MA: Harvard University Press.

Parascandola, J. (1997). The introduction of antibiotics into therapeutics. In J. W. Leavitt & R. L. Numbers (Eds.), *Sickness and health in America: Readings in the history of medicine and public health* (3rd ed.) (pp. 102–112). Madison, WI: University of Wisconsin Press.

Patel, K., & Rushefsky, M. E. (1995). *Health care politics and policy in America.* Armonk, NY: M. E. Sharpe.

Patterson, J. T. (1987). *The dread disease: Cancer and modern American culture.* Cambridge, MA: Harvard University Press.

Pear, R. (1997, April 2). New health insurance rules spell out rights of workers. *New York Times,* p. A15.

Pear, R. (2000, September 24). Forty states forfeit health care funds for poor children. *New York Times,* pp. A1, A26.

Pear, R. (2003, November 26). Sweeping Medicare change wins approval in Congress; President claims a victory. *New York Times,* pp. A1, A18.

Pear, R. (2006, June 11). In Texas town, patients and providers find new prescription drug plan baffling. *New York Times,* p. 30.

Pear, R., & Bogdanich, W. (2003, September 4). Some successful models ignored as Congress works on drug bill. *New York Times,* p. A11.

Perls, T. T. (2004). Anti-aging quackery: Human growth hormone and tricks of the trade—more dangerous than ever. *Journals of Gerontology Series A: Biological Sciences and Medical Sciences, 59*(7), 682–91.

Pernick, M. S. (1985). *A calculus of suffering: Pain, professionalism, and anesthesia in nineteenth-century America.* New York: Columbia University Press.

Petersen, M. A. (1997). Introduction: Health care into the next century. *Journal of Health Politics, Policy and Law, 22,* 291-313.

Poen, M. M. ((1979). *Harry S. Truman versus the medical lobby: The genesis of medicare.* Columbia, MO: University of Missouri Press.

Reinhardt, U. E., Hussey, P. S., & Anderson, G. F. (2004, May/June). U. S. health care spending in an international context. *Health Affairs, 2*(3), 10–25.

Reverby, S. M. (1987). *Ordered to care: The dilemma of American nursing, 1850–1945.* New York: Cambridge University Press.

Risse, G. B. (1999). *Mending bodies, saving souls: A history of hospitals.* New York: Oxford University Press.

Rosenberg, C. E. (1985a). Social class and medical care in 19th century America: The rise and fall of the dispensary. In J. W. Leavitt & R. L. Numbers (Eds.), *Sickness and health in America: Readings in the history of medicine and public health* (2nd ed.) (pp. 273–286). Madison, WI: University of Wisconsin Press.

Rosenberg, C. E. (1985b). The therapeutic revolution: Medicine, meaning, and social change in 19th-century America. In J. W. Leavitt & R. L. Numbers (Eds.), *Sickness and health in America: Readings in the history of medicine and public health* (2nd ed.) (pp. 39–52). Madison, WI: University of Wisconsin Press.

Rosenberg, C. E. (1987). *The care of strangers: The rise of America's hospital system.* New York: Basic Books.

Rosenberg, C. E. (1992). Framing disease: Illness, society, and history. In C. E. Rosenberg & J. Golden (Eds.), *Framing disease: Studies in cultural history* (pp. xiii–xxvi). New Brunswick, NJ: Rutgers University Press.

Rosner, D. (1979). Business at the bedside: Health care in Brooklyn, 1890–1915. In S. Reverby & D. Rosner (Eds.), *Health care in America: Essays in social history* (pp. 117–131). Philadelphia: Temple University Press.

Rosner, D. (1995). Introduction: Hives of sickness and vice. In D. Rosner (Ed.), *Hives of sickness: Public health and epidemics in New York City* (pp. 1–12). New Brunswick, NJ: Rutgers University Press.

Rothstein, W. G. (1996a). Pharmaceuticals and public policy in America: A history. In W. G. Rothstein (Ed.), *Readings in American health care: Current issues in socio-historical perspective* (pp. 375–391). Madison, WI: University of Wisconsin Press.

Rothstein, W. G. (1996b). Trends in mortality in the twentieth century. In W. G. Rothstein (Ed.), *Readings in American health care: Current issues in socio-historical perspective* (pp. 71–86). Madison,WI: University of Wisconsin Press.

Satcher, D., Fryer, G. E., Jr., McCann, J., Troutman, A., Woolf, S., & Rust, G. (2005, March/April). What if we were equal? A comparison of the black–white mortality gap in 1960 and 2000. *Health Affairs, 24*(2), 459–464.

Skocpol, T. (1997). *Boomerang: Clinton's health security effort and the turn against government in U. S. politics.* New York: W. W. Norton.

Slaughter, L. M. (2006, June 1). Medicare Part D—The product of a broken process. *New England Journal of Medicine, 354*(22), 2314–2315.

Smith, C., Cowan, C., Heffler, S., Catlin, A., & the National Health Accounts Team. (2006 January/February). National health spending in 2004: Recent slowdown led by prescription drug spending. *Health Affairs, 25*(1), 186–196.

Sonnedecker, G. (1976). *Kremer's and Urdang's history of pharmacy* (4th ed.). Philadelphia: J. B. Lippincott.

Stage, S. (1979). *Female complaints: Lydia Pinkham and the business of women's medicine.* New York: W. W. Norton.

Starr, P. (1982). *The social transformation of American medicine: The rise of a sovereign profession and the making of a vast industry.* New York: Basic Books.

Starr, P. (1991). The logic of health care reform (The grand rounds press). Knoxville, TN: Whittle Direct Books.

Steinhauer, J. (2000a, June 4). Exotic ills loom large, but what about the flu? *New York Times,* pp. 29–30.

Steinhauer, J. (2000b, February 29). High infant mortality rates in Brooklyn mystify experts. *New York Times,* pp. A1, A23.

Steinhauer, J. (2000c, September 28). States prove unpredictable in aiding uninsured children. *New York Times*, p. A16.

Stevens, R. (1971). *American medicine and the public interest*. New Haven, CT: Yale University Press.

Stevens, R. (1989). *In sickness and in wealth: American hospitals in the twentieth century*. New York: Basic Books.

Stone, D. A. (1997). The doctor as businessman: The changing politics of a cultural icon. *The American Prospect, 22*(2), 533–556.

Tannenbaum, R. (2002). *The healer's calling: Women and medicine in early New England*. Ithaca, NY: Cornell University Press.

Temin, P. (1980). *Taking your medicine: Drug regulation in the United States*. Cambridge, MA: Harvard University Press.

Tesh, S. N. (1988). *Hidden arguments: Political ideology and disease prevention policy*. New Brunswick, NJ: Rutgers University Press.

Tomes, N. (1998). *The gospel of germs: Men, women, and the microbe in American life*. Cambridge, MA: Harvard University Press.

Torrens, P. R. (1989). Historical evolution and overview of health services in the United States. In S. J. Williams & P. R. Torrens (Eds.), *Introduction to health services* (3rd ed.) (pp.3–31). Albany, NY: Thomson Delmar Learning.

Ulrich, L. T. (1990). *A midwife's tale: The life of Martha Ballard, based on her diary, 1785–1812*. New York: Alfred A. Knopf.

U. S. Census Bureau. (2002). *Statistical abstract of the United States*. Washington, DC: Government Printing Office.

U. S. Department of Health and Human Services (DHHS). (1994). *For a healthy nation: Returns on investment in public health*. Washington, DC: Government Printing Office.

U. S. Department of Health and Human Services (1999). *Health: United States 1999*. Washington, DC: Government Printing Office.

Vogel, M. J. (1979). The transformation of the American hospital, 1850–1920. In S. Reverby & D. Rosner (Eds.), *Health care in America: Essays in social history* (pp. 105–116). Philadelphia: Temple University Press.

Wall Street Journal. (2006, June 15). Hospital initiative to cut errors finds about 122,300 lives saved. p. D6.

Warner, J. H. (1997). From specificity to universalism in medical therapeutics: Transformation in the 19th-century United States. In J. W. Leavitt & R. Numbers (Eds.), *Sickness and health in America: Readings in the history of medicine and public health* (3rd ed.) (pp. 87–101). Madison, WI: University of Wisconsin Press.

Weiss, G. L., & Lonnquist, L. E. (2006). *The sociology of health, healing, and illness* (5th ed.). Upper Saddle River, NJ: Pearson Prentice Hall.

White House domestic policy council. (1993). *The President's Health Security Plan*. New York: Times Books.

Young, G., Dasai, K., & Lucas, C. V. (1997). Does the sale of nonprofit hospitals threaten health care for the poor? *Health Affairs, 16(1)*, 137–141.

Young, J. H. (1992). *American health quackery: Collected essays*. Princeton, NJ: Princeton University Press.

Zhang, J. (2006, June 21). Lean times in rich square. *Wall Street Journal*, pp. 1–2.

Health Care Professionals and Interdisciplinary Care

Alice M. Sapienza

Case Scenario

. . . View indispensable drug information for the 150 most commonly prescribed drugs . . . Easy-to-use, menu-driven interface . . . gives you the three-second prescription. . . . Print information for your patients about their prescription. . . . Fits with your favorite Palm application. (www.ephysician.com/product/index)

As you and your colleagues on the intensive care unit (ICU) committee discuss recent budget requests, you recall this advertisement for the "electronic drug reference" that you read over the weekend. One of the physicians had seen it as well, and soon everyone begins to talk about how this and similar innovations might affect not only interdisciplinary collaboration but also pay for performance in critical care.

Your conversation sparks a lively debate about the effects of new technologies (such as broadband communication and the Internet) on health services and the increasingly important role of pharmacists in the provision of quality care. In what ways might this role expand, and why?

The meeting ends. Both a physician and a respiratory therapist set a time to have lunch with you to continue talking about these ideas.

LEARNING OBJECTIVES

Upon completion of this chapter, the student shall be able to:

- be able to define their own characteristics as a pharmacy professional
- have a better understanding of the variety of professionals involved in health care
- be aware of the differences between multidisciplinary care and interdisciplinary care
- begin to appreciate the potential effects of changing technologies—especially information technologies—on the pharmacy professional's career
- begin to appreciate how changing technologies—especially information technologies—might affect health care services more generally

CHAPTER QUESTIONS

1. What distinguishes a profession from an occupation?
2. What do you think is the difference—from the patient's perspective—between multidisciplinary care and interdisciplinary care?
3. What do you think is the difference—from the health care professional's perspective—between multidisciplinary care and interdisciplinary care?
4. How might the professions and health care change as the result of new technologies?

INTRODUCTION

This chapter provides an overview of the principal health care professions, with an emphasis on pharmacists (including pharmacy technicians), physicians (and physician assistants), and nurses. For each profession, background information is provided on training, practice, and compensation. The chapter begins by defining the term *professional* and discussing the special characteristics ascribed to the professional health care provider (that is, the differences between a profession and a job). The next section provides an overview of pharmacists and pharmacy technicians and assistants. (Chapter 3 focuses on the pharmacist.) The third section pays particular attention to physicians, because of their influence on prescribing and on the health care system generally—including how and where physicians are trained and how and where they practice. The fourth section deals with nurses and their role in patient care. The fifth section describes other important members of the health care team, including physical, respiratory, occupational, and recreational therapists; social workers; and dietitians. As suggested by the beginning case, this chapter concludes with some reflections on interdisciplinary care, quality, pay for performance, information technologies, and other issues affecting the future of the health care system.

PROFESSIONALS

What is a professional? As the title of this chapter and the contents of this book suggest, the term *professional* is frequently used in health care to describe the people who provide, directly or indirectly, a vast range of services to the patient. The word has a particular meaning and several implications. Not everyone in health care is a professional. To be described in this way implies that the person has altruistic values (Turner, 1987). In other words, a professional is not expected to be motivated solely (or even primarily) by economics or prestige. Instead, he or she is expected to be motivated by a desire to help, to be of service. In addition, the professional is expected to possess specialized technical knowledge, gained (almost always) in particular schools or educational programs. Finally, the professional is generally licensed to practice by an accepted credentialing body.

In part, the specialized technical knowledge that distinguishes a professional consists of scientific theory. Credentialing organizations typically specify the disciplines and the discipline content that are required for licensure. To gain this theoretical knowledge, the aspiring professional attends tailored programs involving training both inside and outside the classroom. The outside-of-class opportunities provide the hands-on experiences that, in health care, involve patients. At the conclusion of the prescribed course of study and internship/externship, the graduate must satisfactorily pass the program's exams and achieve a requisite score on state or national tests. Only then can a professional practice in his or her chosen field.

Professional training does not end at this point, however. Nearly all professionals are required to demonstrate continued education, usually in the form of so many units or credits per year, to remain credentialed or certified.

PHARMACISTS

> *Pharmacists are assuming greater roles and responsibilities for patient care in the intensive care unit (ICU) and are an integral member of the multidisciplinary ICU team. (MacLaren et al., 2006)*

The pharmacy profession has undergone numerous changes over the past several decades, particularly with regard to philosophy of practice, locations of and opportunities to practice, educational requirements, and ethical codes. Moreover, as the case scenario at the beginning of this chapter suggests, new technologies are broadening the involvement of pharmacists in interdisciplinary care of the most critically ill patients. This section provides an overview of pharmacists in the United States; Chapter 3 discusses the roles and responsibilities of pharmacists in hospitals, managed care settings, and other practice arenas.

Education and Training: Past and Present

Pharmaceutical education has undergone quite an evolution over the last century. In 1905, the state of New York started a critically important trend when it passed a law requiring all new registrants in that state to possess a diploma from a recognized school of pharmacy by 1910. At that time, pharmacy programs entailed at least 2 years of study. More than 50 schools offered 2 years of study, 20 schools offered 3 years, roughly a dozen schools offered a bachelor of science degree after 4 years of coursework, and 4 schools offered a master of science degree following 5 years of study (Higby, 1996).

For the most part, pharmacists at the time were opposed to the idea of mandatory formal education because they believed their apprenticeship system guaranteed basic competency. However, two events took place in 1915 that changed many pharmacists' minds about educational requirements and promoted action. First, the respected reformer of medical school education, Abraham Flexner, declared that pharmacy was not a profession. Shortly thereafter, the U.S. War Department decided that registered pharmacists would not routinely receive commissions because their professional education was so minimal (Higby, 1996).

To help strengthen their position as professionals, pharmacists turned to the best schools and colleges of pharmacy. This reversal in their views set the wheels of professional pharmacy education in motion, as important classes in the sciences were developed. In 1928, the American Association of Colleges of Pharmacy (AACP) adopted the 4-year bachelor of science degree as the minimum course of study, although this mandate did not go into effect until 1932 (Higby, 1996).

Following the results of a comprehensive survey of the profession in the late 1940s, AACP recommended the general adoption of a 5-year bachelor of science degree. Its suggestion was approved, and this degree was the main one offered by most schools of pharmacy from the 1960s through the 1980s. In 1992, AACP recommended that the 6-year doctor of pharmacy (PharmD) degree be the entry-level degree to practice. The state of California was the first to start a PharmD program in 1950, but it seemed too radical at the time for most of the United States (Higby, 1996).

Over time, this view changed, and by 2004, 89 colleges of pharmacy were accredited to confer the PharmD as the first professional degree (i.e., the entry-level degree to practice). The class of 2010 comprises nearly 48,000 students, of whom 64% are female. Of all those students enrolled in 2004 (i.e., for all degrees), approximately 40% are members of a minority race/ethnicity and 67% are female. Total enrollment had been stable or slightly decreasing in the mid-1990s but has increased by an average of more than 5% per year since 2000 (American Association of Colleges of Pharmacy [AACP], 2006). Students in these programs receive instruction in the traditional classroom and spend about one-fourth of their time learning while in a practice setting under the supervision of licensed pharmacists.

In 2004, 67 colleges of pharmacy offered MS or PhD degrees for students who had completed a PharmD program or received a baccalaureate degree. "Many master's and PhD holders do research for a drug company or teach at a university" (Bureau of Labor Statistics [BLS], 2006).

Residencies and fellowships are also available to the motivated pharmacy graduate. Residencies are usually 1 year in length, are practice-based, and traditionally have been located in a hospital setting. The American Society of Health-System Pharmacists accredits residencies and has a "matching" program similar to that of physicians. Currently, more than 700 residency programs are available in the United States. With the increasing emphasis on outpatient care, however, residencies in community and ambulatory care settings are becoming more prevalent. Fellowships generally last 2 years and are research-based; in other words, the pharmacy fellow will likely be engaged in pharmacokinetic, epidemiologic, or other types of research.

Practice

> *Pharmaceutical Care is a patient-centered, outcomes-oriented pharmacy practice that requires the pharmacist to work in concert with the patient and the patient's other health care providers to promote health, to prevent diseases, and to assess, monitor, initiate, and modify medication use to assure that drug therapy regimens are safe and effective. (American Pharmaceutical Association, 2000)*

Like other professions (especially medicine), pharmacy has become much more specialized over the past two decades. Specialties from which a pharmacist may choose include ambulatory care, pharmacy administration, drug information, community practice, industry, geriatrics, managed care, long-term care, home health care, pediatrics, critical care, internal medicine, psychiatry, pharmacokinetics, oncology, and nutrition support.

In addition, as the chapter case suggests, new technologies are influencing both health care practice in general and pharmacy practice in particular. Hospitals are seeking to reduce the average inpatient length of stay by employing diagnostic and treatment technologies that allow patients to be cared for in other locations. As a consequence, pharmacy services are moving to long-term, ambulatory, and home care facilities. In addition, "new opportunities are emerging for pharmacists in managed care organizations, where they analyze trends and patterns in medication use, and in pharmacoeconomics—the cost and benefit analysis of different drug therapies" (BLS, 2006). At the same time, the increasing use of automated technology may serve to limit job growth in some ways.

Nevertheless, employment of pharmacists is expected to grow faster than average, at least through 2014, "because of the increasing demand for pharmaceuticals, particularly from the growing elderly population" (BLS, 2006). Also promoting employment growth are "scientific advances that will make more drug products available, new developments in genome research and medication distribution systems . . . and coverage of prescription drugs by a greater number of health insurance plans and Medicare" (BLS, 2006). In fact, as of April 2006, more than 30 million Medicare beneficiaries had enrolled in the new drug benefit program (Heavey, 2006).

Another change in practice influenced by new technologies is the growth in the number of pharmacy technicians and assistants. Formal education for these positions requires both classroom and laboratory work. The Institute for the Certification of Pharmacy Technicians (ICPT) sponsors The Exam for the Certification of Pharmacy Technicians (ExCPT), and individuals who pass that exam must be recertified every two years. The Pharmacy Technician Certification Board offers another certification exam with similar requirements.

Pharmacists by the Numbers

In 2000, approximately 217,000 pharmacists were employed in the United States (and 7,260 students earned their first professional degree). About 60% worked in community pharmacies, and most of those positions were salaried. More than 4,000 pharmacists taught in schools of pharmacy; others worked for pharmaceutical manufacturers (Midwest Pharmacy Workforce Research Consortium, 2005). Approximately 190,000 pharmacy technicians and assistants were employed in the United States, two-thirds of those in retail pharmacies (BLS, 2002–2003). That same year, 2.9 billion prescriptions were dispensed from approximately 55,000 U.S. pharmacies.

In 2004, approximately 230,000 pharmacists were employed in the United States (and 7,488 students earned a PharmD) and 3.2 billion prescriptions were dispensed from 55,400 retail pharmacies. In the short period from 2000 to 2004, the proportion of pharmacists dispensing more than 160 prescriptions per day increased from 24% to 40%. When asked about the impact of technology on their practice, more than "60% reported that equipment and/or technology increased the level of their productivity and the quality of care . . . [and] increased versus decreased demands on their time in the pharmacy" (Midwest Pharmacy Workforce Research Consortium, 2005).

Compensation

As far as monetary benefits are concerned, full-time pharmacists earned about $44 per hour in 2005. Median annual wages and salary in 2004 were $84,900, with pharmacists in department stores earning the highest average wages and salary (BLS, 2006).

The median hourly wages of pharmacy technicians and assistants increased from $9.93 in 2000 to $11.37 by May 2004. Certified technicians can earn more, and shift differentials (e.g., working evenings or weekends) can increase their level of compensation. To realize higher levels of rewards, technicians must be able to learn and master new pharmacy technologies, such as robotic dispensing machines (BLS, 2006).

PHYSICIANS

Demand for physician services is highly sensitive to changes in consumer preferences, health care reimbursement policies, and legislation. (BLS, 2006)

Physicians have perhaps the longest training period of all the professionals in the health care system. They are the major decision makers, deciding on courses of treatment for patients, admission to (and discharge from) inpatient facilities, medicines prescribed, and other aspects of care. These are tremendous responsibilities, and physicians generally have the greatest influence (and stature) in the health care system.

Education and Training: Past and Present

In the United States, medical education began as a formal system during the early 17th century (Sawin, 1989). There were no medical schools; instead, the educational system was remarkably like the one that prepared the pharmacist—namely, apprenticeship. However, by the mid-1800s, several dozen medical schools had opened their doors, including four that are still in existence (University of Pennsylvania, Columbia, Harvard, and Dartmouth). The curriculum did not yet include basic sciences (e.g., human physiology) but rather focused on techniques (e.g., surgery).

The scale of deaths from infection and (what we today would call) medical inadequacy in the Civil War galvanized an intense reform of medical education. More emphasis was placed on rigorous theoretical and technical preparation, and the medical school curriculum was changed to follow the German model. The Flexner Report of 1910 (by the same author who declared that pharmacists were not professionals) was the culmination of this period of reform.

By 1920, medical education as we would recognize it was essentially in place. Following the creation of the U.S. National Institutes of Health

(NIH) in the 1930s and with greatly expanded funding of biomedical research in the 1950s and 1960s, medical schools became the locus of sophisticated basic and clinical biomedical research programs. By this point, medical schools and their affiliated teaching hospitals had become large, expensive, and complex organizations.

Today, medical education is a post-baccalaureate program that begins with 2 years of in-class study of basic sciences in an accredited medical school. Subjects include anatomy and cell biology, biochemistry, pathology, physiology, and pharmacology. (Medical students' training in pharmacology is much less extensive than that of pharmacy students.) Basic science faculty, mostly PhD holders, teach these courses and are generally part of university science departments rather than the medical school itself.

After this grounding in foundational knowledge, students move to 2 years of clinical training, primarily in teaching hospitals. During this period, they follow prescribed "rotations": periods of several weeks spent learning the rudiments of anesthesiology, dermatology, internal medicine, pediatrics, and so forth. Here, they are taught by clinical faculty, MDs who hold joint appointments at the medical school and the teaching hospital. During this latter portion of their program, medical students decide on a particular area of practice (e.g., pediatrics or thoracic surgery). Regardless of the area of practice that they eventually choose, medical students are exposed to all facets of care—from emergency medicine to neonatology, from routine primary care to intensive care of organ transplant patients, from obstetrics to psychiatry. These 4 years of medical school are the same for all physicians.

Upon successfully graduating from medical school, the degreed physician who intends to practice must now enter a series of required postgraduate years in a hospital setting, beginning with internship. At the end of the fourth year of medical school, medical students list their choice of hospitals in which to train. Hospitals also list their choice of students, as well as the number that they can take per specialty. The sorting process is called "matching" (officially, the National Resident Matching Program, conducted by the Association of American Medical Colleges). Medical school graduates do not necessarily get their first choice of hospital, and hospitals cannot always fill their postgraduate slots. (These positions are important to teaching hospitals because interns and residents provide most of their inpatient care.)

When medical school graduates enter internship and residency programs in hospitals, they are called "house staff." During the internship, doctors take on increasing responsibility for patient care, but always under the guidance of more senior physicians, such as "attendings" or the patients' private physicians. After the internship year, physicians spend 2 years in the hospital, as first-year and then second-year residents, still under the guidance of faculty preceptors. During the residency, the physician does most of his or her work in the selected specialty. The surgeon-in-training rarely delivers babies, and the anesthesiologist-in-training rarely does a psychiatric consult, unlike during their internship year.

Medical education is expensive. In any graduating medical school class, approximately 80% of the students have a large debt to repay. First-year students in 1999–2000 faced a median cost for tuition and fees of $24,000 in public medical schools for out-of-state students and $29,000 in private medical schools (Association of American Medical Colleges, 2000). Those who graduated in 2000 carried about $80,000 in debt. Following big increases in tuition, however, by 2003, "the median amounts for those who have debt [more than 80% of graduates] have enormously increased to more than $100,000. . . . The magnitude and rapidity of these increases have raised serious concerns among affected medical students" (Jolly, 2004).

Physicians are trained in the approximately 120 U.S. medical schools affiliated with about 300 teaching hospitals ("academic medical centers"). Major sources of revenue for these centers include federal research support, primarily through the NIH; subsidies from practice plans; state and local government appropriations; and tuition (which accounts for a minuscule portion of the total).

Pressure to slow the growth of health care costs is of increasing concern to those responsible for medical education. Hospitals are constrained by managed care contracts to reduce costs and streamline services, to reduce patients' length of stay, and to move as much care as possible to outpatient locations. Such changes could have a potentially serious effect on the clinical aspect of medical education.

For example, in teaching hospitals, which provide most of the physician training in the United States, cost-containment efforts must be balanced against the need to retain teaching programs. The shift from charge-based reimbursement to reimbursement based on diagnosis or some other basis (such as capitation) decreases the amount of money available to support those physicians whose role is to provide medical school and postgraduate teaching. Teaching takes time and, therefore, effectively reduces the "productivity" of physicians who must both attend to patients and train students and graduate physicians. This is especially true in the surgical specialties.

Emphasis on decreased length of stay and increased hospital bed utilization affects the clinical portion of medical education as well. Third- and fourth-year medical students serve as part of the "ward team" and perform a variety of patient care tasks. However, their most important tasks involve interacting with patients, learning at the bedside, and following patients over time. As length of stay decreases, students have much less time available for patient interaction. Also, opportunities to expose students to a variety of clinical diseases, technical procedures, and illness and care progression are being compressed.

As medical care becomes increasingly oriented to outpatient facilities, clinical teaching's traditional focus on inpatient services is drawing questions. Some contend that more medical school training must occur in managed care organizations. Physicians who are responsible for the work of third- and fourth-year medical students and interns in such organizations will see fewer patients. In other words, if physicians are to teach students and interns and provide care in the same appointment, they must schedule a longer amount of time for that visit than if they were seeing the patient alone. Productivity—defined as the number of patients seen per day or per week—will therefore be reduced. If physicians see fewer patients, the total cost to the managed care organization will increase. Insurers (other than Medicare) reimburse for care, not for teaching. If physician training moves to these outpatient settings, then managed care may no longer provide a financial advantage to employers, which are worried about the cost of the health care benefit.

The simple fact is that someone must pay for training physicians. How these issues are resolved will, in the long run, affect both the number and quality of physicians.

Practice

> *Opportunities for individuals interested in becoming physicians and surgeons are expected to be very good . . . Unlike their predecessors, newly trained physicians face radically different choices of where and how to practice. (BLS, 2006)*

As previously mentioned, the increased emphasis on primary care in the United States has encouraged more students to become general and family medicine practitioners. "New physicians are much less likely to enter solo practice and more likely to take salaried jobs in group medical practices, clinics, and health networks" (BLS, 2006).

Physicians by the Numbers

Nearly 600,000 physicians practice actively in the United States. Since 1980, approximately 16,000 individuals have graduated each year from medical schools. Representation of women in this profession has increased steadily. In 2004, about half of the entering class (and 45% of the graduates) was female. However, the ratio of men to women faculty in medical schools remains higher, although greater parity exists for the graduating cohort of 1995 (Association of American Medical Colleges, 2005). In other words, as more women graduate from medical school, more women are being employed as faculty to train medical students.

Compensation

A physician's income depends very much on his or her specialty, but it is among the highest of any occupation in the United States. For example, the median total compensation of anesthesiologists with more than one year in that specialty was $322,000 in 2004. Physicians in family practice earned about half that amount, but self-employed physicians "generally have higher median incomes than salaried physicians" (BLS, 2006). Salaries are generally lower in managed care organizations. At the same time, physicians tend to work more predictable hours in such organizations and find that to be a valuable benefit.

PHYSICIAN ASSISTANTS

Employment of PAs is expected to grow much faster than average for all occupations through the year 2014, ranking among the fastest growing occupations . . . ." (BLS, 2006)

The number of physician assistants (PAs) is expected to grow because of the "anticipated expansion of the health care industry and an emphasis on cost containment, resulting in increasing utilization of PAs by physicians and health care institutions" (BLS, 2006). As the health care system expands to meet the needs of the growing elderly population, physician assistants are expected to provide more primary care and assist with medical and surgical procedures. Like pharmacy technicians, physician assistants are cost-effective and productive members of the health care team. New technologies are also expected to encourage growth in the number of these professionals. "Telemedicine—using technology to facilitate interactive consultations between physicians and physician assistants—also will expand the use of physician assistants" (BLS, 2006).

Physician assistants must complete an accredited educational program (most have at least a bachelor's degree). In addition, graduates of such a PA program must pass the Physicians Assistant National Certifying Examination and, to remain certified, must complete 100 hours of continuing medical education every 2 years. Every 6 years, they must pass a recertification exam or accepted alternative.

In 2004, physician assistants held about 62,000 jobs (the number of jobs is larger than the number of physician assistants, because some hold two or more jobs). Median income for PAs in "full-time clinical practice in 2004 was $74,264; median income for first-year graduates was $64,536" (BLS, 2006).

NURSES

As the largest health care occupation, registered nurses held about 2.4 million jobs in 2004 . . . [including] in hospitals, . . . nursing care facilities, home health care services, employment services, government agencies, and outpatient care centers. (BLS, 2006)

Nursing care has deep roots. Long before the age of modern nursing, members of religious orders provided bedside care to the sick. Nursing as a profession perhaps had its origin in the Middle Ages at the time of the Crusades. From Florence Nightingale at Saint Thomas's Hospital in London in the mid-1800s to the trailblazers of today, nurses have been a critical force in caring for the patient holistically—mentally, socially, emotionally, spiritually, and physically. All health professionals have much to learn from the nursing profession's emphasis on caring for the whole patient.

Education and Training: Past and Present

The evolution of nursing education in the United States is similar to that for pharmacists and physicians. The first permanent schools of nursing were established at Bellevue Hospital (in New York), New Haven Hospital, and Massachusetts General Hospital (in Boston) in 1873. These hospital-based programs were called diploma schools, were 3 years in length, and produced well-trained nurses who were in charge of wards by the time they graduated. By 1898, the number of diploma schools had grown to 400, with 10,000 graduates each year (Haglund and Dowling, 1993).

In the 1900s, the professional development of nurses was considered one of the key elements in transforming hospitals into the institutions they are today. Advances in nursing in the early 1900s enhanced the growth of hospitals in two major ways: (1) nurses contributed to the efficacy of treatments, cleanliness, nutritious diets, and formal treatment routines, all of which led to better recovery of patients, and (2) considerate, skilled patient care made hospitals more acceptable for all people—not just the poor (Haglund and Dowling, 1993). The general advancement of hospitals and health care education spurred the development of other nursing programs and degrees.

Over the past few decades, the 2-year associate of science in nursing degree has been the mainstay of nursing education. However, the 4-year bachelor of science in nursing degree (BSN) is becoming increasingly attractive, because graduates are trained in "communication, leadership, and critical thinking, all of which are becoming more important as nursing care becomes more complex" (BLS, 2006). In 2004, nearly 700 nursing programs offered both a BSN and the associate degree in nursing (ADN), and more than 165 programs offered an accelerated ADN-to-BSN program (BLS, 2006).

Nurses also have opportunities to enter postgraduate programs that lead to a master's or doctoral degree. Graduates with a master of science in nursing degree are often clinical nurse specialists in a certain area. In 2004, 417 schools offered master's degrees and 93 offered a doctoral degree. According to the vision of the American Association of Colleges of Nursing, "all new advanced practice nurses in the [United States] will be educated at the doctoral level . . . [which] will put nursing on a par with the other health professions that require a doctorate for the highest level of clinical practice" (Hathaway, 2006).

Today, advanced registered nurse practitioners (ARNPs) are becoming more prevalent in health care institutions and are commonly given limited prescribing privileges. In some states, ARNPs and pharmacists may pursue collaborative prescribing practice. In other states, ARNPs' privileges have raised a bone of contention with pharmacists (who are denied prescribing privileges), because pharmacists are often the ones who teach the pharmacology section of the ARNP curriculum.

The number of certified registered nurse anesthetists has also increased over the past several years. These professionals are required to have experience in the critical care setting before starting specialty training.

Practice

Job opportunities for RNs in all specialties are expected to be excellent. Employment of registered nurses is expected to grow much faster than average for all occupations through 2014, and because the occupation is very large, many new jobs will result. (BLS, 2006)

There are many different areas in which nurses work, including ambulatory care, long-term care, home care, pediatrics, critical care, general medicine or surgery, psychiatry, oncology, labor and delivery, orthopedics, urology, and nutrition support. The emphasis on primary care, as noted earlier in this chapter, has also been a major impetus for nurses to return to school and become ARNPs in some of these specialty areas. Managed care organizations often employ ARNPs, who work as close colleagues with internists in providing primary care.

The profession of nursing is also being affected by the introduction of new technologies. Many procedures that were once performed only in hospitals are now moving to outpatient settings. "Rapid growth [in employment] is expected in hospital outpatient facilities, such as those providing same-day surgery, rehabilitation, and chemotherapy" (BLS, 2006). Hence, nurses will require different skills and training to assist as well as to perform such procedures. "The rapid growth in information technology has already had a radical impact on health care delivery and the education of nurses . . . Nanotechnology will introduce new forms of clinical diagnosis and treatment by means of inexpensive handheld biosensors capable of detecting a wide range of diseases from minuscule body specimens" (National League for Nursing, 2003).

Nurses by the Numbers

Approximately 2.4 million nurses were employed in the United States in 2004. Although employment in hospitals will grow more slowly, "registered nurses are projected to create the second largest number of new jobs among all occupations." Turnover is high in hospital settings, and "all four advanced practice specialties—clinical nurse specialists, nurse practitioners, midwives, and anesthetists—will be in high demand" (BLS, 2006).

Compensation

The median annual earning of registered nurses in 2004 was $52,330. Nurses in employment services earned the most ($63,170) and those in nursing care facilities earned the least ($48,220) (BLS, 2006).

OTHER ALLIED HEALTH PROFESSIONALS

The brevity of the following overview of other allied health professionals is a function of the primary focus of this book. As the chapter case noted, respiratory therapists (as well as physical therapists, occupational and recreational therapists, social workers, and nutritionists) are important members of the health care team.

Physical Therapists

> *Employment of physical therapists is expected to grow much faster than average for all occupations through 2014 . . . [although] the impact of proposed Federal legislation imposing limits on reimbursement for therapy services may adversely affect the short-term job outlook. (BLS, 2006)*

The physical therapist's primary objectives are to help improve the mobility of a person with physical disabilities, to relieve pain, and to prevent or limit the extent of a physical disability. In addition, physical therapists take "a personal and direct approach to meeting an individual's health needs and wants" (American Physical Therapy Association, 2003). Competition for entrance into the accredited physical therapy programs in the United States is intense, and these programs now offer only the master's and higher degrees. In fact, the American Physical Therapy Association accredits 111 programs that offer an entry-level professional doctorate.

Physical therapists held about 155,000 jobs in 2004, although the number of jobs exceeds the number of therapists available (BLS, 2006). Some therapists maintain a private practice and, in addition, work part-time in a health facility. New technologies are affecting this profession in many ways, including the treatments administered by therapists (e.g., sophisticated gait analysis machines). In addition, technologies that enable severe trauma victims to survive are resulting in more patients for therapists to treat.

In 2004, median annual earnings for physical therapists ranged from $42,000 to $88,850. Home health care services accounted for the largest overall employment of these health professionals, offering a median annual salary of $64,650 (BLS, 2006).

Respiratory Therapists

Job opportunities are expected to be very good, especially for respiratory therapists with cardiopulmonary skills or experience working with infants. Employment . . . is expected to increase faster than average for all occupations through the year 2014, because of substantial growth in the numbers of the middle-aged and elderly population . . . . (BLS, 2006)

The Committee on Accreditation for Respiratory Care accredits 51 entry-level and 329 advanced programs in the United States for respiratory therapists. All graduates of either program may take the Certified Respiratory Therapist (CRT) examination. Those who meet additional criteria (educational and experiential) can take a separate exam for the Registered Respiratory Therapist (RRT) credential. (Supervisory and intensive care specialties usually require the RRT.) All states except Alaska and Hawaii require respiratory therapists to be licensed.

In 2004, approximately 80% of the 118,000 practicing respiratory therapists were employed primarily "in hospital departments of respiratory care, anesthesiology, or pulmonary medicine" (BLS, 2006). Median annual earnings in 2004 ranged from $37,650 to $50,860. For those employed in hospitals, median earnings were $43,140 (BLS, 2006).

Occupational Therapists

Employment of occupational therapists is expected to increase much faster than the average for all occupations through 2014. (BLS, 2006)

Occupational therapists help people with physical and emotional difficulties to improve their living and working skills, such as cooking, dealing with public transportation, maintaining a job, and other aspects of daily living. Not only hospitals but also rehabilitation and community facilities (such as schools) employ occupational therapists. In 2004, occupational therapists held about 92,000 jobs in the United States, with 10% working more than one job. All states regulate this profession, and a bachelor's degree is the minimum requirement for entry. Beginning in 2007, however, "a master's degree or higher will be the minimum education requirement" (BLS, 2006). Graduates from an accredited program must also pass a national certification exam to obtain a license. The median annual earnings of occupational therapists were $54,660 in 2004 (BLS, 2006).

Recreational Therapists

Overall employment of recreational therapists is expected to grow more slowly than the average . . . [except] in nursing care facilities. (BLS, 2006)

Recreational therapists provide activities, such as painting and crafts, that help to improve or maintain a person's physical, mental, and emotional well-being. Recreational therapists practice in hospitals and schools, in community-based organizations, and, as the statement above suggests, in long-term care facilities. In 2004, these therapists held about 24,000 jobs, with approximately 60% working in nursing care facilities and hospitals. About 150 programs offer recreational therapy education, and most offer a bachelor's degree. Median annual earnings in 2004 were $32,900 (BLS, 2006).

Social Workers

Although a bachelor's degree is sufficient for entry into the field, an advanced degree has become the standard for many positions. . . . Employment of social workers is expected to increase faster than the average for all occupations through 2014. (BLS, 2006)

Social workers are instrumental in dealing with many psychosocial aspects of care. Social workers focus on the patient's general state (e.g., physical and mental health, finances, possible legal issues, and family problems). They are often called upon to handle "difficult" patients, whose "trouble making" may be the result of conflicting ethical or sociocultural values (Heitman, 1995). Consequently, the social worker's professional relationship draws him or her into the patient's life in a very personal way.

The Council on Social Work Education accredited 442 BSW programs and 168 MSW programs and listed 80 doctoral programs for this profession. In 2004, social workers held about 562,000 jobs, with 90% of those in health care and social assistance industries (as well as state and local government agencies). The median annual salary in 2004 was $40,080 (BLS, 2006).

Dietitians and Nutritionists

Employment of dieticians is expected to grow faster than the average for all occupations through 2014 as a result of increasing emphasis on disease prevention through improved dietary habits. (BLS 2006)

Generally, hospitals and nursing homes employ registered dietitians and nutritionists to supervise, plan, and consult on the nutritional needs of patients. These professionals also practice in a variety of community organizations, including schools and prisons. With the increase in community-based day-care centers for both adults and children, demand for professional dietitians and nutritionists is expected to be high in the future.

The Commission on Dietetic Registration of the American Dietetic Association (ADA) awards the registered dietitian credential to individuals who pass a certifying exam (following academic training). As of 2004, 227 bachelor's and master's programs were approved by the American Dietetic Association. In 2005, the median annual salary for registered dieticians ranged from $44,800 in community nutrition to $60,200 in education and research (BLS, 2006).

IMPORTANT TRENDS AFFECTING HEALTH CARE PROFESSIONALS

Interdisciplinary Care and Quality

The various health care professionals bring much expertise to the service of the patient. However, an important distinction must be made between multidisciplinary care and interdisciplinary care. *Multidisciplinary care* means that many different professionals work for the good of the patient, albeit somewhat independently. *Interdisciplinary care* means that the many different professionals working together for the patient's good also communicate effectively among themselves and with the patient. One factor shifting care from multidisciplinary to interdisciplinary in nature is the "vibrant movement to improve the quality of health care" in the United States (Bodenheimer, 2003).

The Institute of Medicine has defined *quality* as "the degree to which health services for individuals and populations increase the likelihood of desired health outcomes and are consistent with current professional knowledge" (IOM, 2003). Medicare payments to hospitals and other facilities are contingent, among other things, on the facility's meeting quality accreditation standards set by the Joint Commission on Accreditation of Healthcare Organizations. The Joint Commission was formed in 1952 under the aegis of the American Hospital Association and the American Medical Association.

Managed care organizations often seek accreditation by the private National Committee for Quality Assurance (NCQA), showing by "report cards" from the Committee that they meet agreed-upon standards of quality. The mission of the NCQA is "to provide information that enables purchasers and consumers of managed care to distinguish among plans based on quality. . . ." Although accreditation is voluntary, plans usually market themselves on the basis of their "grades," and nearly half of the 650 plans in the United States request accreditation by the NCQA; in fact, 96% of these were accredited in 1998 (Bodenheimer, 2003).

The connection between interdisciplinary care and quality of care has been emphasized by two experts in health care quality: Donald Berwick and Lucian Leape. They insist that meeting quality standards requires a culture of quality. "Physicians, nurses, pharmacists and other care givers cannot individually perform at a . . . [required] level of reliability" (Bodenheimer, 2003). Instead, what is needed to ensure quality care is a redesign of care to support a team approach, or interdisciplinary focus. This revision has been highlighted in the Institute of Medicine's 10 rules for practitioners, which include "shared knowledge and free flow of information" and "cooperation among clinicians" (IOM, 1999).

Four other areas that continue to receive attention and will affect the various health care professionals are patient-focused care, critical pathways, continuous quality improvement (CQI), and pay for performance.

Patient-Focused Care

Patient-focused care in a health care facility is "characterized by decentralization of services, cross-training of personnel from different departments to provide basic care, interdisciplinary collaboration, various degrees of organizational restructuring, simplification and redesign of work to eliminate steps and save time, and an increased involvement of patients in their own care" (Vogel, 1993, p. 2321). All too often, patients in hospitals have had to deal with "employee-focused" care; they have been awakened in the wee hours of the morning to have blood samples drawn, to have a portable chest X ray filmed, or to be given a bath. These procedures have traditionally been performed at the convenience of health care workers. This enables blood and X-ray reports to be ready for physicians when they visit patients and allows nurses to "get their work done," given the responsibilities of particular shifts and the severity of illness of the patients on a ward.

In patient-focused care, these objectives are expanded to include (1) improving patients' perceptions of the quality of care and staff members' job satisfaction and (2) using nonclinical and clinical staff more effectively and efficiently (Vogel, 1993). In providing such care, health professionals work in ward-based teams to increase and improve communication among themselves and with the patient.

Moreover, patients themselves are now being provided with "tools to help them decide among . . . various options" in conjunction with their caregivers. The Agency for Healthcare Research and Quality (AHRQ) provides a set of patient-focused instruments for both patients and clinicians on its website (AHRQ, 2006).

Finally, it should be noted that patient-centered care is one of the hallmarks of the American Nurses Credentialing Center Magnet Recognition Program.

Critical Pathway

A critical pathway (also called a care map or clinical pathway) is an "optimal sequencing and timing of interventions by health care professionals for a particular diagnosis or procedure, designed to minimize delays and resource utilization and maximize the quality of care" (Coffey et al., 1992, p. 45). Although critical pathways are relatively new to health care, project managers in the construction and engineering fields have used them for many years. Goals of critical pathways include (1) providing continuity of care, (2) decreasing the fragmentation of services, (3) guiding the patient and family through the expected treatments and progress, (4) optimizing the cost-effectiveness of health care delivery, and (5) increasing the satisfaction of patients, families, health care professionals, and third-party payers (Kirk, Michael, Markowsky, Restino, and Zarowitz, 1996). As in other fields, critical pathways in health care are usually developed for high-volume, high-risk, or high-cost procedures. They can document pharmacologic as well as nonpharmacologic therapies, interventions, and outcomes throughout the entire course of care from admission to discharge.

To date, critical pathways have been identified for more than 2,000 common disease states or procedures and published in a national directory (Kirk et al., 1996). They require coordinated care from everyone on the health care team and delineate which treatments should be done on each day of the patient's stay. Critical pathways have been shown to reduce variations in the care provided, facilitate achieving expected outcomes, decrease delays, and improve cost-effectiveness (Coffey et al., 1992).

Because of increasing competition within health care, "managers have embraced critical pathways as a method to reduce variation in care, decrease resource utilization, and potentially improve healthcare quality" (Every, Hochman, Becker, Kopecky, and Cannon, 2000).

Continuous Quality Improvement

Continuous quality improvement (also called total quality management or total quality improvement) is another mechanism in which interdisciplinary involvement is crucial. CQI is a method of performance appraisal in which structures, processes, and outcomes are assessed to determine specific areas where improvement is needed. It typically follows the FOCUS-PDCA cycle (Graham, 1995):

F: Find a process to improve.

O: Organize a team that knows the process.

C: Clarify current knowledge of the process.

U: Understand sources of process variation.

S: Select the process improvement.

P: Plan the improvement.

D: Do the improvement, collect data, and analyze data.

C: Check and study the results.

A: Act to hold the gain and to improve the process further.

CQI enables a cross-functional, interdisciplinary team to examine processes that could or should be improved. It brings together a team of health care workers who know that particular procedure well and takes advantage of the fact that employees generally are more receptive to change when they are active participants in the change process.

Pay for Performance

Pay for performance (P4P) is defined by the Centers for Medicare and Medicaid Services (CMS) as "quality based purchasing . . . the use of payment methods and other incentives to encourage high quality and patient focused, high value care" (2006). A report from the Hastings Center described pay for performance as "the next best thing," with a number of pilot programs following the business world's linking of salary to organizational outcomes. Not surprisingly, one push for these programs comes from employers, which "are asking insurers to prove they are worth the money"; in turn, insurers are asking clinicians if their services are, indeed, worth the money (Bayley, 2006).

Perhaps the most prominent insurer, the CMS recently sponsored experiments with this approach. Nevertheless, it cautions, "pay-for-performance programs should be viewed as only one component of a broader strategy of promoting health care quality" (CMS, 2006).

Health Care Services and the Internet

As the chapter case scenario and the previous discussions have implied, both health care services and the professions providing care are influenced by the introduction of new technologies. Technological advances have, made many new procedures and methods of diagnosis possible, as the Bureau of Labor Statistics occupational outlook noted (BLS, 2006). Robots allow cranial and other types of microsurgery; other robotic devices automate drug dispensing; PDAs provide physicians and pharmacists with updated drug information.

One new technology has already had, and is expected to continue to have, a major impact on health and health care: the Internet. The following endorsement comes from a study commissioned by the National Library of Medicine (NLM):

The rapid development of Internet and World Wide Web technologies makes possible the quick, cost-effective distribution and exchange of biomedical information. Progress in telemedicine offers the promise of the cost-effective practice of medicine at a distance. . . . Today, the Internet—

and tomorrow its Next Generation—offers new opportunities for NLM to leverage its resources for strengthening the U.S. and global biomedical information infrastructure. (NLM, 2001)

The health care system in the United States has been characterized as a "trillion-dollar cottage industry." In other words, it includes thousands of hospitals, many thousands of health professionals (e.g., physicians, nurses, pharmacists), and many more thousands of facilities and players. The diversity and size of this industry make it a prime candidate for technologies that can span different sites and caregivers and help to integrate services. The Internet has the potential to accomplish these objectives.

Unfortunately, the same NLM study concluded that many health care organizations are not well equipped to adopt Internet-based technologies and applications. Infrastructure components such as hardware and software are lacking. More importantly, professionals are not yet trained to take advantage of what these technologies can offer them and their patients. Forward-thinking professionals and their organizations are ensuring that their staff members are educated and skilled in this area and that Internet-based resources are provided to patients. As more health care facilities move in this direction, the outcome is expected to be a reduction "in hospital stays and outpatient care, especially in the emergency room . . . [and] better monitoring of wellness, chronic disease, and behavior" (Networking Health, 2000, p. 247).

QUESTIONS FOR FURTHER DISCUSSION

1. Do you think the definition of *professional* will change over the coming years? Why or why not?
2. Has the health care system changed in your experience? How?
3. Do you think all changes are for the better? Why or why not?
4. Why did you choose to become a health care professional? Did your motives conform to the definitions given in the beginning of this chapter?
5. Have you had experience as a patient? If so, do you think you received multidisciplinary care or interdisciplinary care? Why?
6. Has your educational experience been multidisciplinary? Interdisciplinary?
7. If you were to design a pharmacy residency program, how would you ensure that it had an interdisciplinary focus and the appropriate technological sophistication?

KEY TOPICS AND TERMS

Profession
Interdisciplinary
Quality
New technologies

REFERENCES

Agency for Healthcare Research and Quality. (2006). *Research in action: Expanding patient-centered care to empower patients and assist providers.* Retrieved May 8, 2006 from www.ahrq.gov/QUAL/ptcareria.htm

American Association of Colleges of Pharmacy (AACP). (2006). www.aacp.org

American Pharmaceutical Association. (2000). Retrieved May 12, 2006 from www.apa.org

American Physical Therapy Association. (2003). Retrieved May 12, 2006 from www.apta.org/consumer/future

Association of American Medical Colleges. (2000). Retrieved May 12, 2006 from www.aamc.org

Association of American Medical Colleges. (2005). Retrieved May 12, 2006 from www.aamc.org

Bayley, C. (2006). Pay for performance: The next best thing. *Hastings Center Report 36*(1):4. Retrieved January 18, 2006 fromwww.medscape.com/viewarticle/521013_print

Bodenheimer, T. (2003). The American health care system: The movement for improved quality in health care. In P. R. Lee & C. L. Estes (Eds.), *The nation's health* (7th ed.) (pp. 445–452). Sudbury, MA: Jones and Bartlett.

Bureau of Labor Statistics (BLS). (2006). *Occupational outlook handbook.* Retrieved May 12, 2006 from www.bls.gov

Bureau of Labor Statistics (BLS). (2002–2003). *Occupational outlook handbook.* Retrieved May 12, 2006 from www.bls.gov

Centers for Medicare and Medicaid Services (CMS). (2006). *Pay for performance.* Retrieved May 16, 2006 from www.cms.gov

Coffey, R. J., Richards, J. S., Remmert, C. S., LeRoy, S. S., Schoville, R. R., & Baldwin, P. J. (1992). An introduction to critical paths. *Quality Management in Health Care, 1*(1), 45–54.

Every, N. R., Hochman, J., Becker, R., Kopecky, S., & Cannon, C. P. (2000). Critical pathways: A review. *Circulation, 101*(46), 1.

Graham, N. O. (1995). *Quality in health care: Theory, application, and evolution.* Gaithersburg, MD: Aspen Publications.

Haglund, C. L., & Dowling, W. L. (1993). The hospital. In S. J. Williams & P. R. Torrens (Eds.), *Introduction to health care services* (4th ed.) (pp. 135–176). Albany, NY: Delmar.

Hathaway, D. (2006). Introducing the doctor of nursing practice. *Medscape General Medicine, 8*(2), 7. Retrieved April 18, 2006 from www.medscape.com/viewarticle/528446_print

Heavey, S. (2006). US says Medicare drug plan passes 30 million goal. *Reuters Health Information 2006.* Retrieved May 5, 2006 from www.medscape.com/viewarticle/530478_print

Heitman, E. (1995). Institutional ethics committees: Local perspectives on ethical issues in medicine. In R. E. Bulger, E. M. Bobby, & H. V. Fineberg (Eds.), *Society's choices: Social and ethical decision making in biomedicine* (pp. 409–431). Washington, DC: Institute of Medicine, National Academy Press.

Higby, G. J. (1996). From compounding to caring: An abridged history of American pharmacy. In C. Knowlton & R. Penna (Eds.), *Pharmaceutical care* (pp. 18–45). New York: Chapman and Hall.

Institute of Medicine (IOM). (1999). www.iom.edu

Institute of Medicine (IOM). (2003). www.iom.edu

Jolly, P. (2004). Medical school tuition and young physician indebtedness. *Report of the Association of American Medical Colleges,* 23 March.

Kirk, J. K., Michael, K. A., Markowsky, S. J., Restino, M. R., & Zarowitz, B. J. (1996). Critical pathways: The time is here for pharmacist involvement. *Pharmacotherapy, 16*(4), 723–733.

MacLaren, R., Devlin, J. W., Martin, S. J., Dasta, J. F., Rudis, M. I., & Bond, C. A. (2006). Critical care pharmacy services in United States hospitals. *Annals of Pharmacotherapy 40*(4), 612–618. Retrieved May 5, 2006 from www.medscape.com/viewarticle/530059_print

Midwest Pharmacy Workforce Research Consortium. (2005). *Final report of the national sample survey of the pharmacist workforce to determine contemporary demographic and practice characteristics.* Retrieved May 2, 2006 from www.apa.org

National League for Nursing. (2003). Retrieved May 2, 2006 from www.nln.org/nlnjournal/infotrends.htm

National Library of Medicine (NLM). (2001). *Long range plan 2000–2005.* Retrieved May 2, 2006 from www.nlm.nih.gov/pubs/plan/lrp00/goal-3-1.html

Networking Health. (2000). *Prescriptions for the Internet.* Washington, DC: National Academy Press.

Sawin, L. (1989). *Note on the U. S. medical education industry.* Teaching note prepared under the direction of Professor Alice Sapienza, Harvard School of Public Health, Boston, MA.

Turner, B. S. (1987). *Medical power and social knowledge.* London: Sage.

Vogel, D. P. (1993). Patient-focused care. *American Journal of Hospital Pharmacists, 50,* 2321–2329.

The Pharmacist and the Pharmacy Profession

Shane P. Desselle

Case Scenario

You have just completed your educational degree requirements and earned your PharmD degree a few short weeks ago. You are currently working 8 hours per day at WeCare Pharmacy to fulfill your internship requirements, and your appointment to take the board exam the next week is quickly approaching. You have your head buried in books and notes one Wednesday evening before retiring, when suddenly it hits you: "Gosh, if I pass the NAPLEX and jurisprudence examinations, I'll be a registered pharmacist before the end of next month!"

That weekend you make the trip back home to visit with your family for the first time since moving 5 hours away to take the job at WeCare. Your Mom lovingly fires a series of questions your way: "Well, what's it like almost being a pharmacist? Is it what you thought it would be? Have you met any other pharmacists? How do they treat you at your new job? What do you do there, anyway?"

You begin to answer your Mom, one question at a time, but then become puzzled that you are not sure exactly how to answer her. In fact, you had not really thought about these things. What is pharmacy all about anyway? Do you have a "pharmacist's mentality," or does such a thing exist? Did you make the right career and organizational choice? How do you meet other pharmacists in the area? How do you stay apprised of what is going on in the worlds of pharmacy and health care?

LEARNING OBJECTIVES _____

Upon completion of this chapter, the student shall be able to:

- Identify three eras in pharmacy practice and education during the 20th century. Describe the principal forces that shaped the profession.
- Define "pharmaceutical care." Discuss pharmaceutical care as the mission of contemporary pharmacy practice. Identify barriers to this mission and describe where the profession stands in its implementation.
- Discuss the difference between licensure and certification. Discuss opportunities for pharmacists to obtain certification. Identify other postgraduate educational opportunities for pharmacists.
- Describe roles played by professional pharmacy organizations. Identify benefits for pharmacists who join professional pharmacy organizations. Describe the mission and goals of several key professional pharmacy organizations.
- Describe the roles and functions of pharmacy technicians. Discuss the trend toward technician certification and explain what it means to pharmacy.
- Describe how the Internet has affected pharmacy practice. Discuss advantages of and possible threats to patient safety from Internet pharmacy practice. Identify other technologies affecting contemporary pharmacy practice.
- Discuss the implications of the pharmacist workforce for practice and education. Describe factors that affect the pharmacist labor supply. Discuss estimates of the pharmacy workforce for the coming decades.

CHAPTER QUESTIONS

1. How have pharmacists' education and training and the roles they play in society evolved throughout the 20th century?
2. What is "pharmaceutical care"? What are its goals? Why did the pharmacy profession embrace it as a mission? Where does the profession stand in implementing pharmaceutical care? Which barriers might prevent pharmacists from providing pharmaceutical care and how might these be overcome?
3. What are the subdisciplines that constitute pharmacy education and practice? What are some of the postgraduate educational and career options in these areas?
4. What is the difference between certification and licensure? What are some areas in which pharmacists may obtain board certification?
5. What purposes do professional pharmacy organizations serve? What are some of the key organizations that shape pharmacists' practice?
6. What are some trends concerning the roles of pharmacy technicians in practice?
7. What are the advantages and disadvantages of using Internet pharmacies from a patient's perspective? What are some of the public health concerns regarding the proliferation of Internet pharmacies? What steps are government agencies and the pharmacy profession taking to ensure the public's safety?
8. Why is the pharmacy workforce such a critical issue to the profession? What do estimates of pharmacists' labor supply suggest?

INTRODUCTION

Chapter 2 introduced the concepts of professionalism and interdisciplinary care while briefly describing the training, expertise, and professional roles of pharmacists and some of the many health care professionals with whom pharmacists interact with on a regular basis. This chapter examines in greater detail those same aspects of the pharmacy profession, its pharmacist members, and pharmacy education; it is divided into seven major sections.

The first section is an abridged history of the profession and the evolution of current medication use systems. This appropriately leads into the second section, a discussion of pharmacy's mission and philosophy of practice, termed pharmaceutical care. The third section discusses current and expected future trends in practice, emphasizing pharmacist specialization and examining the various settings in which pharmacists practice. A multitude of professional organizations represent pharmacists in each of these settings, as discussed in the fourth section. The fifth section describes the roles of pharmacy technicians, now pharmacists' most important adjuncts in providing pharmaceutical care.

The sixth section examines a phenomenon pervading the delivery of medical care called "cyberpharmacy," or the application of e-commerce to modern medication use systems. Other trends affecting the future of our practice are examined as well, including the projected increase in the number of prescriptions written and dispensed in the United States in the coming decades. This provides a nice segue into the seventh, very critical section of this chapter—the discussion of workforce issues. The labor supply has important implications for the future of pharmacy, including pharmacist education and training; pharmacy laws, rules, and regulations; policy regarding the use of ancillary personnel; pharmacist salaries; and, most importantly, the therapeutic outcomes of patients.

EVOLUTION OF THE PROFESSION AND MEDICATION USE SYSTEMS

Historians of pharmacy have used a variety of methods to categorize the evolution of pharmacy within the context of either "waves" or shifts in educational and industrial forces (Hepler, 1987), stages of professional identity (Hepler and Strand, 1990), or political shifts in the promulgation of our health care delivery system (Broeseker and Janke, 1998). Fortunately, there are a number of commonalties in their descriptions of the forces that have shaped our current method of practice and management of medication use systems. The approach taken here is simply to describe pharmacy practice, pharmacy education, and medication use within three distinct periods of the American 20th century.

Before the 1940s

Pharmacy practice in the United States dates back to shortly after the country's founding. However, aside from the formation of professional associations and the first colleges of pharmacy during the 1800s, the predominant forces shaping pharmacy and medication use today took effect largely during the 20th century. Before this time, pharmacy was primarily an occupation for which its practitioners were trained via apprenticeship, much like participants in other trades. Pharmacy was considered an art that did not require theoretical knowledge and could best be learned "by daily handling and preparing the remedies in common use" (Sonnedecker, 1963, p. 204).

Without any credible standards or enforceable laws regarding the safety of therapeutic agents, the use of patent medicines was the norm. Pharmacists, or "apothecaries," often were engaged in the wholesale manufacture and distribution of such products. The public had to rely on them to ensure that the compounds they sold were pure and unadulterated. Pharmacists came under considerable scrutiny, especially from physicians, when their increasingly profitable trade bred unscrupulous and unknowledgeable practitioners. Many of the patent medicines sold at the time were inefficacious, mislabeled, and even unsafe for consumption.

The first major piece of legislation to affect medication use in the 20th century was the Pure Food and Drug Act of 1906. Because the food and drug product industries were considered to be engaging in interstate commerce, the federal government passed this law to enable authorities to enforce penalties for certain types of misbranding and adulteration. The original statute was not particularly comprehensive or well written, however, so manufacturers, prescribers, and dispensers found many loopholes through which they could evade prosecution. Moreover, the Pure Food and Drug Act of 1906 did little to address the issue of efficacy in drug products.

Pressure continued to mount on the federal government to strengthen the food and drug laws, but, unfortunately, it took a tragedy before more comprehensive measures were taken. During 1937, at least 73 deaths were attributed to ingestion of the toxic "Elixir Sulfanilamide" (Sonnedecker, 1963, p. 200). This scandal provided the necessary impetus for passage of the Food, Drug, and Cosmetic Act of 1938. This act afforded greater authority to the Food and Drug Administration (FDA), the federal agency charged with enforcing it, and with approving new drugs and new indications of drugs before they could be marketed in the United States. The statutes within the act and subsequent regulations issued by the FDA make it easier to enforce standards of safety and efficacy of drug products.

During the early part of this century, pharmacists continued to engage in their roles as drug curators and dispensers. Interestingly, no formal legislation addressed the categorization of drugs into nonprescription and prescription products. Persons typically did not have to visit a physician if they desired a remedy for an ailment. Without such formal restrictions on dispensing, it could be argued that the pharmacist indirectly had some prescribing authority. Additionally, the pharmacist was relied on to provide advice to consumers on compounds he or she prescribed and dispensed (Hepler, 1987). Anecdotally, since pharmacists were—and still are—very accessible and visited frequently by customers, they were often the first source of entry into the health care system, particularly in rural areas that may have been underserved by physicians. They continued to fill this role despite a report published in 1910 by Abraham Flexner, who was appointed to study medical education, in which he contended that pharmacy was not a profession because its only responsibility was to carry out orders given by physicians. In response to this and other reports questioning the standing of pharmacy among other occupations, the American Association of Colleges of Pharmacy (AACP) commissioned a study directed by W.W. Charters. The study ultimately served as the basis for the AACP to require a 4-year baccalaureate degree program to be established by all colleges of pharmacy (Hepler, 1987).

The 1940s to the Early 1970s

The relatively brief period from the 1940s to the early 1970s brought significant changes in how health care was organized, delivered, and financed. This period has previously been described as the "era of expansion" (Relman, 1988, p. 1221). The Hospital Survey and Construction (Hill-Burton) Act of 1946 provided considerable grant monies for the renovation and expansion of existing hospitals as well as the construction of new ones, primarily in underserved inner-city and rural areas (Torrens, 1993; see Chapter 8). Continuously mounting pressure from the growing number of persons who were unable to access the health care system led to the passage in 1965 of the Titles XVIII and XIX amendments to the 1935 Social Security Act, which established the Medicare and Medicaid programs. The result was a significant increase in the number of persons with some type of health coverage and a dramatic rise in the utilization of medical care goods and services. The Medicaid program, in particular, resulted in a dramatic shift in the use of pharmaceuticals and significantly increased the number of prescriptions dispensed (see Chapter 17).

In contrast with the trend of expanding roles for other allied health care professionals during this period, pharmacists began to see their roles in medication use management diminish. Several forces were at play in bringing about these changes. First, large wholesale apothecaries were eventually transformed into large-scale manufacturers of pharmaceutical products. Previously, the majority of products dispensed by pharmacists were the result of their compounding bulk agents. Technological advances in industrial manufacturing and pharmaceutics, coupled with the increasing number of available compounds and societal demand that medicinals become more uniform in their composition, resulted in the ability of and desire by manufacturers to prefabricate drugs in standardized dosage forms such as elixirs, syrups, tablets, and capsules.

The most influential piece of legislation that affected the medication use process in the United States was passed in 1951. The Durham-Humphrey amendment to the Food, Drug, and Cosmetic Act created the prescription or "legend" drug, whose label was required to carry the warning, "Caution: Federal law prohibits dispensing without a prescription." The result was an entirely new class of products that pharmacists did not have the ability to dispense without written orders from a licensed prescriber. At the same time, the profession's code of ethics as derived by the American Pharmaceutical (now Pharmacists) Association stated that "The pharmacist does not discuss the therapeutic effects or composition of a prescription with a patient. When such questions are asked, he suggests that the qualified practitioner is the proper person with whom such matters should be discussed" (Buerki and Vottero, 1994, p. 93). These forces relegated the pharmacist largely to a dispenser of pre-synthesized drug products.

The 1940s to early 1970s period also ushered in tremendous changes in the foci of pharmacy curricula throughout the United States. As part of this reform, many baccalaureate pharmacy programs were expanded to include a fifth year. Many of the extra didactic credit hours in these curricula were devoted to the further inclusion of scientific courses. Hepler (1987) contends that the primary objective of pharmaceutical education was to legitimize faculties, curricula, and ultimately the profession itself. He argues that the pharmaceutical industry encouraged research at pharmacy schools that was oriented toward the drug product. Courses in pharmacognosy gave way to natural products and medicinal chemistry; zoology was transformed into physiology; and Galenical pharmacy evolved into pharmaceutics. In addition, new disciplines, such as pharmacology, biopharmaceutics, and pharmacokinetics, were born from the melding and application of other basic sciences. An argument for inclusion of these courses into curricula is that with the proliferation of new drug discoveries, practitioners required a scientific background to interpret literature and understand the proper use of drug products that would continue to enter the market throughout the pharmacist's career.

Nevertheless, it was argued that pharmacists became "overeducated and underutilized" during this period (Hepler, 1987, p. 537). Brodie (1967) wondered if the profession had lost the mainstream of its practice. A pioneer in pharmacy, he coined the term "drug use control," a mantle he suggested pharmacists carry to use their education to promote patient welfare in the form of drug safety. He defined this term as "that system of knowledge, understanding, judgments, procedures, skills, controls and ethics that assures optimal safety in the distribution and use of medication" (Brodie, 1967, p. 65).

The Early 1970s to the Present

The 1970s ushered in considerable concern over skyrocketing health care costs that were consuming an increasingly larger portion of the U.S. gross national product (GNP). The previous era in health care had resulted in the rapid perfusion of expensive new medications and technologies, professionalization and specialization of health care occupations, and proliferation of medical diagnoses for conditions not previously linked to biomedical origins ("medicalization"), such as alcoholism. Moreover, the orientation of most insurance plans in the form of indemnity rather than service benefits provided incentives for medical care providers and patients to overuse health care services, often resulting in duplication and a loss of continuity in the care provided.

In recent years, several measures have been taken to counter these trends. Although they had existed before that time, the Health Maintenance Organization (HMO) Act of 1973 paved the way for managed care organizations to garner a larger share of the health insurance market. Perhaps even more critical was the implementation of a prospective payment system of diagnosis-related groups (DRGs) by the Health Care Financing Administration (HCFA; now the Centers for Medicare and Medicaid Services) for Medicare patients (Pink, 1991). A DRG is essentially a taxonomy of disease states and conditions for which patients may be admitted into a hospital. Reimbursement to hospitals for treating Medicare patients was set prospectively according to their diagnosis, regardless of the length and intensity of care. This system provided an incentive for hospitals to discharge patients "quicker and sicker" into other less intensive and expensive health care settings.

This period for pharmacy began with two reports that raised concerns among the entire profession. First, the Dichter Institute Study commissioned by the American Pharmaceutical Association (APhA) found that more respondents saw pharmacists as businessmen than as health care providers (Maine and Penna, 1996). With the rapid expansion of large, full-service chain pharmacies that sold many products besides medicines, along with a lack of knowledge of pharmacists' training and expertise, study respondents viewed pharmacists more as extensions of pharmaceutical manufacturers and wholesalers. The blame for patients' lack of awareness of the services that pharmacists could provide rested squarely on the shoulders of the profession and pharmacy academia.

The second study that generated some alarm was the Millis Commission's Report in 1975, *Pharmacists for the Future: The Report of the Study Commission on Pharmacy* (Millis, 1975). This report suggested that pharmacists found themselves inadequately prepared in systems analysis and management skills and had particular deficiencies in communicating with patients, physicians, and other health care professionals. A subsequent report suggested inculcating more of the behavioral and social sciences into pharmacy curricula and encouraged more faculty participation and research in real problems of practice (Millis, 1976).

Before the release of these reports, the American Society of Hospital (now Health-Systems) Pharmacists had published *Mirror to Hospital Pharmacy,* which stated bluntly that pharmacy had lost its way in producing professionals, while noting that the frustration and dissatisfaction of practitioners were beginning to affect students (Hepler, 1987). The clinical pharmacy movement was created to capture the essence of the drug use control concept put forth by Brodie and to promote the pharmacist's role as therapeutic advisor. This movement brought about changes in pharmacy education and practice.

In the late 1960s, the 6-year PharmD degree was introduced, with the additional year being devoted mostly to therapeutics or "disease-oriented" courses and experiential education. Throughout the 1970s, 1980s, and into the early 1990s, an increasing number of colleges of pharmacy began offering the PharmD degree, but primarily as a post-baccalaureate program. Pharmacists who completed such programs secured jobs as "clinical pharmacists," primarily in hospitals where they performed fewer dispensing functions and provided more services such as pharmacokinetic dosing, therapeutic monitoring, and drug information. Eventually, colleges of pharmacy began phasing out their baccalaureate programs. In 1995, the Argus Commission of the AACP recommended the 6-year PharmD as the entry-level degree into the profession. (American Association of Colleges of Pharmacy, 1996).

PHARMACEUTICAL CARE

Initial Conceptualization

Despite the strides made by the profession during the 1970s and 1980s, questions existed about pharmacy's place in society—that is, performing services just for service's sake, without actually serving the welfare of the patient, was by no means a societal mandate and did not necessarily constitute a professional role (Penna, 1990). It was argued that clinical pharmacy, in itself, maintained its focus on products and services and not on the patient. It was also becoming increasingly apparent that medicalization and the proliferated use of drugs had repercussions in addition to benefits. Studies indicating dramatic rises in adverse drug reactions, hospitalizations, and even deaths from "drug misadventuring" grew more common (Manasse, 1989a, p. 936; 1989b, p. 1148). Evidence also demonstrated the pervasiveness of patient noncompliance with drug therapy (Boyd, Covington, Stanaszek, and Coussons, 1974) and its ramifications (Col, Fanale, and Kronholm, 1990).

Linda Strand and her colleagues identified eight categories of problems that could arise and result in poorer health outcomes and drug-related morbidity and mortality of patients: (1) untreated indications; (2) improper drug selection; (3) subtherapeutic dosage; (4) failure to receive drugs; (5) overdosage; (6) adverse drug reactions; (7) drug interactions; and (8) drug use without indications (Strand, Cippole, Morley, Ramsey, and Lamsam, 1990). Hepler and Strand then recognized that many of these problems could be reduced or averted by pharmacists—that pharmacy's raison d'etre should be to serve society by maximizing the benefits and minimizing the untoward effects of drug therapy for patients (Hepler and Strand, 1990). They contended that pharmacy had to change its entire mission and philosophy of practice to promote societal welfare in this fashion and to focus on the patient rather than the product because "drugs don't have doses—people have doses" (Cippole, 1986, p. 881).

This recognition operationally defined pharmacy's mandate for the 21st century: pharmaceutical care as "the responsible provision of drug therapy for the purpose of achieving definite outcomes that improve a patient's quality of life. These outcomes are (1) cure of a disease, (2) elimination or reduction of a patient's symptomatology, (3) arresting or slowing of a disease process, or (4) preventing a disease or symptomatology" (Hepler and Strand, 1990, p. 539). Hepler and Strand further delineated this concept to describe it as a process in which the pharmacist establishes a covenantal relationship with the patient in a mutually beneficial exchange. He or she cooperates with the patient and other professionals in designing, implementing, and monitoring a therapeutic plan that will produce specific outcomes, thereby performing three basic functions: (1) identifying potential and actual drug-related problems, (2) resolving actual drug-related problems, and (3) preventing potential drug-related problems (Hepler and Strand, 1990).

Implementation

The concept of pharmaceutical care set the profession, teachers, and researchers in motion as probably nothing had ever done before. One question that had to be answered, however, was how to put this mission into practice and what specific services pharmacists were to render in providing pharmaceutical care. **Figure 3–1** presents a set of steps that today's pharmacist is to follow in providing pharmaceutical care for the patient.

Pharmacists, in their dispensing roles, have always performed some of these duties, but some of the more critical and novel steps in this process occur in the assessment phase. Whereas software has facilitated the recording of patient information, pharmacists have been notoriously lapse in documenting patient drug therapy problems and any interventions they perform.

The Comprehensive Pharmaceutical Care Process

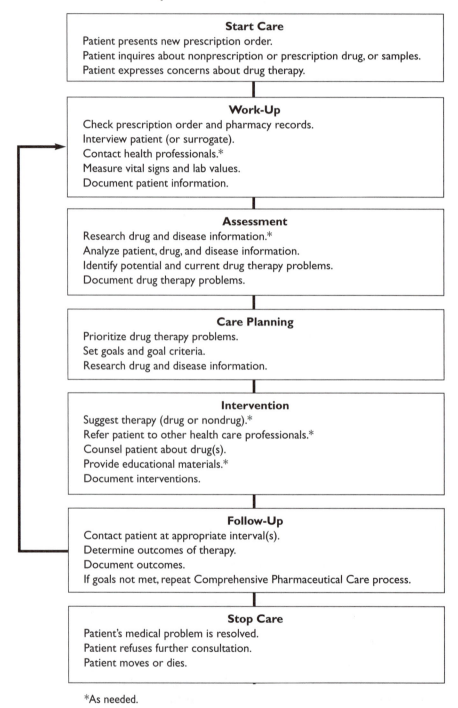

Start Care
Patient presents new prescription order.
Patient inquires about nonprescription or prescription drug, or samples.
Patient expresses concerns about drug therapy.

Work-Up
Check prescription order and pharmacy records.
Interview patient (or surrogate).
Contact health professionals.*
Measure vital signs and lab values.
Document patient information.

Assessment
Research drug and disease information.*
Analyze patient, drug, and disease information.
Identify potential and current drug therapy problems.
Document drug therapy problems.

Care Planning
Prioritize drug therapy problems.
Set goals and goal criteria.
Research drug and disease information.

Intervention
Suggest therapy (drug or nondrug).*
Refer patient to other health care professionals.*
Counsel patient about drug(s).
Provide educational materials.*
Document interventions.

Follow-Up
Contact patient at appropriate interval(s).
Determine outcomes of therapy.
Document outcomes.
If goals not met, repeat Comprehensive Pharmaceutical Care process.

Stop Care
Patient's medical problem is resolved.
Patient refuses further consultation.
Patient moves or dies.

*As needed.

Figure 3-1 The Comprehensive Pharmaceutical Care Process. *Source:* Copyright © 1995 by the American Pharmaceutical Association. Originally published in *American Pharmacy/Pharmacy Today. 35*, (4), April 1995. Reprinted with permission.

Documentation is a necessity for the pharmacist if he or she is to maintain continuity of care for the patient, make adjustments to the patient's care plan, reassess the care being provided to the patient, receive reimbursement for providing these services, and ultimately prove the worth of pharmaceutical care to society at large (Strand, Cippole, and Morley, 1988).

The concept of care planning is not new in the health care arena. Indeed, care planning forms the basis of nursing care. The caring aspect of pharmaceutical care is probably its most significant component. It is through caring that the pharmacist establishes a relationship with the patient that results in the patient providing to the pharmacist the information needed to improve drug-related outcomes. It is through caring that the patient develops trust in the pharmacist as a concerned member of the health care team. Pharmacists need simply to posit a few open-ended questions to patients to establish this caring attitude. Questions such as "How are you feeling?" and "What can I do for you?", when asked at the outset of each patient encounter, can help improve patients' satisfaction with their pharmacy visit. Pharmaceutical care is not merely limited to drug therapy but also incorporates the need for a holistic approach that may involve mental, emotional, and social support (Broeseker and Janke, 1998). Pharmacists would be best served in their endeavor to provide pharmaceutical care by asking the patients other questions. These assessment questions outlined in **Exhibit 3-1** provide a plan for the pharmacist to gather the necessary data from patients.

Early Pharmaceutical Care

Pharmaceutical care has become the rallying cry for leaders in practice, professional organizations, and academia. One does not have to look further than the nearest community pharmacy, however, to see that despite the many strides taken by the profession since Hepler and Strand's landmark paper, pharmaceutical care is not the pervasive modus operandi. This is not to say that most pharmacists are inadequate; indeed, the vast majority of pharmacists are well-trained, hard-working, caring, ethical, and competent professionals. But changing the mission and practice philosophy of an entire profession is not easy, particularly when many barriers exist. Some of these barriers include:

1. Drug product focus: Pharmacists have historically been preoccupied with dispensing drug products.
2. Service focus: Some services provided by pharmacists are distant from the patient and may be performed without regard to the resultant outcomes (e.g., pharmacokinetic dosing calculations).
3. Other health care professionals: Physicians, nurses, and other allied health care professionals may view pharmaceutical care as an infringement on their turf.

4. Lack of incentives: The current methods for paying and rewarding pharmacists center on dispensing volume, not on the care provided.
5. Logistical barriers: Many pharmacies are not designed and equipped properly to provide private consultation, disease monitoring, and dissemination of information—all key to the pharmaceutical care process.

Exhibit 3-1 Pharmacist's Assessment Questions

1. **Does the patient need this drug regimen?**
   - Does the patient have a medical condition? (Misusing drug unintentionally? Addicted? Using for recreation?)
   - Does this condition call for this drug regimen? (Avoidable adverse drug reaction? Nondrug therapy indicated? Duplicate therapy?)
2. **Is this drug/form the most effective and safe?**
   - For the medical condition? (Consider condition onset time, potency, acute/chronic use, oral/topical use, potential adverse reactions)
   - For the patient? (Consider age, gender, pregnancy/lactation, race)
   - With other diseases? (Consider patient's other disease states)
   - With the patient's history? (Refractory condition? Allergic/intolerant?)
   - Considering the cost?
3. **Is this dosage the most effective and safe?**
   - Too low? (Consider weight, patient class, disease states)
   - Too high or changing too fast? (Consider weight, patient class, disease states)
4. **If side effects are unavoidable, does the patient need additional drug therapy for side effects?**
5. **Will drug storage/administration impair efficacy or safety?**
   - Consider lost potency, timing of doses, incorrect dosage technique
6. **Will any drug interactions impair efficacy or safety?**
   - Drug–drug interactions? (Consider presecription and nonprescription drugs, samples, social drugs)
   - Drug–food interactions? (Consider foods affecting drug, drug affecting nutrition)
   - Drug–laboratory interactions?
7. **Will the patient follow this drug regimen?**
   - Is regimen available to patient? (Drug unavailable? Unaffordable?)
   - Is patient physically able to follow regimen? (Cannot swallow/administer drug?)
   - Is patient mentally able/willing to follow regimen? (Cannot remember? Does not know how? Not motivated? Form/dosing disliked?)
8. **Does the patient need additional drug regimen?**
   - For untreated condition? Synergism? Prophylaxis?
9. **Does the patient need any nondrug therapy or information?**
   - Consider other products, referral to health professional or support group, information about disease state.

Source: Copyright © 1995 by the American Pharmaceutical Association. Originally published in *American Pharmacy/Pharmacy Today. 35,* (4), April 1995. Reprinted with permission.

6. Pharmacy ignorance and inertia: "The greatest barrier to pharmaceutical care is ourselves. The success of an idea requires the dedication of people who believe in it and who pledge themselves to its general acceptance and implementation" (Penna, 1990, p. 547).

The last barrier is especially significant because the term "pharmaceutical care" generates ambivalence among many pharmacists. It is difficult to blame individual practitioners for their failure to embrace this notion. For many years, a considerable amount of ambiguity has surrounded the concept. Pharmaceutical care represents an entire philosophy of practice; therefore, identification of the steps involved in preparing and following up on care plans, while useful, is not enough to guide pharmacists in this mission. Pharmacists' interactions with patients are just one component of implementing an effective practice. Other things must be considered, including adequate human, financial, and technical resources, in addition to management, marketing, and legal issues. **Table 3-1** presents a more contemporary view of pharmaceutical care that includes these and other domains. Pharmacists must be competent in each of these areas to maximize their ability to provide effective patient-oriented services.

Taxonomy and Standardization

Researchers and leaders in pharmacy, particularly within professional organizations, have long recognized this problem. Entering an era of assessment and accountability, a significant movement in health care delivery and financing has pushed all members of the health care industry toward benchmarking, quality assurance, and standardization via guidelines, best practices, protocols, and critical pathways (Relman, 1988). Pharmacy has had difficulty in forming consensus on many issues because of the diversity in its practice settings and conflicting goals and objectives among its regulatory bodies and professional organizations. Thus success in reaching an accord on the level of care that should be provided to patients has been elusive.

The APhA has taken on two initiatives to advance quality standards in pharmacy in hopes of expediting pharmaceutical care's widespread implementation. In 1995, it released its *Principles of Practice for Pharmaceutical Care* (American Pharmaceutical Association, 1995), comprising a preamble detailing pharmaceutical care's goals and specific information about how the pharmacist could achieve these goals. The APhA undertook an extensive effort to codify each job responsibility and activity of pharmacists (Kaminsky and Basgall, 1997). The significance of this achievement is that the taxonomy can be used as a basis to establish more specific standards of practice, a tool to help pharmacists manage their practices, a guide to develop performance evaluations of pharmacists, and a simpler means to document activities so that pharmacists can be reimbursed for providing their services. Researchers have

Table 3-1 Pharmaceutical Care Practice Domains

I. Risk Management

- Devise system of data collection
- Perform prospective drug utilization review
- Document therapeutic interventions and activities
- Obtain over-the-counter medication history
- Calculate dosages for drugs with a narrow therapeutic index
- Report adverse drug events to FDA
- Triage patients' needs for proper referral
- Remain abreast of newly uncovered adverse effects and drug-drug interactions

II. Patient Advocacy

- Serve as patient advocate with respect to social, economic, and psychological barriers to drug therapy
- Attempt to change patients' medication orders when barriers to compliance exist
- Counsel patients on new and refill medications as necessary
- Promote patient wellness
- Maintain caring, friendly relationship with patients
- Telephone patients to obtain medication orders called in and not picked up

III. Disease Management

- Provide information to patients on how to manage their disease state/condition
- Monitor patients' progress resulting from pharmacotherapy
- Carry inventory of products necessary for patients to execute a therapeutic plan (e.g., inhalers, nebulizers, glucose monitors)
- Supply patients with information on support and educational groups (e.g., American Diabetes Association, Multiple Sclerosis Society)

IV. Pharmaceutical Care Services Marketing

- Meet prominent prescribers in the local area of practice
- Be an active member of professional associations that support the concept of pharmaceutical care
- Make available an area for private consultation services for patients as necessary
- Identify software that facilitates pharmacists' patient care-related activities

V. Business Management

- Utilize technicians and other staff to free up the pharmacist's time
- Ensure adequate work flow for efficiency in operations

Source: Copyright © 2004 by the McGraw Hill Companies. Originally published in Desselle, S.P. (2004). Pharmaceutical care as a management movement. In S.P. Desselle and D.P. Zgarrick (Eds.), *Pharmacy management: Essentials for all settings* (pp. 3–17). New York: McGraw-Hill.

Pharmaceutical Care ■ 79

also conducted studies using sophisticated focus group (Desselle, 1997) and psychometric (Pitterle, Bond, and Raehl, 1990; Odedina and Segall, 1996) techniques to describe standards or indices of pharmaceutical care practice.

Reimbursement Issues

The profession is making significant strides to address other barriers to the implementation of pharmaceutical care, particularly those concerning pharmacists' recognition as providers and the ability to be reimbursed for providing disease management services. Pharmacists have long had opportunities to become certified as experts in pharmacotherapy, but recognition of those achievements outside the pharmacy profession has been problematic. In the 1990s and early 21st century, state governments aided this quest by beginning to pass legislation expanding pharmacists' scope of practice to include broader pharmacotherapeutic decision making, implementation of home health care services, and provision of immunizations.

Many leaders in pharmacy hailed the passage of the Medicare Prescription Drug Improvement and Modernization Act (MMA) of 2003. While many of its provisions are of concern to pharmacists—particularly in regard to formulary issues, methods used to calculate payment to providers, and the concentration of market power to health plans—the MMA is the most comprehensive federal legislation to date that recognizes the need for medication therapy management services in ambulatory care. The MMA does not strictly govern face-to-face encounters and does not mandate that such services be provided by a pharmacist, but its language does position pharmacy as an obvious choice to fulfill a role in reducing drug-related morbidity and educating older adults on the proper pharmacologic and nonpharmacologic management of comorbid diseases. Of course, providing coverage for prescription medicines for many older adults who previously lacked such insurance also may serve to increase prescription volume and potentially boost profits for pharmacies, which could then invest additional monies into reengineering their practices to provide more patient-oriented services.

Significant breakthroughs are also being realized in the private sector. The Asheville project featured a long-term effort supported by employers to reimburse pharmacists for providing diabetes management services to their employees. The results suggested that pharmacists could help patients in improving both short-term (Cranor and Christensen, 2003) and long-term (Cranor, Bunting, and Christensen, 2003) outcomes, while saving employers money from averted medical costs. Large national chain pharmacies are becoming more frequently involved in providing appropriate resources for their pharmacists to engage in pharmaceutical care services (Tice and Phillips, 2002). Finally, it appears as though some patients may be willing to pay for pharmacists' services out of pocket if necessary (MacKinnnon and Mahrous, 2002).

PHARMACY PRACTICE TODAY AND TOMORROW

One might be tempted to ask, "Well, just where are we now and where are we going?" That question may not be easy to answer, but a few trends are worth noting.

First, the PharmD has replaced the baccalaureate (BS) degree as the entry-level degree in the pharmacy field. Another trend in pharmacy education is the continued efforts by colleges of pharmacy to incorporate more of the social and administrative sciences into their curricula. Colleges of pharmacy were initially slow to respond to the changes proposed in the Millis Commission. The AACP refocused its efforts to encourage a more liberal education for pharmacy students in the 1990s with its Commission to Implement Change in Pharmaceutical Education (1993; American Association of Colleges of Pharmacy, 1996). Among the issues addressed by the commission were the incorporation of specific courses and concepts related to health policy organization, communication, economic analysis, and the understanding of cultural diversity throughout the curriculum. The commission also addressed how courses should be taught, stressing multidisciplinary, problem- or service-based approaches to delivering course content to encourage problem-solving and critical thinking skills in future practitioners.

Other trends related to pharmacy practice concern the proliferation of new and exciting areas of practice, the effects of e-commerce on the profession and the emergence of virtual pharmacies, the use of automated technology and technicians for dispensing functions, and shifts in the pharmacist labor supply.

Licensure Requirements

Pharmacy continues to be one of the more rewarding professions with respect to the starting salaries of its members following completion of the entry-level degree and licensure. In addition to completing the PharmD degree, prospective pharmacists must log a certain number of hours as an intern practicing under the supervision of a licensed preceptor pharmacist; the number of hours required varies across states. The graduate must also successfully complete the North American Pharmacist Licensure Examination (NAPLEX) and his or her respective state's jurisprudence examinations. When the requirements for licensure within a state have been completed, the candidate is qualified to become a registered pharmacist (RPh) who is licensed to practice in that particular state only.

Postgraduate Educational Opportunities

A choice of exciting careers awaits the pharmacy graduate. Some career paths, however, require the student to pursue postgraduate education. Master's and doctoral degree programs are offered at many colleges of pharmacy in the general areas of medicinal chemistry, pharmaceutics, pharmacology/toxicology, and social and administrative sciences, with each college tailoring its specific programs in each of these areas to student needs and faculty interests and backgrounds. Pursuing one of these degrees is ideal for the student who is interested in a career in academia, the pharmaceutical industry, government, or another setting requiring research expertise. Individuals who are interested in advancing their careers in the practice arena may seek one of any number of residencies and fellowships offered through universities, hospitals, and other health care providers throughout the United States.

Specialization through Certification

Other opportunities are available to pharmacists through the process of certification. Certification is recognition by a nongovernment association or agency that an individual has completed predetermined qualifications in a field of specialized knowledge. Pharmacists may become board certified in any of five specialties through programs administered by the Board of Pharmaceutical Specialties (BPS):

Oncology pharmacy. Addresses the pharmaceutical care of patients with cancer. Specialists are closely involved in recognition, management, and prevention of unique morbidities associated with cancer and cancer treatment and recognition of the balance between improved survival and quality of life as primary outcome indicators.

Psychiatric pharmacy. Addresses the pharmaceutical care of patients with psychiatric disorders. The specialist is responsible for optimizing drug treatment and patient care by conducting patient assessments, recommending treatment plans, monitoring patient response, and recognizing drug-induced problems.

Nutrition support pharmacy. Addresses the care of patients who receive specialized nutrition support, including parenteral and enteral nutrition. The specialist has responsibility for promoting maintenance and/or restoration of optimal nutritional status and designing and modifying treatment needs. He or she often functions as a member of a multidisciplinary nutrition support team.

Nuclear pharmacy. Seeks to improve and promote public health through the safe and effective use of radioactive drugs for diagnosis and therapy. A nuclear pharmacist specializes in procurement, compounding, quality assurance, dispensing, distribution, and development of radiopharmaceuticals.

Pharmacotherapy. Assumes responsibility for ensuring the safe, appropriate, and economical use of drugs in patient care. The specialist often has responsibility for direct patient care, may conduct clinical research, and serves as a primary source of drug information for other health care professionals (BPS, 2000).

These programs are rigorous and require extensive work and study. Pharmacists may also complete other certification programs in a wide variety of areas—most notably in the management of certain disease states/conditions, such as diabetes, hypertension, and pain management. Other potential areas of focus include geriatrics, pediatrics, managed care, and management/marketing. These programs are administered by professional or health organizations, such as the American Diabetes Association, and they are often approved by the American Council on Pharmaceutical Education (ACPE), though they do not indicate board certification.

Unlike licensure, certification does not give the recipient any legal privileges. It does offer the recipient many advantages, however. Aside from the implicit value of the knowledge and expertise gained, some job descriptions posted by medical care institutions require certification. In addition, third-party payers may be more likely to reimburse a board-certified specialist or reimburse such a professional for the same services at a higher rate. Board certification also represents a marketing tool that specialists can use to advocate their services. As of 2006, more than 5,000 pharmacists had become certified through BPS alone, with more than half of those certifications in pharmacotherapy (BPS, 2006).

PROFESSIONAL PHARMACY ORGANIZATIONS

A Brief History

The diversity of pharmacists' practice settings is reflected in the large number of professional pharmacy organizations. The first professional pharmacy organization, the APhA, was founded in 1852 for the purpose of establishing national standards of quality for drugs and chemicals. Its founding came in response to criticism of the pharmacy trade by physicians who threatened to regulate the profession. Shortly thereafter, the APhA developed a code of ethics for its member practitioners. During the 1900s, other professional associations developed. Some of them were offshoots from within various sections of the APhA. The number of professional organizations continues to grow as the interests and work environments of pharmacists expand.

The Purpose and Functions of Pharmacy Organizations

Professional pharmacy organizations represent a few of literally tens of thousands of national associations in the United States, not including state and local associations. The primary reason that these organizations exist is to serve the interests of their members. They publish position papers and lobby governments, other professional organizations, and private businesses on behalf of their members. Examples of issues targeted for lobbying efforts include the crafting of specific language beneficial to pharmacists in regulations proposed by federal agencies, reimbursement for cognitive services, and expansion of the scope of pharmacy practice.

Specific benefits and services that professional pharmacy organizations provide include the following:

Information dissemination. Publishing of journals and newsletters to disseminate the results of pertinent studies and updates on professional practice and legal issues. Recently, associations have also initiated weekly e-mail services and regular updates on their Web sites.

Maintenance of practitioners' competency. Codes of ethics, standards of practice, free continuing education, and professional meetings.

Career planning assistance. Posting of jobs in related fields, placement of advertisements in journals by employers, and sponsorship of workshops for career advancement.

Financial benefits. Discount rates on items such as resource materials, credit cards, and insurance policies.

Participation in governance. Members help create and revise organization policies at professional meetings and serve on committees.

Professional Organizations with Pharmacist Membership

Individual pharmacists may enroll as members of some of the organizations that directly or indirectly serve the profession.

The *American Pharmacists Association* (APhA, www.aphanet.org) recently changed its name from the American Pharmaceutical Association to more accurately reflect the importance of its primary constituents: pharmacists. Arguably the most diverse pharmacy-related organization in terms of its membership, the APhA serves pharmacists in all practice settings. Headquartered in Washington, D.C., it is actively involved in lobbying the government on pharmacists' behalf. Its student organization, the Academy of Student Pharmacists (ASP), has more student members than any other professional association. The APhA publishes numerous journals and newsletters including *Pharmacy Today,* to help students and practitioners keep abreast of current issues, and *Journal of the American Pharmacists Association* (*JAPhA*), which features research in the administrative, basic, and clinical pharmaceutical sciences. It also publishes monographs, such as those describing the MMA 2003, which are very helpful to pharmacists.

Formerly the American Society of Hospital Pharmacists, the *American Society of Health-Systems Pharmacists* (ASHP, www.ashp.org) changed its name to reflect the evolution of hospitals into integrated delivery networks. The ASHP is a national accrediting organization for pharmacy residency and pharmacy technician training programs. It publishes numerous educational materials and handbooks, including *American Hospital Formulary System Drug Information* (*AHFS DI*). It also publishes *American Journal of Health-Systems Pharmacy* (*AJHP*) and produces *International Pharmaceutical Abstracts* (*IPA*), a bimonthly abstracting and indexing service. The ASHP promotes guidelines, standards, and best practices in a number of pharmacy practice arenas. Its annual clinical meeting is the largest gathering of pharmacists worldwide.

Founded as the National Association of Retail Druggists, the mission of the *National Community Pharmacists Association* (NCPA, www.ncpanet.org) is to keep the business of pharmacy viable. The NCPA is the voice for America's independent community pharmacists. It provides continuing education through its publication *America's Pharmacist.* The NCPA's Management Institute serves as a clearinghouse for up-to-date management information. The organization also affords to its members the opportunity to join ValuRite, a professional services administration organization, which provides greater purchasing power to community pharmacy owners. The NCPA administers the National Institute for Pharmacist Care Outcomes (NIPCO) program and sponsors the NCPA Foundation, which awards grants intended to promote the profession and pharmacy care outcomes. The NCPA also publishes *NCPA-Pfizer Digest,* which allows independent community pharmacies to assess and compare their financial and clinical performance with indicators for other pharmacies of similar size.

The *Academy of Managed Care Pharmacy* (AMCP, www.amcp.org) serves patients and the public through the promotion of wellness and rational drug therapy by the application of managed care principles. Part of its mission is the advancement of pharmacy practice in managed health care systems. The AMCP publishes *Journal of Managed Care Pharmacy* (*JMCP*), which highlights research on administrative issues and on the rational use of drug therapies, including cost-effectiveness and outcomes studies. This organization has been a leader in efforts to standardize formulary submissions and to improve the quality of formulary decisions made by insurers and institutions. It also provides weekly e-mail and fax-on-demand services that keep its members informed about drug therapy and legislative issues from around the United States.

Membership in the *American College of Apothecaries* (ACA, www.acainfo.org) is open to pharmacists who own or hold shares in a pharmacy, primarily apothecary-style pharmacies with low levels of front-end merchandise. Among its publications are *Guidelines for Improving*

Communication in Pharmacy Practice and *Guidelines for Marketing Your Community Pharmacy Practice.*

Founded to strengthen pharmacy's role in long-term care, the *American Society of Consultant Pharmacists* (ASCP, www.ascp.com) publishes the journal *Consultant Pharmacist,* which features articles on the results of drug utilization reviews and clinical studies, drug information, and managerial aspects of consultant pharmacy. Among its other publications is *Drug Regimen Review: A Process Guide for Pharmacists.*

Founded to advance the practice of clinical pharmacy, the *American College of Clinical Pharmacy* (ACCP, www.accp.com) promotes clinical research, rational drug therapy, and fellowship training. It also publishes educational materials related to pharmacoeconomics and outcomes research. Many faculty members in departments of pharmacy practice are members of the ACCP.

The *National Pharmaceutical Association* (NPhA, www.nphanet.org) is dedicated to representing the views and ideas of minority pharmacists on critical issues affecting health care and pharmacy as well as advancing the standards of pharmaceutical care among all practitioners.

The *National Council on Patient Information and Education* (NCPIE, www.talkaboutrx.org) is dedicated to improving communication between health care professionals and patients. It also makes available the "Talking about Prescriptions Planning Kit" and "Educate Before You Medicate" promotional materials.

Organizations with Corporate Membership

Pharmacists may also be affected by or interact with other organizations of which they are not members. The members of these organizations are corporations, rather than individuals.

Formerly the National Wholesale Druggists Association, the *Healthcare Distribution Management Association* (HDMA, www.healthcaredistribution.org) is the national association of full-service drug wholesalers. This organization's mission is to strengthen relations between wholesalers, their suppliers, and customers, and to sponsor and disseminate research and information on new technology and management practices for wholesalers. Full-service drug wholesalers are typically large companies involved in myriad aspects of drug distribution, including automated dispensing technologies and storage of specialty compounds.

The *Institute for Safe Medication Practices* (ISMP, www.ismp.org) is the United States' only nonprofit organization devoted entirely to medication error prevention and safe medication use. It oversees a voluntary medication error-reporting system and promotes error reduction strategies to the health care community, policy makers, and the public.

The voice of the chain drug store industry, the *National Association of Chain Drug Stores* (NACDS, www.nacds.org) is involved in numerous professional activities, including sponsoring student recruitment programs in high schools, conducting visitation programs for faculty and students to chain store headquarters operations, and awarding grant support for studies in management and administration. It posts positions for pharmacists in chain drug stores throughout the United States on its Web site and, along with organizations such as the NCPA, supports the SureScripts Electronic Prescribing Network to allow for the electronic exchange of information between prescribers and pharmacies.

The *Pharmaceutical Researchers and Manufacturers of America* (PhRMA, www.pharma.org) is a powerful consortium of manufacturers of "brand-name" products that is heavily involved in supporting research and development of new drugs and pharmaceutical delivery systems.

Formerly the Non Prescription Drug Manufacturers Association (NDMA), the *Consumer Healthcare Products Association* (CHPA, www.chpa-info. org) is concerned with issues relevant to makers of over-the-counter (OTC) medications and encourages responsible self-medication practices by consumers. The CHPA conducts a voluntary labeling review service for members and promotes the readability of OTC product labels.

The *Generic Pharmaceutical Industry Association* (GPhA, www.gpha-online.org) represents manufacturers and distributors within the generic drug industry. The GPhA is dedicated to the provision of high-quality, cost-effective equivalents to brand-name prescription drugs. It provides lawmakers, government agencies, regulators, prescribers, and pharmacists with information regarding the safety, effectiveness, and therapeutic equivalence of generic medicines.

Educational and Regulatory Organizations

Some organizations provide services to pharmacists (who may or may not be members of those groups) and regulate their practice and educational requirements.

Society grants pharmacy the power of self-regulation as long as society can reap the benefits of having highly competent and moral professionals serving its interests. The *National Association of Boards of Pharmacy* (NABP, www.nabp.net) assists state boards of pharmacy in protecting the public by developing, implementing, and enforcing uniform standards. The NABP develops and administers the NAPLEX examination and oversees reciprocity of licenses across states.

The *Accreditation Council for Pharmacy Education* (ACPE, www.acpe-accredit.org) is a national agency that provides for the accreditation of professional degree programs in pharmacy and for the approval of providers of continuing pharmaceutical education. The ACPE is an autonomous agency whose board of directors is made up of members of the AACP, APhA, NABP, and American Council on Education (ACE).

The *American Association of Colleges of Pharmacy* (AACP) is a national organization representing the interests of pharmaceutical educators. The AACP is committed to excellence in pharmaceutical education. Both individual faculty members and schools of pharmacy constitute its membership. It publishes *American Journal of Pharmaceutical Education* (*AJPE*), with contributions from pharmacy faculty throughout the United States, to disseminate information on course content, curricula, and innovative teaching strategies.

The mission of the *American Foundation for Pharmaceutical Education* (AFPE, www.afpenet.org) is to advance and support pharmaceutical sciences education at U.S. schools and colleges of pharmacy by awarding scholarships and grants to pharmacy students and faculty.

PHARMACY TECHNICIANS

As the practice of pharmacy evolves, so do the roles of pharmacy technicians. The number of prescriptions dispensed in the United States has increased rapidly in recent years, as has the diversity of settings in which pharmacists practice. To keep up with the rising demand for pharmaceutical products and services, technicians will play a greater role in support of pharmaceutical care. This section examines pharmacy technicians, their expanding roles and responsibilities, and certification and management issues.

The Choice of Pharmacy Technician as a Career

In 2002, approximately 250,000 pharmacy technicians were practicing in the United States (American Pharmaceutical Association, 2003). A national sample of certified pharmacy technicians reported a mean hourly wage of $12.87 for these employees in 2004 (Desselle, 2005), with their exact earnings depending on their location, practice setting, and experience. Technicians receive their training through formal educational programs at vocational or technical schools and community colleges, formal on-the-job training programs sponsored by employers, or informal on-the-job training. An increasing number of nationally accredited technician training programs exist, with the standard for accreditation by the ASHP calling for 600 hours of contact time, extending over at least 15 weeks (American Society of Hospital Pharmacists, 1993).

The jobs of pharmacy technicians were once geared toward clerical and custodial duties. Indeed, the Scope of Pharmacy Practice Project conducted in the early 1990s revealed that pharmacy technicians spent more than 26% of their time collecting, organizing, and evaluating information in assisting pharmacists to serve patients, more than 21% of their time developing and managing medication distribution and control, and a bit less than 7% of their time providing drug information and education (American Society of Hospital Pharmacists, 1994).

Pharmacy Technicians' Expanding Roles and Responsibilities

Today, pharmacy technicians are involved in far more areas of pharmacy practice. **Table 3–2** illustrates the results of a survey of certified pharmacy technicians who indicated their primary areas of work. In addition to assisting with outpatient prescription dispensing, many community pharmacy technicians participate in purchasing/inventory control, billing, and repackaging products. Most hospital pharmacy technicians assist with inpatient medication dispensing, but many also prepare intravenous admixtures and engage in nonsterile compounding, repackaging, purchasing, and billing. A significant minority of the technicians surveyed indicated that they participate in educating and training other technicians.

The Scope of Pharmacy Practice Project report also provided a comprehensive classification of pharmacy technician responsibilities and activities (American Society of Hospital Pharmacists, 1994). It segmented these duties into three main function areas:

Table 3-2 Respondents' Primary Areas of Work

	Total[a] (%) (n = 281)	Community (%) (n = 115)	Hospital (%) (n = 113)	Other[b] (%) (n = 53)
Assisting in outpatient prescription dispensing	58	90	27	55
Assisting in inpatient medication dispensing	42	11	82	21
Preparing IV admixtures	35	2	73	28
Purchasing/inventory	44	51	43	32
Billing	39	46	38	25
Nonsterile compounding	29	18	42	25
Prepackaging/repacking	38	20	61	30
Pharmacy technician educator	15	16	15	11
Other	11	4	10	28

[a]Percentages do not total 100 because multiple responses were permitted.
[b]Includes home health care, long-term care, mail service facility, managed health care, educational/vocational training, pharmaceutical industry, and military.
Source: Copyright © 1999 American Pharmacists Association (APhA). Muenzen, P.M., Greenberg, S., and Murer, M.M. (1999). PTCB task analysis identifies role of certified pharmacy technicians in pharmaceutical care. *Journal of the American Pharmacists Association, 39,* 857–864.

1. *Assist the pharmacist in serving patients.* Receive prescription or medication orders, obtain information from patients and from other health care professionals, collect data, update patient records or profiles, process the medication or prescription order, compound a medication or prescription order, provide medication to the patient, determine and obtain charges for services, communicate with third-party payers, and determine whether counseling by the pharmacist is desired.
2. *Maintain medication and inventory control systems.* Identify drugs, equipment, and supplies to be ordered, place orders, receive goods and verify their receipt against original purchase orders, place received goods into proper storage, perform non-patient-specific distribution of pharmaceuticals (e.g., crash carts and automated dispensing systems), remove expired or recalled products, perform required inventory analyses, perform quality assurance tests on compounded medications, and repackage finished dosage forms for dispensing.
3. *Participate in the administration and management of a pharmacy practice.* Coordinate communications throughout the site, collect productivity information, participate in quality improvement activities, assist with ensuring compliance with regulatory standards, perform routine sanitation and maintenance activities, perform billing and accounting functions, and conduct staff training.

As some work environments shift further toward patient-oriented philosophies, new roles and responsibilities for technicians are emerging:

- Managing an automated pharmacy station (Jackson, Bickham, and Clark, 1998).
- Implementing a prescription assistance program for indigent patients (Mangino, Szajna, Ptachcinski, and Skledar, 1998).
- Triaging patients, processing consults, and managing follow-up appointments in a drug therapy monitoring clinic (Johnson and Yanchick, 1998).
- Monitoring drug use and disease management guidelines in a patient assessment program (Ervin, Skledar, Hess, and Ryan, 1998).
- Conducting pediatric compounding, processing emergency requisitions, emergency operating department setup, and participating in investigational drug studies during the midnight shift at a university hospital (Bedoya, Patel, Bickham, and Clark, 1998).
- Performing duties related to the provision of quality home care services (Ramirez, Jones, and Holmes, 1993).

Pharmacy Technician Certification

The trend toward expansion of pharmacy technicians' roles is reflected in the movement toward voluntary certification of these professionals. A certified pharmacy technician (CPhT) has completed the Pharmacy

Technician Certification Examination (PTCE) sponsored by the Pharmacy Technician Certification Board (PTCB). These rigorous examinations include questions on communication, organizational and interpersonal skills, pharmacy operations, pharmacy law, and calculations. The ExCPT is supported by NACDS and NCPA. The PTCB was founded jointly by the APhA, the ASHP, the Illinois Council of Health-System Pharmacists, and the Michigan Pharmacists Association. As of June 2006, more than 240,000 applicants had become certified through the PTCB (PTCB, 2006), up from slightly more than 48,000 in 1998 (Muenzen, Greenberg, and Murer, 1999).

Certification offers advantages to both the technician and the pharmacist. For technicians, certification may result in an increase in pay or a promotion in title. It may also bring greater job security and give the person an edge when seeking a job or changing jobs. It may also result in expanded job functions and responsibilities and—perhaps most importantly—increased satisfaction on the job. The increased confidence and satisfaction from the technician becoming certified may enhance his or her performance, thereby increasing the pharmacy's productivity. It may also decrease training time and lower the cost of on-the-job training.

Pharmacists have traditionally been reticent to allow technicians to expand their scope of practice, but this reluctance appears to be changing. Today's pharmacists are more secure in their roles and are beginning to see that certified technicians can reduce their workloads and mitigate their stress levels. One study indicated that hospital pharmacy directors believed that such certification would have positive effects by allowing pharmacists to perform more patient-centered activities (Mott, Vanderpool, and Smeenk, 1998).

In addition to addressing the problem of an acute shortage of pharmacists, technician certification has grown more popular because of the progress made in curricula and in the training of technicians, thanks to the development of the Model Curriculum for Pharmacy Technician Training (American Pharmaceutical Association, 2003). Also, a majority of states have revised their pharmacy practice acts in areas related to technicians, and a number of states have liberalized their pharmacist-to-technician ratios. Finally, a few states have begun making certification a requirement for registration or licensure.

E-COMMERCE AND INTERNET PHARMACY

During the latter part of the 1990s, the Internet changed the way that Americans work and play. It has contributed significantly to a booming economy and new heights in productivity never seen before in the United States. As of this writing, it was beginning to leave its mark on the practice of medicine and on the pharmacy profession. It may likely change the landscape of pharmacy care forever, although its precise impact on the industry is unknown.

What Is Internet Pharmacy?

No formal definition exists of "Internet pharmacy," also known as "online pharmacy," "cyberpharmacy," or "e-pharmacy." There are basically three types of Internet pharmacies. One type provides legend pharmaceuticals pursuant to a valid prescription order; it is essentially a mail-order pharmacy whose business address is in cyberspace. Upon receipt of a prescription from a physician who is not affiliated with the Web site, the pharmacist will fill it, mail the product to the patient, and then either bill the patient directly or bill his or her insurance company. The pioneers in this field expanded rapidly to provide many other services. These sites offer a considerable amount of free product, health, and disease management information. They also offer for sale nearly all OTC medications, sundries, and health and beauty aids that are sold at a typical chain or independent community pharmacy.

A second type of Internet pharmacy includes sites that offer free information and counseling for a fee but without the dispensing component. These businesses can be grouped with many other Web sites that offer health information, with or without a fee, but that are not necessarily pharmacies. While some of these sites are legitimate, such as those operated by various professional groups, others are not.

It is the third type of online pharmacy that has drawn the concern of medical professionals, government, regulatory agencies, and society at large. At these sites, consumers log on and complete a survey or questionnaire about their medical problem or make a direct request for a particular prescription drug product. The consumer may be charged a fee for completing the questionnaire, which may be returned or discounted if the physician does not issue a prescription. At legitimate sites of this kind, a physician reviews the data. Many sites, however, pretend to have licensed prescribers and pharmacists "in-house." They have obtained the medications illegally and are selling them to consumers at high prices without regard for the purchasers' safety.

Illegal Pharmacy Operations on the Internet

Illegal pharmacy sites pose a significant health threat to many Americans. One study conducted during 1999 (Armstrong, Schwartz, and Asch, 1999) located 86 sites that offered to deliver sildenafil (Viagra) directly to consumers without a visit to a physician, with 44 of them not requiring an online evaluation. The use of sildenafil as well as many other products in high demand on the Web can be problematic—even lethal—for certain patients who are not under a physician's direct supervision. Another problem is that drugs acquired from certain Internet sources may be adulterated or perhaps even not contain the supposed active ingredient.

Stopping illegal Internet pharmacy operations has been an arduous task for authorities because it is difficult to find their geographic locations. Few enforceable laws govern these types of businesses. Many of them operate on a "fly-by-night" basis; they stay open for only a short period of time (a few days to several weeks), make their money, and then close before the perpetrators are caught. Many sites that exist only to provide information also pose risks to consumers because much of the information and advice are unsubstantiated and may be harmful if followed.

Issues related to Internet pharmacy include re-importation and diversion of pharmaceuticals. As prescription drugs continue to take up a larger portion of the monies spent on health care, many persons are seeking alternatives to traditional means for purchasing prescription drugs. Some, for example, try to purchase medications from pharmacies in Canada and even Mexico to save money. In fact, some state governments have formed cooperatives to arrange for purchase of medications from Canadian pharmacies for state employees or for Medicaid beneficiaries. This contradicts FDA regulations; to date, the federal government has not strictly enforced those rules. There is considerable debate about the authenticity of medications acquired from Canadian Internet sites. The acquisition of drugs from legitimate Canadian operations poses little, if any threat, beyond that normally accompanying medication use without face-to-face counseling with a health professional; however, many Web-based pharmacy operations use a Canadian name or domain name, but are not legally recognized Canadian pharmacies.

What Is Being Done to Curb Fraudulent Operations on the Web?

The NABP responded to illegal online sales of prescription drugs quickly by unveiling its Verified Internet Pharmacy Practice Site program (VIPPS) in February 1999 (Paulsen, 1999). VIPPS is a voluntary program designed to certify each participating online pharmacy's ability to dispense pharmaceuticals. Certification involves documenting licensure from the appropriate state board of pharmacy, ensuring that the pharmacy meets a rigorous 19-point set of criteria, and conducting an on-site review of the pharmacy's written policies and procedures by an NABP-trained inspection team. Certified pharmacies display the VIPPS seal on the home page of their Web site. This seal contains a hyperlink to NABP's home page, where visitors can view information about the online pharmacy.

On a federal level, in December 1999, the Clinton administration announced a $10 million initiative to protect consumers from the illegal sale of pharmaceuticals over the Internet (Food and Drug Administration, 2000). It established federal requirements for all Internet pharmacies to ensure their compliance with state and federal laws, created new civil penalties for the illegal sale of pharmaceuticals, gave federal agencies such as the FDA and the Federal Trade Commission (FTC) new authority to swiftly gather the information needed to prosecute offenders, and launched a public education program about the potential dangers of buying drugs online. Unfortunately, the initiative was never acted upon by Congress and was never funded. While the FDA continues to identify and shut down illegal pharmacy sites, large-scale successes remain elusive.

Some states have also taken measures against illegal online prescription sales. For example, the state of Arkansas passed a law that requires any pharmacy shipping prescription drugs to a resident of the state to have at least one pharmacist licensed to practice by Arkansas's state board (Conlan, 1999). Other states have enacted similar legislation. A few state health departments have successfully identified illegal operations and prosecuted those involved.

Pharmacists should keep abreast of the current events affecting medication distribution systems. In addition to the aforementioned VIPPS program, several organizations have developed voluntary programs through which Web sites may acquire a "seal of approval" based on their compliance with various codes of ethics regarding the reliability and confidentiality of information, including MedCIRCLE (www.medcircle.org), HONcode (www.hon.ch/HONcode) , and TRUSTe (www.truste.org).

Perhaps the most effective means to curb patients' acquisition of medications from specious sources is to improve access to drug therapy. While not a panacea, the MMA greatly improved many seniors' ability to obtain necessary medications and will afford them the opportunity to receive expanded medication therapy management services. Reducing the number of indigent persons without prescription drug coverage will undoubtedly reduce the demand for prescription drugs from alternative sources. Pharmacists working in "bricks-and-mortar" operations can do their part by providing quality service to patients. Although Web-based commerce is preferred by—and even mandated by payers for—a certain proportion of the population, pharmacists may counsel patients that anything short of real-time communication can pose risks. One study found that information provided via "ask the pharmacist" services on the Web was less than optimal, even from trusted sources (Holmes, Desselle, Nath, and Markuss, 2005). Yet another found poor readability and incomplete information for certain drugs on the Web sites of national chain pharmacies (Ghoshal and Walji, 2006).

A Few Last Words about Cybertechnology and Pharmacy

It seems fairly certain that the Internet will serve as yet another medium for the burgeoning prescription and OTC medication markets. It is also providing another venue for direct-to-consumer advertising by pharmaceutical manufacturers and makers of health and beauty products.

Other, similar technologies are also drastically changing the shape of pharmacy care. Telemedicine, for example, has become increasingly widespread. At the time of this writing, nearly every state either had already passed or will soon pass legislation allowing for the electronic data interchange (EDI) of prescriptions from prescribers to pharmacies. This technology allows the prescriber to use either a personal computer or a handheld personal digital assistant (PDA) to transmit prescriptions electronically to the pharmacy. The physician can check for compliance with the patient's insurance formulary and obtain the patient's drug history for drug utilization evaluation (DUE) messaging, all on the same system, before the prescription is even transmitted. Claims can even be pre-adjudicated before the prescription reaches the pharmacy. In such a case, the prescription will not require manual entry by pharmacy personnel. Under this system, pharmacists will have to deal with fewer phone calls to physicians and fewer claims rejections from payers.

Many other technologies will affect pharmacy and medication use systems that are beyond the scope of this chapter. Pharmacists are encouraged to take advantage of the features offered by the Internet, such as assisting them with drug decision support, marketing their services, and obtaining continuing education credits.

PHARMACY WORKFORCE

Implications of Workforce Size for Pharmacy

The final section of this chapter addresses an issue that is intrinsically tied to many of the concepts discussed throughout this text—namely, the number of pharmacists available in the United States as measured in terms of the number of full-time equivalents (FTEs). Maintaining an adequate supply of pharmacists is critical on several fronts.

First, given that the number of prescriptions dispensed annually is expected to continue to increase, an adequate number of pharmacists must be working in community settings to fulfill society's demand for cost-effective pharmaceuticals that are dispensed promptly and accurately.

Second, an adequate supply of well-trained pharmacists is essential to the provision of pharmaceutical care. If the number of FTEs of available pharmacists is unable or minimally able to meet society's need for dispensing, it becomes that much more difficult for the profession to continue along its path of maturation from a product- to a patient-centered focus. One study revealed while the proportion of pharmacies offering any kind of pharmacist care services was increasing, only four services were offered at more than 10% of community pharmacy practices in 2004—specifically, immunizations, smoking cessation, health screening, and diabetes management (Doucette et al, 2006).

Third, an adequate workforce is required to meet the need for public safety. In recent years, medication-related errors and their resultant morbidity and mortality in the hospital setting have come under intense scrutiny. Although pharmacists are not entirely responsible for all of these errors, a number of steps can be taken to mitigate this problem. The lay press has also called attention to the lack of consistency in detecting prescription-related problems in pharmacies across the United States (Knapp, 1999). Part of the problem is that many pharmacies are understaffed or are staffed consistently with "floaters" who do not have a regular site at which to practice.

Pharmacy workforce issues are also important to pharmacy's role in reforming the health care system (Knapp, 1994). As greater emphasis is placed on preventive care, pharmacists may be increasingly called upon to provide services such as healthy lifestyle counseling, disease management, immunizations, and other public health initiatives. Additionally, the government continues to grapple with shortages of primary care practitioners in inner-city and rural areas. One study showed that the presence of pharmacists in combination with other health care professionals such as nurse practitioners in rural areas suffering from a scarcity of physicians can mitigate the problem of diminished access to health care (Knapp, Paavola, Maine, Sorofman, and Politzer, 1999).

The size of the pharmacy workforce is also a source of concern for state boards of pharmacy and the academic community. State boards of pharmacy enforce regulations that affect the number and use of pharmacy technicians. Some state boards have enacted rules limiting the number of technicians who are allowed to work in direct care settings by specifying a maximum ratio of technicians to pharmacists. As mentioned previously, some boards of pharmacy have had to amend these ratios to respond to labor supply shortages.

For their part, schools of pharmacy have the responsibility for continuing to graduate an adequate number of pharmacists to meet the needs of society while maintaining the quality and integrity of their programs. The AACP, the ACPE, and individual schools must keep abreast of supply trends by region and across the United States.

Factors Affecting Pharmacist Labor Supply

As the profession continues to operate within a dynamic health care environment while undergoing comprehensive change, numerous forces appear poised to affect the current and future supply of pharmacists.

First, the demographic composition of pharmacists is shifting toward a greater proportion of female practitioners. Whereas the profession was once virtually all male, by 1991 approximately 32% of pharmacists were female. Women accounted for approximately 46% of the pharmacist supply in 2000 and 50% in 2003 (Gershon, Cultice, and Knapp, 2000). This trend has significant implications because child-bearing women will take at least some time off for maternity leave and women are more likely than men to work part-time for childrearing or other reasons.

Another factor affecting the pharmacist labor supply is the transition from the BS to the PharmD degree as a requirement for practice. The PharmD has typically added an extra year of academic study, resulting in a downturn in applications to some schools of pharmacy. The increased emphasis on pharmacotherapeutics and experiential training also requires additional clinical faculty and preceptors.

Yet another factor reducing the pharmacist labor supply is the dwindling number of independent pharmacies, whose owner pharmacists tend to work more hours than employee pharmacists (Knapp, 1994).

The effects of other factors on pharmacist labor supply are less certain. Pharmacist specialization, while increasing pharmacists' competency to provide pharmaceutical care, may result in their propensity to work in nontraditional settings and reduce their supply in distributive settings. An estimated 6.8% to 13.1% of pharmacists will be certified specialists by 2010 (Knapp and Sorby, 1991). The penetration of managed care into health care markets was once expected to reduce the demand for pharmacists, but studies have shown this not to be the case (Knapp, 1999).

Finally, two factors that directly affect the pharmacy labor supply are pharmacy technicians and automation. Certification of technicians can serve to increase their level of competence and allow these individuals to perform roles that had previously been within the pharmacist's scope of practice only. Automation and other technologies can free up time for pharmacists, allowing them to turn their attention toward patient consultative and disease management activities.

Estimates of the Pharmacist Workforce

Although leaders in the profession agree that workforce issues are important, there has been less consensus on how to measure the labor supply and, therefore, where the profession stands. A variety of methods have been used to quantify the pharmacy labor supply, including worker–population ratios, demand versus supply techniques, the relative income of pharmacists, and the internal rate of return for investing in pharmacy education (Sorkin, 1989). Data on pharmacy manpower are generated primarily from three sources: (1) the Pew Health Professions Commission, (2) the Bureau of Labor Statistics (BLS), and (3) the Bureau of Health Professions.

In 1995, the Pew Health Professions Commission published a report projecting a future surplus of as many as 40,000 pharmacists (Knapp, 1999). Other researchers view this report as inaccurate. Instead, the general consensus forecasts a shortage of pharmacists nationally, with some regions being extremely short of these professionals.

The most comprehensive attempt to measure and predict the future pharmacist labor supply has been the combined effort of professional associations and the BHP in creating the Pharmacy Manpower Project census database (Gershon et al., 2000). This model incorporates the change in the entry-level degree, the opening of new pharmacy schools, the influx of international pharmacy graduates, and separation rates (actuarial estimates of retirement, death, and occupational mobility). It projected a workforce of 196,011 active pharmacists in 2000 and predicts a workforce of 249,086 active pharmacists by 2020. It implies further that the ratio of active pharmacists to the general population will increase by 2020 to a level 76.7 pharmacists per 100,000 population, compared with 68.9 pharmacists per 100,000 population in 1995. The model does not consider FTEs, however, and its primary drawback is that its definition of "active pharmacists" includes a potentially increasing number of practitioners who are working part-time.

Efforts are being made to track the balance of supply and demand forces of pharmacists longitudinally by making survey-based estimates of the amount of difficulty faced by employers in filling open pharmacist positions (Knapp and Livesey, 2002). As of 2001, there was considerable demand in excess of available supply, with the problem being more acute in certain states. This issue is of particular concern as patients experience a number of unmet needs in medication use (e.g., medication counseling and drug therapy monitoring) (Law, Ray, Knapp, and Balesh, 2003) and a sizable portion of pharmacists' work hours are consumed by activities not directly related to patient care (Schommer, Pedersen, Doucette, Gaither, and Mott, 2002). The projected shortage has encouraged a number of new colleges/schools of pharmacy to open across the United States as a response to the unmet need.

CONCLUSIONS

The pharmacy profession has come a long way in a little more than a century. The current pace of change, however, promises more momentous transitions over the next few decades. It is difficult to gauge exactly what pharmacy practice will be like in another century with the profession's renewed focus on patients, the continued specialization of pharmacists in specific disease states, the growing trend of pharmacy technician certification, the rapid diffusion of technology as a facilitator to the provision of care, and a shift in the composition of its workforce. It remains clear, however, that pharmacy will remain an integral part of our health care delivery system and an exciting career choice for its practitioners.

QUESTIONS FOR FURTHER DISCUSSION

1. How will pharmacists' roles continue to evolve over the next 10 to 20 years? What will be the status of pharmaceutical care delivery in 20 years?
2. Should the focus on pharmacist credentialing be on general pharmacotherapy or on further specialization to create experts in managing specific disease states?
3. Why are proportionately fewer pharmacists active in professional associations at a national level compared to physicians and other health care professionals? How has this hindered us as a profession?
4. What is the contribution of each subdiscipline within pharmacy toward practice, education, and research?
5. Should certification of pharmacy technicians be mandated? Why or why not?
6. Will Internet pharmacies threaten the profitability and existence of traditional "bricks-and-mortar" independent and chain pharmacies?
7. What can be done to ensure an adequate supply of pharmacists for the future?

KEY TOPICS AND TERMS

History of pharmacy
Pharmaceutical care
Professional pharmacy organizations
E-commerce
Pharmacy technicians
Pharmacy workforce

REFERENCES

American Association of Colleges of Pharmacy. (1996). Paper from the Commission to Implement Change in Pharmaceutical Education: Maintaining our commitment to change. *American Journal of Pharmaceutical Education, 60,* 378–384.

American Pharmaceutical Association. (1995). *Principles of practice for pharmaceutical care.* Washington, DC: American Pharmaceutical Association.

American Pharmaceutical Association. (2003). White paper on pharmacy technicians (2002): Needed changes can no longer wait. *Journal of the American Pharmaceutical Association, 43,* 93–107.

American Society of Hospital Pharmacists. (1993). ASHP accreditation standard for pharmacy technician training programs. *American Journal of Hospital Pharmacy, 50,* 124–126.

American Society of Hospital Pharmacists. (1994). Summary of the final report of the Scope of Pharmacy Practice Project. *American Journal of Hospital Pharmacy, 51,* 2179–2182.

Armstrong, K. A., Schwartz, J. S., & Asch, D. A. (1999). Direct sales of sildenafil (Viagra) to consumers over the Internet. *New England Journal of Medicine, 341,* 1389–1392.

Bedoya, R., Patel, H., Bickham, P., & Clark, T. (1998). Role of the midnight pharmacy technician. Paper presented at the ASHP Midyear Clinical Meeting, Reno, NV.

Board of Pharmaceutical Specialties (BPS). (2000). *BPS sets new candidate and site records in 2005. BPS News Release #2006-02.* Retrieved May 9, 2006, from http://www.bpsweb.org/News.Releases/NewsReleasesPDFs/2006-02.pdf

Boyd, J. R., Covington, T. R., Stanaszek, W. F., & Coussons, R. T. (1974). Drug defaulting, part 2: Analysis of noncompliance patterns. *American Journal of Hospital Pharmacy, 31,* 485–491.

Brodie, D. C. (1967). Drug-use control: Keystone to pharmaceutical service. *Drug Intelligence, 1,* 63–65.

Broeseker, A., & Janke, K. K. (1998). The evolution and revolution of pharmaceutical care. In R. L. McCarthy (Ed.), *Introduction to health care delivery: A primer for pharmacists* (pp. 393–416). Gaithersburg, MD: Aspen.

Buerki, R. A., & Vottero, L. D. (1994). *Ethical responsibility in pharmacy practice.* Madison, WI: American Institute of the History of Pharmacy.

Cippole, R. J. (1986). Drugs don't have doses—people have doses. *Drug Intelligence and Clinical Pharmacy, 29,* 881–882.

Col, N., Fanale, J. E., & Kronholm, P. (1990). The role of medication noncompliance and adverse drug reactions in hospitalizations in the elderly. *Archives of Internal Medicine, 150,* 841–845.

Commission to Implement Change in Pharmaceutical Education. (1993). Background paper II: Entry-level curricular outcomes, curricular content and educational process. *American Journal of Pharmaceutical Education, 57,* 386–399.

Conlan, M. F. (1999, May 17). It's the law. *Drug Topics, 143,* 72, 74.

Cranor, C. W., Bunting, B. A., & Christensen, D. B. (2003). The Asheville Project: Long-term clinical and economic outcomes of a community pharmacy diabetes care program. *Journal of the American Pharmaceutical Association, 43,* 173–184.

Cranor, C. W., & Christensen, D. B. (2003). The Asheville Project: Short-term outcomes of a community pharmacy diabetes care program. *Journal of the American Pharmaceutical Association, 43,* 149–159.

Desselle, S. P. (1997). Pharmacists' perceptions of a set of pharmaceutical care practice standards. *Journal of the American Pharmaceutical Association, NS37,* 529–535.

Desselle, S. P. (2005). Job turnover intentions among certified pharmacy technicians. *Journal of the American Pharmacists Association. 45,* 676–683.

Doucette, W. R., Kreling, D. H., Schommer, J. C., Gaither, C. A., Mott, D. A., & Pedersen, C. A. (2006). Evaluation of pharmacy service mix: Evidence from the 2004 National Pharmacist Workforce Study. *Journal of the American Pharmacists Association, 46,* 348–355.

Ervin, K. C., Skledar, S. J., Hess, N. M., & Ryan, M. L. (1998). Expanding the scope of clinical pharmacy programs: Technician facilitated patient assessment. Paper presented at the ASHP Midyear Clinical Meeting, Reno, NV.

Food and Drug Administration. (2000). *Online pharmacies frequently asked questions.* Retrieved August 23, 2000, from http//www.fda.gov/oc/buyonline/prfaqs.html

Gershon, S. K., Cultice, J. M., & Knapp, K. K. (2000). How many pharmacists are in our future? The Bureau of Health Professions projects supply to 2020. *Journal of Managed Care Pharmacy, 6,* 298–306.

Ghoshal, M., & Walji, M. F. (in press). Quality of information available on retail pharmacy websites. *Research in Social and Administrative Pharmacy, 2.*

Hepler, C. D. (1987). The third wave in pharmaceutical education: The clinical movement. *American Journal of Pharmaceutical Education, 51,* 369–385.

Hepler, C. D., & Strand, L. M. (1990). Opportunities and responsibilities in pharmaceutical care. *American Journal of Hospital Pharmacy, 47,* 533–543.

Holmes, E. R., Desselle, S. P., Nath, D. M., & Markuss, J. M. (2005). Quality analysis of consumer drug information provided through Internet pharmacies. *Annals of Pharmacotherapy, 39,* 662–667.

Jackson, M. L., Bickham, P., & Clark, T. (1998). Technician management of automation and inventory. Paper presented at ASHP Midyear Clinical Meeting, Reno, NV.

Johnson, I., & Yanchik, J. (1998). Responsibilities of a pharmacy technician in a pharmacist-run drug therapy monitoring clinic in a primary care setting. Paper presented at the ASHP Midyear Clinical Meeting, Reno, NV.

Kaminsky, N. U., & Basgall, J. (1997). "Taxonomy" project moves pharmacy practice closer to a uniform language. *Journal of the American Pharmaceutical Association, NS37,* 629–631.

Knapp, K. K. (1994). Pharmacy manpower: Implications for pharmaceutical care and health care reform. *American Journal of Hospital Pharmacy, 51,* 1212–1220.

Knapp, K. K. (1999). Charting the demand for pharmacists in the managed care era. *American Journal of Health-Systems Pharmacy, 56,* 1309–1314.

Knapp, K. K., & Livesey, J. C. (2002). The aggregate demand index: Measuring the balance between pharmacist supply and demand, 1999–2001. *Journal of the American Pharmaceutical Association, 42,* 391–398.

Knapp, K. K., Paavola, F. G., Maine, L. L., Sorofman, B., & Politzer, R. M. (1999). Availability of primary care providers and pharmacists in the United States. *Journal of the American Pharmaceutical Association, 39,* 127–135.

Knapp, K. K., & Sorby, D. L. (1991). Directions for specialization in pharmacy practice, part 2. *American Journal of Hospital Pharmacy, 48,* 691–700.

Law, A. V., Ray, M. D., Knapp, K. K., & Balesh, J. K. (2003). Unmet needs in the medication use process: Perceptions of physicians, pharmacists, and patients. *Journal of the American Pharmaceutical Association, 43,* 394–402.

MacKinnon, G. E. III, & Mahrous, H. (2002). Assessing consumers' interest in health care services offered in community pharmacies. *Journal of the American Pharmaceutical Association, 42,* 512–515.

Maine, L. L., & Penna, R. P. (1996). Pharmaceutical care—an overview. In C. Knowlton & R. Penna (Eds.), *Pharmaceutical care* (pp. 133–154). New York: Chapman and Hall.

Manasse, H. R. (1989a). Medication use in an imperfect world: Drug misadventuring as an issue of public policy, part 1. *American Journal of Hospital Pharmacy, 46,* 929–944.

Manasse, H. R. (1989b). Medication use in an imperfect world: Drug misadventuring as an issue of public policy, part 2. *American Journal of Hospital Pharmacy, 46,* 1141–1152.

Mangino, M. H., Szajna, J. L., Ptachcinski, R., & Skledar, S. J. (1998). Role of a pharmacy technician in implementing a prescription assistance program for indigent and underinsured patients. Paper presented at the ASHP Midyear Clinical Meeting, Reno, NV.

Millis, J. S. (1975). *Pharmacists for the future: The report of the Study Commission on Pharmacy.* Ann Arbor, MI: Health Administration Press.

Millis, J. S. (1976). Looking ahead—The report of the Study Commission on Pharmacy. *American Journal of Hospital Pharmacy, 33,* 134–138.

Mott, D. A., Vanderpool, W. H., & Smeenk, D. A. (1998). Attitudes of Ohio hospital pharmacy directors toward national voluntary pharmacy technician certification. *American Journal of Health-Systems Pharmacy, 55,* 1799–1803.

Muenzen, P. M., Greenberg, S., & Murer, M. M. (1999). PTCB task analysis identifies role of certified pharmacy technicians in pharmaceutical care. *Journal of the American Pharmaceutical Association, 39,* 857–864.

Odedina, F. T., & Segall, R. (1996). Behavioral pharmaceutical care scale for measuring pharmacists' activities. *American Journal of Health-Systems Pharmacy, 53,* 855–865.

Paulsen, M. (1999). New NABP program combines criteria, inspections to certify online pharmacy quality. *Journal of the American Pharmaceutical Association, 39,* 870.

Penna, R. P. (1990). Pharmaceutical care—pharmacy's mission for the 1990s. *American Journal of Hospital Pharmacy, 47,* 543–549.

Pharmacy Technician Certification Board (PTCB). (2006). *National statistics.* Retrieved May 30, 2006, from http://www.ptcb.org

Pink, L. A. (1991). Hospitals. In J. E. Fincham &·A. I. Wertheimer (Eds.), *Pharmacists and the U. S. healthcare system* (pp. 158–190). Binghamton, NY: Pharmaceutical Products Press.

Pitterle, M. E., Bond, C. A., & Raehl, C. L. (1990). A comprehensive measure of pharmaceutical services: The pharmaceutical care index. *American Journal of Hospital Pharmacy, 47,* 1304–1313.

Ramirez, E., Jones, C. J., & Holmes, D. B. (1993). Expanding roles of the pharmacy technician in promoting quality home care services. Paper presented at the ASHP Annual Meeting, Denver, CO.

Relman, A. S. (1988). Assessment and accountability: The third revolution in medical care. *New England Journal of Medicine, 319,* 1220–1222.

Schommer, J. C., Pedersen, C. A., Doucette, W. R., Gaither, C. A., & Mott, D. A. (2002). Community pharmacists' work activities in the United States during 2000. *Journal of the American Pharmaceutical Association, 42,* 399–406.

Sonnedecker, G. (1963). *Kremers and Urdang's history of pharmacy.* Philadelphia: J. B. Lippincott.

Sorkin, A. L. (1989). Some economic aspects of pharmacy manpower. *American Journal of Hospital Pharmacy, 46,* 527–533.

Strand, L. M., Cippole, R. J., & Morley, P. C. (1988). Documenting the clinical pharmacist's activities: Back to basics. *Drug Intelligence and Clinical Pharmacy, 22,* 63–66.

Strand, L. M., Cippole, R. J., Morley, P. C., Ramsey, R., & Lamsam, G. D. (1990). Drug-related problems: Their structure and function. *DICP Annals of Pharmacotherapy, 24,* 1093–1097.

Tice, B., & Phillips, C. R. (2002). Implementation and evaluation of a lipid screening program in a large chain pharmacy. *Journal of the American Pharmaceutical Association, 42,* 413–419.

Torrens, P.R. (1993). Historical evolution and overview of health service in the United States. In J.S. Williams & P.R. Torrens (Eds.), *Introduction to health services* (4th ed.) (pp. 3–28). Albany, NY: Delmar.

The Patient

Kimberly S. Plake, Peter L. Steere, and Edward Krupat

Case Scenario

Mary is a 63-year-old woman who is greatly concerned about her health. She currently has type 2 diabetes and hypertension, and she knows that she is at least 50 pounds overweight. Lately, Mary has been experiencing symptoms that do not seem to be explained by her current chronic diseases. Because she does not have insurance and has limited access to health services owing to her rural location, she decided to do some research on her symptoms before making an appointment with the physician. Mary became concerned because she found some information on the Internet that indicated that she might have early signs of arthritis. She started taking Tylenol (McNeil) when she saw a commercial indicating that it can be used for her symptoms. However, it did not seem to be controlling all of her pain.

Mary decided that she must go to a physician because she can no longer stand the pain. Before meeting with her physician, she talked to her neighbor, Mrs. Johnson, who suffers from arthritis. After learning of Mary's suspicions, Mrs. Johnson gave her an article about arthritis from a women's magazine. A couple of pages after the article, Mary saw an advertisement for Celebrex (Searle Pfizer Pharmacia) and planned to talk with her physician about this medication.

At her appointment, Mary asked the physician about the information she obtained from the Internet and about Celebrex. In addition, she brought a list of her current symptoms. The physician, sensing that Mary would like to be an active participant in her health care, answered her questions, prompted her to provide information he thought was pertinent to her care, and then talked about her treatment options. After discussing her alternatives with her physician, Mary decided to begin taking Naprosyn for her arthritis and to start a weight reduction program to help treat her osteoarthritis.

LEARNING OBJECTIVES

Upon completion of this chapter, the student shall be able to:

- Describe factors that influence the health care system's focus on the treatment of diseases rather than the prevention of them
- Identify and describe services and programs for individuals with limited financial resources or limited access to health care services
- Explain the impact of the Internet on patients' access to health information
- Define and explain direct-to-consumer advertising
- Compare and contrast health practitioners' opinions of direct-to-consumer advertising to those of the pharmaceutical industry
- Explain the following models of the practitioner–patient relationship and their application when interacting with patients:
  a. Szasz and Hollender's models of care
  b. Consumer model of care
  c. Patient-centered model of care
- Describe the role that patient autonomy plays in patient–practitioner relationships
- Compare and contrast the biomedical and biopsychosocial models of care
- Explain the following health behavior models:
  a. Locus of control
  b. Health belief model
  c. Theory of reasoned action
  d. Theory of planned behavior
  e. Social cognitive theory (self-efficacy)
  f. Transtheoretical model (stages of change)
- Explain patient attitudes and behavior using the models described in the chapter when presented with a patient
- Develop an approach to facilitate behavior change and indicate your rationale for the selected approach when given a patient case

CHAPTER QUESTIONS

1. In what ways is the current crisis in health care financing a result of past successes of America's health care system?
2. How different are the opinions of health care payers and providers from the opinions of consumers about the purpose of the country's medical system? Why?
3. How have patient expectations of and experiences in the health care system changed in the past several years?
4. How do the models of health care delivery address some of the classic issues of patient–practitioner relations (the balance of power, patient autonomy, and patient satisfaction)?

INTRODUCTION

As reforms in health care occur, corresponding changes are also seen in patients, health professionals, and the health care environment. Although the health care system always seems to be in a state of flux, the focus remains on restoring sick patients to health. Health care professionals, health institutions, and insurance companies are interested in patients and their behaviors. Along with this interest is the desire to work with patients and to improve their care and satisfaction with services. This chapter explores topics related to the patient, including the shift in focus of care from acute to chronic diseases, the health care environment, patient expectations of care, models of care, and health care behaviors.

DEFINITIONS

Being a "patient" perhaps at one time suggested that an individual was under the care of a physician. It suggested illnesses, and a process of healing and recovery. While this definition still holds true, being a patient today may mean that a person is receiving services from a pharmacist, nurses, therapists, and other Western practitioners, as well as from providers of therapeutic massage, acupuncture, or a variety of other complementary services.

This multidisciplinary approach is a change in—and perhaps even in some ways, a return to—the manner in which individuals seeking care find services they feel are necessary for healing. This shift comes despite the fact that medical technology is, in the United States, at its highest-ever level of sophistication. While the introduction of new medical technologies has certainly changed patients' expectations and experiences, just as important are the effects that the economics of this evolving system of health care will have on the United States' financial ability to provide a reasonable standard of care for every patient.

DEMOGRAPHICS

The "graying of America" and its far-reaching implications are exerting serious pressure on the United States' health care systems. The rapid acceleration in the aging of the population (according to the U.S. Census Bureau, the median age increased by nearly 8 years between 1970 and 2000) and the use of medical services by the elderly, when combined, threaten to bankrupt America's health care reimbursement programs. By 2030, 20% of Americans will be age 65 or older (National Center for Health Statistics, 2004). Although the general population is growing at a rate of less than 1%, the number of "old" elderly—those older than 85 years—is growing at an even more rapid rate (see **Table 4–1**). Further,

Table 4-1 Shifts in American Population (thousands) as of July 1 for Each Year

	2005	2003	2000	1998	1996
Total population	296,410	290,850	282,193	270,248	265,229
5 to 13	36,087	36,764	37,051	35,396	34,604
14 to 44 years	130,391	129,714	128,464	120,462	119,826
65 to 84 years	31,694	31,236	30,791	30,336	33,957
85 years and older	5,095	4,716	4,286	4,049	3,800

Source: Adapted from U.S. Census Bureau.

the number of individuals aged 100 years or older has swelled by 33% since 1995 (United States Bureau of the Census, 2000).

This success at extending longevity is at least partly attributable to the United States' effective public health policy, including improvements in sanitation and nutrition and the development of immunizations. In the early 1900s, a person could expect to live 50 years (Tebbe, 1998), whereas someone born in 2003 can anticipate 75 or more years of life (Arias, 2006). In the early 20th century, Americans had to deal with then-fatal diseases such as smallpox, malaria, yellow fever, and tuberculosis (Leavitt and Numbers, 1997), which often prevented afflicted persons from living long enough to enter the years where more chronic diseases might be expected to be present.

Because advances in technology have helped to find treatments and cures (e.g., immunizations and antibiotics) for many of the more acute forms of illness, much of the current effort in health care focuses on the management of chronic conditions (Boult and Pacala, 1999). Diabetes, hypertension, cancer, cystic fibrosis, human immunodeficiency virus (HIV) infections, and other long-term (lifelong), multisystem diseases have replaced scarlet fever, measles, and whooping cough as targets of the country's health care system. Mary is an example of this phenomenon—she has several chronic conditions to be managed.

TREATMENT VERSUS PREVENTION

The U.S. system of health care, despite significant investments and experimentation with managed care and related wellness programs, remains largely a system designed to care for the sick. Many of the initiatives aimed at educating the public about ways it can avoid illness have met with only marginal success. Programs such as mandatory employer support of managed care benefits and Healthy People (the federal government's prevention agenda) are helping to focus attention on the objective of increased wellness. Nevertheless, individuals have been slow to embrace many of the suggested "wellness" behaviors, and programs targeting such behavioral changes are difficult to fund when dollars marked for health care are so quickly consumed by sick care.

Changing consumer behavior and community responsibilities to promote wellness, despite clear messages of the dangers of not doing so, is a slow and difficult task (Knowles, 1997). Cigarette smoking, for example, has long been recognized for its ability to cause cancer but remains a frequent behavior, despite community, state, and national efforts that apply financial and cultural pressures to stop.

In addition, compliance with positive contributors to health such as consumption of a proper diet and engaging in exercise are often seen as difficult, tedious, or simply overly mundane. The relationship between such practices and actual wellness is too unclear for many to appreciate. As a consequence, many individuals who are at risk for sedentary lifestyle diseases often experience them.

Further, while many illnesses caused by environmental factors (e.g., poor sanitation) have been eliminated or at least minimized in the United States, many of the current preventive practices responsible for reducing chronic disease are provided by health care professionals. Using diagnostic tools such as blood pressure screening, bone density testing, and prostate examinations adds costs to the health care system. However, the reduction in future costs (money that would otherwise be spent on more acute care) can often be accomplished by making an investment in preventive measures. Ideally, such an investment would come from insurers, at-risk providers, and consumers.

Unfortunately, these groups appear hesitant to make this investment in preventive care. Consumers frequently say they would be willing to pay more for a more satisfying health care system, yet reject options such as new taxes and/or higher insurance premiums to do so (Barnard, 2000). In addition, price sensitivity for health care suggests that the return would be small and too far in the future if insurers shouldered the financial burden of prevention programs. Often insurance companies do not see any of the benefits of preventive care. As people age and change jobs, their health insurance may change as well. Therefore, the insurance company that provided the preventive care may never see any cost savings from the provided service. For example, an infant vaccination burdens the parent's insurance company with the expense, while the insurance company of the middle-aged former infant reaps the benefit.

INSURANCE ISSUES

Although medical technology plays a significant role in society's ability to fight and cure disease, so, too, does having access to insurance that might cover its treatment. The United States has evolved a number of systems for ensuring patient access to health care. Although generally similar in their objectives, it is the differences between these systems that are at least partly to blame for the variations in services offered.

Most Americans have some form of private insurance (69%), either indemnity based or involving varying levels of managed care, including 69 million (23%) individuals who belong to HMOs (National Center for Health Statistics, 2005). (See **Table 4-2**.) Other individuals—chiefly, the country's elderly, disabled, or poor—have their care paid for through public funding (Medicare and Medicaid; see Chapters 20 and 21). The government maintains two somewhat separate systems for its active military and veteran groups. The remaining segments of the population are underinsured or uninsured (Lyons and Zanetti, 1999; National Center for Health Statistics, 2005).

Despite the U.S. government's heavy investment in these multiple health care systems and their widespread availability, a disproportionate number of uninsured individuals, like Mary in the chapter's case scenario, are found in the United States relative to other industrialized nations (Saver and Doescher, 2000). The large number of unemployed individuals places great pressure on publicly funded health care in this country, as do the swelling ranks of the "working poor" and the growing part-time employment base. Although the latter individuals are employed, their employers do not necessarily offer health care benefits. In the case of part-time employees, their employers are not required to offer health care coverage, so many go without insurance. If the employer provides benefits, they are sometimes not comprehensive, which leaves employees underinsured. Not considered in these figures are the 8.4 million children (11% of all children in the United States) who were uninsured in 2003 (Federal Interagency Forum on Child and Family Statistics, 2005). Interestingly, a growing segment of the uninsured are wealthier-than-average individuals, often young professionals, who perform their own cost-benefit analysis of their risk of illness or impairment and opt against buying insurance (Lyons and Zanetti, 1999).

Table 4-2 Health Insurance Statistics for U.S. Population (thousands), 2004

Private indemnity-based coverage	198,262
Employment based	174,174
Government	79,086
Medicare	39,745
Medicaid	37,514
Military	10,680
Not covered	45,820

Source: Adapted from U.S. Census Bureau (*www.census.gov/hhes/www/hlthins/historic/hihistt1.html*).
Note: The estimates of coverage are not mutually exclusive; people can be covered by more than one type of health insurance during the year.

PATIENTS AND THE HEALTH CARE ENVIRONMENT

Changing Needs of Society

Patient demands on America's health care system have been moving from a more acute model of need to one in which chronic disease services are required. Because of prior investments, the health care system is finding it painful to shift from being largely a hospital-centered structure to one that delivers community-based care. Although the demand for hospital beds is down relative to the balance of all of health care provided, when institutional care is needed, the patient is typically sicker and requires more intensive care (Johnson, Coons, Hays, and Pickard, 1999).

The movement away from hospital and sickness-based care has also been a struggle for many patients. Although 1946's Hospital Survey and Construction Act (Hill-Burton Act; see Chapters 1 and 8) provided funds for the creation of new health care facilities and promoted the concept of "a hospital for every community," changes in the way and amount that hospitals are paid are now causing fewer hospitals to be available to consumers (Stuifbergen, 1999). In addition, many patients do not fully understand the movement toward wellness and realize what is expected of them in practicing healthy behaviors, so they continue to use an increasingly wellness-based health care system for sick services.

Patients, however, are adjusting nicely to receiving care in new settings with new practitioners. Mail-order pharmacy, surgical centers, geriatric day care, and other programs have changed the way people access services they need. Through managed care restrictions and even the disappearance of traditional systems of care, a slow forced acceptance of new models has emerged (Greeno, 1999). Outpatient surgery, for example, has replaced all but the most invasive procedures provided by hospitals. Such a shift has forced patients and families to take a more active role in postsurgical recovery and care.

Access Issues

In places where economics limits the availability of health care services, patients are confronted with new challenges. Although residents in rural sections of the United States (like Mary) have geographical issues to contend with, both rural and poorer urban patients often have access to lower-quality health care relative to their wealthier urban counterparts (Stuifbergen, 1999).

This issue creates a paradox: When members of these communities seek out treatment for their illness, their care frequently is more emergent and expensive than if better access had been available in the first place (Greeno, 1999). Even when one considers the historical discrepancies in reimbursement leveling off (Ray et al., 2000), finding an appropriate set of qualified practitioners in either rural or urban settings who are willing to provide health care to the poor is very difficult. The differences between public and private health care reimbursement levels historically not only have determined the quality of care one can expect to receive, but also weigh heavily on its accessibility. For example, lower levels of payment in these communities has tended to mean health care for patients often is less readily available and of poorer quality. In the case of Mary, she delayed seeking treatment until she could no longer stand the pain. One of the reasons for her delay was that she had limited access to physicians because she lived in a rural area.

Perceptions of Managed Care

It is interesting to researchers how dissatisfied both providers and patients seem to be with the practices of managed care. Typically, market forces shape the product desired by consumers, yet managed care frequently is criticized for its failure to meet the expectations of either group (Westman and Tomlin, 1999).

A key concept behind managed care is that patients should be held responsible for practicing wellness behaviors, including not smoking, exercising regularly, and maintaining a nutritious diet (Westman and Tomlin, 1999). As part of America's public health initiative, these healthy living patterns are being promoted to help reduce the cost of treating lifestyle-related illnesses. To date, public health campaigns promoting health behaviors have resulted in small, gradual reductions in unhealthy behaviors, such as cigarette smoking (National Center for Health Statistics, 2005). Although there have been some successes, many Americans continue to exhibit unhealthy habits (despite understanding at a very early age the values of such practices) and to consume significant resources when treating the results of their behavior.

In the case of smoking, 16% of 12th graders report smoking on a daily basis (Federal Interagency Forum on Child and Family Statistics, 2005). Although members of this group recognize the dangers of smoking, they begin to smoke for a variety of reasons and eventually develop a dangerous habit. It is not until 30 to 50 years pass that the former teenagers realize the consequences of a habit obtained in their youth, when they begin to develop lung cancer, emphysema, and related cardiac diseases. These diseases are expensive to treat and consume a large amount of health care resources.

Because of the growing disconnect between lower levels of reimbursement, patient needs, and the financial risk being pushed toward health care providers, certain services are coming under heavier scrutiny within managed care organizations. To maintain quality, providers argue, they must make decisions as to which services they will offer and to whom. Patients, meanwhile, often perceive the reduction in time spent with the physician and restrictions placed on services as an unsatisfactory level of care.

Although the transition from indemnity-based insurance to managed care is usually not terribly traumatic for younger, healthier individuals, it can be difficult for older enrollees who are accustomed to the flexibility of traditional insurance based on episodes of illness. This change has been troubling for managed care organizations as well, making the costs associated with caring for individuals who logically need more frequent services difficult to leverage. As a result, many managed care companies have begun disenrolling older patients and discontinuing their products for seniors (Nelson et al., 1996).

Public Programs

Entitlement-based health care programs—specifically Medicare and Medicaid—have been slower than indemnity services to move toward physician-directed care. Unlike in the physician-as-gatekeeper systems used by managed care organizations to control utilization of services, Medicare and Medicaid patients tend to establish their own network of providers (Lyons and Zanetti, 1999), choosing their physicians and ancillary health professionals. For some, this means that health care services continue to be provided on a sickness basis. The failure to coordinate care sometimes leads to an environment in which early and proper diagnosis is unlikely to occur, perpetuating a cycle of expensive, more urgent care rather than a system characterized by patient education and management.

Although Medicare and Medicaid have been slow to change in general, there is interest in expanding "insurance" options to beneficiaries in an effort to control costs and improve the quality and coordination of care. Some states have applied to the federal government and received managed care waivers for their Medicaid programs. The use of these waivers has enabled several states to test a variety of managed care models, and it is helping to facilitate a transition from the traditional fee-for-service Medicaid to one that operates more like commercial managed care organizations (see Chapter 22).

In addition, a managed care option has been available to Medicare beneficiaries since the 1970s. In 1997, the role of private plans in Medicare was expanded by the Balanced Budget Act under Medicare + Choice (Kaiser Family Foundation, 2005). In 2003, the Medicare Prescription Drug Improvement and Modernization Act (MMA) renamed the program to Medicare Advantage. In 2005, 12% of the Medicare population was covered under the Medicare + Choice/Advantage program (Kaiser Family Foundation, 2005).

Programs for the Indigent

Many of the uninsured people in the United States are younger than 35 years of age. In 2004, for example, 40% of the uninsured were between the ages of 19 and 34 (Hoffman, Carbaugh, Moore, and Cook, 2005).

This high percentage becomes more understandable when one considers the student status, terminated or changing employment, and part-time employment often found in this age group. However, many of these individuals simply cannot afford insurance. Sixty-five percent of the U.S. families with the lowest incomes (less than 200% of federal poverty level) were uninsured in 2004 (Hoffman, Carbaugh, Moore, and Cook, 2005).

Because they lack insurance, many of these individuals do not seek proper medical care or do so only when they require urgent care. To accommodate the costs of treating these patients, states have allowed hospitals to access special funding. For example, in Massachusetts, an uncompensated care pool has been established for this purpose (Neighborhoodlaw.org, 2003). This pool of dollars is meant to shift monies from those facilities that do not provide a substantial amount of free care to those that do. Other mechanisms for treating the uninsured population include free clinics and the goodwill of practitioners.

To ensure access to medications and help patients and providers pay for pharmaceutical care when financial resources are limited, the Omnibus Reconciliation Act of 1990 (OBRA '90) mandated rebates from the drug manufacturing industry in exchange for coverage by Medicaid programs of their products. Further, to make drug therapies more affordable to agencies such as U.S. Public Health Service (USPHS) grantees and other drug-assistance programs, drug makers must discount their products or relinquish coverage of their products under Medicaid reimbursement programs for all eligible patients. Because the lack of continued access to quality drug therapy is such a critical element in the management of uninsured patients' disease, significant resources are now being applied to make such products available, including those offered by municipal, county, state, and federal government programs (outside of Medicaid), as well as by charitable organizations, private donors, and healthcare providers themselves.

Medication assistance programs (MAPs), also known as patient assistance programs, are an example of programs intended to increase lower-income patients' access to prescription medications. In these programs, patients who meet the eligibility criteria receive brand-name medications from pharmaceutical companies at no or very little cost to patients. Eligibility criteria vary across programs, but often include income limitations and lack of or limited prescription insurance coverage. Although the programs provide accessibility to medications, patients may have to complete a complex application process and may have to apply to multiple programs, depending on their medication regimens (Chisholm, Reinhardt, Vollenweider, Kendrick, and Dipiro, 2000; Chauncey, Mullins, Tran, McNally, and McEwan, 2006).

PATIENTS' EXPECTATIONS: CONSUMERISM

Health care is different from most consumer products and services offered in the marketplace. When buying a car, a consumer can go to the car dealership and test drive a car before deciding to purchase it. Of course, a patient cannot test drive surgery. Instead, patients rely on health professionals to advise them about the most appropriate procedure or decision.

Although the patient may rely on health professionals' advice on appropriate decisions, consumers are becoming increasingly more active participants in the health care process. In the past, health care professionals seemed to have all the knowledge related to health and well-being. Patients visited the physician or other health professional to obtain this information. The physician would advise, and the patient would (in theory) comply.

Today, however, a wealth of information is available. Patients can watch television and learn about medications available for various conditions. They can "surf the Web" to find resources and information on diseases, treatments, and medications. For example, Mary found information on arthritis through the Internet and learned of the use of Tylenol to treat this condition while watching television. Patients are becoming informed consumers. As a consequence, the dynamic of the relationship between health care professionals and patients is changing.

Instead of the physician telling the patient what to do, a more collaborative relationship between physician and patient is evolving. In this relationship, the patient asks questions and becomes an active participant in making health care decisions; in a sense, the health care professional and patient become partners in the care process. In some cases, the patient may actually ask the physician for a specific product or treatment for a condition based on personal research. For example, Mary went to her physician's appointment armed with specific questions about arthritis and Celebrex. (The "Models of Care" section in this chapter discusses this phenomenon in more detail.)

ACCESS TO HEALTH INFORMATION

Internet

Although the Internet is not a new invention, its household use is a recent development. Originally, the Internet was developed by U.S. academic institutions, with the U.S. defense agencies funding the start-up of this research network (Briggs and Early, 1999). In the early 1990s, it was extended so that the system could be accessible to the general public. Since then, use of the Internet has grown dramatically, with 68.7%

of U.S. households now being online (Internet World Stats, 2006). More than 20,000 Web sites focus on health and medical issues (Guadagnino, 2000), and approximately 95 million American adults use the Internet to obtain at least some health or medical information (Pew Internet and American Life Project, 2005).

With the increased accessibility to the Internet comes an increased volume of information. With one click of a mouse button, patients can obtain data on a wide variety of topics, including information about diseases, medications, and therapies. Of Internet users surveyed in a 2004 study, 63% indicated they had used the Internet to research a specific disease or medical problem. In addition, more than 50% of respondents had looked for information regarding a medical treatment or procedure. More than 51% of Internet users reported searching for information on diet and nutrition, vitamins, and nutritional supplements. Forty percent had searched for information on prescriptions and over-the-counter medications, and 30% had looked for alternative treatments or medicines (Pew Internet and American Life Project, 2005).

By using the Internet, patients like Mary can easily acquire information that is written in a layperson's terms. They can go online at any time of day or night—information is immediately available around the clock. Besides finding information, patients can identify support systems through online advocacy groups, chat rooms, and message boards (Sennett, 2000; Levy and Strombeck, 2002). Compare this ready accessibility and ease of use to the maze that must be navigated to reach many health care practitioners, and it is easy to see why patients might turn to the Internet for help.

Of course, the information presented on Web sites varies in terms of its accuracy and relevance. More than 86% of the Internet users surveyed in 2000 indicated that they were concerned about getting health information from an unreliable source. However, 52% of users who had visited health sites thought "almost all" or "most" health information retrieved from the Internet was credible (Pew Internet and American Life Project, 2000). Health professionals are, in turn, being asked by their patients about the information they obtain from online sources. With the anticipated increase in the use of the Internet as a source for health information, patients' questions to practitioners about this information will likely become more frequent. For this reason, health care practitioners should be aware of how to retrieve information from the Internet as well as how to evaluate the credibility of Web sites.

As mentioned in Chapter 3, growing concern exists about the access to prescription medications through online pharmacies or Web sites. Many Web-based pharmacies offer legitimate services and opportunities for counseling. These pharmacies may increase the access to medication for some patients, although their prices and their acceptance of insurance plans vary from site to site. Although many such Internet pharmacies are legitimate and dispense medication appropriately, others operate on the fringes of U.S. law (Bloom and Iannacone, 1999).

In the past, there have been reports of individuals obtaining medications that they should not have received (e.g., a child obtaining Viagra online). In addition, some pharmacies rely on a "snapshot" of the patient history and may be unable to detect drug–drug and drug–disease interactions, owing to the lack of pertinent patient-specific information. In fact, some patients have obtained prescription medications without a proper prescription. Some U.S. citizens have obtained prescription medications from Web sites originating from other countries; these sites do not necessarily follow U.S. regulations and laws. Over the next few years, online pharmacies will continue to be a topic of interest to patients, health care practitioners, and the government (see Chapter 3).

Direct-to-Consumer Advertising

In 1997, the Food and Drug Administration (FDA) offered new guidelines for direct-to-consumer (DTC) advertising in the form of broadcast television commercials for prescription drugs (Wilkes, Bell, and Kravitz, 2000). These guidelines allowed drug manufacturers to advertise pharmaceutical products and their indications without stating all the risks. In such a case, the advertisement had to include a statement describing where additional information can be obtained about the medication (e.g., Web sites, physicians, and pharmacists).

As a consequence of the FDA's decision, television advertisements for medications have proliferated (Wilkes et al., 2000). When watching television, a patient can learn of many different products available with or without a prescription. These commercials range from a description of a health problem/disease to an explanation of a particular brand-name product, such as Nexium or Vytorin. In addition, print advertisements may be found in magazines and newspapers. In the chapter-opening case, Mary used information from both television and print advertisements. She tried to self-treat her arthritis with the Tylenol that she learned about from a television advertisement. She learned about Celebrex from a magazine ad. What is the impact of DTC advertising on patients? Do they pay attention to what they have seen or heard from these advertisements?

In a survey conducted by *Prevention* magazine and the American Pharmacists Association (APhA) in 1997, 63% of respondents recalled seeing an advertisement for a prescription medication (*Prevention*/APhA, 1997). Almost one-fourth of these patients then asked their physician for a prescription for the medication. When this study was repeated a few years later, 85% of respondents indicated that they had seen or heard an advertisement for a prescription medication (*Prevention*, 2000–2001).

In another study, 30% of participants stated they had asked their physician about a medication they saw advertised in the past. Of those who asked about the medication, 44% stated that the physician provided the prescription discussed, indicating that about 13% of Americans have received a specific prescription medication due to a prescription advertisement (Kaiser Family Foundation, 2001).

From these surveys, it appears that pharmaceutical companies may, indeed, be influencing consumer demand for a medication. Drugs that are heavily advertised to patients are some of the best-selling medications (General Accounting Office, 2002). Many companies advertise their products in this way as part of their strategy for dealing with an increasingly competitive marketplace—that is, in an attempt to increase the demand/market share for their products (Wilkes et al., 2000). In fact, recent studies suggest that DTC advertising increases drug utilization and sales (General Accounting Office, 2002; Kaiser Family Foundation, 2003).

As with any controversial issue, both supporters and detractors of DTC advertising exist. Proponents suggest that such advertising enables consumers to become better informed by learning about new products and alternative treatment options. Critics of DTC advertising claim that this practice promotes inappropriate prescribing, strains the patient–provider relationship, increases the costs of care, and distorts the physician's professional role (Wilkes et al., 2000). Despite these concerns, it appears that DTC advertising will continue in the future and be a part of the health care dynamic.

Self-Care

Self-health care is "a range of behavior undertaken by individuals to promote or restore health" (Dean, 1989, p. 119). In other words, it consists of actions that individuals take to treat or prevent an illness. These actions can include self-medicating with nonprescription products and seeking advice from family and friends.

When individuals become ill, they go through an appraisal process of their symptoms. Is it serious? Is it getting better? Is it disruptive? Depending on the results of their assessment, patients may believe that they are sick and assume the sick role. As a part of this transformation, they begin to investigate what is occurring. They may talk to friends and family for their advice, take medication, and consult alternative health practitioners. For example, Mary talked to her friend Mrs. Johnson about arthritis. In addition, patients may assume a "wait and see" attitude or they may take action. When patients perceive the illness as serious or life-threatening are they prompted to go to the physician (Lubkin, 1990; Suchman, 1965; see Chapter 6)? In the case of Mary, she did not seek attention from the physician until she could no longer stand the pain and it became disruptive to her life.

In the last several years, pharmacies and pharmacists have played a larger role in helping patients manage their self-care. Pharmacists have implemented disease management programs for a variety of chronic diseases, including diabetes (Baran et al., 1999; Nau and Ponte, 2002), hyperlipidemia (Bluml, McKenney, and Cziraky, 2000), and hypertension (Park, Kelly, Carter, and Burgess, 1996). An example of a diabetes disease management program is the Asheville Project, in which pharmacists in Asheville, North Carolina, have been providing diabetes services since March 1997. The pharmacists in the 12 participating community pharmacies receive reimbursement for the cognitive services they provide to their patients. These services include patient education and training, clinical assessment, monitoring, follow-up, and referrals (Cranor and Christensen, 2003).

In addition, preventive and screening services are being implemented in pharmacies, both chain and independent. Vaccination programs to administer the influenza vaccine can be found in community pharmacies in several states. Similarly, many pharmacies offer diabetes, hypertension, and osteoporosis screening programs. As pharmacists become more intimately involved in patient care, learning about models of care and health behavior theory is important to improve their interactions with patients and to facilitate health behavior change.

MODELS OF CARE

Szasz and Hollender's Three Models of Care

Two physicians, Thomas Szasz and Marc Hollender (1956), described three models of physician–patient relations. These models, which are now recognized by many as the standard in the field, relate the nature of the patient's illness to the patient's capacity for meaningful dialogue and/or independent action. Each model of care is analogous to the relationship between parents and their children at different stages in their lives (infant, adolescent, and adult).

The activity–passivity model is characterized by an active practitioner and a passive patient; it is analogous to the relationship parents have with an infant child. This model of care is typically used in emergency situations, when the patient has been severely injured and is incapable of coherent communication and/or independent action (e.g., trauma, delirium, or coma). Szasz and Hollender described this form as the oldest type of practitioner–patient relationship; by definition, this model does not include much, if any, interpersonal communication. In this model, the patient is simply a recipient—the object of the practitioner's actions.

The guidance–cooperation model is used in situations in which the patient is capable of interpersonal communication and is actively involved in the relationship. Szasz and Hollender considered this form to be the most commonly used approach to care. Under this model, patients have more power of independent action than in the activity–passivity model of care, but still require professional attention and defer to medical expertise. This relationship is analogous to the relationship between parents and an adolescent child, and it typically applies to patients who are seeking help for some acute condition (e.g., infection or a broken bone).

The third model, mutual participation, applies most commonly when patients have some type of chronic disease (e.g., diabetes, heart disease, or arthritis). This model assumes that the patient and the practitioner are equally powerful and interdependent. Their mutual power comes from their relatively equal yet distinct knowledge bases: The practitioner possesses medical expertise, and the patient has personal experiences gained by living with the condition. In this way, both parties are interdependent: They share with and learn from each other to achieve an ongoing, successful treatment program. The patient and the practitioner relate to each other as two adults. For example, Mary and her physician exchanged information; her physician presented Mary with treatment options, and she made the decision as to which option she would try.

Szasz and Hollender described these three models of care as operating in a dynamic fashion, applied as the patient's situation dictates. That is, much as a parent's relationship with a child changes as the child gains independence, so, too, might a practitioner's relationship change with a patient. If a patient's condition evolves from traumatic to acute to chronic, as in an accident with enduring health effects, the practitioner's model of care would likewise evolve to accommodate these changes. Nonetheless, Szasz and Hollender acknowledged that (at least in the 1950s) the balance of power in physician–patient relations was significantly tipped toward physicians, with guidance–cooperation being the standard mode of practice, and mutual participation being least common.

As is suggested by the parent–child analogies of these models, the traditional imbalance of power has often been characterized as paternalistic (Beisecker and Beisecker, 1993; Emanuel and Emanuel, 1992; Parsons, 1951; President's Commission, 1982). However, as pointed out by Reeder (1972), societal changes beginning in the 1960s fostered a shift in this traditional imbalance, with patients becoming increasingly less deferential.

The Consumer Model of Care

Reeder suggested a consumer model of care that was eventually elaborated on by others (Haug and Lavin, 1981, 1983; Roter and Hall, 1992). The consumer model is characterized by greater patient autonomy in decision making, where the traditional authority of physicians has become increasingly challenged. As the word "consumer" suggests, patients are perceived as increasingly informed and skeptical buyers of medical care, whereas physicians are sellers who respond to the needs of the patient. In this conceptualization, the traditional emphasis on the physician's rights (to direct) and the patient's obligations (to follow) are essentially reversed to emphasize the patient/buyer's rights and the physician/seller's obligations. This dramatic shift in power has led some to criticize this model as going too far, by emphasizing conflict and mistrust while discrediting medical expertise.

As with most representations, the three Szasz and Hollender models and the consumer model reflect some significant proportion of reality—in this case, emphasizing the balance of power within the physician–patient relationship. This has been a popular topic, with the nature of the relationship being represented in various ways (see, for example, Childress and Siegler, 1984; Emanuel and Emanuel, 1992; Roter and Hall, 1992; Veatch, 1972). Some observers, however, have shifted the emphasis away from issues of power and disease as the focus of the medical encounter; instead, they consider the manner in which practitioners and patients relate to each other in terms of how they define the problem at hand.

The Patient-Centered Model of Care

The patient-centered model is often contrasted with the disease-centered perspective of patient care (Balint, Hung, Joyce, Marinker, and Woodcock, 1970; Byrne and Long, 1976; Henbest and Stewart, 1990; Levenstein et al., 1989; Mishler, 1984). In the disease-centered models, the presenting problem is understood with scientific detachment; the focus is on organic pathology and accurate diagnosis.

The patient-centered orientation shifts the focus from just the body to the person as a whole. Practitioners who adopt this model are encouraged to view the illness through the patient's eyes by considering four key elements: (1) understanding the patient's ideas about what is wrong; (2) eliciting the patient's feelings (especially fears) about the illness; (3) assessing how the problem affects the patient's daily life; and (4) discovering what expectations the patient has regarding treatment (Weston, Brown, and Stewart, 1989). With these considerations in mind, the dialogue between practitioner and patient takes on different characteristics. Instead of the traditional closed-ended, disease-centered questions, phrased to keep the patient's responses brief and focused on pathology, a patient-centered dialogue asks open-ended questions that facilitate the patient's feedback and explore the meaning of the problem from the patient's point of view.

Consider the contrast between these two models as they are depicted in the following examples. We begin with the disease-centered interview.

> **Doctor:** Hello, Pat. What seems to be the problem that's brought you here today?

Patient: I've been getting these stomach cramps lately, and I thought I ought to come and find out what's going on.

Doctor: I see. How long have you been having the cramps?

Patient: A couple of weeks.

Doctor: Have you been constipated?

Patient: Yes, I have.

Doctor: How about diarrhea?

Patient: That, too. It goes from one to the other.

Doctor: I see. How long does the diarrhea last?

Patient: About three days at a time.

Doctor: And then you get constipated?

Patient: That's right.

Doctor: What kinds of foods have you been eating?

Patient: For a while I was eating pretty much nothing except junk food, but since this has happened I've been laying off the Big Macs, and it's still no better.

Doctor: Have you tried any self-medication?

Patient: My roommate said I ought to take Pepto-Bismol, but I decided not to.

Doctor: That's good. You shouldn't take anything unless you consult first with a doctor. Are you on any medication regimen now?

Patient: No, I'm not taking anything at all.

Doctor: Yes, I see. Well, I'll have to examine you and do some tests before I can give any definite diagnosis. It's too early to tell what it could be.

Patient: What could it be? When will I know?

Doctor: As I said, I can't tell you anything significant without test results, but I should have something more definitive soon. The tests will rule out some possibilities and get me closer to an answer.

Patient: I guess I'll just have to wait.

Doctor: That's right. I'll have something for you soon. Is there anything else wrong that I can take care of now?

Patient: That's all for now. I'll be in touch with you soon, doc.

Now consider how a patient-centered interview with the same patient might go.

Doctor: Hi, Pat. How are you doing?

Patient: Pretty well. I'm on spring break now.

Doctor: Really? How much longer until you're done with classes?

Patient: Finals are in early May, and then I'll be back home again.

Doctor: That's good to hear. What can I do for you today?

Patient: I've been getting these stomach cramps lately, and I thought I ought to find out what's going on.

Doctor: Sounds tough. What about them have you noted?

Patient: Sometimes I get these real bad bouts of diarrhea, and sometimes I get constipated. I'm a real mess.

Doctor: It sounds as if you don't know whether you're coming or going. What do you think is the problem?

Patient: I'm not sure. For a while I was pretty much eating only junk food, but since this has happened I've been laying off the Big Macs, and it's still no better.

Doctor: So it hasn't made much of a difference? Is there anything else you've tried?

Patient: My roommate said I ought to take Pepto-Bismol, but I decided not to try it.

Doctor: I think you made a good decision. Are things going well at school? Have you been under a lot of stress?

Patient: This has been a hard semester, and I have been having a hard time keeping my grades up.

Doctor: Well, that might have something to do with it, but that's only one possibility. I'll have to examine you and do some tests before I can tell you anything for sure. Is there anything else on your mind?

Patient: No, that's all that's on my mind for now, but I really am concerned.

Doctor: It certainly is enough to get anyone upset, but I want you to know that these kinds of symptoms are not uncommon and, of the several possible things it could be, most are quite treatable. I hope you're not letting this ruin your life at school.

Patient: It's been tough. I run track, but this was not my idea of practicing the dash.

Doctor: I'll bet not. Well, within the next week when the tests come back, I think we'll be able to come up with a number of good suggestions. Are you comfortable with the plan of attack we've set out? Is there anything else I can do for you?

Patient: Yeah, that's all for now. I'll be in touch with you soon, doc.

If one were to assume the role of the patient while reading these brief exchanges, the first example might ring truer to most experiences with medical practitioners, whereas the second example might seem more satisfying. A review of the research strongly suggests that patients generally express greater satisfaction with their care when treated as a whole person rather than simply as a medical problem (Hall and Dornan, 1988a, 1988b).

Another form of patient-centered care also emerged from the general dissatisfaction with the traditional disease-centered model of care for terminally ill persons. That is, once cure is no longer possible, the disease-centered model ceases to serve patients' needs. Several years ago, care for the dying (such as hospice care) began to shift toward the patient-centered model. In this case, the model shifts power farther away from physicians, who serve as members of an interdisciplinary team (including nurses, social workers, chaplains, and volunteers) that provides palliative (comfort) care. Rather than physicians being in charge, patients and their families control the care provided during their remaining time together (Barton, 1977; Mesler, 1995; Torrens, 1985).

The Biopsychosocial Model of Care

Although paternalistic disease-centered models of care may still be the norm, in recent years there has been a general movement away from these perspectives and toward the consumer and patient-centered models. In this context, it seems appropriate to mention one more way of conceptualizing models of care that reflects this era of change. Similar to the perceived movement from disease-centered to patient-centered care, some observers have noted a broad shift in Western medicine away from the standard biomedical model and toward a more inclusive biopsychosocial model (Engel, 1978, 1979, 1980; Stroebe and Stroebe, 1995).

Thanks to its scientific roots in molecular biology, the standard biomedical model evolved to emphasize mind–body dualism; biochemical deviation became the sole basis of disease, and psychosocial matters were relegated to nonmedical status. Because the biomedical model served our purposes so well during eras in which the major killers were acute, infectious diseases (e.g., influenza, tuberculosis, and gastroenteritis), it became accepted as the standard model of patient care. As life expectancy began to increase and chronic diseases became the major killers (e.g., heart disease, cancer, and cerebrovascular disease), the scope of the biomedical model has been viewed as overly narrow and less satisfactory given our current needs. Today, psychosocial issues such as poverty, place of residence, environmental pollution, diet, exercise, and stress are recognized as increasingly significant variables in understanding what ails us. George Engel succinctly expressed the problem with the biomedical model:

> *The crippling flaw of the model is that it does not include the patient and his attributes as a person, a human being. Yet in the everyday work of the physician the prime object of study is a person, and many of the data*

necessary for hypothesis development and testing are gathered within the framework of an ongoing human relationship and appear in behavioral and psychological forms, namely, how the patient behaves and what he reports about himself and his life. (1978, p. 536)

The biopsychosocial model takes into account health and illness as a product of a person's physical and social context as well as his or her emotional and psychological state. Thus this model adds behavioral and other psychosocial data into the equation with biochemical processes for scientific analysis and understanding of illness. If we are to understand how individual behaviors and the meanings that people attach to their symptoms can and do affect health, we need to consider more broad-based models in treating patients.

HEALTH BEHAVIOR MODELS

Given that there appears to be a desire to move toward a more comprehensive patient care model, health care professionals should be aware of how to help patients change their health behaviors and comply with recommended therapies. The following models attempt to explain and predict health behaviors and behavior change based on a variety of factors.

Locus of Control

Locus of control has it origins in Rotter's social learning theory, which states "the potential for a behavior to occur in a given situation is a function of expectancies that the behavior will lead to a particular outcome and the extent to which an outcome is valued" (AbuSabha and Achterberg, 1997, p. 1125). Although it may sound similar to some of the models discussed later in this chapter, locus of control specifically refers to whether an individual feels that attainment of a particular outcome is within his or her control or outside of it. If we think that health outcomes are within our control, we are considered to have an internal locus of control. In other words, we think that what we do (or do not do) determines the outcome of our health. If we think that outcomes are outside of our control, we are said to have an external locus of control. In other words, we believe that forces outside of our control determine health outcomes.

External locus of control can be further divided into two categories: (1) powerful others and (2) chance (AbuSabha and Achterberg, 1997; Levenson, 1974; Wallston, Wallston, and Devellis, 1978). Individuals who believe that other people, such as health care professionals and family members, determine health outcomes are said to have a powerful others orientation. Those with a chance orientation believe that their health outcomes and other events are attributable to fate or chance.

Health Belief Model

The Health Belief Model is used to understand the successes and failures of health behavior change. Rosenstock and colleagues initially developed this model to explain why people practice preventive behavior, but it has since been used to explain such behaviors as compliance with drug therapy and other disease management practices (Clark and Becker, 1998; Rosenstock, 1974; Salazar, 1991).

This model focuses on the likelihood that an individual will take action or change his or her behavior. According to this model, the perceived susceptibility and severity of the disease determine the perceived threat of the disease to the individual and contribute to the likelihood of changing behavior. Susceptibility is an individual's perception of his or her risk for contracting the disease; severity is the seriousness of a disease if left untreated (Clark and Becker, 1998; Salazar, 1991).

In addition to susceptibility and severity, the perceived benefits and barriers contribute to the likelihood of taking action. Benefits are the individual's beliefs that changing the behavior will reduce the disease threat. These are weighed against the barriers to change or the negative aspects (e.g., money, effort) of such a change in behavior, which act as deterrents to behavior change. If an individual believes that he or she has a high susceptibility to a severe/serious disease, the perceived threat is high enough so he or she may see the benefits of changing behavior (Clark and Becker, 1998; Salazar, 1991). Conversely, if the susceptibility and/or severity of the disease is low, the perceived threat is low and, therefore, the behavior change may not be perceived as providing sufficient benefits. In this case, the person is unlikely to change the behavior.

Demographic (age, gender, ethnicity), sociopsychological (personality, social class, peer and reference group pressure), and structural variables (knowledge about the disease, prior contact to the disease) may influence how someone perceives the susceptibility, seriousness, and threat of the disease. In addition, cues to action can influence how an individual perceives the threat of disease. These cues might include mass media campaigns, advice from others, reminder postcards from a physician, illness of a family member or friend, or a newspaper or magazine article (Clark and Becker, 1998; Salazar, 1991).

Finally, self-efficacy may play a role in the health belief model. In brief, self-efficacy or efficacy expectation pertains to a person's confidence in his or her ability to take action or change a behavior. In other words, an individual must feel competent to overcome the barriers to positive behavior change (Strecher and Rosenstock, 1997). Self-efficacy is described in more detail in the "Social Cognitive Theory" section later in this chapter.

According to the Health Belief Model, for an obese person to lose weight, the individual would need to believe that he or she is susceptible to the negative effects of obesity as well as the possibility of severe effects from the disease. For example, for a behavior change to occur, the person needs to believe that he or she is more susceptible to suffering a cardio-vascular event because of being overweight. In addition, the individual needs to believe that the cardiovascular event is serious to perceive a threat from developing the disease. The patient may see the benefits of enrolling in a weight reduction program, but if the barriers are greater than the benefits, he or she still may not take action. In addition, modifying factors, such as social support or cues to action (e.g., an obese family member having a heart attack) may influence the likelihood that the individual will actively try to lose weight. Besides the modifying factors, the person must believe in his or her ability to overcome the barriers to losing weight (self-efficacy) before the patient will attempt the weight loss regimen.

Social Cognitive Theory

Social Cognitive Theory, like the other theories/models discussed in this chapter, was developed to help predict behavior. Bandura identified two types of expectations that influence behavior: (1) outcome expectations and (2) efficacy expectations (Bandura, 1977). Outcome expectations are the individual's expectation or belief that a particular behavior will result in a particular outcome. For example, a person may believe that exercise can help him lose weight. Efficacy expectations are the individual's expectations that he or she has the ability to accomplish this behavior, such as participating in an exercise routine to lose weight.

According to Social Cognitive Theory, the key lies in the individual's perceptions of the outcomes and efficacy in performing these behaviors—not his or her true capabilities (Clark and Becker, 1998). That is, a person might begin an exercise program to lose weight because she believes that exercise will result in a weight loss and that she can perform this activity. In addition, expectations are specific for particular behaviors (AbuSabha and Achterberg, 1997; Clark and Becker, 1998). In other words, just because a person believes that that he can undertake an exercise program, it does not mean that he believes that he can decrease his caloric intake or diet. His outcome and efficacy expectations may be different for a diet as compared to an exercise program.

Efficacy expectations are learned through four mechanisms: (1) performance accomplishments, (2) vicarious experience, (3) verbal persuasion, and (4) physiological state (Bandura, 1977, 1986; Clark and Becker, 1998). Performance accomplishments refer to an individual's attempt at a particular behavior that is perceived to be difficult. The experience of success in accomplishing this difficult behavior increases self-efficacy. For example, if a person fears going on a diet, yet attempts to make this lifestyle change and experiences success, then her self-efficacy will improve.

Vicarious experiences refer to the modeling of behaviors by others and the individual observing such behaviors. To improve self-efficacy, it must be seen that the model achieved success through overcoming difficulties (as compared to being easy) and the model must be similar in characteristics (gender, age) to the observer. Perhaps a friend is successful in achieving weight loss by dieting. By observing his friend's weight loss and the difficulties in succeeding in this task, a person may feel more capable of attempting this same change.

Verbal persuasion encourages the individual to continue to make attempts in behavior changes, such as a pharmacist encouraging a patient to continue or advising him or her to attempt an exercise regimen or diet. The final mechanism that influences efficacy expectations pertains to the physiological state of the individual. High physiological arousal, such as tension and agitation, increases the likelihood of failure. For instance, a person who feels fatigued or experiences pain after exercising may believe that he cannot accomplish the behavior.

Theory of Reasoned Action and the Theory of Planned Behavior

According to the Theory of Reasoned Action (TRA), a determinant of a person's behavior is one's behavioral intention, or the likelihood of performing the behavior. Two factors are hypothesized to lead to an individual's behavioral intention: (1) the attitude toward performing the behavior and (2) the subjective norm associated with the behavior.

With the first factor, the likelihood of performing a behavior is influenced by the person's beliefs about the behavior and the outcome(s) associated with it. The value associated with the outcome—whether positive or negative—is another important component of one's attitude toward the behavior (Clark and Becker, 1998; Madden, Ellen, and Ajzen, 1992; Montano, Kasprzyk, and Taplin, 1997). For example, an individual who believes that losing weight is associated with positive outcomes will have a positive attitude toward the behavior change needed to lose weight.

The second factor, subjective norm, refers to what other "important" individuals think about the person's behavior change or of his or her desire to perform the behavior. In other words, do others approve or disapprove of the performance of the specific behavior? As part of this evaluation of others' beliefs, the individual also is affected by his or her desire or motivation to comply with others' wishes (Clark and Becker, 1998; Madden et al., 1992; Montano et al., 1997). For example, if an individual believes that others want him to lose weight and is motivated by these beliefs or expectations, he has a positive subjective norm. Both positive attitudes and a positive subject norm will increase the likelihood of performing the behavior or carrying through on the behavioral intention.

TRA fails to address the issue of the person's degree of control over the behavior. Control refers to factors, both personal and external, that influence the behavior such as a workable plan, skills, knowledge, time, money, willpower, and opportunity. However, the degree of control or factors could influence both behavioral intention and the performance of a behavior. The Theory of Planned Behavior (TPB) is an extension of TRA in which perceived behavioral control is added to the TRA model to address those cases in which a person does not have a high degree of control over the behavior (Clark and Becker, 1998; Madden et al., 1992; Montano et al., 1997).

Perceived behavioral control is determined by control beliefs, which refers to the presence or absence of resources for and the barriers to the performance of the behavior. In addition, the perceived power of each resource and barrier to promote or deter behavior is considered. For example, if an individual has a strong belief about the existence of resources to encourage the behavior, then she has a high perceived control over the behavior. By contrast, if an individual believes that factors can deter her from performing the behavior, such as the lack of time to exercise, the person is said to have low perceived control and is less likely to perform the behavior (Clark and Becker, 1998; Madden et al., 1992; Montano et al., 1997).

Transtheoretical Model of Change

The Transtheoretical Model of Change was developed by Prochaska in the 1970s and 1980s to determine why the attempts to change behavior failed or succeeded. Commonly referred to as the readiness to change model, it theorizes that a patient progresses through five stages before a change in behavior, such as quitting smoking or losing weight, occurs. These stages are (1) precontemplation, (2) contemplation, (3) preparation, (4) action, and (5) maintenance (Berger, 1997; Prochaska and Velicer, 1997).

Patients in the precontemplation stage have not thought of changing a specific behavior, and such a change is not expected to occur in the foreseeable future (the next 6 months). Patients are in the precontemplation stage for a variety of reasons, including being uninformed or underinformed about the outcomes of their behaviors and being discouraged about their ability to change because of past failures. In addition, this category includes individuals who are unwilling to change their behaviors. Individuals in this stage of change avoid talking, reading, or thinking about the needed behavior change. Often they are perceived as unmotivated and as unprepared for action-oriented intervention programs (Berger, 1997; Prochaska and Velicer, 1997).

Unlike individuals in the precontemplation stage, patients entering the contemplation are beginning to consider a change in their behavior and intend to make that change within the next 6 months. These individuals recognize the benefits of changing, but also realize the costs or negative aspects of behavior change. For this reason, patients may become stuck in this stage because of their ambivalence about the benefits versus the costs of change. In other words, they have no plan for action and are not entirely ready to commit to a change (Berger, 1997; Prochaska and Velicer, 1997).

In the preparation stage, patients plan to take action, usually within the next month. In many cases, they have already taken some small steps toward action within the past year and are ready to make a change. These individuals are prepared to engage in an action-oriented intervention, such as a smoking cessation program (Berger, 1997; Prochaska and Velicer, 1997).

Patients in the action stage are in the process of changing their behavior and have taken specific steps to do so over the past 6 months (Berger, 1997; Prochaska and Velicer, 1997). In the maintenance stage, individuals do not use change processes as frequently as in the action stage. Instead, they focus on triggers (e.g., environment, friends, and family) that may make them susceptible to their old habits. The goal during this stage is to prevent relapse into the old behavior. People in this stage need help to control or become aware of these triggers for relapse. Despite the temptation, patients are more confident that they will not return to their old behaviors. The maintenance stage can last anywhere from 6 months to 5 years (Berger, 1997; Prochaska and Velicer, 1997).

According to the Transtheoretical Model of Change, interventions to change patient behavior should be specific to the patient stage. If someone is overweight and in the precontemplation stage, the desired intervention should be promoting awareness rather than enrolling him or her in a weight reduction plan, such as Weight Watchers. The weight reduction plan will not be successful for this individual because he or she has no intention to change at this point. By comparison, a person in the preparation stage is ready to make a change and has already taken small steps toward weight reduction. He or she is more likely to be successful in a weight reduction program.

Besides focusing on appropriate interventions based on the patient's stage, the health care professional should facilitate movement through this model. For example, if someone is in the precontemplation stage, the pharmacist should use interventions and techniques geared toward moving the patient into the contemplation stage. These interventions and techniques, which are called processes of change (**Table 4-3**), can be used to help patients move toward the action and maintenance stages of change.

Table 4-3   Processes of Change

Process of Change	Definition	Example	Stage Emphasized
Conscious raising	Increasing awareness about the causes, consequences, and cures for a problem behavior or diseases	Education, pamphlets, media campaigns	Precontemplation Contemplation
Dramatic relief	Arousing an emotional response with a subsequent reduced effect if action can be taken	Personal testimonies, media campaigns, role-playing	Precontemplation Contemplation
Self-reevalution	Assessing one's self-image with and without unhealthy habit	Smoker assessing what it would be like to be a non-smoker	Contemplation
Environmental reevaluation	Assessing how a behavior impacts the social environment	Smoker assessing how his or her smoking impacts spouse, children, etc.	Precontemplation Contemplation
Self-liberation	Believing that one can change and committing to the change	New Year's resolution or telling others of changes	Preparation
Counterconditioning	Substituting healthier behaviors for unhealthy ones	Nicotine replacement, fat-free foods	Action Maintenance
Stimulus control	Removing cues for unhealthy behaviors and adding prompts for healthy behaviors	Removing high-fat foods from home, keeping exercise equipment in car for easy access	Action Maintenance
Contingency management	Using rewards to encourage behavior change	Praise, group recognition, purchase of new clothes after weight loss	Action Maintenance
Helping relationships	Receiving and using support from others	Buddy systems for exercise, weight loss, family involvement in change	Action Maintenance

Source: From *The Handbook of Health Behavior Change,* 2e, S.A. Schumaker, E.B. Schron, J.K. Ockene, and W.L. McBee (eds.), 1998. Reproduced with the permission of Springer Publishing Company, LLC, New York, 10036.

CONCLUSIONS

Patient care is currently undergoing a transition toward increased collaboration between health care professionals and patients. Given the increasing knowledge patients have about their health, providers will need to take a different approach to care other than telling the patient what to do and expecting unquestioning compliance. Of course, not all patients are alike. They have their own unique issues and characteristics that affect their interactions with health care professionals as well as determine their impact on the health care system and the health care system's impact on them.

As the health care system continues to try to change patient health behaviors, the models described in this chapter provide a basis for the development of effective interventions. Through the questioning of patients, health care practitioners can determine patients' beliefs regarding the numerous factors that influence their behaviors. By using these models, practitioners can use the information gained from patients to target specific behaviors with specific interventions.

QUESTIONS FOR FURTHER DISCUSSION

1. Would you suggest other models of care, or variations on the models discussed in this chapter, based on a pharmacist–patient interaction rather than a physician–patient interaction?
2. How do your personal experiences relate to the health behavior models discussed in this chapter?
3. Do pharmacists need to make changes in the various practice settings to improve delivery of health care to patients? Why or why not?

KEY TOPICS AND TERMS

Health insurance
Preventive health
Health information
Health behavior models
Models of patient care

REFERENCES

AbuSabha, R., & Achterberg, C. (1997). Review of self-efficacy and locus of control for nutrition and health-related behavior. *Journal of the American Dietetic Association, 97*(10), 1122–1133.

Arias, E. (2006). United States life tables, 2003. *National Vital Statistics Reports, 54*(14), 1–6.

Balint, M., Hung, J., Joyce, D., Marinker, M., & Woodcock, J. (1970). *Treatment of diagnosis: A study of repeat prescription in general practice.* Toronto, Ontario: J. B. Lippincott.

Bandura, A. (1977). Self-efficacy: Toward a unifying theory of behavioral change. *Psychological Review, 84,* 191–215.

Bandura, A. (1986). *Social foundations of thought and action.* Englewood Cliffs, NJ: Prentice-Hall.

Baran, R. W., Crumlish, K., Patterson, H., Shaw, J., Erwin, W. G., Wylie, J. D., & Duong, P. (1999). Improving outcomes of community-dwelling older patients with diabetes through pharmacist counseling. *American Journal of Health-System Pharmacists, 56,* 1535–1539.

Barnard, A. (2000, August 26). Clinics market scans for the symptom-free. *Boston Globe,* pp. A1, A10.

Barton, D. (Ed.). (1977). *Dying and death: A clinical guide for caregivers.* Baltimore: Williams and Wilkins.

Beisecker, A. E., & Beisecker, T. D. (1993). Using metaphors to characterize doctor–patient relationships: Paternalism versus consumerism. *Health Communications, 5,* 41–58.

Berger, B. A. (1997). *Readiness for change: Improving treatment adherence.* Durham, NC: Glaxo, Inc., and Clean Data.

Bloom, B. S., & Iannacone, R. C. (1999). Internet availability of prescription pharmaceuticals to the public. *Annals of Internal Medicine, 131,* 830–833.

Bluml, B. M., McKenney, J. M., & Cziraky, M. J. (2000). Pharmaceutical care services and results in Project ImPACT: Hyperlipidemia. *Journal of the American Pharmaceutical Association, 40,* 157–165.

Boult, C., & Pacala, J. (1999). Integrating healthcare for older populations. *American Journal of Managed Care, 5*(1), 45–52.

Briggs, J. S., & Early, G. H. (1999). Internet developments and their significance for healthcare. *Medical Informatics, 24*(3), 149–164.

Byrne, P. S., & Long, B. E. L. (1976). *Doctors talking to patients.* London: Royal College of General Practitioners.

Chauncey, D., Mullins, C. D., Tran, B. V., McNally, D., & McEwan, R. N. (2006). Medication access through patient assistance programs. *American Journal of Health-System Pharmacy, 63*(13), 1254–1259.

Childress, J. F., & Siegler, M. (1984). Metaphors and models of doctor–patient relationships: Their implications for autonomy. *Theoretical Medicine, 5,* 17–30.

Chisholm, M. A., Reinhardt, B. O., Vollenweider, L. J., Kendrick, B. D., & Dipiro, J. T. (2000). Medication assistance reports medication assistance programs for uninsured and indigent patients. *American Journal of Health-System Pharmacy, 57*(12), 1131–1136.

Clark, N. M., & Becker, M. H. (1998). Theoretical models and strategies for improving adherence and disease management. In S. A. Shumaker, E. B. Schron, J. K. Ockene, & W. L. McBee (Eds.), *The handbook of health behavior change* (2nd ed.) (pp. 5–32). New York: Springer.

Cranor, C. W., & Christensen, D. B. (2003). The Asheville Project: Short-term outcomes of a community diabetes care program. *Journal of the American Pharmacists Association, 43*(2), 149–159.

Dean, K. (1989). Conceptual, theoretical, and methodological issues in self-care research. *Social Science and Medicine, 29*(2), 117–123.

Emanuel, E. J., & Emanuel, L. L. (1992). Four models of the physician–patient relationship. *Journal of the American Medical Association, 267,* 2221–2226.

Engel, G. L. (1978). The biopsychosocial model and the education of health professionals. *Annals of the New York Academy of Sciences, 310,* 169–181.

Engel, G. L. (1979). The need for a new medical model: A challenge for biomedicine. *Science, 196,* 129–136.

Engel, G. L. (1980). The clinical application of the biopsychosocial model. *American Journal of Psychiatry, 137,* 535–544.

Federal Interagency Forum on Child and Family Statistics. (2005). *America's children: Key national indicators of well-being, 2005.* Washington, DC: U.S. Government Printing Office.

General Accounting Office. (2002, October) *FDA oversight of direct-to-consumer advertising has limitations.* Retrieved July, 2006 from http://www.gao.gov/new.items/d03177.pdf

Greeno, R. (1999). Perspectives on the evolving hospitalist model. *Managed Care Interface, 12*(4), 80–84.

Guadagnino, C. (2000, July). Using medical information on the Internet. *Physician News Digest.* Retrieved July, 2006 from http://www.physiciansnews.com/spotlight/700.html

Hall, J. A., & Dornan, M. C. (1988a). Meta-analysis of satisfaction with medical care: Description of research done in and analysis of overall satisfaction. *Social Science and Medicine, 26,* 637–644.

Hall, J. A., & Dornan, M. C. (1988b). What patients like about their medical care and how often they are asked: A meta-analysis of the satisfaction literature. *Social Science and Medicine, 27,* 935–939.

Haug, M. R., & Lavin, B. (1981). Practitioner or patient—Who's in charge? *Journal of Health and Social Behavior, 22,* 212–229.

Haug, M. R., & Lavin, B. (1983). *Consumerism in medicine: Challenging physician authority.* Beverly Hills, CA: Sage.

Henbest, R. J., & Stewart, M. (1990). Patient-centeredness in the consultation, 2: Does it really make a difference? *Family Practice, 7,* 28–33.

Hoffman, C., Carbaugh, A., Moore, H., & Cook, A. (2005). *Health insurance coverage in America: 2004 data update.* Washington, DC: Kaiser Commission on Medicaid and the Uninsured.

Internet World Stats. (2006). *American Internet usage and population statistics.* Retrieved July, 2006 from http://www.internetworldstats.com/stats2.htm

Johnson, J., Coons, S., Hays, R., & Pickard, A. (1999). Health status and satisfaction with pharmacy services. *American Journal of Managed Care, 5*(2), 163–170.

Kaiser Family Foundation. (2001, November). *Understanding the effects of direct-to-consumer prescription drug advertising.* Washington, DC: Kaiser Family Foundation.

Kaiser Family Foundation. (2003, June). *Impact of direct-to-consumer advertising on prescription drug spending.* Washington, DC: Kaiser Family Foundation

Kaiser Family Foundation. (2005, September). *Medicare: Medicare advantage fact sheet.* Washington, DC: Kaiser Family Foundation.

Knowles, J. H. (1997). *Doing better and feeling worse: Health in the United States.* New York: Norton Press.

Leavitt, J. W., & Numbers, R. L. (1997). Sickness and health: An overview. In J. W. Leavitt & R. L. Numbers (Eds.), *Sickness and health in America: Readings in the history of medicine and public health* (3rd ed.) (pp. 3–10). Madison, WI: University of Wisconsin Press.

Levenson, H. (1974). Activism and powerful others: Distinctions within the concept of internal-external control. *Journal of Personality Assessment, 38,* 377–383.

Levenstein, J. H., et al. (1989). Patient-centered clinical interviewing. In M. Stewart & D. Roter (Eds.), *Communicating with medical patients* (pp. 107–120). Beverly Hills, CA: Sage.

Levy, J. A., & Strombeck, R. (2002). Health benefits and risks of the Internet. *Journal of Medical Systems, 26*(6), 495–510.

Lubkin, I. M. (1990). *Chronic illness: Impact and interventions* (2nd ed.). Sudbury, MA: Jones and Bartlett.

Lyons, W., & Zanetti, L. (1999, March/April). The uninsured in the context of an experimental approach to health care reform. *American Journal of Health Behavior, 23*(2), 83–94.

Madden, T. J., Ellen, P. S., & Ajzen, I. (1992). A comparison of the theory of planned behavior and the theory of reasoned action. *Personality and Social Psychology Bulletin, 18*(1), 3–9.

Mesler, M. A. (1995). Negotiating life for the dying: Hospice and the strategy of tactical socialization. *Death Studies, 19,* 235–255.

Mishler, E. G. (1984). *The discourse of medicine: Dialectics of medical interviews.* Norwood, NJ: Ablex.

Montano, D. E., Kasprzyk, D., & Taplin, S. H. (1997). The theory of reasoned action and the theory of planned behavior. In K. Glanz, F. M. Lewis, and B. K. Rimer (Eds.), *Health behavior and health education* (pp. 85–112). San Francisco: Jossey-Bass.

National Center for Health Statistics. (2004). *NCHS data on aging.* Hyattsville, MD: National Center for Health Statistics.

National Center for Health Statistics. (2005). *Health, United States, 2005 with chartbook on trends in the health of Americans.* Hyattsville, MD: National Center for Health Statistics.

Nau, D. P., & Ponte, C. D. (2002). Effects of a community pharmacist-based diabetes patient-management program on intermediate clinical outcome measures. *Journal of Managed Care Pharmacy, 8*(1), 48–53.

Neighborhoodlaw.org. (2003). Nelson, L., Gold, M., Brown, R., et al. (1996). Access to care in Medicare managed care: Results from a 1996 survey of enrollees and disenrollees. *Physician Payment Review Commission Selected External Research Series #7.* Washington, DC: Physician Payment Review Commission.

Nelson, L., Gold, M., Brown, R., et al. (1996). *Access to care in Medicare managed care: Results from a 1996 survey of enrollees and disenrollees. Physician Payment Review Commission Selected External Research Series #7.* Washington, DC: Physician Payment Review Commission.

Park, J. J., Kelly, P., Carter, B. L., & Burgess, P. P. (1996). Comprehensive pharmaceutical care in the chain setting. *Journal of the American Pharmaceutical Association, NS36*(7), 443–451.

Parsons, T. (1951). *The social system.* Glencoe, IL: Free Press.

Pew Internet and American Life Project. (2000, November). *The online health revolution helps Americans take better care of themselves. Summary of findings: Influence on "health seekers."* Retrieved July, 2006 from http://www.pewinternet.org/reports/toc.asp?Report=26

Pew Internet and American Life Project. (2005, May). *Health information online.* Retrieved July, 2006 from http://207.21.232.103/pdfs/PIP_Healthtopics_May05.pdf

President's Commission for the Study of Ethical Problems in Medicine and Biomedical and Behavioral Research. (1982). *Making health care decisions: The ethical and legal implications of informed consent in the patient–practitioner relationship* (Vol. 1). Washington, DC: U. S. Government Printing Office.

Prevention/American Pharmaceutical Association (APhA). (1997). *Navigating the medication marketplace: How consumers choose.* Washington, DC: *Prevention*/APhA.

Prevention Magazine. (2000–2001). *International survey on wellness and consumer reaction to DTC advertising of prescription drugs.* (report, 2000/2001).

Prochaska, J. O., Johnson, S., & Lee, P. (1998). The transtheoretical model of change. In S. A. Schumaker, E. B. Schron, J. K. Ockene, and W. L. McBee (Eds.), *The handbook of health behavior change* (2nd ed.). New York: Springer (p. 59-84).

Prochaska, J. O., & Velicer, W. F. (1997). The transtheoretical model of health behavior change. *American Journal of Health Promotion, 12*(1), 38–48.

Ray, G., Lieu, T., Weinick, R., Cohen, J., Fireman, B., & Newacheck, P. (2000). Comparing the medical expenses of children with Medicaid and commercial insurance in an HMO. *American Journal of Managed Care, 6*(7), 753–760.

Reeder, L. G. (1972). The patient-client as a consumer: Some observations on the changing professional–client relationship. *Journal of Health and Social Behavior, 13,* 406–412.

Rosenstock, I. M. (1974). Historical origins of the health belief model. *Health Education Monographs, 2,* 328–335.

Roter, D. L., & Hall, J. A. (1992). *Doctors talking with patients—Patients talking with doctors.* Westport, CT: Auburn House.

Salazar, M. K. (1991). Comparison of four behavioral theories: A literature review. *AAOHN Journal, 39*(3), 128–135.

Saver, B., & Doescher, M. (2000). To buy or not to buy: Factors associated with the purchase of nongroup, private health insurance. *Medical Care, 38*(2), 141–151.

Sennett, C. (2000). Ambulatory care in the new millennium: The role of consumer information. *Quality Management in Health Care, 8*(2), 82–87.

Strecher, V. J., & Rosenstock, I. M. (1997). The health belief model. In K. Glanz, F. M. Lewis, & B. K. Rimer (Eds.), *Health behavior and health education* (pp. 41–59). San Francisco: Jossey-Bass.

Stroebe, W., & Stroebe, M. S. (1995). *Social psychology and health.* Pacific Grove, CA: Brooks/Cole.

Stuifbergen, A. (1999). Barriers and health behaviors of rural and urban persons with multiple sclerosis. *American Journal of Health Behavior, 23*(6), 415–425.

Suchman, E. A. (1965). Stages of illness and medical care. *Journal of Health and Human Behavior, 6,* 114–128.

Szasz, T., & Hollender, M. (1956). A contribution to the philosophy of medicine: The basic model of the doctor-patient relationship. *Archives of Internal Medicine, 97,* 585–592.

Tebbe, J. (1998). Health care delivery in America: Historical and policy perspectives. In R. L. McCarthy (Ed.), *Introduction to health care delivery: A primer for pharmacists* (p. 18). Gaithersburg, MD: Aspen.

Torrens, P. R. (1985). Development of special care programs for the dying: A brief history. In P. R. Torrens (Ed.), *Hospice programs and public policy* (pp. 3–29). Chicago, IL: American Hospital Publishing.

United States Bureau of the Census (USBOC). (2000). Retrieved August, 2000 from www.census.gov/population/estimates/nation/intfile2-1.txt

Veatch, R. M. (1972). Models for ethical medicine in a revolutionary age. *Hastings Center Report, 2,* 5–7.

Wallston, K. A., Wallston, B. S., and Devellis, R. (1978). Development of the multidimensional health locus of control (MHLC) scales. *Health Education Monographs, 6,* 160–170.

Westman, E. C., & Tomlin, K. F. (1999, March/April). Implementing a Patients' Bill of Rights with the personal health organizer. *American Journal of Health Behavior, 23*(2), 128–133.

Weston, W. W., Brown, J. B., & Stewart, M. (1989). Patient-centered interviewing.,Part I: Understanding patients' experiences. *Canadian Family Physician, 35,* 147–151.

Wilkes, M. S., Bell, R. A., & Kravitz, R. L. (2000). Direct-to-consumer prescription drug advertising: Trends, impact, and implications. *Health Affairs, 19*(2), 110–128.

Drug Use, Access, the Pharmaceutical Industry, and Supply Chain in the United States

Peter L. Steere, Michael Montagne, and Dana P. Hammer

Case Scenario

During a strategic planning meeting, Beeker Pharmaceutical's senior management reflected on the early success of its decision to limit the channel of distribution for its cystic fibrosis medication. The drug, Aperaire, is a self-administered injectable product discovered 8 years ago using molecular modeling technologies; it represents the first commercial use of this development method by the company.

Beeker found that the more specific modeling format for therapy development enabled the company to move faster through early testing stages than did the somewhat dated trial-and-error mode of discovery. The company concluded that the accelerated drug identification and patent registration period would allow additional time for Aperaire to gain market share while remaining free of generic competition.

In gaining U.S. Food and Drug Administration (FDA) approval, however, Beeker had to ensure that patients using Aperaire would have access to laboratory monitoring services due to the product's adverse affects on the liver in a minority of cases, as well as to self-injection training and education by capable health care professionals. Furthermore, the FDA was concerned about storage of the product, as the chemical was sensitive to degradation under warmer conditions.

Pricing considerations aside, Beeker faced the risk that the FDA might not approve Aperaire for marketing unless the company could ensure complete compliance with the agency's safety requirements.

Most commonly, pharmaceuticals are distributed through drug wholesalers, which serve as "middlemen" between the manufacturers and the hospitals, drugstores, and clinics that purchase those manufacturers' drugs. Beeker sold nearly all of its other products through this well-developed process but worried about its suitability for Aperaire, given the drug's education, storage, and safety limitations. As the company considered its alternatives, it realized that most of its customers were patients seen at comparatively few, but highly specific, medical clinics. What's more, these patients were reasonably well networked through support groups and national associations and, because of their multiple prescription needs, sought services from a small group of highly qualified pharmacy providers.

Two pharmacies in particular—MedsAtHome and ChroniWellness—served large segments of the cystic fibrosis market, mostly through mail-order mechanisms.

Because the population of patients was small but the number of potential retailers very large, Beeker thought a more restrictive distribution channel would allow access while enabling the company to adhere to all quality and safety standards. Accordingly, it developed a three-step plan for making Aperaire available in the marketplace.

First, Beeker would establish a relationship with the two mail-order pharmacies that were currently serving the needs of large groups of patients with cystic fibrosis. The company would ensure that the pharmacies had access to third-party contracts that would allow most—if not all—needy patients to receive Aperaire under a prescription benefit plan. By choosing only two vendors, the company would reduce the risk of improper storage that was inherent when many wholesaler warehouses inventoried the medication. By selling directly to the contracted vendors, Beeker would also be able to substantially reduce its distribution costs and to better control production as a result of a closely managed sales plan. In addition, this early-stage distribution plan would consolidate the number of pharmacists who would be providing detailed drug education services to patients and make training of the pharmacists a far more efficient process than blanketing the nation's drugstores with corporate educators.

The second stage of Beeker's plan to distribute Aperaire was intended to ensure that patients who wanted to receive their maintenance doses from a different or more local pharmacy could do so. The two original contract pharmacies, MedsAtHome and ChroniWellness, would be required to identify wholesaler organizations that would distribute the drug to local pharmacies at patients' requests. By developing this phase of channel distribution, Beeker would avoid the added costs of shipping to multiple wholesalers, yet would be able to maintain a national infrastructure that could accommodate most patients whose needs might best be met by local providers.

The third stage of channel development would be to open up the wholesaler component of drug delivery and allow pharmacy access in a more traditional way, once the product was in later stages of marketing and its safety and storage needs were more universally understood.

The early results of the team's decision to develop this novel delivery system appeared promising. The contract pharmacies were doing a very good job of making sure that all requirements were met, including comprehensive patient education and coverage by third-party insurance carriers. More important, however, was the report of strong satisfaction from the prescriber and patient communities regarding the ease of use and effectiveness of Aperaire.

LEARNING OBJECTIVES

Upon completion of this chapter, the student shall be able to:

- Discuss the various attitudes and expectations consumers have toward the use of pharmaceutical products
- Describe the four stages or steps in the U.S. drug approval process
- Describe the four phases of clinical testing of a new drug product
- Explain the various methods used by manufacturers to market their products
- Discuss significant factors that contribute to the growth in cost and use of pharmaceuticals in the United States
- Describe major steps in the pathway medications take from the manufacturer, through various distribution channels, to the consumer
- Discuss alternative channels of distribution and vulnerabilities of the system

CHAPTER QUESTIONS

1. What different types of drug-taking behavior do consumers exhibit, and which type is dominant in American society?
2. What important social factors influence drug development and drug use in American society?
3. How has the pharmaceutical industry changed the ways in which it discovers, manufactures, and markets its new products?
4. What changes in the pharmacy profession are redefining the role of the pharmacist in drug use and patient care?

INTRODUCTION

The U.S. pharmaceutical market provides some of industry's most interesting examples of supply, demand, and pricing strategy and demonstrates the importance of the search for an appropriate balance in health care policy development. It is, by almost any standard, an industry with a history marked by great success, entrepreneurial growth, and important advances in the fight against and prevention of disease. It is also an industry that has come under fire, at least from certain segments of the public, because of the cost of its products, the large profits generated, and the methods by which it promotes its products. Much of this criticism stems from the nature of the industry itself: Most health care providers offer goods and services on the basis of a somewhat altruistic motivation in helping patients, whereas the pharmaceutical industry operates in a significantly more business-like model.

This is not to suggest that drug makers are insensitive to the needs of individuals with cancers or infections or any other syndrome or illness. They must balance these needs with the risks and costs involved in drug discovery, including, the time, expense, and process of testing; the regulations of the drug approval process; and the sale and marketing of products in a complex health care and payment system.

Chronic diseases that affect large populations, such as hypertension, diabetes, and hyperlipidemia, are of interest to drug manufacturers due to the potential rewards available from a product's success. Markets for pharmaceuticals that treat less common diseases are more difficult to predict, so companies are careful in proceeding with such products so as to minimize their business risk.

The Beeker example suggests that the company's strategy of developing products for a needy population while minimizing its risk was to modify how it distributed Aperaire. Limited distribution affects consumers, the manufacturer, the pharmacy supply chain, health policy, and other components of the medication distribution channel. It also could affect how patients perceive, select, and use the drug.

A discussion about drug distribution and use must include not only the makers of medications but also the methods by which these products are accessed and the attitudes of these consumers. This chapter explores some of these issues, including how perceptions of drugs influence demand, how drug manufacturers respond to meet this demand, what steps are taken between the discovery and sale of a drug, how pharmacists fit into this complicated system of drug use, and what trends and concerns are currently affecting this process.

DRUGS AS REMEDIES, POISONS, OR MAGICAL CHARMS

Substances that produce a change in cellular or physiological functioning of humans are called drugs, but there is more to these chemicals than their pharmacologic activity (Montagne, 1996). In most economically developed countries, many drug products have become social commodities. In other cultures, the perception and use of plant-based medicines and even synthetic pharmaceuticals can be based on social values.

The Greek term for drug is *pharmakon*, and it has three meanings: remedy, poison, and magical charm. Substances used in a medical or healing context are thought of as remedies, although many such substances also can induce negative effects (side effects, adverse reactions) and toxic episodes. In such a case, the drug, instead of a remedy, is thought of as a poison. Throughout history, remedies and poisons also have been thought to possess magical properties. Even today we sometimes refer to drugs, especially newer ones, as "magic bullets"—a phrase first used by Ehrlich when trying to find a cure for syphilis that would destroy the syphilis bacterium without affecting human tissue (Wikipedia, 2006).

Manufacturers focus on a drug's therapeutic effect. That is, they attempt to optimize the biochemical activity of the molecule, increase its specificity, and reduce or limit its negative effects. This mindset is very similar to the perspective of health professionals, who often focus on treating their patients with a drug that has a single main effect. Because providers realize that individual patients might respond differently to the same drug, they also search for the most active drug that works for a specific patient.

By contrast, patients and consumers may focus on a number of different effects that they think a drug can produce. They may hone in on a drug's reported therapeutic effect and demand this drug from their prescriber. Or they may be more concerned about a drug's side effects than its therapeutic effect and be discouraged from using that particular medication. Interestingly, some drugs have been used specifically because they produce a certain side effect—consider minoxidil, which was first used to lower blood pressure, but was found to grow hair as a side effect.

Unique and innovative drugs can restructure our perceptions and actions regarding states of health and illness. As biology and technology continue to dominate medicine and health care, health and illness behaviors are often defined solely in biological or biochemical terms. "Medicalization" is the redefining or relabeling of a personal or social problem as a medical condition, thus necessitating treatment in the health care system (Conrad and Schneider, 1980). Many conditions such as anxiety, depression, insomnia, attention-deficit disorder, and eating disorders do have physical pathologies, but they may also involve more complex mental, emotional, and social processes that may not be effectively treated with medications.

Individual and societal beliefs about drugs and their effects form the basis for their use; the social context of drug use can influence or modify these beliefs. Consumer beliefs are often very different from the beliefs held by health professionals. This difference can create tension between the patient and the health care provider in the search for a solution to health problems.

USE OF DRUG PRODUCTS FROM A CONSUMER PERSPECTIVE

The long history of self-care in the United States dates back to the widespread, largely unregulated use of patent medicines and herbal remedies in the 19th century (Young, 1961, 1967). Self-care was also the norm in areas where there were neither health care providers nor manufactured products to purchase. In fact, self-care really was the first type of medical drug use, being practiced by ancient peoples before designated healers became a part of structured societies. Before laws and regulations were promulgated in the 20th century, drugs such as opiates, cocaine, cannabis, and other substances from a variety of plant sources were popular and effective ingredients in many medicinal products.

Consumer Actions in Response to Health Problem Situations

From the consumer perspective, drug use is not solely a function of the biochemical action of a substance. Consumers' perceptions of current or potential symptoms, along with their social knowledge, may suggest to them the presence of a health problem (see **Figure 5-1**). They may then take a specific action in response to this problem. They may not recognize fully the symptoms as an illness, or they may ignore them or simply choose to do nothing about them. For about one third of all health problems, consumers take no action. In the other two thirds of such cases, consumers decide to act and choose an approach to resolve their problems (Heller, 1992; Montagne and Basara, 1996).

When consumers do take action, they contact the health care system only about one fourth of the time, and two out of three patients who visit a doctor leave with a prescription (National Association of Chain Drug Stores [NACDS], 2005). In most cases, however, consumers tend to self-diagnose and self-treat their health problems; indeed, most medical drug use in the United States involves self-care with nonprescription drugs and herbal remedies, rather than the use of prescription drugs (Montagne and Basara, 1996). Consumers generally view nonprescription medications, herbal remedies, and any substance they can obtain without a prescription as safer, easier to use, and less expensive.

American use of "nondurable medical products," which the U.S. Department of Health and Human Services, Centers for Medicare and Medicaid Services, defines as nonprescription products and medical sundries, is extensive, with almost $32.3 billion spent by U.S. consumers on these products in 2004 (Centers for Medicare and Medicaid Services, 2006a). More than one third of American adults also report using some form of complementary or alternative medicine (CAM), with total visits to CAM providers each year now exceeding those to primary-care physicians (Centers for Medicare and Medicaid Services, 2006b). An estimated 15 million adults take herbal remedies or high-dose vitamins along with prescription drugs. The various expenditures add up to annual out-of-pocket costs for CAM that are estimated to exceed $27 billion in the United States (Institute of Medicine and Board of Health Promotion and Disease Prevention, 2005).

Interestingly, spending for prescription drugs increased 8.2% in 2004, which was a slower growth rate than the 10.2% growth seen in 2003 and the 14.3% growth observed in 2000–2002. In 2004, spending growth for prescription drugs was similar to that of overall health spending growth, and prescription drugs accounted for 11% of overall health costs (Centers for Medicare and Medicaid Services, 2006c).

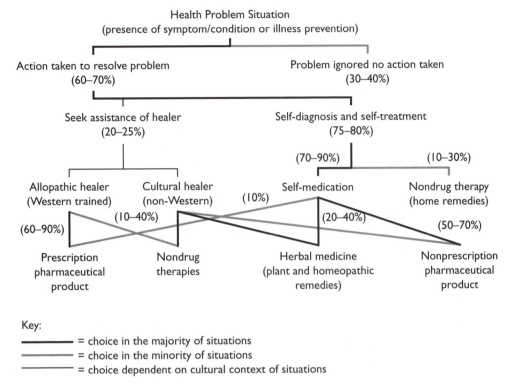

Figure 5-1 Actions Taken in Response to Health Problem Situations

Consumers' Sources of Drug Products

The consumer's ability to obtain and use certain drug products is controlled by laws and regulations. "Prescription" and "nonprescription" are actually legal terms, as are "approved" and "unapproved" with regard to indications of use in therapy, and "illicit" with regard to substances that tend to be used for presumably nonmedical reasons. Differences between prescription and nonprescription products reflect issues related to their safety and habit-forming potential. Safety is a major issue when a manufacturer seeks to switch a drug from prescription to nonprescription status, because there are fewer mechanisms for monitoring drugs' use and effects once they are used as over-the-counter (OTC) products.

The source of drug products for most consumers is the pharmacy. Consumers obtain their prescription drugs from pharmacies, but purchase their OTC drugs from a variety of sources. In 2004, 38.3% of OTC products were purchased from drugstores, 25.1% from mass merchandisers, 21.4% from food stores, and 15.1% from other outlets such as dollar stores and online retailers (Kline & Company, 2005). Convenience is the primary reason for choosing a particular pharmacy, followed by low prices, which is the most important reason for using alternative sources such as the Internet. Once obtained, drug products also can be disseminated through a population as people share or exchange them with their relatives and friends.

DRUG USE FROM THE HEALTH PROFESSIONAL'S PERSPECTIVE

Health professionals are involved in diagnosing and treating health problems. Some of these professionals—especially pharmacists—may suggest or recommend a course of action to the consumer (e.g., self-care with a nonprescription drug). Prescribed treatments usually include a drug component, although a physician or other health professional may also prescribe specific diets or nutritional changes, surgery, lifestyle changes, or other types of nondrug therapies. For patients in the traditional U.S. health care system, however, drug therapy is the mainstay of prescribed treatments.

Prescribers

The ritual of interacting with a physician and receiving a prescription usually involves a strong symbolic healing component (Pellegrino, 1976). The act of taking a drug fulfills an ingrained habit: the need to take action when confronted with illness. The healer's act of prescribing a drug enhances and solidifies the interaction, reinforces the healer's power to cure, and provides the patient with a sense of satisfaction. The process of prescribing can reduce uncertainty and frustration for both patient and prescriber by identifying a possible solution for the health problem.

In 2004, more than 3.2 billion prescriptions were filled in retail pharmacies—a 62% increase since 1994 (NACDS, 2005). For chain pharmacies, 68.3% of total sales were from prescriptions, while nonprescription drugs accounted for 8.1% of sales. Independent pharmacies typically derive greater than 90% of their sales from prescriptions (National Community Pharmacists Association [NCPA], 2005).

Prescribing behaviors are influenced by a number of factors (Raisch, 1990a, 1990b; Soumerai, McLaughlin, and Avorn, 1989):

- Education, especially additional training in pharmacotherapeutics and preceptors' prescribing behavior
- Promotional campaigns, especially drug advertising
- Colleagues, or those health professionals who are part of the prescriber's social network
- Control and regulatory mechanisms (e.g., drug laws, formularies, triplicate prescriptions)
- Demands from patients and society

Dispensers

Pharmacy has evolved significantly as a profession, and is poised to undergo even more changes, as expanded educational and clinical experience suggest pharmacists' readiness for a greater role in health care delivery such as providing medication therapy management (MTM) under Medicare Part D. Although the majority of existing clinical opportunities for pharmacists are found in managed care, hospital, benefits management, and other work settings, consumers continue to identify with the image of the community pharmacist when considering the profession.

The relationship consumers maintain with their pharmacists has changed over time. While not necessarily held in the same clinical esteem as physicians, pharmacists were, at one time, perhaps more involved with the social and non-health care aspects of their patients' lives. Over the years, as volume and regulatory pressures have mounted, pharmacists have been able to spend increasingly less time on activities other than filling prescriptions. Even though they are highly trained to offer valuable clinical oversight, pharmacists have become concerned that their prescription-filling responsibilities are precluding them from performing more valuable and patient-centered services (McDaniel and DeJong, 1999).

Partly in response to this dissatisfaction, the dispensing element of pharmacy practice is currently undergoing rapid change, particularly through the increase in technologies that allow pharmacists to be less involved in the manual process of counting and labeling medications. While an increase in the use and certification of pharmacy technicians has helped to remove the pharmacist from many of these technical functions, the complete drug-handling capabilities of robotics and counting equipment are also working to make pharmacies more efficient and patient centered. Similarly, while prescription writing, patient management, and billing systems were at one time pen-and-paper based, computer systems have all but replaced the paper profiles and accounting required to operate a pharmacy, and e-prescribing is becoming much more commonplace. Computer and online systems also perform sophisticated screening of potential drug-related problems, adherence monitoring, and adjudication of claims during the filling process. (See Chapter 3.)

Hospitals and other institutional pharmacies seeking to better manage personnel costs while maintaining quality and improving patient safety are also paying close attention to dispensing productivity. Robotics and increased technician responsibilities for filling and preparing medication orders in the central pharmacy, as well as sophisticated dispensing technologies (such as Pyxis machines) on patient care units, allow pharmacists to spend more time on reviewing, recommending, and monitoring patient therapies. (See Chapter 6.)

DRUG DEVELOPMENT AND DISTRIBUTION SYSTEMS

The concept of chemotherapy began a new era in therapeutics at the turn of the 20th century. As Paul Ehrlich stated, "Substances able to exert their final action exclusively on the parasite harbored within the organism would represent, so to speak, magic bullets which seek their target of their own accord" (cited in Himmelwert, 1960, p. 22). "Miracle" drugs of the 1940s and 1950s were antibiotics; they were followed by newer "miracles"—psychotropic drugs—in the 1950s and 1960s. Gene therapy and many products of biotechnology represent our contemporary "magic bullets."

Pharmaceutical Development and Regulation

Drugs developed and approved for the market originate with the manufacturer; they are stored and distributed throughout the system in wholesale operations and at the points of distribution (dispensers) until they are acquired by drug users (see **Figure 5-2**). The pharmaceutical industry focuses its efforts on chemical manufacturing, raw material supply, and pharmaceutical production, all of which involve quality assurance processes. Drug distribution involves wholesalers, whereas drug dispensing occurs mostly in pharmacies. Management, regulation, and financing are important aspects of the development and distribution systems. Transfer of drug products to and from legitimate distribution occurs at points of manufacture, wholesaling, dispensing, and consumer use; it is at these same points where drug diversion can occur.

Regulation of pharmacy practice and professionals occurs mostly at the state level, but regulation of drug products is the federal government's responsibility. The U.S. Food and Drug Administration reviews new drug products for safety and effectiveness, including substances that will be made available as nonprescription or OTC drugs. Drugs cannot be legally marketed or sold until they have acquired FDA approval. The FDA performs five functions as part of this process:

1. The premarketing clearance of all new drug products on the basis of purity, safety, and effectiveness
2. Regulation of all labeling, including advertising, of prescription drug products
3. Regulation of manufacturing, along the guidelines of good manufacturing practices and instituting recalls of unacceptable products
4. Regulation of bioequivalence standards
5. Conducting postmarketing surveillance (after a drug is on the market) to detect unanticipated adverse reactions and other problems associated with the use of that drug

Once a drug product has been approved for the market, the FDA has few powers to determine how it is ultimately used. The agency has little

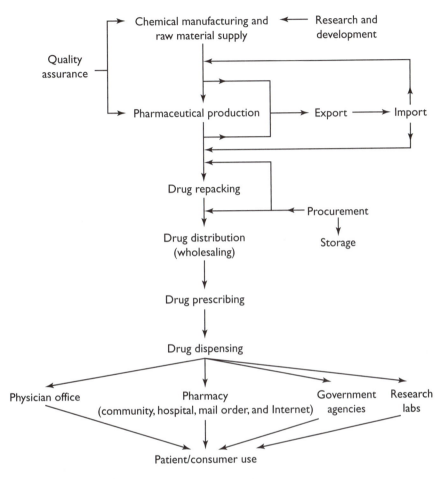

Figure 5-2   Pharmaceutical Development and Distribution Systems

control over the medication use behaviors of patients or the prescribing behaviors of health professionals, who may choose to prescribe FDA-approved drugs for non-FDA-approved ("off-label") indications.

Behind most drug control legislation is a certain philosophy—namely, that, given the refinements of science and modern technology, the safety and effectiveness of a drug product can be measured and determined absolutely and completely. The language of many laws and the perceptions of many consumers are couched in absolute terms. They are based on the assumption that all scientific matters, such as those in medicine and health care, can be decided as ultimate truths. Safety and effectiveness, however, mean different things to different people and, unfortunately, there are no absolutes. What results is a political process with continual discussions and disputes among researchers, clinicians, federal authorities, industrial personnel and managers, the media, and consumers. The FDA makes most of the decisions in the drug approval process, and in the final analysis, it may determine what is scientific fact, even while basing its decision on industry-based data. In the Beeker Pharmaceutical example, safety concerns over Aperaire and the risks it posed to FDA approval prompted Beeker's development of creative methods of distribution in an effort to control the drug's use.

Pharmaceutical Research and the Drug Approval Process

Modern drug development has evolved into a complex process that involves a number of components (Basara and Montagne, 1994). The process of drug discovery starts with basic scientific characterization of a newly identified or synthesized molecule, then charts a course through pharmacologic and toxicologic evaluation in animals, formulation development, clinical pharmacology studies, evaluation of safety and efficacy in humans, the regulatory process, marketing, manufacture and supply, postmarketing surveillance, and international development. While basic pharmaceutical research may create useful compounds, their beneficial applications are ultimately demonstrated through clinical research.

The drug development process includes four major steps. Drug development begins with the identification of potentially useful compounds through preclinical research. Of every 5,000 to 10,000 compounds that are created by pharmaceutical companies, only 250 may make it into preclinical testing (Pharmaceutical Research and Manufacturers of America [PhRMA], 2006). Compounds that show promise in the preclinical testing phase and that a pharmaceutical company wishes to explore are approved for further study (clinical testing) by the FDA. Only 5 compounds of the 250 that undergo preclinical clinical testing typically make it to this stage (PhRMA, 2006). The drug's sponsor (usually the manufacturer or potential marketer) then submits an investigational new drug application (INDA) to the FDA for approval. Once the INDA is approved, clinical testing occurs in four phases, three of which take place before the drug is finally approved for sale in the market. The final steps of drug development involve review and approval of the drug, marketing it to the public, and follow-up postmarketing studies (Bleidt and Montagne, 1996).

Clinical Research and Evaluation of New Drugs

The first phase of clinical testing is directed at determining the drug's safe dosage range, the preferred administration route, the mechanisms of absorption and distribution in the body, and possible toxicities. These tests usually are conducted in a small number (fewer than 100) of normal, healthy volunteers and require less than 12 months to complete. A majority (50–70%) of compounds tested in Phase 1 are abandoned because of problems with safety or efficacy.

The second phase of clinical testing attempts to learn more about the drug's safety and efficacy in treating a certain disease or symptom. These studies still involve a small number of subjects (typically a few hundred), but these people suffer from the disease or symptom for which the drug seems to be effective. Phase 2 trials may take as long as 2 years. If the studies show that the drug is useful in a particular disease, and preclinical animal data show no unwarranted harm, the sponsor can proceed to Phase 3. According to the FDA, only about one third of new drug entities in Phase 2 continue on to Phase 3.

Phase 3 studies assess safety, efficacy, and appropriate dosage range for the drug in treating a specific disease in an expanded group of patients. The number of patients involved can range from several hundred to several thousand, depending on the drug. During Phase 3 studies, the drug is used by patients under physicians' care in a manner similar to the way in which the drug would be used if it were on the market. On average, only 25% of all new drug entities introduced into Phase 3 testing successfully complete this phase. The Pharmaceutical Research and Manufacturing Association notes that only one of the five compounds beginning clinical testing actually moves on for approval (PhRMA, 2006).

After clinical testing of the new drug, the manufacturer is required to submit a new drug application (NDA) to the FDA before it can be approved for marketing. The FDA has 60 days to determine whether it will fully review an NDA; it can refuse to review an application that is incomplete. The FDA's Center for Drug Evaluation and Research (CDER) expects to review and act on at least 90% of NDAs for standard drugs no later than 10 months after the applications are received. The review goal is 6 months for higher-priority drugs (United States Food and Drug Administration, 2002).

After a drug is approved for marketing, the sponsor must continue to submit information to the FDA on a regular basis. In the Beeker example, the company found an unanticipated advantage in its distribution model for meeting this expectation, in that the company needs to collect data from a substantially smaller number of prescribers and pharmacies due to its tight controls. Such data requirements are considered Phase 4 clinical trials and are a part of postmarketing surveillance of the drug product. Since the early 1970s, the FDA has been responsible for monitoring the safety and quality of drugs. Physicians, pharmacists, nurses, and other health care professionals are asked to report adverse drug reactions or other concerns about a product to the FDA by using an online form or by calling the FDA directly if the reaction is life-threatening or dangerous. Another part of Phase 4 studies involves clinical trials of the drug in various subgroups of patients, such as children or women.

A drug's sponsor submits a supplemental NDA (sNDA) to the FDA when it requests approval to promote an existing drug with either a new indication or a new labeling, or when manufacturing procedures have changed. An abbreviated NDA (ANDA) is filed by a generic manufacturer that wishes to produce an existing drug whose patent protection has expired. The generic manufacturer must scientifically demonstrate that its product is bioequivalent (i.e., performs in the same manner as the existing drug). Once approved, the generic company may "manufacture and market the generic drug product to provide a safe, effective, low cost alternative to the American public" (United States Food and Drug Administration, 2006).

Exhibit 5-1 reviews the steps in the drug approval process. Attempts to facilitate and improve this process have included accelerating the drug development and approval process; seeking innovations from newer, smaller companies; changing drug laws and regulations; reducing potential drug product liability; standardizing the development and approval process; and eliminating trade barriers. U.S. pharmaceutical industry exports are about equal to the country's drug imports, with most exports going to Japan, Germany, Canada, and Italy, and with most incoming products being manufactured in the United Kingdom, Germany, Switzerland, and Japan. Differences in national regulatory schemes and other factors that influence pharmaceutical pricing are having a major effect on the U.S. pharmaceutical industry (Milne and Lasagna, 2002). These differences also are affecting U.S. drug consumers, who are increasingly seeking nontraditional sources of drug supply (e.g., exports, personal travel to bordering countries).

Following discovery of a new drug, the supply chain for the pharmaceutical industry includes several segments, from manufacturing to retailing and from marketing new products to managing the economics of prescriber activities. Each step offers interesting career opportunities for pharmacists, including many positions that have come into existence only recently, such as those occupied by the highly disease-specific Internet- and mail-order-based professionals handling Beeker's product and patients. At the industrial end, a variety of professionals are involved in the study, development, testing, and manufacture of medications. Specialists are needed to determine the need and marketability of chemicals and to obtain approval from the FDA. Upon a drug's release to the public, new roles emerge that begin to touch on other supply chain segments, including marketing or sales activities to prescribers and consumers, contracting with insurance vendors for coverage of the product, advertising, distribution, and large-scale manufacturing.

Research Productivity, Marketing, and Cost

In 2005, the FDA approved 79 NDAs, although some of these were reformulations of or new combinations with existing approved drugs. Twenty-eight of these NDAs were for new compounds (PhRMA, 2006), and most were approved in less than 6 months. PhRMA reported that the cost

Exhibit 5-1   Drug Review Steps

1. Preclinical (animal) testing.
2. An investigational new drug application (IND) outlines what the sponsor of a new drug proposes for human testing in clinical trials.
3. Phase 1 studies (typically involve 20 to 80 people).
4. Phase 2 studies (typically involve a few dozen to about 300 people).
5. Phase 3 studies (typically involve several hundred to about 3,000 people).
6. The pre-NDA period, just before a new drug application (NDA) is submitted. A common time for the FDA and drug sponsors to meet.
7. Submission of a new drug application is the formal step asking the FDA to consider a drug for marketing approval.
8. After an NDA is received, the FDA has 60 days to decide whether to file the NDA it so it can be reviewed.
9. If the FDA files the NDA, an FDA review team is assigned to evaluate the sponsor's research on the drug's safety and effectiveness.
10. The FDA reviews information that goes on a drug's professional labeling— that is, guidance on how to use the drug.
11. The FDA inspects the facilities where the drug will be manufactured as part of the approval process.
12. FDA reviewers will approve the drug or find it either "approvable" or "not approvable."

Source: United States Food and Drug Administration (FDA). The FDA's Drug Review Process: Ensuring Drugs Are Safe and Effective. *FDA Consumer Magazine.* 2002; 36(4): Pub No. FDA05-3242. Retrieved December 11, 2006 from http://www.fda.gov/fdac/features/2002/402_drug.html.

of developing one new medicine now amounts to approximately $800 million over a 10- to 15-year period (PhRMA, 2006). Estimated biopharmaceutical research and development (R&D) expenditures for PhRMA member companies totaled $39.4 billion in 2005. This number increased to $51.3 billion when other U.S. biotechnology companies were included "that are not PhRMA members but are often supported through business ventures and funding from PhRMA member companies" (PhRMA, 2006, 4). This dollar figure represents 15.8% of the total sales for biopharmaceutical companies.

The pharmaceutical industry has come under intense scrutiny for the promotion and marketing of its products, as well as for the increasing prices of medications. The business argument suggests that the pharmaceutical industry is like any other industry and, as such, should establish prices that the market will bear and aggressively advertise and promote its products. The health care sector argues that promotion and advertising may undermine evidence-based care and increase overall health care spending. Whichever side one supports, it is important to understand promotion and pricing in greater detail.

The promotion of prescription pharmaceuticals can include direct-to-consumer (DTC) advertising (i.e., advertisements in journals, magazines, television, radio, and other media), samples of medications provided to health care facilities, information and materials provided by sales force members directly to providers ("detailing," which may include promotional gifts such as pens, mugs, or clocks), and sponsorship of meetings, events, and speakers. It is difficult to find conclusive data on the total amount spent on the promotion of pharmaceuticals, but it has been reported that more than $11 billion was spent on promotional activities in 2005 (IMS Health, 2005). This figure did not include sponsorship of meeting or events, but more than one third of this amount ($4.2 billion) was attributed to DTC advertising.

Direct-to-Consumer Advertising

The FDA regulates pharmaceutical product advertising under the Food, Drug and Cosmetic Act. Prior to 1997, regulations required that accurate information was presented that fairly balanced risks and benefits, and that adequate provision was made for information in a brief summary included in the package labeling relating to side effects, contraindications, and effectiveness. In 1997, the FDA clarified "adequate provision" as meaning that consumers should be offered several venues by which to get additional information about the product: (1) a toll-free phone number; (2) printed brochures easily accessible in appropriate locations such as doctors' offices, pharmacies, grocery stores, and public libraries; (3) an Internet site; and (4) contact with health care providers such as physicians or pharmacists (United States Food and Drug Administration, 1999). Interestingly, the amount of DTC advertising has increased significantly since 1997 (United States General Accounting Office [U.S. GAO], 2002).

Research about the effects of DTC advertising has shown mixed results. One report noted that 40% of physicians believe that it has had a positive effect on their patients and practice, 30% say it has had a negative effect, and 30% see no effect at all (Berndt, 2005). Other studies have reported concerns that greater advertising of drugs leads to increased expenditures rather than more effective or efficient care (Wilkes, Bell, and Kravitz, 2000). PhRMA notes that DTC advertising helps to educate consumers about their conditions and symptoms, can increase compliance with medications, and can enhance communications between patients and physicians (PhRMA, 2006). PhRMA has also published *Guiding Principles on Direct to Consumer Advertisements About Prescription Medicines*, a stricter set of guidelines than that currently required by the FDA (PhRMA, 2006).

Interestingly, as of 2002, only the United States and New Zealand allowed DTC advertising. Regardless of whether they agree with DTC advertising, pharmacists need to be aware of these advertisements and be prepared to answer questions from consumers and other health care providers about these advertised products and the conditions that they treat.

Drug Pricing

The pricing of pharmaceuticals and resulting prescriptions is incredibly complex, so much so that a full discussion is beyond the scope of this chapter. Suffice it to say that many people do not understand how prescriptions are priced. Prices for pharmaceutical products are determined by their manufacturers; actual consumer out-of-pocket prescription medication costs are determined in many instances by the consumer's insurance plan. The ultimate costs reflect the manufacturers' costs, the wholesalers' costs, and the dispensing pharmacies' costs. In the community pharmacy arena, many owners and managers have watched their prescription profits shrink (especially for brand-name products), while the profits of manufacturers, wholesalers, and pharmaceutical benefits managers (PBMs) for insurance companies continue to increase. Unfortunately for dispensing pharmacies, many consumers blame them for the high prices owing to a lack of understanding of where the costs come from. For this reason, education of consumers on these issues can be very helpful.

It is worth further exploring pharmacy benefit management as a component of the drug supply chain not just because of the role it plays in drug reimbursement and formulary development, but also because of the volatility, rapid expansion, and controversy that it has engendered in the market. Organizations such as Prescription Card Services (PCS) and PAID—two early innovators in establishing benefit programs—have found that they can play vital roles in the provision of pharmaceutical services by networking at various stages in the insurance, manufacturing, and retailing industries. PBMs began by distributing credit-card-like cards that would identify patients as covered by a given health insurance company. They soon moved from negotiating pharmacy discounts to, most recently, administering sophisticated online services for chronic disease, pharmacoeconomic, and compliance management. PBMs also create, implement, and enforce the use of their own formularies.

At various times during the 1990s, drug manufacturers sought to acquire PBMs, which in some cases were associated with wholesalers, hoping to leverage their contracts with insurance companies for increased drug sales. Chain drug vendors also sought PBMs, seeking to control market share and, eventually, prescription reimbursement rates. PCS was involved in two such ventures. At one time, it was a division of McKesson HBOC, a national drug wholesaler; it was then sold, first to Eli Lilly, a drug maker; then to Rite Aid, a chain drugstore corporation; then to Advance Paradigm, another pharmacy benefit manager and service provider; and most recently to Caremark, another PBM. (See Chapter 16.)

Channels of Distribution and Pharmaceutical Systems

In the United States, consumers usually obtain prescription medications by visiting a prescriber, obtaining a prescription for a medication, and getting that prescription filled at a local pharmacy. Patients may also get their prescriptions filled from mail-order pharmacies. By contrast, consumers can purchase nonprescription medications in hundreds of thousands of retail or mail-order outlets throughout the United States, many of which do not employ a health care provider to help consumers make decisions on their purchases. Pharmacies obtain their medications (and chemicals needed for compounding) either from wholesalers or directly from manufacturers or other distributors. Wholesalers obtain their medications directly from manufacturers or other distributors. These channels are examined in greater detail later in this chapter.

The drug wholesaling industry dates back decades in various forms and has evolved into the predominant distribution channel for medications in the United States. When independent community pharmacies were more prevalent and administered the major share of prescription services, wholesalers served to centralize the purchasing and sale of drugs from the manufacturer, although many pharmacies maintained direct accounts with the larger drug makers. It was more efficient and economical for individual pharmacies to obtain the bulk of their inventory from a wholesaler, rather than from individual manufacturers. When chain drugstore networks expanded rapidly in the 1970s and 1980s, wholesalers saw some of their core market erode, because the chains often negotiated for and warehoused their own products. Today, chain store management seems to believe that such practices are an unnecessary duplication of costs and is returning to the major wholesalers for supplies.

The dispensing of pharmaceuticals takes place in a variety of settings, including hospitals; independent, chain, supermarket, and mass-merchandiser pharmacies; and mail-order, clinic, and Internet-based pharmacies (a type of mail-order pharmacies). It is the responsibility of these pharmacies to provide patient education, monitoring, and access to pharmaceuticals. While varying widely in the way they operate and the efficiencies they are capable of achieving, pharmacists are still responsible for ensuring safe and appropriate drug therapy in each setting. Some providers are experimenting with technologies such as automated teller machines (ATMs) to dispense medication to consumers.

Alternatives to these channels of distribution may emerge in special situations, such as when manufacturers need to safely accommodate the sophisticated requirements of some new biotechnology-based pharmaceuticals. Some drug manufacturers have sought out disease specialty pharmacies to ensure that laboratory-monitoring services, needle disposal, or counseling take place. Others, when selling products that treat conditions with a small population of patients such as hemophilia and cystic fibrosis, seek to limit costs associated with selling products on a national scale. In the chapter-opening case, Beeker's product distribution was limited for both of these reasons, as well as to ensure that its potential for safety problems would not prevent the drug from being marketed at all. Under these case scenarios, pricing, availability, insurance coverage, and patient expectations are all affected, depending on whether the medication is available locally, through the mail, in the physician's office, or by accessing Internet-based sole-source vendor pharmacies.

Other restricted channels of distribution may become necessary when a drug has been abused. Consider the case of pseudoephedrine, which has been a popular nonprescription decongestant for many years. Pseudoephedrine is a precursor for methamphetamine, and abuse of home-made methamphetamine has increased dramatically in the last few years. This powerful addiction is devastating to the addict, his or her family and friends, and the community at large. Because of this rise in abuse, products containing pseudoephedrine went from unregulated nonprescription status to "behind-the-counter" status in some states, and even back to prescription status or designation as a scheduled, controlled substance in other states.

Importation and Counterfeiting

There has been much concern recently over international channels of distribution related to product fraud, lack of evidence of safety and efficacy, lack of medical need, and cost. Part of this debate involves the ability of U.S. citizens to purchase prescription medications in other countries at much cheaper prices. The FDA currently bans any "drug importation" of products, although it permits a personal 3-month supply to be acquired as long as the patient has a valid U.S. prescription, is under the care of a U.S. health care provider, and provides this documentation when asked (Blumberg, 1998).

Related to the drug importation problem is the acquisition of counterfeit products by unknowing pharmaceutical wholesalers and distributors, which then sell the drugs to pharmacies for dispensing to the public. Most often these products' packages, labeling, and dosage forms are identical to those of the original products. The implications for patient harm are immeasurable, whether patients consume unknown chemicals that may harm them in some way or whether they are taking a medication to prevent a life-threatening condition such as blood clots or asthma attacks but actually receive only placebo. A February 2006 World Health Organization (WHO) report estimated that counterfeit pharmaceuticals account for more than 10% of the global drug market, and possibly 25% of medications consumed in developing countries (World Health Organization, 2006). The U.S.-based Center for Medicine in the Public Interest (CMPI) predicts that counterfeit drug sales will reach $75 billion by 2010, a 92% increase from sales in 2005 (Center for Medicine in the Public Interest [CMPI], 2006).

In response to this growing problem, the FDA formed the Counterfeit Drug Task Force in July 2003 to study the issues. Its first report, which was published in February 2004, identified a fourfold increase in the number of counterfeit investigations undertaken from the late 1990s to 2004 (United States Food and Drug Administration, 2004). Some examples cited in the report included counterfeit Epogen and Procrit (products that stimulate red blood cell production for patients with cancer and/or anemia) and Lipitor (a popular cholesterol-lowering product) found in pharmacies and consumed by patients, as well as counterfeit Ortho Evra contraceptive patches (with no active ingredient) being sold online by a company based in India. The Counterfeit Drug Task Force has since submitted two additional reports, with the most recent being published in June 2006.

The Task Force has recommended that the FDA implement regulations by December 1, 2006, that would require pharmaceutical manufacturers, wholesalers, and distributors to use radiofrequency identification (RFID) technology for the verification and tracking of individual dosage units, as well as a "pedigree" documentation system that would allow for tracking these units as they move through the pharmaceutical supply chain. Although this recommended deadline has passed without formal FDA implementation, some manufacturers are already employing this technology with their most vulnerable products—Pfizer has taken this step with Viagra, for example.

The National Association of Boards of Pharmacy (NABP) is also taking active steps to help curb the counterfeit problem. The organization recently released *Model Rules for the Licensure of Wholesale Distributors* to help state boards of pharmacy revise their own regulations with regard to wholesalers (NABP, 2006). These rules include language that describes the use of technology and a pedigree system to "authenticate, track, and trace" prescription drugs. These updated rules work in concert with the organization's Verified-Accredited Wholesale Distributors (VAWD) program, which began in 2004 as an effort to help protect the public against counterfeit pharmaceuticals. The VAWD program "provides assurance that the [wholesale distribution] facility operates legitimately, is validly licensed in good standing, and is employing security and best practices for safely distributing prescription drugs from manufacturers to pharmacies and other institutions."(NABP, 2005)

Related to these initiatives, the Partnership for Safe Medicines (PSM) serves as a "Clearinghouse of information on counterfeit drugs, fake medicines, and ways to stay safe" (PSM, 2006). PSM includes member organizations from all over the world to share information both regionally and globally. Two of its North American members, the Healthcare Distribution Management Association (HDMA; formerly the National Wholesale Drug Association), which represents drug wholesalers, and the American Pharmacists Association (APhA) recently testified before the U.S. House of Representatives' Committee on Government Reform, Subcommittee on Criminal Justice, Drug Policy, and Human Resources regarding counterfeits and the pharmaceutical supply chain (Gray, 2006; Winckler, 2006). APhA's testimony made recommendations for Congress to act upon, and outlined three roles that pharmacists could play in protecting the public from counterfeit pharmaceuticals:

- Be prudent purchasers of products to stock in their pharmacies.
- Educate patients about the potential risks associated with imported medications and those purchased through nontraditional means.
- Report any suspected counterfeit products to the FDA or other appropriate agency.

A related concern to importation and counterfeiting is the aggressive advertising and widespread availability of very popular prescription medications (e.g., sexual enhancers, sleep aids, antidepressants, pain relievers) through online outlets. Much of the "spam" received on seemingly any type of e-mail account consists of this sort of advertisement. It is unknown how often consumers respond to these solicitations, but many of the solicitations advertise "no prescription required" for consumers to obtain the desired product. Not only is the lack of medical supervision a concern for consumers who may be obtaining and using these products, but the possibility of the products themselves being counterfeit raises concerns. (See Chapter 3.)

FUTURE CHANGES IN THE PHARMACEUTICAL SECTOR

With the advance of genomic science and biotechnology, health care is entering into an era of "personalized medicine," in which prescribers use a patient's genetic traits and pharmacogenomic markers to select therapies most appropriate for a particular individual (PhRMA, 2006). For example, use of the breast cancer drug trastuzumab and individualized dosing of warfarin therapy are both based on genetic variation. Additionally, much-needed new drugs are being developed for underserved disease states. According to PhRMA (2006), the top ten areas of new drug development are

- Cancer
- Neurologic disorders
- Infections
- Cardiovascular disorders
- Psychiatric disorders
- HIV/AIDS
- Arthritis

- Diabetes
- Asthma
- Alzheimer's disease and dementia

Because of the increased competitive pressure to get products on the market, and because of the relatively brief patent life span that such new drugs are allowed to enjoy before facing generic competition, drug companies are expected to continue to comarket or merge in an effort to realize greater efficiencies in their operations (Koberstein, 2000). In the mid- to late 1990s, a number of biotechnology research companies emerged that had developed promising new compounds but lacked marketing and distribution experience. These organizations may be inclined to network on a contract basis for marketing expertise or to gain such advantages more formally through mergers as part of their quest to bring their products to market.

The pharmacy care provider segment is expected to grow, given the new-store initiatives undertaken by most of the nation's chain drugstore operators (Carroll, 1998), even while the number of companies continues to decline because of market consolidation. New systems of delivery will take form, as bricks-and-mortar institutions develop or link up with alternative distributive processes including mail-order, pharmacy benefit management, and Internet-based services.

In all of these settings, as well as in new practice alternatives, pharmacists will be expected to play increasingly larger clinical and financial roles, using their pharmacoeconomic skills to influence the costs of prescribing and outcomes. Patient and prescriber education will become more central to pharmacists' roles, as they step away from the more manual functions of prescription filling. Such services will likely be reimbursed separately from the prescription payment, in recognition of the pharmacist's growing ability to influence the quality of care. In particular, the provision for possible reimbursement for MTM services as part of Medicare Part D may help to advance pharmacists' clinical role.

New distribution networks may also include remote, vending machine-like technologies, detached from a traditional pharmacy, where patients play more active roles in the procurement of their medicines. Pharmacy practice in this environment will be the result of many things, including volume pressures on pharmacists as the country's baby boomers age into their sixties, seventies, and eighties. The next generation, however, because of its lifelong exposure to certain technologies, and because of an increase in self-care and wellness practices, will likely receive many pharmacy services and products over the Internet or via sophisticated dispensing technologies.

To accommodate this shift, boards of pharmacy will begin to recognize the advantages of using dispensing equipment in novel settings and will place increased distribution responsibilities on pharmacy technicians, thereby separating the information and drug delivery portions of dispensing. These efforts may also help pharmacists to evolve their clinical role in the health care system.

CONCLUSIONS

Health care, drug development, and pharmacy professionals and systems continue to evolve. Today's trend toward greater consumer activism is leading patients outside the traditional health care system in search of the newest "magic bullet." Consumer drug use directs the pharmaceutical sector in terms of discovering new drug products and determining the type of health professional who should educate and monitor people about medication use.

The drug discovery, distribution, and use process in the United States is one of the most complex but also one of the most sophisticated. Evolving roles of pharmacists are necessary to continue to improve patient medication use to improve overall health outcomes while reducing costs.

QUESTIONS FOR FURTHER DISCUSSION

1. Why is the pharmacist the best health professional for monitoring and advising consumers on their drug use? What changes in pharmacy education and practice are needed for pharmacists to maintain and enhance their roles as drug consultants?
2. What are some current examples of the symbolic and social aspects of drug and medication use where you live, and what influence do they have on drug effects and use? (*Hint:* Examine the mass media, and talk to patients, consumers, and health professionals.)
3. What is the importance of power and control in the patient–health professional relationship, and how does it affect self-medication? Are there drug-use situations in which the consumer should not make the final decision? Should health professionals offer their advice in all cases? How does a society control and regulate drug use to the benefit of all?
4. How might pharmacy careers vary in the following practice settings: pharmacy benefit manager (PBM), community independent pharmacy, community chain pharmacy, hospital, government agency services (FDA)?
5. What must change in American society for patients to take a more active role in receiving and administering their drug therapies?

KEY TOPICS AND TERMS

Alternative health therapy
Brand-name drug product
Clinical testing of new drugs
Community chain pharmacy
Community independent pharmacy
Consumer drug use
Counterfeiting
Direct-to-consumer (DTC) advertising
Dispenser
Drug wholesaler
Generic drug product
Institutional pharmacy
Internet pharmacy
Investigational new drug (IND)
Mail-order pharmacy
Medicalization
New drug application (NDA)
Nonprescription (over the counter, OTC)
Off-label drug use
Patent registration
Pharmaceutical manufacturer
Pharmaceutical marketing
Pharmaceutical research and development (R&D)
Pharmaceutical Research and Manufacturers Association (PhRMA)
Pharmakon
Postmarketing surveillance
Prescriber
Prescription
Self-care
U.S. drug approval process
U.S. drug development process

REFERENCES

Basara, L. R., & Montagne, M. (1994). *Searching for magic bullets: Orphan drugs, consumer activism and pharmaceutical development.* New York: Haworth Press.

Berndt, E. R. (2005). To inform or persuade? Direct-to-consumer advertising of prescription drugs. *New England Journal of Medicine, 352*(4), 325–328.

Bleidt, B., & Montagne, M. (Eds.). (1996). *Clinical research in pharmaceutical development.* New York: Marcel Dekker.

Blumberg, M. A. (1998). *Information on importation of drugs prepared by the Division of Import Operations and Policy, FDA.* Retrieved December 11, 2006 from http://www.fda.gov/ora/import/pipinfo.htm.

Carroll, N. V. (1998). The effects of managed care on the retail distribution of pharmaceuticals. *Managed Care Interface.* Retrieved December 11, 2006 from www.

medicomint.com/MCI/Details.asp?SUBJECT=The+Effects+of+Managed+Care+ on+the+Retail+Distribution+of+Pharmaceuticals&ISSUE=199811.

Center for Medicine in the Public Interest. *Mission Statement.* Retrieved December 13, 2006 from http://cmpi.org/CMPI_Mission.pdf.

Centers for Medicare and Medicaid Services. (2006a). *Category definitions for health care expenditures.* Retrieved December 11, 2006 from http://www.cms. hhs.gov/NationalHealthExpendData/downloads/quickref.pdf.

Centers for Medicare and Medicaid Services. (2006b). *Table 10: Personal health care expenditures by type of expenditure and source of funds: Calendar years 1998– 2005.* Retrieved December 11, 2006 from http://www.cms.hhs.gov/NationalHeal- thExpendData/downloads/tables.pdf.

Centers for Medicare and Medicaid Services. (2006c). *Health expenditures by spon- sors: Business, household and government.* Retrieved December 11, 2006 from http://www.cms.hhs.gov/NationalHealthExpendData/downloads/highlights.pdf.

Conrad, P., & Schneider, J. W. (1980). *Deviance and medicalization: From badness to sickness.* St. Louis, MO: Mosby.

Gray, J. M. (2006). *John M. Gray, President and CEO, HDMA, testifies before House Subcommittee on Criminal Justice, Drug Policy, and Human Resources.* Retrieved December 13, 2006 from http://www.healthcaredistribution.org/gov_ affairs/testimony/2006-07-11_gray_supplychain.asp.

Heller, H. (1992). *Health care practices and perceptions: A consumer survey of self-medication.* Washington, DC: The Proprietary Association.

Himmelwert, F. (Ed.). (1960). *The collected papers of Paul Ehrlich.* London: Pergamon.

IMS Health Inc. (2005). *Total U.S. promotional spend by type, 2005.* Retrieved December 11, 2006 from http://www.imshealth.com/ims/portal/front/arti- cleC/0,2777,6599_78084568_78152318,00.html.

Institute of Medicine and Board of Health Promotion and Disease Prevention, Com- mittee on the Use of Complementary and Alternative Medicine by the American Public. (2005). *Complementary and alternative medicine in the United States.* Washington, DC: National Academies Press.

Kline & Company, Inc. (2005). *Nonprescription drugs USA 2005.* Retrieved Decem- ber 11, 2006 from http://www.klinegroup.com/brochures/cia6d/brochure.pdf.

Koberstein, W. (2000). Team AHP—Parting the clouds: Chairman John Stafford and his top executives answer bad press with good news. *Pharmaceutical Exec- utive, 20*(12), 46–68.

McDaniel, M. R., & DeJong, D. J. (1999). Justifying pharmacy staffing by presenting pharmacists as investments through return-on-investment analysis. *American Journal of Health-Systems Pharmacists, 56,* 2230–2234.

Milne, C. P., & Lasagna, L. (Eds.). (2002). The cost and value of new medicines in an era of change. *Pharmacoeconomics, 20*(Suppl. 3), 1–108.

Montagne, M. (1996). The pharmakon phenomenon: Cultural conceptions of drugs and drug use. In P. Davis (Ed.), *Contested ground: Public purpose and private interest in the regulation of prescription drugs* (pp. 253–294). New York: Oxford University Press.

Montagne, M., & Basara, L. R. (1996). Consumer behavior regarding the choice of prescription and non-prescription medications. In M. C. Smith and A. I. Wert- heimer (Eds.), *Social and behavioral aspects of pharmaceutical care.* Bingham- ton, NY: Pharmaceutical Products Press.

National Association of Boards of Pharmacy. (2005). *VAWD program overview.* Retrieved December 11, 2006 from http://www.nabp.net/.

National Association of Boards of Pharmacy. (2006) Model rules for the licensure of wholesale distributors, June 2006. Retrieved December 11, 2006 from http://www.nabp.net/ftpfiles/NABP01/WholesalerModelRules.pdf.

National Association of Chain Drug Stores Foundation (NACDS). (2005). *The chain pharmacy industry profile 2005.* Alexandria, VA: NACDS.

National Community Pharmacists Association (NCPA). (2005). *NCPA-Pfizer digest 2005.* Alexandria, VA: NCPA.

Partnership for Safe Medicines (PSM). *SafeMedicines.org: A clearinghouse of information on counterfeit drugs, fake medicines, and ways to stay safe.* Retrieved December 13, 2006 from http://www.safemedicines.org/.

Pellegrino, E. (1976). Prescribing and drug ingestion, symbols and substances. *Drug Intelligence Clinical Pharmacy, 10,* 624–630.

Pharmaceutical Research and Manufacturers of America (PhRMA). (2006). *Pharmaceutical industry profile 2006.* Washington, DC: PhRMA.

Raisch, D. W. (1990a). A model of methods for influencing prescribing: Part I. *DICP: Annals of Pharmacotherapy, 24,* 417–421.

Raisch, D. W. (1990b). A model of methods for influencing prescribing: Part II. *DICP: Annals of Pharmacotherapy, 24,* 537–542.

Soumerai, S., McLaughlin, T. J., & Avorn, J. (1989). Improving drug prescribing in primary care: A critical analysis of the experimental literature. *Milbank Quarterly, 67,* 268–317.

United States Food and Drug Administration. (FDA). (1999). *Guide for industry: Consumer-directed broadcast advertisements.* Retrieved December 11, 2006 from http://www.fda.gov/cder/guidance/1804fnl.pdf.

United States Food and Drug Administration (2002). The FDA's drug review process: Ensuring drugs are safe and effective. *FDA Consumer Magazine.* 2002; 36(4): Pub No. FDA05-3242. Retrieved December 11, 2006 from http://www.fda.gov/fdac/features/2002/402_drug.html.

United States Food and Drug Administration. (2004). *Combating counterfeit drugs: A report of the Food and Drug Administration.* Retrieved December 11, 2006 from http://www.fda.gov/oc/initiatives/counterfeit/report02_04.pdf.

United States Food and Drug Administration. (2004). *Drugs@FDA Glossary of Terms.* Retrieved December 11, 2006 from http://www fda.gov/cder/drugsatfda/Glossary.htm#S.

United States General Accounting Office (U. S. GAO). (2002, October). *Report to Congressional requesters: Prescription drugs—FDA oversight of direct-to-consumer advertising has limitations.* (GAO-03-177). Washington, DC: U.S. Government Printing Office.

Wikipedia. (2006). *Magic bullet.* Retrieved December 11, 2006 from http://en.wikipedia.org/wiki/Magic_bullet.

Wilkes, M. S., Bell, R. A., & Kravitz, R. L. (2000). Direct-to-consumer prescription drug advertising: Trends, impact, and implications. *Health Affairs (Millwood), 19,* 110–128.

Winckler, S. C. (2006). *Statement of the American Pharmacists' Association submitted to the House Committee on Government Reform Subcommittee on Criminal Justice, Drug Policy, and Human Resources.* Retrieved December 13, 2006 from http://www.aphanet.org/AM/Template.cfm?Section=News_Releases1&template=/CM/ContentDisplay. cfm&ContentID=5918.

World Health Organization (WHO). *Counterfeit medicines.* Retrieved December 11, 2006 from http://www.who.int/mediacentre/factsheets/fs275/en/.

Young, J. H. (1961). *The toadstool millionaires.* Princeton, NJ: Princeton University Press.

Young, J. H. (1967). *The medical messiahs.* Princeton, NJ: Princeton University Press.

ORGANIZATIONAL ASPECTS OF HEALTH CARE DELIVERY

Hospitals

Catherine N. Otto and William W. McCloskey

Case Scenario

Frank is a 60-year-old retired Army officer with a history of hypertension and angina. One evening he complains of a severe tightness in his chest. His wife calls 911, and Frank is rushed to the emergency department at a 250-bed community hospital affiliated with a medical school. After evaluation, Frank is admitted to the cardiac care unit for treatment of an acute myocardial infarction (MI).

While Frank is hospitalized, a pharmacist specializing in cardiology introduces herself to him as part of the medical team. The pharmacist explains that one of the drugs for hypertension he was taking before admission is not on the hospital "formulary," but that he will be given a very similar medication. Frank also notices that his medications are prepared in tiny blister packs, not in the prescription vials with which he is familiar.

Upon discharge, an individual describing himself as a "pharmacy resident" reviews with Frank those medications he will be taking at home. After discharge, Frank will receive follow-up care at the hospital's cardiac clinic.

LEARNING OBJECTIVES

Upon completion of this chapter, the student shall be able to:

- List and describe four factors that have influenced the role and function of the modern hospital
- Summarize how hospitals have adapted to changes in financing of health care and competition
- Compare and contrast horizontal and vertical integration
- Describe how hospitals are classified
- Describe and give examples of general and specialty hospitals; federal and nonfederal government hospitals; nongovernment, not-for-profit, and investor-owned hospitals
- Discuss the three sources of managerial authority in a hospital
- Describe the purpose of hospital accreditation
- Explain the roles and responsibilities of the following professionals: pharmacy director, staff/clinical pharmacist, pharmacy technician
- Explain what unit dose distribution is, and describe two advantages of its use
- Compare and contrast centralized and decentralized drug distribution systems
- Describe how automation is utilized to support drug distribution
- Identify four nondistributive pharmacy services provided by a hospital pharmacist
- Define *hospital formulary*
- Summarize the purpose of a pharmacy residency program

CHAPTER QUESTIONS

1. What are the characteristics of hospitals?
2. How have hospitals adapted to changes in the delivery of health care?
3. What types of drug distribution systems are found in hospitals?
4. What is the role of the pharmacist in providing clinical services in the hospital?

INTRODUCTION

Since their origins as charitable institutions, hospitals have adapted to a variety of social, technological, and political forces to become the center of the health care delivery system. This chapter explains how hospitals have evolved over time and discusses the challenges that they face. In addition, it introduces the role of the hospital pharmacist.

HISTORICAL PERSPECTIVE

The role and function of the modern hospital are a result of hospitals' adaptations to a number of significant developments that occurred in the first half of the 20th century. The Flexner report was one of the first factors that imposed a structural change on the hospital. In 1910, Abraham Flexner, funded by the Carnegie Foundation, conducted a survey of all medical schools in the United States and Canada. His evaluation assessed their admissions requirements, curricula, and financial basis, and estimated the projected need for physicians and medical schools based on the size of the population. Flexner's recommendations included reducing the number of medical schools from 150 to 31, changing their admissions requirements to a minimum of a baccalaureate degree, and incorporating the scientific method as the foundation for medical education (Meites, 1995).

After the American Medical Association adopted the recommendations of the Flexner report, medical education in the United States was transformed into a system based on the scientific method. The scientific method bases diagnosis and treatment of disease on hypothesis formulation, experimentation, and conclusions. In response, hospitals became teaching and research centers for the practice of medicine. As medical practice increasingly came to rely on scientific principles, the use of technology became ever more important to the diagnosis and treatment of disease. It followed that the hospital became a center for technological innovations developed by researchers (see Chapter 1).

Health insurance provided financial stability for hospitals. Before the advent of such insurance, individuals paid for their hospital care with their own resources. Under that financing system, many individuals went without hospital care because it was unaffordable; others who received hospital care found it difficult or impossible to pay their bills. As a consequence, hospitals were at a significant risk for incurring large debts and possibly suffering bankruptcy. Once health insurance became widespread, hospitals no longer had to assume the financial risk and potential losses when patients could not pay their bills. Health insurance created a steady cash flow to hospitals and was critical for the funding of new technologies.

Because health insurance removed the financial barriers to hospital care for patients, the demand for health care increased. That is, health care was no longer limited by the individual's ability to pay. In addition, because health insurance initially covered only inpatient care, it provided a financial incentive to admit patients to the hospital to administer tests and procedures. Many of these admissions were unnecessary—routine diagnostic evaluation could have easily been performed on an outpatient basis. However, the availability of services in the hospital, coupled with the removal of the financial risk with health insurance, increased the demand for hospital beds, hospital services, and health care in the United States.

The Hospital Survey and Construction Act of 1946 (also known as the Hill-Burton Act) is credited with expanding the infrastructure of the health care delivery system by creating federal funding sources to build new hospitals, expand and renovate facilities, increase bed capacity, and add emerging technology. This legislation was particularly instrumental in supporting the building of hospitals in rural areas and small cities. Although Hill-Burton was not considered to be successful, it resulted in an increase in the number of beds in many hospitals and the incorporation of new technology, such as that currently used in emergency departments and intensive care units.

Finally, there has been a change in the types of diseases that are prevalent in the U.S. population. During the first half of the 20th century, infectious diseases were the most common types of illnesses warranting health care interventions. Because these disease processes were acute, hospitalizations were singular events. With the advent of preventive measures (such as immunizations and antimicrobial agents) and improvement in the water supply and general sanitation, morbidity resulting from infections has declined in recent decades. As a result, chronic diseases are now the most prevalent types of disease. Thus hospitalizations are no longer singular events. Treatment for chronic diseases requires more than hospital care; it requires a continuum of care including ambulatory, acute, and long-term care.

Each of these factors has contributed to the development and modernization of the hospital and the U.S. health care delivery system. Adaptations made in the past continue to affect hospitals' reactions to the social, technological, and political forces.

HOSPITALS IN THE NEW CENTURY

Impact of Diagnosis-Related Groups

Over the years, the hospital adapted its structure and function so that it could remain a viable entity in the health care delivery system. The 1980s and 1990s brought dramatic and continuous changes to the hospital environment. One of the first significant events hospital administrators had to contend with was the diagnosis-related group (DRG) payment mechanism for the hospitalization component (Part A) of the Medicare program. Congress instituted DRGs in 1983 as a method to control increases in Medicare spending.

Although hospital administrators perceived DRGs and the other prospective payment systems to be a detriment to their facilities' financial success, DRGs actually created new incentives for hospitals and other segments of the health care delivery system. Efficiency, utilization review, and evaluation of diagnostic procedures for appropriateness became important—if not vital—for hospitals to survive. Under the retrospective fee-for-service payment method, providers had an incentive to perform more procedures and keep patients in the hospital as long as possible. By contrast, the prospective payment mechanism of the DRG program created new incentives that ran contrary to those under fee-for-service: Hospitals were motivated to perform fewer procedures and to discharge patients as quickly as possible. In the past, patients with acute MIs like Frank were often hospitalized for several weeks. Under a DRG reimbursement system, uncomplicated MI patients are discharged after a few days because reimbursement to the hospital is independent of the services provided or the length of stay.

Hospitals adapted to the shift in the payment mechanism by "unbundling"—that is, separating out—the services included in the DRG payment scheme. For example, presurgical diagnostic procedures were performed on an outpatient basis instead of as a component of the hospital stay. In addition, the recovery period following surgical procedures was removed from the hospital stay by transferring the patient to a rehabilitation unit or facility. These unbundled services no longer were included in the DRG prospective payment, but were billed separately under the Medicare Part B fee schedule. Thus the Medicare DRG payment mechanism resulted in decreased lengths of stay: It reimbursed only the acute phase of the illness or surgery, leading to higher acuity of inpatients—no longer was there a mixture of patients requiring limited to complex nursing and medical care—and it provided less financial support for uncompensated hospital care—there were fewer opportunities to absorb these costs from the hospital stays requiring less complex medical care.

Competition

By the 1990s, it seemed as if all the forces that had helped to elevate the hospital to the center of the health care delivery system had converged to cause its failure. It was as if all of the players and components of the health care delivery system underwent radical changes simultaneously, leaving the hospital to adapt by modifying both its structure and its function.

First, following implementation of the DRG payment method, other prospective, capitated (i.e., the provider is paid a fixed amount per capita regardless of the type or number of services delivered) methods of financing health care began replacing the predominant retrospective, fee-for-service form of financing. Second, health insurance companies began adopting the cost-containment mechanisms used in managed care, such as using prior approval mechanisms for hospital admissions and procedures, requiring second opinions for expensive procedures, and using primary-care providers as gatekeepers. As a result, the supply of specialty-care providers exceeded demand, and there was a shortage of the primary-care clinicians required to implement a managed care type of financing and delivery system. Third, as competition for patients grew fiercer, hospitals began advertising on radio, television, billboards, and in newspapers. Hospitals created special services and programs for targeted populations, such as homelike birthing rooms for maternity patients instead of the aseptic hospital atmosphere of labor and delivery rooms.

Horizontal Integration

Although inter-hospital competition continued, hospitals began to form affiliations with one another to improve efficiency and to secure better opportunities for purchasing equipment and supplies. Affiliations were created between two or more hospitals; these hospitals combined some services and usually created managerial efficiency by employing one managerial staff for both institutions (Massachusetts Hospital Association, 1995). *Horizontal integration* is the term used to describe these types of affiliations between hospitals. Sometimes the services provided by the two affiliated hospitals were similar. Often each hospital provided one or more services not provided by the other. Frequently, a partnership was formed between a smaller community hospital and a large, urban, tertiary care hospital; the urban hospital provided sophisticated technological procedures not available in the community hospital.

Vertical Integration

In addition to integrating horizontally, hospitals began to integrate vertically. An organization is vertically integrated when it provides a continuum of services. Hospitals began to expand to offer services other than acute care, such as outpatient services, home health care, rehabilitation services, and nursing home care (Massachusetts Hospital Association, 1995). Vertically integrated hospitals did not have to depend solely on the declining revenues from acute care. For example, in the chapter-opening case study, the hospital was able to participate in Frank's care post-discharge because it had an outpatient cardiac clinic. Further, by integrating vertically, hospitals were prepared to provide managed care organizations with a variety of services.

Hospitals have responded to the current social, political, and technological forces by integrating their acute care services with other services in the delivery of health care. Reactions to these driving forces have provided an unintended benefit, as hospitals undergoing vertical integration have laid the foundation of a structure for providing a continuum of care—an integrated health care delivery system.

HOSPITAL CHARACTERISTICS

Hospitals are classified by length of stay, type of service provided, and ownership. Given that these classifications are not mutually exclusive, all three categories are used to classify a hospital (Health Forum, 2005). A number of other characteristics that do not fit neatly into these three categories are also used in the literature to describe hospitals—for example, community/noncommunity hospitals, teaching/nonteaching hospitals, number of beds, and multihospital chains.

Length of Stay

Classifying hospitals by the average length of stay differentiates hospitals that provide acute care from those that provide long-term care. Acute care hospitals (also referred to as short-term hospitals) have an average length of stay of fewer than 30 days. Long-term hospitals have an average length of stay of 30 or more days (Health Forum, 2005).

Type of Service

Hospitals are also classified by the type of service provided. General hospitals provide a variety of services, including general medical and surgical services. Well-known general hospitals include the Massachusetts General Hospital and the San Francisco General Hospital Medical Center. Specialty hospitals, by contrast, concentrate on one disease process (e.g., psychiatric diseases or cancer) or on one segment of the population (e.g., children's hospitals or veterans' hospitals). Noted specialty hospitals include McLean Hospital, a psychiatric hospital in Massachusetts; Memorial Sloan-Kettering Cancer Center in New York; and Shriners' Hospitals for Crippled Children, located in many cities throughout the country.

Ownership

Hospitals are further characterized by their ownership and control: federal government, nonfederal government (both also referred to as public hospitals), nongovernment and not-for-profit, and investor owned (for-profit) (Health Forum, 2005).

The federal government operates a number of hospitals for specific populations: veterans, military personnel, and Native Americans. Examples of hospitals under the jurisdiction of the federal government include Veterans Affairs Medical Centers throughout the nation and the Walter Reed Army Medical Center in Washington, D.C.

Nonfederal government hospitals include hospitals owned and operated by city, county, or state governments. Most nonfederal government hospitals are general hospitals. State governments are primarily responsible for specialty care provided in psychiatric hospitals and caring for patients with mental retardation.

Non-government-owned hospitals are divided into two groups: (1) not-for-profit (nonprofit) hospitals and (2) investor-owned (for-profit) hospitals. A number of differences exist between a nonprofit and a for-profit hospital, but the primary difference concerns what the organization does with any excess revenues at the end of the fiscal year. A nonprofit organization reinvests its excess revenues in the organization, usually in the form of capital, new equipment, remodeling, or new buildings. A for-profit organization uses its excess revenues in a similar manner; however, a portion of the excess is paid to the organization's investors in the form of a dividend. Nonprofit hospitals include those operated by the government, religious organizations, and other community hospitals.

Community Hospitals

Hospitals are described as either community or noncommunity hospitals. Community hospitals, such as the one to which Frank was admitted, include all nonfederal hospitals, short-term general, and specialty hospitals that are available to the public (Health Forum, 2005). Noncommunity hospitals are not open to the general public; they include federal hospitals for military personnel and the Veterans Affairs (VA) Medical Centers. Because Frank was a veteran of the armed services, he would have been eligible to go to a VA Medical Center if one was available in his area.

Teaching Hospitals

Hospitals are also classified as teaching or nonteaching hospitals. The designation of "teaching hospital" refers to the teaching and practice of medicine (Raffel and Raffel, 1989). Although a hospital may serve as a clinical training site for students in pharmacy, nursing, clinical laboratory, and any of the other allied health professions, it is not considered a teaching hospital unless it serves as a clinical training site for physicians. A teaching hospital may be expressly associated with a medical school, or it may have an affiliation with a medical school, serving as a site for physicians' residencies.

A teaching hospital can also be classified in another way, such as a community hospital—Frank received his medical care in this type of hospital. A teaching hospital can be a nonprofit, general, community hospital, such as Massachusetts General Hospital, or it can be a federal, general, teaching hospital, such as the many VA Medical Centers.

Number of Beds

American hospitals typically have fewer than 200 beds; indeed, 71.7% of U.S. hospitals fit this criterion (Health Forum, 2005). Larger hospitals are found in major urban areas, whereas smaller hospitals are found in the rural sections of the country. Depending on the size of the hospital, the percentage of occupancy varies. As the hospital size increases, the average occupancy rate increases: Smaller hospitals (those with fewer than 200 beds) have an average occupancy rate ranging from 34% to 65%;, whereas larger hospitals (those with more than 200 beds) have an average occupancy rate ranging from 69% to 76% (Health Forum, 2005).

Multihospital Chains

Multihospital systems emerged as a response to the changes in the health care environment in the 1990s through mergers, acquisitions, or other legal arrangements. Multihospital systems are frequently national in scope, with hospitals being located in one or more geographic areas of the country. Not only do these national multihospital systems gain purchasing power with vendors, but they also have an advantage when competing for managed care contracts for businesses located in more than one state. HCA is an example of a large multihospital system.

HOSPITAL MANAGEMENT

Three sources of managerial authority and power exist in the hospital: the board of trustees, the hospital administration, and the medical staff.

The primary source of authority is the board of directors (in for-profit hospitals) or trustees (in nonprofit hospitals). The board is composed of members of the community who often have knowledge and skills specific to health care delivery. Its purpose is to determine the mission and goals of the hospital and to develop policies. It delegates more specific duties to the other two sources of managerial authority, the hospital administration and the medical staff (Raffel and Raffel, 1989).

Daily operations are the responsibility of hospital administration. The hospital administrator or chief executive officer is either a physician or an individual with an advanced degree in health administration or business. The hospital administration is responsible for implementing the policies developed by the board of trustees. The hospital management structure is usually a pyramid-like structure in which managers of departments report to assistants to the hospital administrator, who then report to the hospital administrator.

The medical staff is composed of staff physicians and community-based physicians who have staff privileges to admit and treat patients in the hospital. The medical staff is a self-governing body responsible for the quality of the medical services provided to hospitalized patients.

The organizational structure of hospitals follows the function or service provided. Direct patient care services include nursing, emergency department, urgent care, ambulatory care, surgery, and labor and delivery. Ancillary services include pharmacy, laboratory, and diagnostic imaging. Support services include housekeeping, dietary, laundry, purchasing, materials management, and security.

AMERICAN HOSPITAL ASSOCIATION

The American Hospital Association (AHA), founded in 1898, is composed of hospitals, health care systems, and individuals. Its purpose is to provide education and resource material, collect statistics regarding its members, conduct research, and represent the point of view of hospitals in the legislative process (AHA, 2006).

HOSPITAL ACCREDITATION

The American College of Surgeons developed the first hospital standards in 1918. Those standards required hospitals to offer laboratory and radiology services for diagnostic purposes, to hold medical staff meetings to review clinical practices, and to maintain medical records (Roberts, Coale, and Redman, 1987).

The Joint Commission on Accreditation of Healthcare Organizations (Joint Commission) is a national organization founded in 1951 by the American Medical Association, American Hospital Association, American College of Physicians, and American College of Surgeons. Its purpose is to set standards and to subsequently accredit hospitals based on those standards. It accredits approximately 15,000 healthcare organizations and programs in the United States (Joint Commission, 2006). In addition to the four founding organizations, the American Dental Association is represented on its board of commissioners. The Joint Commission, as its name suggests, accredits more than hospitals: It also accredits behavioral health facilities, long-term care facilities, assisted living facilities, ambulatory care facilities and laboratory services (Joint Commission, 2006).

Joint Commission accreditation is based on voluntary compliance with the standards. However, that accreditation has become critical for fulfilling state licensure requirements and essential for receiving reimbursement in the Medicare and Medicaid programs.

The Joint Commission's mission is to improve the quality of health care in the United States. Its initial standards focused on the structure and the processes of health care delivery. However, because the environment of the health care delivery system has changed, the Joint Commission has begun to change the focus of its standards to include clinical processes and outcomes of care. In particular, standards of accreditation will no longer be based solely on the structural inputs of the health care delivery system, such as physicians' qualifications (Auxter, 1997).

THE FUTURE OF HOSPITALS

Predicting the future of hospitals is difficult and perhaps foolish. However, considering the continuing trend of health care cost containment and the focus on the outcomes of the services delivered, some directions for change can be anticipated. Hospitals will continue to try to provide state-of-the-art services and technology while operating within limited budgets. This balancing act will be coupled with greater use of health care services resulting from the aging of the American population. Limited hospital budgets will likely be exacerbated by changes in the reimbursement policies of Medicare, Medicaid, and managed care organizations (Institute for the Future, 2000).

As more individuals seek health care, an increasing percentage of that care will be delivered in an outpatient setting. To contend with this trend, hospitals will continue to diversify their services, to operate clinics, and to offer other diagnostic and therapeutic services on an outpatient basis.

The change in the pattern of the delivery of care and budgets limited by capitated reimbursement policies will probably precipitate more hospital closures and mergers. To remain viable, hospitals will compete for managed care contracts, physicians, and patients.

One can expect that the trends that affected hospitals in the 1990s will become even more significant in the 21st century, as the U.S. population continues to age. Hospitals, along with the entire health care delivery system, must continue to adapt and evolve.

THE PHARMACIST'S ROLE IN A HOSPITAL-BASED PRACTICE

Most hospital pharmacies have an organizational structure that consists of a director of pharmacy, an associate or assistant director, pharmacy managers or supervisors, and pharmacists with clinical and/or distributive responsibilities. Depending on the size of the department, some pharmacists may be solely dedicated to providing clinical services in a specialized area such as infectious diseases or critical care. In addition to professional personnel, the pharmacy department includes technical and support staff who may assist with product preparation, distribution, and purchasing.

Director of Pharmacy

Based on what is expected of this position, the director of pharmacy has one of the most complex jobs within the hospital (Nold and Sander, 2004). The director of pharmacy must satisfy a variety of leadership and management responsibilities, including overseeing both personnel and department budget issues. The director justifies and develops job descriptions for new pharmacy positions and generally manages the recruitment and interview process.

A major challenge facing hospital pharmacy directors today is managing the drug budget in the face of escalating medication costs. While a formulary system (as described later in the chapter) may help control costs, it is often difficult to anticipate how the cost of a new drug will affect the overall drug budget. The inability to contain drug budget costs may have a negative impact on the personnel budget and result in the loss of existing positions or failure to get approval for new ones.

In addition to leadership and fiscal responsibilities, the director often serves as the department representative on a number of multidisciplinary hospital committees. The director is also responsible for setting quality standards for the department, evaluating policies and procedures, implementing new programs, and ensuring compliance with regulating agencies such as the Joint Commission, Department of Public Health, and Board of Registration in Pharmacy.

In hospitals with larger pharmacy departments, an associate or assistant director may assist the director with these responsibilities. In addition, managers or supervisors may be responsible for specific areas of the department such as sterile product formulation, outpatient services, or clinical services (Abramowitz and Mork, 1992). By comparison, in smaller hospitals, the pharmacy director may have to provide some staffing as well. Such directors are often referred to as "working directors." In some very small institutions (fewer than 50 beds), the director may be the only full-time pharmacist and would be generally supported by part-time or per-diem personnel.

Staff and Clinical Pharmacists

The staff and clinical pharmacists provide the daily distributive and clinical services for the department of pharmacy. Since many hospital pharmacists provide a combination of both distributive and clinical services, they may not be characterized as either a "staff pharmacist" or a "clinical pharmacist." However, some institutions may still use these terms to distinguish pharmacists whose primary responsibility may be in one area or the other. Staff pharmacists are generally more involved with routine pharmacy operations (e.g., order entry/verification, checking medication carts, sterile product preparation), and they supervise the activities of the technicians and other support staff who help with these activities. Clinical pharmacists are generally more involved with patient-care-related activities, including rounding with medical teams, obtaining medication histories, providing discharge counseling, managing adverse drug reaction programs, and responding to drug information inquiries.

Because hospitals operate "24/7," an appropriate number of professional staff must be available to provide continuous pharmaceutical services. Joint Commission standards require that a qualified pharmacist be on call or available at another institution to answer questions or provide any medications that are not readily accessible to nonpharmacist personnel (Joint Commission, 2004). Effective July 1, 2006, only pharmacists should be allowed into a pharmacy after it is closed; nurses or other non-pharmacist personnel should not be able to gain access to the pharmacy to secure medications after hours.

Joint Commission standards also require that a pharmacist review all medication orders before they are dispensed unless a licensed independent practitioner (e.g., a physician) controls the ordering, preparation, and administration of the order, or if a delay would result in patient harm. If a pharmacist is not available 24 hours a day, then a qualified health care professional (e.g., a nurse) must review the order and a pharmacist must conduct a retrospective review as soon as he or she is available (Joint Commission, 2004).

Technical and Support Staff

The technical personnel of a hospital pharmacy department comprise pharmacy technicians. These personnel have received special training in drug distribution, either from the hospital or from a school, such as a community college, that offers technician training programs. Pharmacy students who are fulfilling internship requirements may perform some of the tasks of a technician. Under the supervision of the pharmacist, technicians perform many of the distribution functions within the pharmacy department such as filling unit-dose cassettes, preparing IV admixtures, and monitoring and restocking inventory within the pharmacy and on the nursing stations.

Two national voluntary technician certification programs have been established: The Exam for the Certification of Pharmacy Technicians (ExCPT), sponsored by the Institute for the Certification of Pharmacy Technicians (ICPT) and the Pharmacy Technician Certification Exam (PTCE), sponsored by the Pharmacy Technician Certification Board (PTCB). Certification encourages technicians to expand their knowledge and skill base, and it provides technicians with formal national recognition of their training (Murer, 1996). The expanding role of the technician allows the pharmacist to concentrate on more direct patient care or clinical activities (see Chapter 3). A technician was most likely responsible for initially preparing Frank's medications, which were then checked by the pharmacist.

In addition to technicians, the support staff of the pharmacy department may include clerical personnel and individuals responsible for inventory management.

RESPONSIBILITIES OF THE HOSPITAL PHARMACY

The hospital pharmacy is responsible for the safe and effective use of drug therapy for the entire institution. Its duties include drug product selection, procurement, and distribution. The pharmacy is also responsible for ensuring that medications are prescribed appropriately and that guidelines for proper drug administration are followed (Black and Nelson, 1992).

DRUG DISTRIBUTION SYSTEMS

Floor-Stock Distribution

Floor-stock distribution was the traditional method of drug distribution for many years. This system involves supplying the nursing staff units with a predetermined number of dosage forms, which are stored in a separate drug room on each patient care area. Nurses dispense the medications to any number of patients from this supply, and then they reorder from the pharmacy as needed.

Two major problems have been identified with floor-stock distribution. First, the pharmacist does not have the opportunity to review the physician's order for accuracy or potential drug interactions before the medication is administered to the patient. Second, the pharmacist does not have the chance to review the patient's profile to monitor drug therapy for safety and efficacy.

Although floor-stock distribution may be sometimes used to provide bulk supplies such as powders, some basic intravenous solutions (e.g., D_5W and normal saline), and selected emergency medications, the unit-dose distribution system is the distribution system of choice in hospital pharmacies.

Unit-Dose Distribution

The unit-dose distribution system was developed in the mid-1960s to encourage the pharmacist to become more actively involved in the patient's drug therapy (Barker and Heller, 1963). A recent survey of more than 1,000 hospital pharmacy directors indicated that more than 80% of the hospitals dispensed more than 75% of oral doses and approximately 65% of parenteral doses to non-critical care patients as unit doses (Pederson, Schneider, and Scheckelhoff, 2006). The number of hospitals reporting that they use a unit-dose distribution system has increased steadily since 1999.

The unit-dose distribution system consists of two key elements. First, a pharmacist reviews all physicians' orders for appropriateness and potential drug interactions before medications are dispensed. Second, medications are dispensed in "unit doses," where each dose of medication is separately packaged and labeled with the drug name, strength, lot number, and expiration date in a ready-to-administer form (like the one that Frank received). Products may be purchased in unit-dose forms or repackaged from bulk dosage forms. The Food and Drug Administration (FDA) bar-code rule may explain the recent increase in repackaging reported by hospitals (Pederson et al., 2006). This rule requires bar codes on all labels of thousands of drugs and biological products (FDA, 2004), but may have resulted in decreased availability of drugs in unit-dose forms (Pederson et al., 2006).

With the unit-dose distribution system, each patient has an assigned drawer that is typically filled with a 24-hour supply of medication. For instance, if a patient is getting a medication every 8 hours, three doses of the drug would be supplied in that person's drawer. Patients' drawers are part of a medication cart for a specific patient care area; the drawers are exchanged at a predetermined time every day so they can be replenished by the pharmacy. In manual unit-dose distribution systems, the medication fill process is generally performed by a technician and verified by a pharmacist, although some hospitals may use technicians to check other technicians (Woller et al., 1991). Approximately 15% of hospitals have a robotic distribution system that automates the cart fill process, with larger hospitals being more likely to rely on such technology (Pederson et al., 2006). This percentage also has steadily increased over the past few years, despite the fact the robotic systems are relatively expensive.

For new orders or medication changes, an alternative delivery system must be used to ensure that patients get their medication in a timely fashion. Either the pharmacy or another department is responsible for regular medication runs to patient care areas.

More than 40% of hospitals surveyed in one study reported using automated dispensing systems (ADS) to deliver "stat" doses of medications in between routine scheduled cart exchanges (Pederson et al., 2006). ADS devices, such as Pyxis, are available in patient care areas, and they dispense medications after the pharmacist reviews the order. These systems offer some potential advantages over traditional, manually processed cart exchange methods and "stat" deliveries, including reduced drug delivery time and better inventory control. These devices also provide emergency doses of medications in the absence of 24-hour pharmacy services. If Frank had required an emergency medication for his heart condition, that drug would have been readily available in the cardiac care unit. ADS may also free up the pharmacist to engage in more patient-care-related activities.

The advantages of the unit-dose system include fewer medication errors, because the pharmacist reviews the medication order before dispensing. In addition, inventory costs are reduced by significantly cutting back on floor-stock supplies. However, labor costs are higher because more personnel are required to fill unit-dose drawers. In addition, sometimes it is necessary to prepare medication in unit doses that are not commercially available. Another drawback to the unit-dose system is the potential for delays in getting the medication to patients, because drugs are not stocked in the patient care area. For this reason, "emergency kits" that contain drugs used in situations such as cardiac arrest are routinely available in patient care areas for immediate access. Despite these minor limitations, the unit-dose system remains the preferred drug distribution system owing to its potential for improved patient care and better cost-effectiveness (Black and Nelson, 1992).

CENTRALIZED VERSUS DECENTRALIZED PHARMACY SERVICES

Hospital pharmacy services may be provided either from a centralized area or from two or more satellite locations.

Centralized pharmacy services originate from a single location within the hospital. This scheme is the distribution system most commonly utilized by hospital pharmacies, although many hospitals are switching to a more decentralized function (Pederson et al., 2006). Because all pharmacy services are provided from a single location, fewer professional and technical resources are required than with decentralized services (John, Burkhart, and Lamy, 1976). In addition, inventory remains more consolidated, which reduces overall drug and supply costs. Survey data indicate that the use of a particular type of distribution system is dependent on the number of beds in the facility, with centralized drug distribution systems being more common in smaller hospitals than in larger ones (Pederson et al., 2006).

Some hospital pharmacies provide pharmacy services from satellite locations in patient care areas or specialized areas, such as the operating room or emergency department. At a minimum, these decentralized services perform first-dose dispensing and pharmacist order review. Most satellites are supported by a centralized pharmacy that generally fills medication carts and performs other distributive functions. For example, Frank's first doses were provided from a satellite pharmacy in the cardiology unit to which he was admitted, but all subsequent doses were prepared in the central pharmacy. Decentralized services offer the primary advantage of having a pharmacist's presence in a patient care area, such as the pharmacist Frank encountered who specialized in cardiology. The major drawbacks of decentralization are the duplication of inventory and the additional professional and technical personnel needed to staff satellites, which increase the overall costs. A recent survey found that pharmacy directors are split evenly over the type of system they foresee for their institutions in the future, with larger hospitals (more than 400 beds) more likely to consider decentralized systems (Pederson et al., 2006).

One method suggested to improve prescribing practice is the use of computerized prescriber order entry (CPOE), although only a small number of hospitals (5%) reported using it in a recent survey (Pederson, Schneider, and Scheckelhoff, 2005). Larger hospitals are far more likely to have such systems in place than smaller hospitals (Pederson et al., 2005). Some evidence indicates that CPOE may enhance patient care by reducing medication errors, although the successful implementation of the system is a complex process requiring input from a variety of health care professionals (Shane, 2002).

Bar coding is another technology that can be used to scan and verify the correct patient and medication. Although it is not widely utilized by many hospitals at present, survey data indicate that use of this approach is increasing (Pederson et al., 2006).

INTRAVENOUS ADMIXTURE SERVICES

Pharmacy personnel often prepare sterile dosage forms of medications. This requires special training in aseptic technique to ensure product integrity and to reduce infectious complications. Hospitals and other organizations that compound sterile products must be in compliance with new standards set by the *U.S. Pharmacopeia* (USP Chapter <797>). These standards define how all sterile products should be prepared based on risk level. The risk level—low, medium, or high—is determined by factors such as how many manipulations are involved in compounding the final product and whether it is prepared from sterile or nonsterile ingredients (United States Pharmacopeial Convention, 2004).

Intravenous admixture services include the preparation of large-volume parenteral medications such as parenteral nutrition solutions and electrolyte replacement preparations (e.g., potassium chloride infusions), as well as small-volume parenteral medications such as antibiotics. Hospital pharmacies generally maintain special, environmentally controlled facilities, such as a clean room or laminar flow workbenches, in which to prepare sterile products. Such facilities are designed not only to protect the product from contamination, but also to protect the person preparing the product from potential exposure to hazardous or toxic products (e.g., chemotherapy). Some hospital pharmacies may outsource bulk compounding of parenteral solutions (e.g., parenteral nutrition solutions) to an agency that specializes in sterile product preparations if this approach is more cost-effective (Gates, Smolarek, and Stevenson, 1996). During his hospitalization, Frank required several large-volume intravenous solutions that were prepared by the pharmacy department in compliance with USP Chapter <797>.

NONDISTRIBUTIVE PHARMACY SERVICES

Drug Therapy Monitoring

In addition to being responsible for drug distribution, hospital pharmacists provide a wide variety of direct patient care services. The focus of most clinical pharmacy practice is drug therapy monitoring, to promote the safe and effective use of medications within the institution. Drug therapy monitoring involves verifying drug, dose, and route of administration and monitoring for medication-related problems to optimize drug therapy. Some pharmacists, like Frank's cardiology specialist, may routinely participate in patient care rounds with the medical staff to assess the patient's status and provide point-of-care input into the patient's therapy. Pharmacists may also conduct admission drug histories to ensure that the patient continues to receive a chronic medication during hospitalization or to evaluate the situation based on the potential for drug-induced problems.

Given the cost constraints so prevalent in health care, pharmacists must consider both the fiscal implications and the clinical impact of each drug order. For example, can a less expensive therapeutic alternative be prescribed, or can the patient receive the medication orally rather than intravenously? During his hospitalization, Frank's cardiology pharmacist was able to suggest a cost-effective oral antiplatelet therapy for him.

In-Service Education

Pharmacists serve as a valuable drug therapy resource to physicians, nurses, and other health care personnel within the hospital. They may also counsel patients on their medications before discharge or in the ambulatory clinics of the institution. Pharmacists often provide in-service education programs on issues related to drug therapy to physicians, nurses, and other interested parties. They may participate with other members of the health care team on daily patient care rounds, during which the status of patients is evaluated and changes are made to their therapeutic regimens. During these rounds, the pharmacist has the opportunity to provide input on drug therapy before the order is written. To support these educational endeavors, many hospital pharmacies publish a newsletter to help update the hospital community on a new drug, pharmacy service, or other related topic.

Medication-Utilization Evaluation

Medication-utilization evaluation (MUE) is a multidisciplinary quality assurance program that was incorporated into the Joint Commission's standards in 1992. Current standards do not require a specific method be used, but rather focus on the quality improvement aspect of MUE (Joint Commission, 2004).

MUE programs objectively evaluate the use of selected drugs in the hospital by comparing them to specific criteria established for these medications, including medication-related activities such as dispensing and administration. MUE criteria typically include justification for use, monitoring parameters that should be followed, and outcome measures to determine efficacy. Results of the MUE are reviewed, opportunities for improvement are noted, and corrective actions are taken to improve drug use.

MUE programs may focus on a specific medication, a particular class of medications, or an outcome or a component of the medication use process. Drugs may be selected for MUE because of their potential risk if used inappropriately or because of their high cost compared to alternative therapies. For example, inappropriate use of an expensive antibiotic may not only increase overall drug costs to the institution but also result in the development of drug-resistant pathogens. The pharmacy department may dictate which medications should undergo MUE (e.g., expensive medications or potentially toxic drugs) and work in collaboration with other health care disciplines to establish the criteria for their use.

In addition to performing data collection and analysis, the pharmacy may direct the efforts to correct any deficiencies in drug use found during the MUE process. Such efforts may include in-service educational programs and pharmacy newsletters.

Adverse-Drug-Reaction Monitoring

Adverse-drug-reaction (ADR) monitoring is another quality assurance activity in which the pharmacy department participates. The major focus of ADR monitoring is the reduction of preventable ADRs within the hospital. Suspected ADRs are reviewed by the pharmacy to determine the likelihood of an untoward event from a medication. In addition, the pharmacy can alert the medical staff to ADRs that may be associated with drugs that have recently been made available within the hospital.

Specialized Clinical Pharmacy Services

Pharmacists may specialize in an area of practice such as infectious diseases, nutrition support, critical care, or cardiology, such as the pharmacist on Frank's medical team. These specialists are responsible for monitoring drug therapy in a more selective patient population. For example, the infectious disease specialist may focus his or her efforts on appropriate antibiotic selection; the critical care pharmacist may be responsible for patients in the medical or surgical intensive care units of the hospital; the nutrition support specialist may monitor patients receiving parenteral nutrition; and the cardiology specialist may be responsible for monitoring anticoagulation therapy. Certification or credentialing in the area of specialization may be strongly encouraged or required for pharmacists in these positions (see Chapter 3).

Some specialized clinical pharmacy services are provided as part of a formal consultation service, and the clinical activity is performed following the written order of a physician. Pharmacokinetic consultation services are provided by many hospital pharmacies to optimize therapy using serum drug concentrations. In some cases, pharmacies may be reimbursed by third parties for such consultation services.

Although all pharmacists are responsible for providing basic drug information, some hospitals have established formal drug information (DI) services. Pharmacists with special training in drug literature retrieval and evaluation generally provide these DI services. A recent survey of more than 150 DI centers in the United States reported that 73% of the funding for drug information centers has been provided by hospitals, with the remainder coming from colleges or universities (Rosenberg et al., 2004). This percentage is significantly lower than that reported in 1986 (88%) and may reflect the cost constraints that hospitals are faced within the current health care environment.

HOSPITAL FORMULARY SYSTEM

The purpose of a hospital formulary system is to help ensure appropriate drug therapy and control drug costs. The formulary itself is only one component of the overall system. The formulary is a "continually revised compilation of pharmaceuticals that reflects the current clinical judgment of the medical staff" (American Society of Hospital Pharmacists [ASHP], 1983). Whereas the formulary is essentially a list of medications routinely stocked in the pharmacy, the formulary "system" involves the overall process of evaluating and selecting medications to be included in the formulary. Consequently, only certain representatives of a class of drugs may be available. The decision to add or delete a drug from the formulary is based on the relative clinical benefit and cost of the medication as compared to other agents within a similar therapeutic class, or to nonpharmacotherapeutic options such as surgery.

In a hospital with a "closed" formulary system, physicians are directed to prescribe only those agents that are on the formulary unless the patient's medical condition dictates that a nonformulary drug is necessary. The prescriber typically has to document the reason why the alternative drug is required before the pharmacy will obtain it. As was the situation with Frank, nonformulary drugs are not routinely available within such a system and a therapeutically equivalent agent may need to be substituted for it. Under an "open" formulary system, although physicians are encouraged to prescribe formulary drugs, nonformulary medications are generally more readily available.

The advisory group that determines which drugs are included in the hospital formulary is typically called the pharmacy and therapeutics (P&T) committee. The P&T committee is a multidisciplinary committee made up of members of the medical, pharmacy, and nursing departments, as well as hospital administration. Pharmacy members generally include the director of pharmacy, who often is responsible for setting the committee agenda, and a drug information or other clinical pharmacist, who prepares an objective review of each agent requested for addition to the formulary. This review is presented to P&T committee members along with background material provided by the individual requesting the drug for formulary addition. The pharmacist's review provides an impartial perspective of the requested drug's potential benefits as compared to similar medications.

Some agents may be added to the formulary on a "conditional" basis; these drugs are reevaluated after a period of time to determine whether they should remain on the formulary based on clinical experience with the drug. In some cases, a drug may be added with "restriction," meaning that the agent may be prescribed only by selected individuals. For example, an infectious disease specialist may have to approve an order for certain antibiotics before the pharmacy can distribute these drugs. Such restrictions usually apply to drugs that are very expensive or whose potential risks warrant that they be prescribed only by physicians who are very familiar with their appropriate use.

PURCHASING AND INVENTORY CONTROL

The pharmacy department is primarily responsible for drug management in the hospital, including purchasing and inventory control. Once the formulary status of a drug is determined, the decision regarding the brand of product acquired is ultimately made by the pharmacy; factors such as quality of manufacturer, cost, and dosage forms available all play a role in this decision.

Group-Purchasing Agreements

Many hospitals participate in group-purchasing agreements. Under such agreements, hospitals can collaborate with other institutions to negotiate more favorable pricing with pharmaceutical manufacturers.

Investigational Drugs

The pharmacy is also responsible for controlling the use of investigational drugs within the hospital. The pharmacist must be knowledgeable about investigational protocols being used within the hospital, including drug information, pharmaceutical data, recordkeeping procedures, and proper administration techniques. In institutions that conduct a great deal of drug-related research, a specific investigational drug pharmacist is often responsible for coordinating these activities.

RESIDENCY PROGRAMS

A pharmacy residency is an organized, directed, postgraduate training program designed to develop competencies in a defined area of pharmacy practice (Lazarus and Letendre, 1992). Most residency programs last 12 months and are now referred to as PGY1 (postgraduate year 1) residency training. Unlike undergraduate training programs such as internships, a residency is designed to develop skills beyond those required by the state board of pharmacy for licensure. A residency is distinguished from a fellowship, another type of postgraduate program, by its preparation of the pharmacist for practice rather than independent research (see Chapter 3). Pharmacy residents typically engage in patient-care-related activities, such as counseling Frank from the chapter-opening case study on his discharge medications.

Some residency programs may offer training at an advanced level and are referred to a PGY2 programs. These programs require that the trainee complete a PGY1 program first.

In response to an increased need for qualified hospital pharmacy practitioners, the American Society of Hospital Pharmacists (ASHP) established the first accredited, postgraduate training program in 1962 (Lazarus and Letendre, 1992). The ASHP (now the American Society of Health-System Pharmacists) program was the first to assess compliance with minimal standards for postgraduate training by an external review process. Programs that are ASHP-accredited have been reviewed by a team of individuals from outside the hospital who determine whether the institution complies with the minimal training standards established by the ASHP.

Hospital pharmacy residency programs may be either oriented toward general pharmacy practice or concentrated in a specific area of pharmacy practice (such as primary care or drug information). If someone is interested in pursuing a career in hospital pharmacy, doing a residency is strongly suggested.

CONCLUSIONS

The changing health care environment presents significant challenges as well as opportunities for hospitals. Those institutions that adapt most quickly to these changes will position themselves more favorably to succeed in the future. Pharmacists play a significant role in the delivery of health care within the institutional setting. Individuals who wish to practice in the hospital may be advised to pursue postgraduate training experience.

QUESTIONS FOR FURTHER DISCUSSION

1. Describe the hospital of the future. Will hospitals exist as they are currently configured?
2. What role should hospitals play in the continuum of care?
3. What opportunities will be available in the future for hospital pharmacists? Will their roles expand?
4. How will automation affect drug delivery and the pharmacist's role in the hospital?

KEY TOPICS AND TERMS

Adverse drug reaction (ADR)
American Hospital Association
Centralized pharmacy services
Decentralized pharmacy services
Diagnosis-related group (DRG)
Drug therapy monitoring
Drug-utilization evaluation (DUE)
Floor-stock distribution
Formulary
Horizontal integration
Joint Commission on Accreditation of Healthcare Organizations
Length of stay
Unit-dose distribution
Vertical integration

REFERENCES

Abramowitz, P. W., & Mork, L. A. (1992). The hospital and the department of pharmaceutical services. In T. R. Brown (Ed.), *Handbook of institutional pharmacy practice* (3rd ed.) (pp. 19–29). Bethesda, MD: American Society of Hospital Pharmacists.

American Hospital Association (AHA). (2006). *About the AHA.* Retrieved May 10, 2006, from http://www.aha.org/aha/about/index.html

American Society of Hospital Pharmacists (ASHP). (1983). American Society of Hospital Pharmacists statement on the operation of the formulary system. *American Journal of Hospital Pharmacy, 40,* 1384–1385.

Auxter, S. (1997). JCAHO announces new accreditation process. *Clinical Laboratory News, 23*(4), 1, 4.

Barker, K. N., & Heller, W. M. (1963). The development of a centralized unit dose dispensing system. Part one: Description of the UAMC experimental system. *American Journal of Hospital Pharmacy, 20,* 568–579.

Black, H. J., & Nelson, S. P. (1992). Medication distribution systems. In T. R. Brown (Ed.), *Handbook of institutional pharmacy practice* (3rd ed.) (pp. 165–174). Bethesda, MD: American Society of Hospital Pharmacists.

Food and Drug Administration. (2004). *FDA issues bar-code regulation.* Retrieved May 8, 2006, from www.fda.gov/oc/initiatives/barcode-sadr/fs-barcode.html.

Gates, D. M., Smolarek, R. T., & Stevenson, J. G. (1996). Outsourcing the preparation of parenteral nutrient solutions. *American Journal of Health-System Pharmacy, 53,* 2176–2178.

Health Forum. (2005). *AHA hospital statistics 2005 edition.* Chicago, IL: Health Forum (American Hospital Association).

Institute for the Future. (2000). *Health and health care 2010: The forecast, the challenge.* San Francisco: Jossey-Bass.

John, G. W., Burkhart, V. D., & Lamy, P. P. (1976). Pharmacy personnel activities and costs in decentralized and centralized unit dose distribution systems. *American Journal of Hospital Pharmacy, 33,* 38–43.

Joint Commission on Accreditation of Healthcare Organizations. (2004). *Comprehensive accreditation manual for hospitals.* Oakbrook Terrace, IL: Joint Commission on Accreditation of Healthcare Organizations.

Joint Commission on Accreditation of Healthcare Organizations. (2006). *Facts about the Joint Commission.* Retrieved May 10, 2006, from http://www.joint-commission.org/AboutUs/joint_commission_fact.htm

Lazarus, H. L., & Letendre, D. E. (1992). Residency programs in pharmacy practice. In T. R. Brown (Ed.), *Handbook of institutional pharmacy practice* (3rd ed.) (pp. 39–43). Bethesda, MD: American Society of Hospital Pharmacists.

Massachusetts Hospital Association. (1995). *Vision 2000: Caring for people into the 21st century.* Burlington, MA: Massachusetts Hospital Association.

Meites, S. (1995). Abraham Flexner's legacy: A magnificent beneficence to American medical education and clinical chemistry. *Clinical Chemistry, 41*(4), 627–632.

Murer, M. M. (1996). Technician certification leads to recognition, better patient care. *Journal of the American Pharmaceutical Association, 36*(8), 514, 519–520.

Nold E. G., & Sander, W. T. (2004). Role of the director of pharmacy: The first six months. *American Journal of Health-System Pharmacy, 61,* 2297–2310.

Pedersen, C. A., Schneider, P. J., & Scheckelhoff, D. J. (2005). ASHP national survey of pharmacy practice in hospital settings: Prescribing and transcribing. *American Journal of Health-System Pharmacy, 62,* 378–390.

Pedersen, C. A., Schneider, P. J., & Scheckelhoff, D. J. (2006). ASHP national survey of pharmacy practice in hospital settings: Dispensing and administration—2005. *American Journal of Health-System Pharmacy, 63,* 327–345.

Raffel, M. W., & Raffel, N. K. (1989). *The U. S. health system: Origins and functions* (3rd ed.). New York: Delmar.

Roberts, J. S., Coale, J. G., & Redman, R. R. (1987). A history of the Joint Commission on Accreditation of Hospitals. *Journal of the American Medical Association, 258*(7), 936–940.

Rosenberg, J. M., Koumis, T., Nathan, J. P., et al (2004). Current status of pharmacist-operated drug information centers in the United States—2003. *American Journal of Health-System Pharmacy, 61,* 2023–2032.

Shane, R. (2002). Computerized physician order entry: Challenges and opportunities. *American Journal of Health-System Pharmacy, 59,* 286–288.

United States Pharmacopeial Convention. (2004). Pharmaceutical considerations—sterile preparations (general information chapter 797). In *The United States pharmacopeia* (26th rev.)/*National formulary* (22nd ed.) (pp. 2350–2370). Rockville, MD: United States Pharmacopeial Convention, Inc

Woller, T. W., Stuart, J. S., Vrabel, R., et al. (1991). Checking of unit dose cassettes by pharmacy technicians at three Minnesota hospitals. *American Journal of Hospital Pharmacy, 48,* 1952–1956.

Ambulatory Care

David M. Scott

Case Scenario

As a consultant to George, a 45-year-old pharmacist, you have been asked to provide him with some advice about whether he should integrate pharmaceutical care into his community pharmacy practice. Over the past 20 years, George has developed a thriving independent community pharmacy practice in a rural community of 2,000 persons in a Midwestern state. However, the trend toward third-party prescription payment, greater managed care penetration (which is expected to continue in the next five years), and an increasing number of prescriptions being transferred to mail-order pharmacies and Web-based pharmacies has created financial difficulties for George's business.

To counter this economic pressure, George is considering developing a pharmaceutical care practice. If he decides to pursue this route, George plans to market the pharmaceutical care program initially to his private-pay patients, and by the second year, to managed care organizations. Common disease states that are most prevalent in this rural community are hypertension, diabetes, and asthma. George has maintained an adequate level of prescription care, but he realizes that a high-level pharmaceutical care practice does require a major shift in his practice.

What would you advise him to do? When formulating your answer, consider the trends in ambulatory care, the impact that pharmaceutical care has made on community pharmacy practice, and the training and workforce changes that George must incorporate to implement this change in his practice.

LEARNING OBJECTIVES _____

Upon completion of this chapter, the student shall be able to:

- Explain what is meant by the term ambulatory care
- Describe what settings provide ambulatory care
- Describe the concept of primary care
- Explain how managed care is affecting ambulatory care
- Describe the contributions the Indian Health Service has made in pharmaceutical care
- Depict the pharmacist's role in ambulatory care

CHAPTER QUESTIONS

1. What settings provide ambulatory care services?
2. How is managed care altering ambulatory care?
3. What contributions did the Indian Health Service make in pharmaceutical care?
4. How is pharmaceutical care affecting ambulatory care?

INTRODUCTION

Ambulatory care services have rapidly evolved and expanded in the past two decades. Managed care has spirited the change away from the inpatient side of hospitals to less costly forms of services provided in the outpatient settings. As costs of health care continue to rise, employers, insurance companies, and policy makers are continually searching for new ways to provide care that maintain quality, yet are accessible and cost-effective. This chapter will examine the settings that provide ambulatory care, depict how managed care is affecting ambulatory care, and describe the pharmacist's role in ambulatory care.

GROWTH OF AMBULATORY CARE

Ambulatory care is care for "an individual presenting for personal health services, who is neither bedridden, nor currently admitted to any health care institution" (Schappert, 1992). Ambulatory care services have greatly expanded in recent years because of the rapid growth of managed care and the greater emphasis placed on outpatient hospital care. One significant event underlying this change in focus was the 1983 introduction of the Medicare Prospective Payment System (PPS) for inpatient hospitalizations. PPS stimulated hospitals to change from rendering more services to providing shorter lengths of stay and getting patients out of the hospital faster and sicker. These changes encouraged the development of ambulatory care programs and are referred to in the case scenario.

Common Problems

What types of problems are seen in ambulatory care settings? The National Ambulatory Medical Care Survey (NAMCS) is an ongoing survey of ambulatory care. **Table 7-1** lists the distribution of office visits in the United States by common primary diagnosis groups. Most of the common disease states require routine primary care. Therapeutic services summarized in **Table 7-2** show the important roles that medication therapy and patient counseling have in medical management (e.g., acute

Table 7-1   Distribution of Office Visits in the United States by Primary Diagnosis Groups, 2002

Primary Diagnosis Group	Total Visits		Percent Distribution	
	N (1,000)	Total	Female	Male
All visits	889,980	100.0	100.0	100.0
Essential hypertension	46,180	5.4	5.4	5.4
Routine infant or child health check	35,935	4.0	3.2	5.2
Acute upper respiratory infections, excluding pharyngitis	30,141	3.4	3.1	3.7
Diabetes mellitus	24,877	2.8	2.3	3.5
Arthropathies and related disorders	23,725	2.7	2.8	2.4
General medical examination	22,362	2.5	2.5	2.6
Spinal disorders	20,444	2.3	2.3	2.3
Rheumatism, excluding back	17,766	2.0	1.9	2.1
Normal pregnancy	17,585	2.0	3.3	0.0
Otitis media and Eustachian tube disorders	16,702	1.9	1.6	2.2
Malignant neoplasms	15,651	1.8	1.5	2.1
Chronic sinusitis	14,197	1.6	1.6	1.6
Allergic rhinitis	14,101	1.6	1.7	1.4
Asthma	12,692	1.4	1.5	1.3
Gynecological examination	11,883	1.3	2.2	0.0
Lipid disorders	11,767	1.3	1.1	1.6
Heart disease, excluding ischemic	11,670	1.3	1.2	1.5
Ischemic heart disease	10,970	1.2	0.8	1.9
Acute pharyngitis	10,090	1.1	1.1	1.2
Follow-up examination	9,995	1.1	1.0	1.2
All other	509,248	57.2	57.7	56.5

Note: Numbers may not add to totals because of rounding.

Source: National Ambulatory Medical Care Survey. Hyattsville, MD: National Center for Health Statistics, 2002.

Table 7-2 Distribution of Office Visits by Medication Therapy in the United States, 2002

Medication Therapy[a]	Number of Visits		Percent Distribution	
	N (1,000)	Total	Female	Male
All visits	889,980	100.0	100.0	100.0
Drug visits[b]	577,075	64.8	65.5	63.9
Visits without mention of medication	312,906	35.2	34.5	36.1
Number of medications prescribed or provided by the physician				
All visits	889,980	100.0	100.0	100.0
0	312,906	35.2	34.5	36.1
1	239,750	26.9	28.9	27.0
2	146,236	16.4	16.6	16.2
3	76,317	8.6	8.8	8.3
4	39,594	4.4	4.4	4.5
5	23,309	2.6	2.8	2.3
6	51,671	5.8	6.0	5.5

Note: Numbers may not add to totals because of rounding.

[a.] Medications include prescription drugs, over-the-counter preparations, immunizations, and desensitizing agents.

[b.] Drug visits are visits at which one or more medications is prescribed or provided by the physician.

Source: National Ambulatory Medical Care Survey. Hyattsville, MD: National Center for Health Statistics, 2002.

respiratory tract infections, hypertension, and diabetes). Nearly two thirds of physician visits result in one or more medications prescribed by the physician. As summarized in **Table 7-3,** commonly cited prescribed drugs include Lipitor, albuterol, amoxicillin, and Synthroid. **Table 7-4** lists the distribution of drug visits by physician specialty. Prescription drugs were prescribed most commonly by the physician in the specialty area of family practice, followed by internal medicine, pediatrics, and obstetrics and gynecology.

In ambulatory care settings, most of the diagnoses and prescribed drugs come from a few disease states. For this reason, primary-care providers and pharmacists should receive extensive training in the management of these common diseases.

Primary-Care Providers

Primary-care providers include physicians, midwives, nurse practitioners (NPs), and physician assistants (PAs). Although training programs and practice responsibilities vary among states, the primary-care capabilities are similar. Scheffler and colleagues have estimated that NPs

Table 7-3 Distribution of Drug Mentions for the 20 Most Frequently Prescribed Drugs at Office Visits in the United States, 2002

Entry name of the drug[b]	Number of mentions[a]		Therapeutic Classification[c]
	N (1,000)	Percentage of Total	
All drug mentions	1,347,312	100.0	—
Lipitor	18,842	1.4	Hyperlipidemia
Albuterol	15,442	1.1	Asthma
Amoxicillin	14,690	1.1	Penicillins
Synthroid	14,525	1.1	Thyroid
Lasix	14,004	1.0	Diuretics
Celebrex	13,763	1.0	Nonsteroidal anti-inflammatory
Tylenol	12,919	1.0	Analgesics/antipyretics
Vioxx	12,650	0.9	Nonsteroidal anti-inflammatory
Augmentin	11,995	0.9	Penicillins
Norvasc	11,853	0.9	Calcium-channel blockers
Zyrtec	11,573	0.9	Antihistamines
Zocor	11,429	0.8	Hyperlipidemia
Acetysalicylic acid	10,670	0.8	Analgesics/antipyretics
Prednisone	10,422	0.8	Adrenal corticosteroids
Allegra	10,420	0.8	Antihistamines
Coumadin	10,090	0.7	Anticoagulants
Atenolol	9,694	0.7	Beta blockers
Claritin	9,208	0.7	Antihistamines
Paxil	9,118	0.7	Antidepressants
Prevacid	8,981	0.7	Acid/peptic disorders
All other	1,105,025	82.0	—

Note: Numbers may not add to totals because of rounding.

[a] Number of drug mentions divided by total number of visits multiplied by 100.

[b.] Entry made by the physician on the prescription or other medical records. This may be a brand name, generic name, or desired therapeutic effect.

[c] Therapeutic class based on the standard drug classification used in the *National Drug Code. Directory*, 1995 edition.

Source: National Ambulatory Medical Care Survey. Hyattsville, MD: National Center for Health Statistics, 2002.

and PAs can perform about three fourths of services that physicians perform in adult practices and about 90% of services in pediatric practices (Scheffler, Waitzman, and Hillman, 1998). At both the federal and state levels, there is interest in increasing the number of these practitioners, especially in underserved areas (Mezey, 1999; see Chapter 2).

Table 7-4 Distribution of Drug Visits by Physician Specialty in the United States, 2002

Physician Specialty	Drug Visits	
	N (1,000)	Percentage of Total
All specialties	577,075	100.0
General and family practice	165,371	28.7
Internal medicine	115,219	20.0
Pediatrics	80,814	14.0
Obstetrics and gynecology	34,355	6.0
Ophthalmology	25,066	4.3
Dermatology	21,292	3.7
Psychiatry	17,901	3.1
Cardiovascular diseases	15,889	2.8
Orthopedic surgery	14,293	2.5
Urology	8,352	1.4
Otolaryngology	8,033	1.4
Neurology	5,799	1.0
General surgery	4,773	0.8
All other specialties	59,919	10.4

Note: Numbers may not add to totals because of rounding.
Source: National Ambulatory Medical Care Survey. Hyattsville, MD: National Center for Health Statistics, 2002.

TYPES OF MEDICAL PRACTICES

Two major types of medical practices exist. The predominant form is care provided by private-practice physicians in solo, partnership, and private group practice settings on a fee-for-service basis. The second form, which has experienced dramatic growth in recent decades, is ambulatory care provided in organized settings that have an identity independent of that of the physicians practicing in it. This second category includes managed care programs such as health maintenance organizations (HMOs) and preferred provider organizations (PPOs).

Solo Practice

Traditionally, solo medical practice has attracted the largest number of physicians. In recent years, however, the number of solo practitioners has been rapidly decreasing, largely because of managed care pressures. From a physician's perspective, solo practice offers an opportunity to avoid organizational dependence and to be self-employed. Primary-care services provided by solo practitioners include family practice, internal medicine, pediatrics, and obstetrics and gynecology. These solo practitioners care for patients in office space owned or leased by the physician or in the physician's home. When patients are hospitalized, the physician sees them and provides care for them in the hospital.

Group Practice

Besides solo practice, office-based practice includes group practice. Group practice is an affiliation of three or more providers, usually physicians who share income, expenses, facilities, equipment, medical records, and support personnel, and who provide services through a formal organization (Roemer, 1981). Although other definitions exist, the essential elements are formal sharing of resources and distribution of income. The first successful non-industrial group practice was the Mayo Clinic in Rochester, Minnesota. The Mayo Clinic was organized as a single-specialty group practice in 1887; later it was broadened into a multiple-specialty group that showed that group practice was feasible in the private sector.

Advantages of group practice from a physician's perspective include shared operation, joint ownership, centralized administrative functions, and availability of a professional business manager. From a financial viewpoint, the group practice relieves the provider of having to scare up the large initial investment often required to establish a practice. Disadvantages of group practice from a provider's perspective include less individual freedom, less income, weak provider–patient relationships, and greater restrictions on referral practices (Williams, 1993).

MANAGED CARE

Managed care is the use of a planned and coordinated approach to providing health care, with the goal being delivery of quality care at the lowest cost, including emphasis on preventive care. With HMOs, the provider usually receives prepayment for services on a per-member, per-month basis. Thus a provider is paid the same amount of money every month for a member regardless of whether that member receives services and how much those services cost (a service contract). Types of managed care organizations (MCOs) include staff model HMOs, group model HMOs, network HMOs, independent practice association (IPA) model HMOs, point-of-service model HMOs, and PPOs. This classification scheme is based on how the MCO links providers (e.g., physicians, pharmacists, and hospitals) together. These distinct types have "blurred" considerably, and today's MCOs are often hybrids of two or more specific types.

Managed care utilizes a network of providers formed to offer cost-effective services. An HMO is a prepaid (capitation) health plan in which enrollees pay a fixed fee (often with a co-payment) for designated health services. A PPO is an insurance plan in which the MCO contracts with health providers to provide health services under a discounted-fee schedule. This health care plan is prepaid, and the member or family is enrolled usually for one year and is entitled to certain agreed-upon services. Health care services usually include physician visits, hospital services, prescription drugs, mental health services, and home health care services.

Typically, a primary-care physician (gatekeeper) is chosen or assigned to coordinate an individual or family's health care services. When a specialist referral or hospital service is required, the gatekeeper physician must approve these services. If an individual or family goes outside the plan for these services, these services are usually not fully reimbursed or may not be reimbursable at all. Strong incentives are built in to encourage members to stay within the system (see Chapter 16).

HOSPITAL-RELATED AMBULATORY SERVICES

Hospital Clinics

Hospital clinics developed as American dispensaries in the 1700s and were intended to serve the urban poor and individuals who did not require inpatient care. Dispensaries were often free-standing buildings, so indigent care did not mix with the paid hospital patients. The first U.S. dispensary was established in Philadelphia in 1786, followed by facilities in New York City, Boston, and Baltimore. A physician and/or apothecary who provided minor surgery, extracted teeth, and prescribed medications generally staffed the dispensary. By the mid-1850s, larger dispensaries had both a physician and a pharmacist. Financial support was meager and reliant on private donations. Most physicians volunteered their services without compensation. Free-standing dispensaries grew to about 100 by 1900 (Roemer, 1981).

By 1916, public health dispensaries' clinics experienced rapid expansion and numbered 1,300 sites, including about 500 for tuberculosis, 400 for baby hygiene, 250 for school children, and 150 for other purposes. Clinics maintained their preventive orientation, and clientele were usually limited to low-income groups. Private medical practitioners increasingly saw dispensaries as competitive and spoke of the "abuse of the dispensary" by patients who could properly afford private medical care. Since the end of World War I, private medical practice and hospitals have continued to flourish, causing the steady decline and closure of charitable dispensaries (Roemer, 1981). Hospital clinics have continued to provide health care for poor persons, although very little free care remains. Those patients not covered by Medicare, Medicaid, or commercial insurance usually pay according to a means-tested sliding fee scale. In some states, "a free-care pool" exists to offset the costs of providing unreimbursed care.

Teaching Hospital Clinics

In response to the managed care movement, teaching hospitals have reorganized their clinics to function more as group practices. Many teaching hospitals now have three groups of clinics: (1) medical, (2) surgical, and (3) others. General medical clinics approximate a family practice or general internal medicine clinic, but may also include other medicine areas, such as dermatology and cardiology. Surgical clinics generally include general surgery, urology, orthopedics, and plastic surgery, and they provide follow-up care for these patients. The "other" category of clinics includes pediatrics, obstetrics and gynecology, and other specialties, such as rehabilitation medicine (Mezey and Lawrence, 1995).

As the managed care movement casts its net even farther, hospitals will become more responsive to community needs and move toward organizing medical care in a model that Madison (1983) has described as community-oriented primary care. Within this model, greater attention will be paid to common disease states and the primary-care practitioner will play an even more important role (Mezey and Lawrence, 1995). Academic health centers (AHCs), for example, have been aggressively developing primary-care networks to maintain their missions of clinical research, resident and student training, and patient care. AHCs have constructed new facilities, bought existing practices, or created partnerships with other hospitals to increase their primary-care clinic base. For instance, the University of Nebraska Medical Center (a public, state-owned teaching hospital) merged with Clarkson Hospital (private, nonprofit) in Omaha, Nebraska, to expand its network of primary-care clinics.

Veterans Affairs Medical Centers (VAMCs) have been among the leaders in the expansion of pharmacists' roles in ambulatory care. Pharmacists have participated in VA primary-care clinics' initiatives to improve blood pressure and increase medication compliance. Pharmacists have also become involved in pharmacist-managed anticoagulation clinics, where they have provided benefits over usual care in the form of desired therapeutic control with fewer adverse effects (Alsuwaidan, Malone, Billups, and Carter, 1998). Foss reported that two thirds of clinic patients were within the therapeutic range following such interventions, and the percentage of thromboembolic complications was one-third that of usual-care patients (Foss, Shoch, and Sintek, 1999).

The Impact of Managed Pharmaceutical Care on Resource Utilization and Outcomes in Veterans Affairs Medical Centers (IMPROVE) study has been one of the largest studies to date to examine the outcomes with pharmaceutical care. Nine VAMCs participated in this study, in which a total of 1,054 patients were randomized to either an intervention group ($n = 523$) or a control group ($n = 531$). After identifying patients at high risk for developing drug-related problems, pharmacists documented a total of 1,855 contacts in the intervention group and implemented 3,048 therapy-specific interventions over the 12-month study period. Following these interventions, hemoglobin A_{1c} measurements were found to be improved in the intervention group compared with the control group (Carter et al., 2001).

The IMPROVE study also examined the impact of ambulatory pharmacist interventions in management of dyslipidemias in older adults. In addition to usual medical care, clinical pharmacists were responsible for providing pharmaceutical care for patients in the intervention group. The control group received usual medical care only. The change in total cholesterol and the reduction in low-density lipoprotein (bad cholesterol) levels were found to be significantly greater in the pharmacist intervention group than in the control group (Ellis et al., 2000).

With the growth of the pharmacist roles in ambulatory care, guidelines have been developed outlining the minimum requirements for the operation and management of pharmaceutical services for patients in the ambulatory care setting. Clinical practice guidelines are being developed and increasingly incorporated into health information systems. Murray and colleagues, for example, reported on a study to measure the effects of the electronic display of guideline-based, patient-specific treatment suggestions on pharmacist work patterns (Murray, Loos, Eckert, Zhou, and Tierney, 1999). The results showed that a dramatic change in work patterns occurred when pharmacists were provided with an electronic display of guidelines. In comparison with the control group, pharmacists with access to treatment suggestions spent less of their time preparing and filling prescriptions and more of their time functioning in an advisory role with patients, physicians, and nurses. Pharmacists in the intervention group also spent more of their time solving problems (Murray et al., 1999).

Ambulatory Surgery Centers

Response to the prospective payment system and managed care pressures on hospitals has led to the establishment of ambulatory surgery centers. Ambulatory surgery centers can be housed in hospital-based settings or in a free-standing ambulatory surgical center. Many surgeries that in the past required lengthy hospital stays can now be done in outpatient surgery centers in less time and at a lower cost. Patients having surgeries such as hernia repair are often admitted by 8:00 A.M. and discharged before noon. In fact, many third-party payers require surgical procedures to be done on an ambulatory basis unless evidence suggests that the procedure would be unsafe for the patient. As a consequence, the majority of surgical procedures are now done on an outpatient basis. Generally, surgery centers report a high level of patient satisfaction, and patients think that the quality of care is good.

Other Outpatient Services

Other outpatient services include free-standing diagnostic imaging centers, home intravenous services, and home care services. Additional ambulatory services will undoubtedly emerge as government and MCOs continue to seek delivery of care at a reduced cost (see Chapter 10).

EMERGENCY SERVICES

Hospital Emergency Services

Approximately 93% of community hospitals in the United States have emergency departments. Misuse of the emergency department has drawn intense scrutiny because it leads to routine care being delivered in expensive facilities at high costs.

Weinerman and colleagues (1966) defined three categories of cases presenting to the emergency departments: (1) nonurgent, (2) urgent, and (3) emergent cases. An "emergent" case is a condition requiring immediate medical attention where any time delay would be potentially threatening to life or function. An "urgent" case involves a condition that requires attention within a few hours, but is not necessarily life-threatening. A "nonurgent" condition is non-acute or minor in severity, and emergency service is not required. A review of cases entering emergency departments found that of all patients using emergency services, 5% are emergent, 45% are urgent, and 50% are nonurgent (Jonas et al., 1976). Consequently, most of the "nonurgent" conditions presenting at emergency departments involve delivery of costly services that could be provided at a less expensive venue, such as a clinic, emergi-center, or physician's office. For this reason, some managed care systems require enrollees to get prior approval before authorizing emergency services.

Medicaid patients often seek care from an emergency department because it is the only option available when they believe they need immediate attention. After some states implemented Medicaid managed care programs, they showed substantial declines in emergency department use (American College of Healthcare Executives, 1993).

Emergency Medical Services

Federal legislation has stipulated the creation of greatly improved emergency medical services (EMS) throughout the United States. The National Highway Safety Act of 1966, for example, established performance criteria that required states to submit their EMS plans for federal approval. The Emergency Medical Services System Act of 1973 authorized funding over 3 years to states, counties, and nonprofit agencies in an effort to expand and modernize their emergency medical services. Components of these services were expected to include a uniform emergency telephone number (911) and modernization of ambulance design from a hearse-type vehicle to a light van with equipment to provide cardiopulmonary resuscitation (CPR). Ambulance attendants were given emergency medical training so they could provide life support services and trauma treatment en route to the hospital. Thanks to the improved training and equipment, EMS has increased survival rates for victims of both traumatic injuries and myocardial infarction (Hoffer, 1979; Roth, Stewart, Rogers, and Cannon, 1984; Sherman, 1979).

The same legislative acts that set the EMS standards also established community trauma centers and developed trauma teams to handle emergencies. Level I trauma centers offer around-the-clock care including medical and surgical specialists, diagnostic imaging, and operating rooms staffed by personnel in well-equipped, well-trained, intensive care units (Mezey, 1999).

Emergi-centers

Emergency centers (emergi-centers) are designed to provide medical care 24 hours a day, 7 days a week. Another type of facility called an urgi-center provides emergency services, but is open approximately 12 hours a day, 7 days a week. Both centers are designed to provide care for urgent and nonurgent problems. Most do not receive ambulance cases or serve emergent cases, however.

In comparison to services provided at the emergency department, costs are generally lower at emergi-centers. Advantages of these centers include the convenience of and access to services without appointments and long delays, and that health insurance carriers generally prefer them to emergency department treatment (Mezey, 1999).

GOVERNMENT PROGRAMS

Health Department Services

In large European cities, boards of health were established in the 1800s and 1900s to halt the spread of communicable diseases such as plague, cholera, and typhus. Generally, these bodies were temporary boards—once the disease was eradicated, they were dissolved.

In the United States, Massachusetts set up the first state department of health in 1869. In the early days, U.S. health departments dealt largely with the prevention of tuberculosis. Another health department initiative dealt with the reduction of infant mortality by establishing "milk stations" where mothers who could not breastfeed could obtain clean cow's milk to feed their babies. Later, this initiative was expanded to provide advice to low-income mothers on the care of infants; it also established child health clinics and the Visiting Nurses Association.

As an outgrowth of two federal acts passed in the 1920s, maternal and child health (MCH) grants were provided to states for the development of well-baby clinics. In the late 1920s, however, a conservative antigovernment wave swept over the country, led by the American Medical Association (AMA), which attacked these MCH grants as socialistic programs. As a result, the U.S. Congress ended this program in 1929. It was reactivated during the Great Depression as part of Title V of the 1935 Social Security Act (Roemer, 1981).

Most public health agencies in the early 1900s were devoted to environmental problems, sanitation, and collection of statistics on communicable diseases. The 1929 stock market crash and the massive poverty during the 1930s led to a resurgent American public health movement. Currently, four major categories of public health services exist: (1) communicable disease control, (2) MCH services, (3) chronic diseases, and (4) general ambulatory care.

Communicable disease control, the first major category, involves the control of contagious diseases and sexually transmitted diseases (STDs) such as acquired immune deficiency syndrome (AIDS). Immunizations against diseases such as diphtheria, pertussis (whooping cough), tetanus, polio, and measles are given to infants as part of well-baby clinics and other health department-sponsored activities.

The second major category encompasses the maternal and child health clinics that have risen and fallen based on funding provided at federal, state, and local levels. Federal funding for MCH services has generally come from Title V of the Social Security Act and supports local health department services for babies and pregnant women. MCH services are provided to low-income families, while families with moderate to high income are referred to private physicians. As part of President Lyndon Johnson's Great Society Program, comprehensive health care (treatment and prevention) was also established under Social Security Act amendments that authorized grants for maternal and infant care clinics and "children and youth" (C&Y) clinics.

In 1976, the author of this chapter established clinical and distributive pharmaceutical services in an ambulatory C&Y clinic serving low-income families in south Minneapolis (Scott and Nordin, 1980). Instead of filling prescriptions from a prescription blank, the prescriptions were filled from the patient's chart. The pharmacy was located inside the primary patient care area, so the pharmacist could consult with the appropriate health professional or refer the patient for more extensive evaluation. As part of the patient counseling program, the pharmacy staff also administered the first dose of medication prescribed for pediatric patients, including liquid preparations (e.g., antibiotics), ophthalmic drops, and ointments and otic preparations. As part of the clinic's interdisciplinary team, pharmacists provided therapeutic and pharmacokinetics consultations, drug monitoring, drug information, educational programs for the community, and poison prevention services. The pharmacy closed in 1984 because of federal and state funding cutbacks. However, such pharmaceutical care services are possible in clinic settings, community health centers, staff model HMOs, and other ambulatory care settings.

The third major category of public health services focuses on chronic (noncommunicable) diseases—for example, the cancer detection clinic. Other efforts have targeted smoking reduction, Pap smears for cervical cancer detection, breast examinations, and hypertension screening.

The fourth major category of public health services consists of generalized ambulatory care clinics. In the mid-1960s, health departments influenced by the "War on Poverty" movement expanded the scope of these clinics from preventive functions to the provision of general ambulatory care. These clinics were predominantly found in low-income neighborhoods, but the prevailing policy was to turn no one away on grounds of inability to pay. Patients with complex problems were typically referred to a contracted hospital outpatient department. Today, public health clinics are vulnerable to governmental funding priorities and organized medicine pressures to eliminate or reduce the services offered there. Accordingly, health departments generally provide services in areas where most physicians are not interested in working (Roemer, 1981).

Neighborhood and Community Health Centers

In 1965, Congress funded the Neighborhood Health Center (NHC) Act to provide comprehensive health care to low-income populations in urban and rural areas of the United States in an attempt to stimulate societal growth and decrease poverty (Mezey and Lawrence, 1995). The first NHC established in 1965 was the Gouverneur Health Center, which served poor persons from New York's Lower East Side. Other early health center projects were developed in Boston, Chicago, and south-central Los Angeles. Evaluations of these initiatives concluded that NHC program performance was generally equal, and sometimes superior, to that of other established providers of health care (Morehead, Donaldson, and Servavelli, 1971; Sparer and Anderson, 1975). In 1973, the entire NHC program under the Office of Economic Opportunity (OEO) was ended, and the NHC facilities were transferred to the U.S. Public Health Service (PHS) and were designated as Community Health Centers (CHC) (Roemer, 1981).

In 1974, Congress passed the Community Health Centers Act, which defined the scope of CHC services that must be offered to warrant receipt of federal grants. The criteria defining "underserved areas" were quantified and included poverty level as defined by local per-capita income, an excessive infant mortality rate, and a shortage of primary-care physicians. Mandated services in these federally supported CHCs were diagnostic treatment, consultation, and other services by a physician or physician extender; laboratory and X-ray services; dental services; social services; and pharmaceutical services (Roemer, 1981). Currently, 650 CHC organizations operate 2,500 clinics in the United States and serve more than 11 million underserved patients. The 1978 amendments to Sections 329 and 330 of the Public Health Services Act changed the "supplemental" services designation and made pharmacy a "primary" service in CHCs. All CHCs are required to provide prescription drugs for their patients either through on-site licensed pharmacies or through a contracted arrangement with an off-site pharmacy.

The Siouxland Community Health Center (SCHC) is an example of a CHC that provides in-house pharmacy services. SCHC is located in Sioux City, Iowa. The city has become more racially mixed and culturally diverse over the past 20 years, in part because of the changing demographics of the meat packing industry workforce. Hispanics account for more than one half of the minority population, followed by a significant number of Asian Americans, African Americans, and Native Americans. SCHC manages more than 50,000 patient visits per year, and the majority of clients are at or below 100% of the federal poverty level. SCHC facilities include 18 exam rooms, 2 minor procedure rooms, 8 dental operatories (dental chairs), a basic lab, and a pharmacy. The major health concerns encountered by the center's practitioners are diabetes and hypertension. The on-site pharmacy fills more than 300 prescriptions per day.

A number of colleges/schools of pharmacy are developing partnerships with CHCs to integrate clinical pharmacy services in CHCs and to provide training sites for pharmacy students. SCHC, in conjunction with the University of Nebraska's College of Pharmacy, was one of the first seven CHCs to receive funding from the U.S. Health Resources and Services Administration's (HRSA) Clinical Pharmacy Demonstration Projects (CPDP) to develop and deliver clinical pharmacy services. The project objective was to determine whether provision of education services by the clinical pharmacist working with the SCHC team would improve glycosylated hemoglobin (A_{1c}) levels and quality of life for patients with diabetes in an intervention group, as compared to members of the control group (who received standard care) (Scott, Boyd, Stephans, Augustine, and Reardon, 2006). Based on a national evaluation, the SCHC project was deemed a successful CPDP project: It was one of only two CPDPs in which the regression analysis showed significantly better health outcomes than the average project. It reached and retained patients in its diabetes disease management program better than most, and it has been sustained since the end of the grant period in August 2003. The Siouxland project used an intensive program of mostly individual diabetes counseling, along with incentives as a means to encourage patient retention (Mathematic Policy Research, 2004).

In another study, Leal and colleagues assessed the improvement that a clinical pharmacist at a CHC can make as a provider for patients with diabetes and comorbid conditions (hypertension and hyperlipidemia) by using a medical staff-approved collaborative practice agreement. Although this study did not include a comparison group, the intervention at the El Rio Health Center in Tucson, Arizona, produced a statistically significant 2% drop in mean A_{1c} in 199 patients as compared to baseline. Regarding attainment of treatment goals, the pharmacist managed service showed an almost sevenfold increase in the number of patients at target A_{1c} levels (Leal, Glover, Herrier, and Felix, 2004).

Indian Health Service

Treaties signed between Native American tribes and the U.S. government stipulated that Native Americans would be provided certain medical and hospital services, and this obligation continues to the present day. Management of the Indian Health Service (IHS) is provided by the U.S. Department of Health and Human Services' PHS. Currently, the majority of IHS pharmacists are members of the PHS Commissioned Corps. Health care and pharmacy services are provided to 1.5 million Native Americans and Alaska Natives living on or near reservations in 34 states. IHS programs are carried out through 49 hospitals and 545 ambulatory health centers. Although they are distributed throughout the country, most of these facilities are concentrated in the western and southwestern areas of the continental United States.

Pharmacists were first assigned as PHS officers to hospitals in 1953 to establish dispensing policies and practices. During the 1960s, several IHS innovations set the stage for a more active clinical role for pharmacists. The first innovation was that the patient's medical record replaced the traditional prescription blank as the primary document used to fill all prescriptions. By accessing the patient's chart, the pharmacist could provide a concurrent review of prescribed drug therapy for appropriateness before dispensing. The second innovation was that IHS pharmacists were the first to use private consultation rooms and provide patient counseling to every patient receiving prescriptions.

The third major innovation was the provision of primary care to ambulatory patients with both acute and chronic health problems. This program began as pharmacists independently initiated and extended drug therapy. The primary-care program has now progressed to where pharmacists take histories, do physical assessments, and prescribe treatment including prescription medication. These programs were developed under the leadership of Dr. Allen J. Brands, an IHS pharmacist from 1955 through 1981, and they remain an important part of pharmacy practice today.

Since 1972, IHS pharmacists have obtained didactic and clinical training that enables them to become certified as pharmacist practitioners (Copeland and Apgar, 1980). These trained pharmacists perform physical assessments and manage both acute and chronic disease states using protocols (Apgar, 1978). The protocols provide guidelines for pharmacists, including the requirement that complex and severe cases be referred to physicians. The notion of the pharmacist as a primary-care provider similar to a PA or NP is more comprehensive in the IHS than the roles found in most ambulatory care settings. This unique conception of the pharmacist's primary-care role was originally evolved to counteract a physician undersupply and the unmet needs of the underserved Native American population, but it is also well suited for many other rural areas. Although the pharmaceutical care role has recently been advocated in the ambulatory setting, most of these innovations were first developed in the IHS (see Chapter 15).

MISCELLANEOUS PROGRAMS

School Health Clinics

The vast majority of children older than age 5 attend school in the United States; when first aid is needed or acute illness occurs, schools must provide at least limited services for these children. School health services in the United States can be traced back to 1840, when William Alcott, a distinguished educator, called for periodic visits to schools by physicians who would see children referred by teachers (Roemer, 1981). The first permanent school medical officer was appointed in New York City in 1892, followed by one in Boston, to ensure that school children with contagious diseases were identified, removed from school, and treated. School nursing services were brought into schools in New York City in 1902 and later adopted in other U.S. cities.

A wide disparity of nursing services exists in U.S. schools because communities have different socioeconomic levels, and local property taxes are usually the schools' major financial support. Ambulatory services vary between education levels because health needs change from childhood to young adult years (Roemer, 1981).

At the elementary school level, three components are ideally addressed: (1) health education of the child, (2) maintenance of a safe and healthy school environment, and (3) personal health services. To control communicable diseases, immunizations are required for entrance into school. Personal health services include health status appraisals (examinations), first aid to trauma cases, referral for needed medical care, psychological services, and dental care. School nurses are the most commonly employed school health personnel, although the number working in full-time and part-time positions is unavailable.

Secondary schools require a different pattern of health services than in elementary schools to serve adolescent needs. Passage through puberty requires programs for sexuality, STDs, premarital pregnancy, substance abuse prevention and treatment, violence prevention, and sports medicine. The pharmacist as a health educator is well trained to provide accurate and appropriate information on alcohol, tobacco, and other drug usage. Some colleges of pharmacy have speakers' bureaus that give presentations on a variety of substance abuse topics (e.g., smoking prevention and cessation, alcohol use, anabolic steroid use, amphetamines, marijuana, and diet pills). Health education programs on STDs and birth control can be given at the school and then augmented at the community pharmacy level.

The first school health clinic was developed at a high school in St. Paul, Minnesota. Since then, clinics have been established in other schools throughout the country. Students can receive personal health services at school health clinics, which are especially important in underserved population areas.

Prison Health Services

The U.S. Department of Justice operates a system of federal prisons or penitentiaries through its Federal Bureau of Prisons. Federal prisons' capacities range from 200 to more than 2,200 inmates, and prisons are linked to more than 28 hospitals, each with a clinic for ambulatory care. Larger prisons are staffed by the PHS with full-time salaried physicians, and smaller prisons are staffed by part-time private physicians working under contract (Roemer, 1981). As part of the PHS, more than 100 pharmacists work in the Bureau of Prisons. Practice settings range from ambulatory care sites to 500-bed hospitals. Responsibilities of the pharmacist include distributing drugs, performing pharmacy interventions, and providing patient education.

Voluntary Agencies and Free Clinics

Many voluntary health agencies exist in the United States, including those run by the American Red Cross, the Salvation Army, and some overseas church missions that provide ambulatory care services in developing countries.

Another voluntary health service was the "free clinic movement," a dramatic innovation in ambulatory care. Its first facility was the Haight-Ashbury Free Medical Clinic, which opened in a bohemian section of San Francisco, California, in the summer of 1967. These clinics opened without substantial grants from the federal government and were planned and supported by consumers, who were usually groups of young adults. Other free clinics opened in Cincinnati, Detroit, Seattle, and Minneapolis. By 1971, about 175 free clinics had been established throughout the country, with the greatest concentration in California. Roemer (1981) suggested that the rationale for these clinics was the feeling of distrust by socially alienated youth ("hippies") of the establishment in the American health care system.

These alienated youth generally did not want to go to hospital outpatient departments and public health clinics. Free clinics were often located in vacant stores, old houses, and church basements, and they were open to everyone who came—at no charge—although donations were welcomed.

Jerome Schwartz (1971) defined free clinics as having seven characteristics: (1) a physical facility; (2) trained health personnel; (3) other health staff or volunteers; (4) direct provision of medical, dental, or psychological service, including treatment of drug abuse; (5) availability to everyone without eligibility tests; (6) specified hours of service; and (7) no set payment required, although small fees might be charged for specified services and donations might be requested (Schwartz, 1971). Services are provided predominantly by volunteer physicians, nurses, pharmacists, and paraprofessionals.

Free clinics provide professional and community service opportunities to pharmacy, medical, dental, and nursing students. The author of this chapter participated as a pharmacy student at the Union Gospel Mission Free Clinic in St. Paul, Minnesota, from 1970 through 1973. Services provided at this free clinic included medical care, dental care, nursing care, and pharmaceutical care. Clientele included homeless men, women, and children, and runaway youth. Many homeless men had a variety of medical problems, including alcoholism. A pharmacist oversaw distribution of medications when possible, although a volunteer pharmacist was not always at the site. Consequently, a pharmacy student dispensed medication and provided counseling under the supervision of a volunteer physician. Medical students diagnosed and prescribed following consultation with the pharmacist and physician. Medications were generally donated to this free clinic by community hospitals and by some drug companies. Opportunities to provide pharmaceutical care increased as pharmacists and pharmacy students gained further insight and skills.

Free clinics' major obstacles are continual financial crises and staffing by voluntary health professionals. Since the 1971 Schwartz study, no general survey has been conducted of the free clinic movement (Roemer, 1981). Undoubtedly some free clinics remain, although most of them have changed their names to community clinics, and some have evolved into community health centers as described earlier.

AMBULATORY PHARMACY SERVICES

Hospital Outpatient Clinics

Since 1983, community hospitals in the United States have experienced a significant reduction on the inpatient side and a significant increase in outpatient visits. To compensate for the loss of inpatient revenue, most community hospitals have moved toward expansion and modernization of ambulatory care clinics (Iglehart, 1993).

Clinical pharmacy is evolving from primarily an inpatient hospital focus to a greater concentration on ambulatory care. To meet the mandatory counseling requirements of OBRA '90 (covering Medicaid) and state-passed legislation (extension to non-Medicaid patients), outpatient hospital pharmacies are undergoing layout redesign by incorporating semiprivate consultation areas and patient consultation rooms. Pharmacist participation in the management of specific disease states (e.g., anticoagulant therapy, hypertension, asthma, and diabetes) has already been described. Pharmacists and physicians working together have developed practice guidelines for pharmacists' management of patients with these chronic disease states (Reinders, 1986). Thanks to the pharmacist's contribution in these clinics, patient compliance with both medication therapy and future clinic appointments has improved.

Primary-Care and Family Practice Clinics

Carter and Helling (1992) have described pharmacy services in primary-care clinics and family practice clinics, and some of the following review is based on their description. Pharmaceutical care services have been reported in clinics associated with Appalachian Regional Hospitals, especially clinics for patients with specific diseases. As members of an interdisciplinary team, pharmacists lend their expertise to physicians and other health care professionals who are caring for their patients. Typically, the pharmacist performs physical assessments, orders laboratory tests, and changes medication regimens (Carter and Helling, 1992). Clinical pharmacists' participation in physician group practices in Area Health Education Centers (AHEC) and in North Carolina and South Carolina has also been documented (Eichelberger, 1980; Johnston and Heffron, 1981; Robertson and Groh, 1982).

Pharmacists' interventions have been shown to improve care. Morse and colleagues showed that blood pressure control could be improved and its cost reduced by pharmacy interventions (Morse, Douglas, Upton, Rodgers, and Gal, 1986). In a clinic for diabetic patients, intensive monitoring and follow-up by the pharmacist resulted in improved compliance, improved control, and reduced hospitalizations (Sczupak and Conrad, 1977).

After passage of California Assembly Bill 717 in 1977, some California pharmacists were allowed to prescribe medications after participating in a specific training program (Stimmel and McGhan, 1981). Pharmacists who completed the training program came from ambulatory care settings such as mental health centers, anticoagulation clinics, county clinics, and offices of private practice physicians. McGhan and colleagues (1983) compared the quality of pharmacists' ($n = 2$) and physicians' ($n = 3$) drug prescribing for ambulatory hypertensive patients in a California HMO. They found that more of the patients had controlled blood pressure in the pharmacists group than the physicians group (96.8% versus 78.1%) (McGhan, Stimmel, Hall, and Gilman, 1983).

Pharmacist-managed anticoagulation clinics have shown that better anti-coagulation control results in fewer hospitalizations and improved management of patients (Garabedian-Ruffalo, Gray, Sax, and Ruffalo, 1985). In an economic evaluation, Garabedian-Ruffalo and colleagues found that the hospitalization rate was 3.2 days per patient-treatment-year in the control group and only 0.05 day in the pharmacist study group. The net savings in hospitalizations was estimated to be $11,776 per year in the pharmacist-managed group (Gray, Garabedian-Ruffalo, and Chretien, 1985).

Chrischilles et al.'s cost-effectiveness analysis of pharmacy services' effects on family practice identified pharmacy services as improving physician efficacy, reducing adverse reactions, improving compliance, and improving the quality of care (Chrischilles, Helling, and Rowland, 1984a, 1984b). Given their expanding role in ambulatory care settings, pharmacists should aggressively pursue these practice opportunities, document their effectiveness, and publish these findings after developing good research designs (Carter and Helling, 1992).

Community Pharmacy

Pharmacists are in a unique position in the health care system: They are the most accessible of health care professionals, and they are highly regarded by their patients. Pharmacists know that their everyday activities benefit patients. They are responsible for saving money for patients and third-party payers, improving therapeutic regimens, and averting therapeutic failures. Recent Gallup Public Opinion Polls shows that pharmacists are listed among the most trusted individuals in society. This trust, along with the fact that most people visit their pharmacist several times for every visit they make to their physician, means that the pharmacist plays a crucial role in providing pharmaceutical care and improving patient outcomes.

Many independent pharmacies have survived by diversifying their revenue bases, including consulting with skilled nursing facilities, selling durable medical equipment (DME), and building home health care businesses. Chain pharmacies have also been faced with declining revenues as they compete with mail-order pharmacies, Web-based pharmacies, supermarket pharmacies, and super-drugstores (mass merchants). Part of chain pharmacies' acceptance of lower margins on prescriptions reflects the thought that pharmacy departments generate more foot traffic through their stores; thus the lower margins on prescriptions are thought to be more than offset by increases in nonprescription and sundry sales and/or increased prescription volume (Tootelian and Gaddeke, 1993).

One way that community pharmacies have diversified is though the development of mini-clinics or "Minute Clinics." The mini-clinic is located in retail stores such as grocery stores and drugstores (e.g., CVS and Rite Aid) and offers relatively inexpensive, convenient care for minor ailments (e.g., colds, strep throat, bronchitis, and minor rashes).

Mini-clinics are usually staffed by nurse practitioners, who (in most states) can write prescriptions and conduct basic medical exams and procedures. Not surprisingly, such clinics have met with some resistance from competing health providers (family practitioners and emergicenters) and are seen as providing limited service competition. Critics suggest that they present problems in areas of continuity of care, quality of care, referral, and insurance issues. Nevertheless, the cost of a mini-clinic visit is typically about one-half the cost of a physician visit, so mini-clinics are drawing interest from both health insurance companies and employers, which are constantly seeking innovative ways to reduce health care costs (Kher, 2006).

Another way that community pharmacists have diversified is through the provision of pharmaceutical care. Hepler and Strand (1990) define pharmaceutical care as "the responsible provision of drug therapy for achieving specific outcomes that improves a patient's quality of life." The four possible outcomes include (1) cure of a disease, (2) elimination and reduction of a patient's symptomatology, (3) arresting or slowing of the disease process, and (4) preventing a disease or symptomatology. Traditionally, pharmacists have been primarily concerned with the process of care—that is, what they do when the patient receives care (whether the correct drug and the right dose at the right time are provided). With the focus on outcomes, the pharmacist also takes responsibility for what happens to the patient when the drug is given (the outcome of care). Examples of outcome criteria include increased patient knowledge of the specific disease, improved medication compliance, improved medication therapy, decreased adverse reactions, decreased misuse and abuse, and higher patient satisfaction levels (see Chapter 3).

Given that more independent community pharmacies are facing the threat of closure because of steadily declining gross margins and increasing competition by high-volume pharmacies and mail-order centers, an increasing impetus exists for pharmacists to adopt the pharmaceutical care role. As managed care programs continue to lower prescription drug reimbursements, pharmacists should investigate other revenue sources, such as providing cognitive services.

To assume this role, community pharmacists must be trained to provide pharmaceutical care. The emphasis in such training programs is to encourage the community pharmacist to assume the role of the drug therapy expert and to be responsible for the reduction of drug-related problems. This training should include documenting clinical and financial successes rather than "assuming" savings. These programs also assume that getting the pharmacist more involved in patient care will result in improved treatment outcomes and reduce utilization of more expensive services, such as hospitalization and unnecessary physician visits, thereby reducing the overall cost of health care.

The University of Minnesota's College of Pharmacy was one of the pioneers in development, training, and support of community pharmacists in the pharmaceutical care role. Purdue University was another early developer of pharmaceutical care training programs for community pharmacists. A third example can be found in Iowa, where the two colleges of pharmacy (University of Iowa and Drake University) and the Iowa Pharmacists Association came together to promote pharmaceutical care training and development in community pharmacy practice settings. Presently, some national pharmacy organizations (e.g., American Pharmacists Association, American Society of Health Systems Pharmacists) and a number of state organizations offer pharmaceutical care training programs. For example, training programs have been developed in the areas of anticoagulation, asthma, diabetes, dyslipidemias, and hypertension.

Although the pharmacist's role in pharmaceutical care is promoted by pharmacy academia and organizational leaders, the concept of pharmaceutical care is not yet widely accepted by consumers, physicians, and health insurance carriers. Before insurance carriers begin reimbursing pharmacists for pharmaceutical care services, they are requesting evidence that the programs are cost-effective (Scott and Miller, 1997). Some of the research supporting their effectiveness is presented next.

Pharmacists in the Asheville Project in North Carolina have been providing services to patients with diabetes since 1997. Pharmacists in 12 participating community pharmacies receive reimbursement from two local employers in North Carolina for providing cognitive services (e.g., patient education, clinical assessment, monitoring, follow-up, and referral). This project is assessing the short-term clinical, economic, and humanistic outcomes of pharmaceutical care services. When compared to a control group, the pharmaceutical care group's glycosylated hemoglobin (A_{1c}) concentrations were found to be significantly reduced and the satisfaction with pharmacy services improved significantly (Cranor and Christensen, 2003). This study demonstrates the value of pharmaceutical care provided by the community pharmacist.

In a randomized trial, Tsuyuki reported on the impact of community pharmacists' ($n = 54$ pharmacies) intervention on the process of cholesterol risk management in patients at high risk for cardiovascular events. The pharmacist intervention group received education and a brochure on risk factors, point-of-care cholesterol measurement, physician referral, and follow-up for 16 weeks. In the intervention group, pharmacists faxed a form to the primary-care physician listing risk factors and suggestions. Usual-care patients received the same brochure and general advice with only minimal follow-up. Among the 675 patients enrolled in this study, the primary endpoint was reached in 57% of intervention patients versus 31% of usual-care patients, and the results were statistically significant. The cholesterol risk management program demonstrates the value of community pharmacists working in collaboration with physicians (Tsuyuki et al., 2002).

However, not all studies have demonstrated the value of pharmaceutical care programs. For instance, Weinberger and colleagues (2002) assessed the effectiveness of a pharmaceutical care program for patients with asthma or chronic obstructive pulmonary disease (COPD). These investigators conducted a randomized controlled trial involving 898 patients who were monitored over 12 months at 36 community drug stores in Indianapolis, Indiana. The pharmaceutical care program ($n = 447$) provided pharmacists with patient-specific clinical data (peak expiratory flow rates [PEFRs], emergency department [ED] visits, hospitalizations, and medication compliance), training, patient education materials, and resources to implement the program. The PEFR monitoring group ($n = 363$) received a peak flow meter, instructions about its use, and monthly calls to elicit PEFRs. The usual-care group ($n = 303$) did not receive the same items as the monitoring group. At 12 months, patients receiving pharmaceutical care had significantly higher peak flow rates than the usual-care group, but not higher than the rates seen in the PEFR monitoring control group. Asthma patients receiving pharmaceutical care had significantly more breathing-related ED or hospital visits than the usual-care group. The researchers concluded that this program increased patients' PEFRs compared with usual care, but provided little benefit compared with peak flow monitoring alone. While pharmaceutical care increased patient satisfaction, the investigators found that it also increased the amount of breathing-related medical care sought (Weinberger et al., 2002).

As Posey (2003) has reported, not all pharmaceutical care projects and evaluations have enjoyed the success that the Asheville Project did. This author's Medline search conducted in January 2003 using the term "pharmaceutical care" yielded 607 published articles. Of these, only 28 of these studies were randomized, controlled evaluations, and only 11 studies had been conducted in community pharmacies (Posey, 2003). While the Asheville Project did not use randomized controlled evaluations, the project does provide evidence suggesting that pharmaceutical care is working. According to Posey, there were only 11 studies that provide the best evidence on whether pharmaceutical care is an effective means in making a difference in patients' health.

In 2006, the Centers for Medicare and Medicaid Services (CMS) implemented the Medicare Prescription Drug Benefit (Part D) for seniors. As part of this program, some Medicare beneficiaries will receive Medication Therapy Management (MTM) services. The intention of this program is to ensure that seniors who have annual prescription costs of $4,000 or more, have multiple chronic disease states, and are taking multiple chronic prescription medications receive management assistance with their medication regimens, thereby ensuring that their drugs are used safely, effectively, and within a reasonable cost range.

While MTM is a requirement of the regulations, the actual level of pharmacist involvement in this program has not yet been determined. While MTM presents a wonderful opportunity for pharmacists, it may be performed by other providers, or it may be a program that a pharmacy benefit manager decides to provide through a consultant service. Some MTM programs are already being planned and implemented at the state and community pharmacy level. For instance, the University of Iowa is partnering with researchers and pharmacists in seven states (Iowa, Minnesota, North Dakota, South Dakota, Montana, Nebraska, and Wyoming). The initial phase of this partnership, which is being funded by the Community Pharmacy Foundation, will establish a network of pharmacists and pharmacies in the Midwest region that will be able to provide MTM services to seniors (see Chapter 20).

While community pharmacists have made valuable inroads into patient care, Posey suggests that pharmaceutical care to the average patient remains an enigma, primarily because it is not provided on a broad scale and in an identifiable manner in the community pharmacies where most people encounter pharmacists (Posey, 2003). National and state pharmaceutical organizations, community pharmacists, and researchers need to work together to demonstrate the impact of pharmaceutical care programs before the concept will be broadly accepted. In the case study, for example, George is considering whether he should integrate pharmaceutical care into his community pharmacy practice.

CONCLUSIONS

Ambulatory care services have undergone rapid development and expansion during the past two decades. With managed care being established as the pinnacle of health care reform, continued emphasis will be placed on developing innovative and cost-effective services.

QUESTIONS FOR FURTHER DISCUSSION

1. What pharmaceutical care innovations from the Indian Health Service can be adapted for use in community pharmacy practice?
2. Several ambulatory care services have developed in the past decade. What new services do you envision in the next decade?
3. Contrast ambulatory medical practice in rural and urban areas in your state.
4. Contrast ambulatory pharmacy practice in rural and urban areas in your state.

KEY TOPICS AND TERMS

Ambulatory care
Community health centers
Community pharmacy
Emergency services
Health department
Hospital clinics
Indian Health Service
Managed care
Pharmaceutical care
Primary care

REFERENCES

Alsuwaidan, S., Malone, D. C., Billups, S. J., & Carter, B. L. (1998). Characteristics of ambulatory care clinics and pharmacists in Veterans Affairs Medical Centers. *American Journal of Health-Systems Pharmacy, 55,* 68–72.

American College of Healthcare Executives. (1993). *Managed care in Medicaid: Lessons for policy and program design.* Melrose Park, IL: Health Administration Press.

Apgar, D. A. (1978). Clinical role in Indian Health Service (letter).

Carter, B. L. (1992). Ambulatory care. In T. R. Brown (Ed.), *Handbook of institutional pharmacy practice* (pp. 367–373). Bethesda, MD: American Society of Hospital Pharmacists.

Carter, B. L., & Helling, D. K. (1992). Ambulatory care pharmacy services: The incomplete agenda. *Annals of Pharmacotherapy, 26,* 701–708.

Carter, B. L., Malone, D. C., Billups, S. J., Valuck R. J., et al. (2001). Interpreting the findings of the IMPROVE study. *American Journal of Health-Systems Pharmacy, 58,* 1330–1337.

Chrischilles, E. A., Helling, D. K., & Rowland, C. R. (1984a). Clinical pharmacy services in family practice: Cost-benefit analysis. I: Physician time and quality of care. *Drug Intelligence in Clinical Pharmacy, 18,* 333–341.

Chrischilles, E. A., Helling, D. K., & Rowland, C. R. (1984b). Clinical pharmacy services in family practice: Cost-benefit analysis. II: Referrals, appointment, compliance and cost. *Drug Intelligence in Clinical Pharmacy, 18,* 436–441.

Copeland, G. P., & Apgar, D. A. (1980). The pharmacist–practitioner training program. *Drug Intelligence in Clinical Pharmacy, 14,* 114–119.

Cranor, C. W., & Christensen, D. B. (2003). The Asheville Project: Short-term outcomes of a community pharmacy diabetes care program. *Journal of the American Pharmacists Association, 43,* 149–159.

Eichelberger, B. N. (1980). Family practice clinical pharmacy opportunities in the community setting. *American Journal of Hospital Pharmacy, 37,* 740–742.

Ellis, S. L., Carter, B. L., Malone, D. C., Billups, S. J., et al. (2000). Clinical and economic impact of ambulatory care clinical pharmacists in management of dyslipidemias in older adults. *Pharmacotherapy, 20,* 1508–1516.

Foss, M. T., Shock, P. H., & Sintek, C. D. (1999). Efficient operation of a high-volume anticoagulation clinic. *American Journal of Health-Systems Pharmacy, 56,* 43–48.

Garabedian-Ruffalo, S. M., Gray, D. R., Sax, M. J., & Ruffalo, R. L. (1985). Retrospective evaluation of a pharmacist-managed warfarin anticoagulation clinic. *American Journal of Hospital Pharmacy, 42,* 304–308.

Gray, D. R., Garabedian-Ruffalo, S. M., & Chretien, S. D. (1985). Cost justification of a clinical pharmacist-managed anti-coagulation clinic. *Drug Intelligence in Clinical Pharmacy, 19,* 575–580.

Hepler, C. D., & Strand, L. M. (1990). Opportunities and responsibilities in pharmaceutical care. *American Journal of Hospital Pharmacy, 47,* 533–542.

Hoffer, E. (1979). Emergency medical services. *New England Journal of Medicine, 301,* 1118.

Iglehart, J. K. (1993). The American health care system: Community hospitals. *New England Journal of Medicine, 329,* 372–376.

Johnston, T. S., & Heffron, W. A. (1981). Clinical pharmacy in family practice residency programs. *Journal of Family Practice, 13,* 91–94.

Kher, U. (2006, March 20). Get a check-up in Aisle 3. *Time,* pp. 52–53.

Leal, S., Glover, J. J., Herrier, R. N., & Felix, A. (2004). Improving quality of care in diabetes through a comprehensive pharmacist-based disease management program. *Diabetes Care, 27,* 2983–2984.

Madison, D. L. (1983). The case for community oriented primary care. *Journal of the American Medical Association, 249,* 1279–1282.

Mathematic Policy Research, Inc. (2004, November 30). Evaluation of HRSA's clinical pharmacy demonstration projects. Final report, volume II: Case studies, chapter II. *Siouxland Community Health Center Network,* pp. 11–20.

McGhan, W. F., Stimmel, G. L., Hall, T. G., & Gilman, P. M. (1983). A comparison of pharmacists and physicians on the quality of prescribing for ambulatory hypertensive patients. *Medical Care, 21,* 435–444.

Mezey, A. P. (1999). Ambulatory care. In S. Jonas & A. R. Kovner (Eds.), *Health care delivery in the United States* (pp. 183–205). New York: Springer.

Mezey, A. P., & Lawrence, R. S. (1995). Ambulatory care. In A. R. Kovner (Ed.), *Jonas's health care delivery in the United States* (pp. 122–161). New York: Springer.

Morehead, M. A., Donaldson, R. S., & Servavelli, M. R. (1971). Comparisons between OEO neighborhood health centers and other health care providers of ratings of the quality of health care. *American Journal of Public Health, 61,* 1294–1306.

Morse, G. D., Douglas, J. V., Upton, J. H., Rodgers, S., & Gal, P. (1986). Effect of pharmacist intervention and control of resistant hypertension. *American Journal of Hospital Pharmacy, 43,* 905–909.

Murray, M. D., Loos, B., Eckert, G. J., Zhou, X., & Tierney, W. M. (1999). Work patterns of ambulatory care pharmacists with access to electronic guideline-based treatment suggestions. *American Journal of Health-Systems Pharmacy, 56,* 225–232.

Posey, L. M. (2003). Proving that pharmaceutical care makes a difference in community pharmacy. *Journal of the American Pharmaceutical Association, 43,* 136–139.

Reinders, T. P. (1986). Clinical services and ambulatory care. In T. R. Brown and M. C. Smith (Eds.), *Handbook of institutional pharmacy practice* (pp. 509–515). Baltimore, MD: Williams and Wilkins.

Robertson, D. L., & Groh, M. (1982). Activities of the clinical pharmacist in a private family practice. *Journal of Family Practice Research, 1,* 188–194.

Roemer, M. (1981). *Ambulatory health services in America*. Rockville, MD: Aspen Systems.

Roth, R., Stewart, R. D., Rogers, K., & Cannon, G. M. (1984). Out of hospital cardiac arrest: Factors associated with survival. *Annals of Emergency Medicine, 13,* 237–243.

Schappert, S. M. (1992). *1990 summary: National ambulatory medical care survey. Advanced data from vital and health statistics, no. 213.* Hyattsville, MD: National Center for Health Statistics.

Scheffler, R. M., Waitzman, N. J., & Hillman, J. M. (1998). The productivity of physician assistants and nurse practitioners and health force policy in the era of managed care. *Journal of Allied Health, 25,* 207–217.

Schwartz, J. L. (1971). Preliminary observations of free clinics. In D. E. Smith, D. J. Bentel, & J. L. Schwartz (Eds.), *The free clinic: A community approach to health care and drug abuse* (pp. 144–206). Beloit, WI: Stash Press.

Scott, D. M., & Nordin, J. D. (1980). Pharmacist role in projects for children and youth. *American Journal of Hospital Pharmacy, 37,* 1339–1342.

Scott, D. M., & Miller, L. G. (1997). Reimbursement for pharmacy cognitive services: Insurance company assessment. *Journal of Managed Care Pharmacy, 2,* 699–714.

Scott, D. M., Boyd, S. T., Stephans, M., Augustine, S. C., & Reardon T. P. (2006). Outcomes of pharmacist-managed diabetes care services in a community health center. *American Journal of Health-Systems Pharmacy, 63:21,* 116-22.

Sczupak, C. A., & Conrad, W. F. (1977). Relationship between patient-oriented pharmaceutical services and therapeutic outcomes of ambulatory patients with diabetes mellitus. *American Journal of Hospital Pharmacy, 34,* 1238–1242.

Sherman, M. A. (1979). Mobile intensive care units: An evaluation of effectiveness. *Journal of the American Medical Association, 241,* 1899–1901.

Sparer, G., & Anderson, A. (1975). *Cost of services at neighborhood health centers: A comparative analysis.* Washington, DC: Office of Economic Opportunity.

Stimmel, G. L., & McGhan, W. F. (1981). The pharmacist as prescriber of drug therapy: The USC pilot project. *Drug Intelligence of Clinical Pharmacy, 15,* 665–772.

Tootelian, D. H., & Gaddeke, R. M. (1993). *Essentials of pharmacy management.* St. Louis, MO: Mosby-Yearbook.

Tsuyuki, R. T., Johnson, J. A., Teo, K. K., Simpson, S. H., et al. (2002). A randomized trial of the effect of community pharmacist intervention on cholesterol risk management: The study of cardiovascular risk intervention by pharmacists (SCRIP). *Archives of Internal Medicine, 162,* 1149–1155.

Weinberger, M., Murray, M. D., Marrero, D. G., Brewer, N., et al. (2002). Effectiveness of pharmacist care for patients with reactive airways disease: A randomized controlled trial. *Journal of the American Medical Association, 288,* 1594–1602.

Weinerman, E. R., et al. (1966). Yale studies in ambulatory medical care: Determinants of use of hospital emergency services. *American Journal of Public Health, 56,* 1037–1056.

Williams, S. J. (1993). Ambulatory health care services. In S. J. Williams and P. R. Torrens (Eds.), *Introduction to health services* (4th ed.) (vol. 1, pp. 108–113). Albany, NY: Delmar.

Long-Term Care

Kimberly S. Plake, Kristin B. Meyer, and Ernest J. Dole

Case Scenario

In the past year, Betty, a 76-year-old widow, has experienced a decline in her health. Until recently, she was an active and reasonably healthy woman. One morning in January, she slipped on some ice in her driveway, fell, and broke her hip. During her recovery, Betty received rehabilitative care while residing at a local nursing home. After a period of time, she was discharged and moved into her daughter's residence.

Tracy, her 44-year-old daughter, works full-time as a real estate agent. In addition, she has a son in high school and a daughter in college. Initially, Tracy did not have too much difficulty in caring for her mother. Although her mother had experienced a serious injury, she was recovering well and, for the most part, was still able to care for herself. Unfortunately, Betty experienced a setback when she had a heart attack later in the year. It became more challenging for Tracy to balance her work and family responsibilities, yet she needed to continue to work full-time to support her family.

When her mother continued to have difficulty caring for herself—dressing, bathing, and toileting—Tracy talked to her mother about care alternatives. Costs associated with alternative care options were a concern. Because of her age, Betty is covered by Medicare. She also has a Medigap insurance policy. Neither of these plans covers the type of care that Betty needs—that is, custodial care rather than skilled nursing care. As a consequence, most of the bills were paid with Betty's limited financial resources.

Ultimately, Tracy and Betty decided on a nursing home close to Tracy's home. Betty paid the bills until her financial resources were depleted. At that time, she qualified for Medicaid, which pays for her nursing home stay.

LEARNING OBJECTIVES

Upon completion of this chapter, the student shall be able to:

- Define *long-term care*
- Compare and contrast Medicare and Medicaid regarding their coverage of long-term care services
- Explain the reasons patients face financial difficulties in paying for long-term care services
- Identify and explain the types of institutional and community-based long-term care services available to patients and their families
- Describe the types of patients who use long-term care services
- Explain why there is a need for extended-care services
- Distinguish between the philosophies of institutional and community-based long-term care
- Define *aging-in-place*
- Compare and contrast DRR, DUE, and DUR
- List the opportunities for pharmacist involvement in the care of residents in long-term care facilities
- Describe the benefits of pharmacist involvement in the care of residents in long-term care facilities
- Identify resources available to consultant pharmacists who wish to further develop their patient care skills

CHAPTER QUESTIONS

1. What factors have led to the increasing need for long-term care (LTC) facilities?
2. What opportunities are available for pharmacists in the LTC setting?
3. What are the financing mechanisms available to persons who use LTC services?
4. What types of patients use LTC services?

INTRODUCTION

In the United States, many types of health care services are available. One type of care whose use is increasing is called extended care or long-term care (LTC). LTC is defined as a "set of health, personal care, and social services delivered over a sustained period of time to persons who have lost or never acquired some degree of functional capacity" (Kane and Kane, 1987). In addition, it is defined as "health, social, and residential services provided to chronically disabled persons with functional or cognitive impairments" (Liu, 1994, p. 477). Primarily, LTC assists people who have limitations in performing activities of daily living (ADLs) such as bathing, dressing, and toileting, or instrumental activities of daily living (IADLs) such as shopping and food preparation. For example, Betty had problems with dressing, bathing, and toileting and needed additional care beyond the capabilities of her family. It was at this time that she entered the nursing home.

Many people assume that LTC refers only to nursing home care. In reality, people may receive LTC in both community and institutional settings. Of those individuals who receive LTC, one third are in institutional settings and two thirds reside in the community either at home or with others (Williams, 1995). The determination of the type of care received is based on the individual patient's needs. The factors determining the type of LTC needed include the level of disability, availability of informal caregivers, financial circumstances, availability of public programs, and other personal circumstances (Liu, 1994). The main risk factors for institutionalization include advanced age, diagnostic condition, and living alone. Other risk factors include problems with ADLs, mental status, ethnicity (minorities are generally at a lower risk), low social support, poverty, outpatient admission, and hospital admission.

This chapter addresses many of the LTC options available to individuals in the United States, including institutional services (such as nursing homes and psychiatric institutions), community-based services (such as home health care and hospice), and community facility services (such as adult day care). In addition, it examines the role of pharmacy and pharmacists in these health care environments.

PATIENTS WHO MAY REQUIRE LONG-TERM CARE SERVICES

Elderly Patients

Although the majority of elderly persons are not seriously impaired and do not need LTC services, the primary users of these services are individuals older than age 65. In general, the need for LTC services increases with age. As people age, they are more likely to develop chronic diseases and incur disabilities similar to Betty's. Approximately 80% of people older than age 65 have at least one chronic disease, and 50% have two such conditions (He, Sengupta, Velkoff, and DeBarros, 2005). In addition, 19.7% of older persons experience limitations in their ability to perform self-care or manage household activities (He et al., 2005).

For people with low levels of disability, LTC services may be provided by family and friends—often called informal caregiving—as was the case initially with Betty (Scanlon, 2000). Although friends may contribute to care, spouses as well as adult children and their spouses are the primary providers of LTC in the home (National Alliance for Caregiving and American Association of Retired Persons, 1997; Scanlon, 2000) (**Exhibits 8–1** and **8–2**).

Exhibit 8-1   The Spectrum of the Long-Term Care Environment

Hospital-based nursing facility	Community-based care
Subacute care	Adult congregate living
Nursing facility	Adult day care
Psychiatric hospital	Home health care
Intermediate care facility for the	Community mental health center
mentally retarded	Hospice
	Senior center
	Retirement housing
	Correctional facility
	Home care
	Independent community living

Source: Reprinted with permission from W. Simonson, Pharmacy Practice in the Long-Term Care Environment, *Journal of Managed Care Pharmacy, 3,* (2), p. 190, © 1997.

Exhibit 8-2   Terminology Describing Community-Based Care Environments

Residential care facility	Leisure care facility
Assisted living home	Retirement home
Board and care home	Adult care facility
Chronic custodial care	Life care–continuing care
Congregate care	retirement community
Domiciliary care	Catered housing
Home for adults	Personal board and care
Residential home	Sheltered care
Rest home	Subsidized apartment building
Sheltered home	Residential board and lodging
Group home for mentally	facility
retarded persons	Senior apartment building
Adult foster home	Personal care home
Community-based care facility	

Source: Reprinted with permission from W. Simonson, *Consultant Pharmacy Practice,* (2nd ed.), 1996, p. 49.

In the case of informal caregiving, the average caregiver is a woman who is 46 years old, has some college education, and cares for her mother approximately 20 hours per week (National Alliance for Caregiving and American Association of Retired Persons, 2004). Although the perception is that only women provide care, over the last several years men have been increasingly providing care: 39% of caregivers are men and 61% are women (National Alliance for Caregiving and American Association of Retired Persons, 2004). However, female caregivers often spend more time providing care as compared to their male counterparts (National Alliance for Caregiving and American Association of Retired Persons, 2004) . In addition, females are more likely to provide "hands-on" care or handle some of the most difficult caregiving, such as bathing, toileting, and dressing. Men are more likely to provide caregiving by assisting with finances and arranging care (National Alliance for Caregiving and American Association of Retired Persons, 2004).

At any given time, 4.5% of the elderly population will reside in a nursing home; as individuals age, however, this percentage increases. Approximately 18% of persons age 85 and older live in a nursing home setting (Hetzel and Smith, 2001). In 1999, nearly 90% of the 1,628,300 U.S. nursing home residents were older than age 65. The majority of these residents were female (71.9%) and white (85.6%) (Jones, 2002). Approximately 75% of elderly nursing home residents received assistance with three or more ADLs. Only 3% did not need assistance performing any ADL. The majority of residents needed help with bathing (94%), dressing (87%), and toileting (56%). In addition, 47% needed help with eating (Jones, 2002). Conditions that are commonly found in elderly nursing home residents include incontinence, mental health conditions, and diseases of the circulatory system, such as essential hypertension, heart disease, and cerebrovascular diseases (Gabrel, 2000).

The use of long-term care services is expected to increase in coming years, primarily because of the aging of the baby-boomer population. According to current predictions, there will be two to four times more elderly persons with disabilities in 2030 than there are today. In 2011, the first of the baby boomers will reach age 65. Given that LTC use is more predominant in persons 85 years of age and older, demand for LTC is expected to grow even more after 2030, when the first of the baby boomers turn 85 years old (Scanlon, 2000, 2001; Walker, 2002).

Patients with Chronic Diseases

Although the elderly are the primary users of LTC, others also use these services. Some patients younger than age 65 who live with chronic diseases and terminal illnesses require assistance beyond the informal caregiving provided by family and friends. Besides nursing home care, these patients often receive services from hospice, home health care, and other community-based care providers. Because of the progressive nature of chronic disease, these patients may require assistance in performing daily activities and complying with their health care regimens. Diagnoses commonly associated with LTC services include cancer, stroke, femur fracture, depression, and diabetes (Nielson, Henderson, Cox, Williams, and Green, 1996).

Alzheimer's disease is an example of a chronic disease that often requires LTC services. People with this disease begin to lose their memory. Not only do they forget friends and family members, but they also may not remember how to eat, dress, or go to the bathroom. In addition, these patients have a tendency to wander from their homes or rooms and may not be able to return. They become disoriented and often cannot provide information, such as their name or the address where they live. These patients and their families typically require assistance in daily activities (such as toileting and dressing) and the provision of health care (such as medication), regardless of whether they reside in the home or in an institution.

Alzheimer's disease generally strikes individuals 50 years or older, but other illnesses requiring LTC services can occur in individuals much younger. Any disease that can limit physical functioning to a significant extent can increase the likelihood that the affected individual will need some type of LTC services, regardless of his or her age. For example, individuals who have severe head or spinal injuries as the result of an accident often require LTC.

Patients with Rehabilitative Needs

Like Betty with her broken hip, some patients may need LTC services for a short time. These patients generally require additional time to recover before returning home after discharge from a hospital or some type of rehabilitative services. Because of the emphasis on cost containment, patients frequently are released from the hospital earlier—and sicker—than in past years. If they are not ready to return to their homes, they may be discharged for additional care in a nursing home setting. Other patients may be ready to return home but need assistance there (such as patients recovering from a broken hip, other broken bones, or major surgery). In such cases, home health care may be provided. As stated earlier, the type of service used depends on the level of care required, the availability of informal caregivers (such as family and friends), and the patient's insurance coverage and other financial resources.

Patients with Terminal Illness

Patients who are terminally ill include individuals whose prognosis is poor and are thought to be close to death. For these patients, hospice care is often used to help with physical, social, and spiritual aspects of their illnesses. Although some institutional hospice facilities exist, hospice services do not necessarily require institutionalization of the patient. Instead, they may allow patients to remain at home with family and friends while receiving palliative ("comfort") care.

FINANCING LONG-TERM CARE

This section provides a brief description of the types of financing available to individuals to pay for LTC services. Extended care services are financed in four major ways: (1) Medicare, (2) Medicaid, (3) private insurance, and (4) out-of-pocket resources.

Medicare is a federally operated insurance program primarily intended for individuals older than age 65. In addition, younger persons with disabilities may have coverage through Medicare. Eligibility for these individuals depends on the status or length of the person's disability and sometimes on the type of disability. For instance, renal dialysis patients automatically qualify for Medicare coverage.

Medicare provides limited benefits for LTC institutional services such as skilled nursing care in residential homes. In 2000, approximately 10% of nursing home care was paid for by Medicare (Pastor, Makuc, Reuben, and Xia, 2002). For Medicare to reimburse these services, the patient must be hospitalized for three or more consecutive days, must be admitted to a skilled nursing facility (SNF) within 30 days of discharge, and must require rehabilitation or skilled nursing on a daily basis for a hospital-treated condition. Medicare will pay for covered services for the first 20 days of care (Centers for Medicare and Medicaid Services, 2006b). For days 21 through 100, the patient must pay a specific amount for each day the service is used. For example, patients paid $119 per day in 2006. After 100 days, patients are expected to pay the full costs associated with their care in a SNF. In addition, Medicare reimburses home health care and hospice services (Centers for Medicaid and Medicare Services, 2006a). Although Medicare pays for skilled nursing care, it usually does not pay for custodial care (e.g., help with bathing, dressing, using the bathroom, or eating) or other residential care services that elderly people like Betty need (see Chapter 17). These services are primarily financed by Medicaid, private insurance, or private out-of-pocket resources.

With the advent of Medicare Part D (i.e., the prescription drug benefit for Medicare beneficiaries), there is now an added level of payment complexity for those receiving LTC services. For Medicare beneficiaries receiving LTC services, the type of service or the setting in which it is delivered determines who pays for the prescription medications (Administration on Aging, 2006). For example, if a patient receives skilled nursing care in a nursing home within his or her benefit period, then Medicare Part A pays for the patient's prescription medications. Once the benefit period offered through Medicare Part A ends, the patient's prescriptions are paid for by Medicare Part D (if the patient is enrolled in the program). (Chapter 17 describes the Medicare program in detail.)

Medicaid is a federally regulated, public welfare program for the poor. Although the program is regulated by the federal government, it is financed by both the federal and state governments. Medicaid is administered by the states, however. As a consequence, Medicaid programs vary from state to state; different qualifications for eligibility exist (usually based on income and assets) and different services are provided. Currently, all 50 states include some type of benefits for LTC services for participants in the program (Schneider, Fennel, and Keenan, 1999; see Chapter 17). Because custodial care is not reimbursed by Medicare, Medicaid often is the primary payer for nursing home care in many, if not all, states. In 2004, 43% of nursing home care was paid by Medicaid (Kaiser Family Foundation, 2006).

In the past, much of the LTC paid for by Medicaid was institutional care or nursing home care. Today, however, there is increasing interest in community-based services. In fact, Medicaid expenditures for home and community care have been growing over the last several years, with 37% of LTC expenditures going to this type of care in 2005. This represents an increase from 14% in 1991 (Kaiser Family Foundation, 2006). Community-based care is likely to become even more popular in the future, given the desire of individuals to remain in the community and the lower costs associated with this type of care as compared to nursing home care.

Patients also use private insurance to finance their care. Many older individuals have policies that pay for those charges that Medicare does not cover. These policies are called Medigap insurance policies because they fill in the "gaps" in Medicare reimbursement. Depending on the policy, benefits may include payment of Medicare deductibles, Medicare co-payments, outpatient prescription medications, and extended home health care services. Like Medicare itself, many of these policies do not include custodial or residential care benefits.

Because a gap exists in many general insurance plans' reimbursement of long-term health care, there is interest in LTC insurance (Feder, Komisar, and Niefeld, 2000; Scanlon, 2000). This private insurance provides financial assistance in the event that a person needs to enter an LTC facility. Some policies also assist individuals in paying for home health care and hospice care. Other popular benefits include case management services, homemaker services, and some medical equipment. Limits to these LTC policies are based on the expense, scope, and duration of benefits, and exclusion of high-risk applicants.

In addition, some policies do not provide inflation protection (Scanlon, 2000), which would allow the benefit paid to increase as inflation increases. If a policy does not have such a clause, the benefit paid is the one stated at the time of purchase. At first, this may not seem like a problem. If a person buys a policy at age 50 and does not need to use the policy until he or she is 70, however, there will be a significant difference in the benefit paid and the actual cost of care. Of course, inflation protection can greatly increase the premium, rendering some policies unaffordable. In addition, it is not certain that everyone will need this type of policy, which makes it difficult for consumers to decide whether to purchase one. Also, policies are generally less expensive when purchased at a younger age. This purchase decision is more difficult for younger consumers, however, because they do not know whether they will need LTC or LTC insurance benefits.

LTC insurance policies have been improving over the past several years, and some now include lifetime benefits, coverage for home health care, short deductible periods, and inflation protection. Nevertheless, this type of insurance is not as tightly regulated as Medigap policies are, and it may be confusing to some consumers. Consumers should compare policies and identify the benefits of these policies before purchasing (Scanlon, 2000).

If a patient does not have private insurance that covers LTC or if they do not qualify for Medicaid, the costs of care must be paid from the patient's and the family's financial resources. Considering that the cost for nursing home care can average $74,095 per year depending on the location of the nursing home, family resources may be quickly depleted (MetLife Mature Market Institute, 2005). Indeed, nursing home care for a sustained period of time can prove catastrophic to a patient's financial stability. In such cases, patients may have to spend down their assets to qualify for Medicaid. Betty paid for her own nursing home bills until her assets were exhausted.

Paying for LTC services often can exhaust some families' financial resources. Recognizing this possibility, some seniors are seeking creative financing options and the advice of estate planners. An example of a financing option for seniors needing additional health care services is the reverse mortgage. Many seniors are homeowners, and a reverse mortgage allows them to receive a lump-sum payment, monthly payments, or a line of credit, thereby enabling the individual to remain in his or her own home despite a cash flow crunch (Stucki, 2005). The borrower never owes more than the value of the home, and the loan comes due when the borrower moves, sells the home, or dies.

INCREASING NEED FOR FACILITIES

Originally, the United States adopted 65 years as the age to begin receiving Social Security. Thus the elderly population was defined as 65 years old or older (U.S. Senate Special Committee on Aging, 1982). Today's elderly can be divided into three categories: (1) the "young old"—aged 65 to 74; (2) the "middle old"—aged 75 to 84; and (3) the "old old"—85 years old and older (Rosenwaike, 1985). In 1997, 13% of the U.S. population was 65 years of age and older (Kramarow, Lentzer, Rooks, Weeks, and Saydah, 1999). A rapid increase in the number of elderly is expected between 2010 and 2030, when the first baby boomers will reach age 65. By 2030, approximately 20% of Americans will be age 65 years or older (U.S. Census Bureau, 2004b). The fastest-growing segment of the elderly population consists of those 85 years and older. By 2040, the number of people 85 years and older will more than triple to over 14 million (U.S. Census Bureau, 2004b). In addition, life expectancy has been increasing, such that the average life expectancy was 80.1 years for women and 74.8 years for men in 2003 (National Center for Health Statistics, 2005). For babies born today, 82% will likely live to 65 years of age, with 35% surviving to 85 years (He et al., 2005).

Not only is America aging, but the demographics of the population are also changing. In 2004, 67.4% of the population was recognized as non-Hispanic white (NHW), 13.4% as African American, 14.1% as Hispanic, 4.8% as Asian American, and 1.5% as American Indian (some people identified themselves as belonging to more than one ethnic group) (U.S. Census Bureau, 2004a). The U.S. Census Bureau estimates that by 2010, approximately one third of the U.S. population will be people of color, with Hispanics constituting the largest ethnic group. By 2050, NHW Americans will account for approximately 50% of the country's population (U.S. Census Bureau, 2004a).

The older population is currently less diverse then the population of the United States as a whole. In 2004, it was estimated that 18.5% of people 65 years and older were minorities, with African Americans representing the largest minority group at 8.4% (Federal Interagency Forum on Aging-Related Statistics, 2006). Over time, however, the trend seen in the national population of increasing diversity is expected to occur in the older population as well, with minorities predicted to account for 40.0% of the elderly population in 2050 (Federal Interagency Forum on Aging-Related Statistics, 2006). The changing demographics of the older population, along with the cultural expectations within various minority groups, will undoubtedly influence the provision of LTC services.

In addition, the roles of women are changing. This trend is of prime importance to the delivery of LTC services because wives, daughters, and daughters-in-law provide much of the caregiving in the home. One of a woman's primary roles is as a mother. The nature of the life cycle does provide some insulation against a woman's shouldering the responsibilities for aging parents and child care responsibilities at the same time. In recent decades, however, some women have postponed childbearing until their late twenties and thirties. Because of this delay in starting their own families, they may have to balance the dual responsibilities of caring for parents and children as Tracy did. In addition, some women have assumed responsibility for raising their grandchildren (Boyd and Treas, 1989; National Alliance for Caregiving and American Association of Retired Persons, 1997; Administation on Aging, 2005). In addition to their familial responsibilities, many women, like Tracy, work outside the home; this makes it difficult to care for an elderly parent. Women who must bear the double burden of performing paid work and caregiving for a parent deal with the situation in a variety of ways, such as leaving the workforce or making changes at work or home (Boyd and Treas, 1989;

National Alliance for Caregiving and American Association of Retired Persons, 1997, 2004). In addition, they may consider using LTC services to care for their family members.

The growth and increased interest in extended care have been primarily driven by the changing economics of health care. Between 1976 and 1987, U.S. spending for medical care exceeded inflation by approximately 80%. In 1987, national health expenditures were 11.1% of the gross national product and totaled $500 billion. Spending for federal Medicaid and Medicare programs grew from $70 billion in 1982 to $111 billion in 1987 (Schneider and Guralnik, 1990). In 1993, the average daily private room rates for skilled nursing care and unskilled nursing care in extended care facilities were $111 and $96, respectively (Marion Merrell Dow, 1994). In the same year, the average charge for one day of hospitalization ranged from $700 to $1,000 (Brooks, 1994).

Costs have continued to spiral upward. In 2004, U.S. national health expenditures were 16.0% of the country's gross domestic product, amounting to more than $1.8 trillion. Spending by the federal government for health care totaled $600 billion, and state and local expenditures for health care amounted to $247.3 billion (Centers for Medicare and Medicaid Services, 2006c). In 1999, the average rates for private-pay residents were $146 for skilled care, $114 for intermediate care, and $101 for residential care (Jones, 2002).

Although extended care facilities are more economical than hospitals, their cost is still a major concern. National health expenditures for nursing home care totaled $115.2 billion in 2004 (Centers for Medicare and Medicaid Services, 2006c). Approximately 60% of these services were paid by Medicare and Medicaid, with Medicaid paying for the majority of these costs (Pastor et al., 2002; Kaiser Family Foundation, 2006).

The Congressional Budget Office has projected that LTC expenditures will increase 2.6% annually between 2000 and 2040. If these forecasts prove correct, LTC expenditures will almost double in 25 years (Scanlon, 2000). The aging of America coupled with a stressful economic climate makes it necessary to construct creative solutions to funding extended care.

INSTITUTIONAL SERVICES

As defined earlier, LTC or extended care is care that is delivered over extended time. LTC is not environment specific; it encompasses a spectrum of care levels ranging from acute hospitalization to ambulatory, home-based health care (Simonson, 1997). LTC facilities offer continuity of care and services to optimize a patient's recovery. In addition, LTC facilities are based on an interdisciplinary philosophy of care (Simonson, 1997).

Nursing Facilities

Nursing facilities (NFs) encompass a wide spectrum of care, with nursing homes being the most recognizable form. Since the passage of the Omnibus Budget Reconciliation Act of 1987 (OBRA, 1987), nursing homes have been referred to as nursing facilities.

Although the average length of stay in a nursing home was 892 days in 1999, the length of stay in an NF can vary greatly. Approximately 27% of the admissions into NFs are "short-stayers" who remain in the facility less than 6 months. Short-stayers can be further classified into residents who enter the NF extremely ill and with a short life expectancy and residents who enter the NF for short-term rehabilitation. Residents who will be in the NF longer than 6 months are referred to as "long-stayers." As many as 25% of residents remain in the NF for 3 years or longer. Long-stayers can be further classified into residents with impairments primarily of cognitive function (such as ambulatory patients with dementia) or impairments of physical function (such as residents with severe degenerative joint disease or end-stage heart failure) or residents with both impairments (Ouslander, 1989; Jones, 2002).

The most medically and therapeutically intensive of the NFs are the skilled nursing facilities (SNFs), which are regulated by the federal government. SNFs provide medical and nursing care in addition to restorative therapy, physical therapy, and occupational therapy. SNFs that are associated with a hospital are referred to as acute-affiliated nursing facilities (AANFs) (Simonson, 1996).

AANFs are designed for patients who need clinical and rehabilitative services and for patients who need continuous care that may not be available in all NFs. Patients with clinical conditions, such as postcerebrovascular accident or chronic obstructive pulmonary disease, and patients who require parenteral nutrition and postsurgical wound care may use AANFs. The average stay in these facilities is 12 days.

Approximately 15% of AANFs offer some kind of special care unit. For example, specially designed Alzheimer's disease units can allow patients to walk around in a protected environment. Additionally, the use of specifically trained personnel and protocols designed to address the needs of patients with Alzheimer's disease has a positive impact on the behavioral problems associated with this disease (Williams, Doyle, Feeney, Lenihan, and Salisbury, 1991).

Psychiatric Hospitals

Psychiatric hospitals provide a distinctive environment for a pharmacist's practice. Although little of the literature has focused on this practice site, pharmacists in these settings can provide medication reviews, clinical psychopharmacology consultations, individual patient consultations, and forensic consultations, and they can operate group patient medication clinics. Pharmacists also can participate in interdisciplinary team conferences regarding the therapy of patients, and they can contribute to pharmacy and therapeutics committees, quality assurance activities, and activities to ensure that the facility meets the standards set by the Joint Commission on Accreditation of Healthcare Organizations (D. Smith, personal communication, 1997). For more information on this subject, see Chapter 9.

Correctional Facilities

Correctional facilities often provide long-term health care to their residents. As the general population ages, so does the inmate population. Elderly inmates have chronic diseases and medical problems, just like the general population. The need for pharmaceutical care in this population offers a unique practice opportunity for pharmacists (Simonson, 1996).

Specialized Institutional Care

Patients with cognitive deficits are a distinct population that is often overlooked in the LTC setting. Secondary to their specialized needs, these patients may reside in intermediate care facilities for patients with cognitive deficits, foster homes, group homes, assisted living facilities, and state homes. Pharmacists working with these patients can offer many of the same services found in psychiatric hospitals and in general LTC facilities (Hegland, 1991; Sirroco, 1987).

Hospice Care

The word *hospice* comes from the Latin root for "hospitality" and "hospitable" (Storey, 1996). The focus of hospice care is the humane and compassionate management of patients with noncurable diseases. The goal of therapy is to maintain the quality of the patient's life rather than to cure the patient's disease. Growth in hospice care has been spurred on by its transformation from an alternative health care choice to a Medicare-reimbursable benefit with the 1985 enactment of the Medicare Hospice Benefit program. For a patient to be eligible for hospice under Medicare, death must be imminent (expected within 6 months) and the patient must agree to have all curative efforts halted and to focus solely on palliative efforts, or "comfort care" (Riley, 1996). Although services provided to patients may vary from organization to organization, services available to Medicare recipients include physician services, regular home visits by registered and licensed practical nurses, home health aides and home-maker services to help patients with ADLs, social work and counseling, medical equipment (e.g., hospital beds), medical supplies, medications for symptom control and pain relief, volunteer support for the patient and family, physical therapy, speech therapy, occupational therapy, and dietary counseling (National Hospice and Palliative Care Organization, 2003).

The National Hospice and Palliative Care Organization (NHPCO) estimates that there were more than 3,650 hospice programs in the United States in 2004 serving 1,060,000 patients. Although the majority of hospice patients are 65 years and older, approximately 18% are younger than 65. Forty-six percent of patients are admitted with a cancer diagnosis. The rest are admitted with noncancer diagnoses such as end-stage heart disease, dementia, debility, lung disease, and end-stage renal disease. In 2004, the average length of stay in hospice care was 57 days; the median was 22 days (National Hospice and Palliative Care Organization, 2004).

In 2002, 50% of hospices were independent, free-standing agencies; 32% were hospital based; 18% were home-health agency based; and fewer than 1% were based in LTC facilities (Connor, Tecca, LundPerson, and Teno, 2004). In 2002, Medicare covered 81% of hospice patients, 11% had private insurance coverage, and Medicaid covered 5% (National Hospice and Palliative Care Organization, 2004). More than 90% of hospice care days are provided in patients' homes, thereby avoiding more expensive hospitalizations (National Hospice and Palliative Care Organization, 2000). In 1995, it was estimated that for every dollar Medicare spent on hospice care, a savings of $1.52 was realized in Medicare Part A and B expenditures (National Hospice and Palliative Care Organization, 2003).

Working with hospice programs offers the pharmacist the opportunity to become an expert in the management of patients' pain. Few pharmacists are recognized as pain management experts, despite the fact that pharmacists are pharmacotherapy experts. Pharmacists can also participate in patient and family education about medications, review and manage patients' medication therapy, and ensure compliance with state, local, and federal regulations.

COMMUNITY-BASED CARE

Community-based care (CBC) is care that falls between institutional LTC and care for the ambulatory patient. In other words, the patient is not so debilitated as to need nursing home care, yet he or she cannot live completely independently. To help these individuals, CBC often includes a combination of housing, health care, and social support (Somers, 1993). In addition, it provides suitable conditions for patients who need some degree of assistance with their ADLs, such as eating, dressing, bathing, and transferring (Schneider and Guralnik, 1990).

CBC relies on the concept of a "managed risk environment": With increased independence of the patient comes increased risk to the patient, as well as increased responsibility. By accepting a certain degree of risk and weighing the options to try to meet the needs of each patient and the family members, a balance between risk and quality of life can be maintained (Simonson, 1996, 1997). Given this fact, much of the care provided in CBC is provided by nonlicensed personnel who may not have an adequate understanding of medications.

Adult Day Services

Adult day care services are "community-based group programs designed to meet the needs of functionally and/or cognitively impaired adults through an individual plan of care" (National Adult Day Services Association, 2000). Often patients enrolled in adult day care are functionally impaired and need to be cared for in a supervised environment. The care focuses primarily on maintenance and rehabilitation. Patients reside in their own or their families' homes and travel to a central location for services. The individual's family can continue their daily activities, such as work, because their loved one can be cared for in a supervised setting. In some cases, the adult day center also may offer health-related services and provide day care staff trained in patient care.

In 2001–2002, there were 3,407 adult day centers in the United States (Cox, Starke, and Holmes, 2001–2002). Many adult day centers are affiliated with or part of larger organizations, such as home health care agencies, skilled nursing facilities, medical centers, or senior citizen centers. Although no federal regulations exist for these centers, consultant pharmacists can provide staff, patient, and family education; advice on medication use and storage; maintenance of medication profiles; and drug-utilization review (DUR).

Assisted Living Facilities

Group residential settings are available in the community. Assisted living communities provide supportive, individualized, and personal services in a residential setting. In general, the level of care is not as extensive or as skilled as that found in a nursing home setting, even though assisted living facilities may house people who are disabled enough to qualify for nursing home care. Individuals usually "live and receive service in self-contained, unfurnished apartments in complexes that offer a full range of personal care, nursing services, housekeeping, and congregate meals" (Kane, 1995). This can vary, however, depending on the community and the needs of the residents. Some rooms may have kitchenettes with stoves and refrigerators; others may not. The goal of assisted living communities is to "encourage independence, privacy, and dignity . . . [and to keep] the persons involved and as active and empowered as possible"

(Buss, 1994, p. 60). As of 2004, there were 35,451 licensed assisted living residencies with 937,601 units or beds in the United States (Mollica and Johnson-Lamarche, 2005).

Board and Care Facilities

A board and care facility is defined "as a nonmedical, community-based living arrangement for elderly and people with mental/physical disabilities" (Mead, 1994, p. 738). Generally, these facilities house 3 to 16 residents who are unrelated to the operator. The facility provides shelter, board, 24-hour supervision, and personal care services. Currently, 34,000 licensed homes and an estimated 28,000 unlicensed homes provide these services (Hawes, Wildfire, and Lux, 1993; HHS Press Office, 1995).

Adult foster care is a variation on these board and care facilities. Foster family care "approximates the normal living environment, with the added dimension of supervision" (Dunkle and Kart, 1990, p. 241). In foster care, private residences are used for an unrelated person who needs supervision and/or assistance in performing daily activities.

FUTURE OF LONG-TERM CARE

Because the accessibility and affordability of long-term care are major concerns, the federal government and state governments are beginning to explore alternative financing and care options. Such alternatives include expanding home and community-based services, encouraging the purchase of long-term care insurance, developing programs to support informal caregivers, and integrating acute and long-term care services (Cubanski and Kline, 2002).

In looking for alternatives, the idea of "aging-in-place" has gained momentum. Aging-in-place refers to the "ability [a patient has] to receive services in the same setting as the person's needs change" (Mollica, 2003, p. 177). This approach seeks to maintain a level of independence "by continuing a certain degree of competence and degree of control over one's environment" (Cutchin, 2003, p. 1081). In 1999, the Supreme Court ruled that "under the Americans with Disabilities Act (ADA), states must serve people with disabilities (including the elderly) in the setting most appropriate to their needs, whether institutional or community-based" (Cubanski and Kline, 2002). Known as the Olmstead decision, this ruling seems to fit with the aging-in-place philosophy of care. As a consequence of this decision, states and consumers believe that a broader range of care alternatives may become available, including those endorsing the philosophy of aging-in-place. For example, many states are applying for Home and Community-Based waivers to Medicaid to allow them greater flexibility in providing extended care services to their elderly residents (Mollica, 2003).

One of the fastest-growing types of senior housing is the continuing care retirement community (CCRC). CCRCs are based on the aging-in-place philosophy and provide a continuum of independent living, assisted living, and skilled nursing care on a single campus. As a senior's health status changes, he or she can move among the different levels of care without having to relocate from the "campus." Between 2003 and 2004, there was a 32.2% increase in the number of CCRC facilities in the United States (American Seniors Housing Association, 2004).

Another example of an aging-in-place approach is PACE (Program of All-Inclusive Care for the Elderly). PACE's roots lie in San Francisco, where the On Lok Senior Services "developed a comprehensive, community-based approach to maintaining frail elders in the home" (Pierce, 2002, p. 173). On Lok initiated a Medicare demonstration project in 1976, which produced positive results. With the hopes of expanding this model, On Lok created PACE in 1986. In 1997, the Balanced Budget Amendment Act authorized Medicare coverage for PACE initiatives and allowed it as a Medicaid-reimbursable option. The core components of PACE include acute care, an adult day health center, durable medical equipment, home care, long-term care, meals and nutrition services, medical specialty care, multidisciplinary case management, pharmacy, primary care, restorative therapies, social services, and transportation (Pierce, 2002).

PHARMACY SERVICES IN LONG-TERM CARE

Pharmacy services in long-term care can be divided into two categories: distribution services and consultant services. Medications can be provided to residents in a facility from a pharmacy in a variety of unit-dose packaging systems, according to the needs of the facility. In addition to medications, the pharmacy may provide other distribution-related services, forms, and reports and be involved in the development of policies and procedures (see **Exhibit 8-3**).

In the case of consultant services, a consultant pharmacist may be employed by the distribution pharmacy, may be employed by a network of LTC facilities, or may be an independent consultant who contracts individually with a facility. Pharmacy consulting offers the practitioner many special opportunities (**Exhibit 8-4**), and many pharmacists have found a rewarding practice niche in this area. In this setting, the pharmacists are hampered only by their imagination. Pharmacists provide special pharmaceutical care services such as drug-regimen review (DRR) as well as monitoring for patient outcomes of care, identifying and resolving drug interactions, selecting cost-effective medications, using pharmacokinetic dosing principles to ensure proper dosing, following good formulary management practice, conducting DURs, educating health care providers, and providing case management to

Exhibit 8-3 Distribution Pharmacy Functions

Drug Distribution
Initial screening of medication orders
Drug packaging and labeling
Drug delivery (routine and emergency)
Medication reordering
Audit system for controlled medications
Emergency medication supply
Monitoring of proper storage of medication

Other
Policy and procedure development
Drug information
Durable medical equipment
Medical/surgical supplies
Enteral products
Intravenous services

Provision of Forms and Reports
Computer-generated patient medication
    profile
Medication administration record
Treatment records
Patient cardex
Physician order forms
Automatic stop orders
Treatment records
Patient care plans
Drug utilization reports
Billing statements

Source: Reprinted with permission from W. Simonson, *Consultant Pharmacy Practice,* (2nd ed.), 1996, p. 71.

Exhibit 8-4 Selected Pharmacist Activities in the Long-Term Care Environment

Drug regimen review (DRR)
Nutrition assessment and support
    services
Durable medical equipment (DME)
Surgical appliance fitting
Clinical research programs
Pharmacokinetic dosing services
Pain management counseling
Patient counseling
Intravenous therapy services
Therapeutic drug monitoring
Formulary development
Medication pass observation
Committee participation
Resident assessment and care
    planning
Drug use evaluation (DUE)

Drug information
In-service education programs
Enteral feeding products
Outpatient compliance packaging
Home diagnostic services
Laboratory test ordering and
    interpretation
Specialized medication delivery
    systems
Medical and surgical supplies
Quality assurance programs
Computer generated forms and
    reports
Infection control
Participation in state survey process
Specialized clinical activities
Drug utilization or use review (DUR)

coordinate medication use as a patient moves through various case settings (Gore, 1994; Simonson, 1997). Additional opportunities may exist in some settings for creating collaborative practice agreements with physicians for disease state management services in areas such as anticoagulation, asthma, diabetes, hypertension, lipid management, pain management, and smoking cessation.

Both skilled nursing facilities and intermediate care facilities are governed at the federal level by the Centers for Medicare and Medicaid Services (CMS). CMS develops and periodically updates guidelines to help nursing facility staff and consultant pharmacists provide the best care possible to the residents of the facilities they serve. These regulations and interpretive guidelines can be found in the State Operations Manual (SOM; see http://www.cms.hhs.gov/Manuals/IOM/itemdetail.asp?filter Type=none&filterByDID=-99&sortByDID=1&sortOrder=ascending&itemI D=CMS019027). Historically, as part of OBRA 87, federal legislation was enacted to address quality and care issues of nursing home residents. An important concept in the OBRA 87 requirements was that outcome indicators should be measurable and objective. In particular, this law mandated the use of a resident assessment instrument (RAI) to provide comprehensive, accurate, standardized, and reproducible assessments of each resident's functional capacity.

Assessment of the resident is the essential first step in the care planning process. This process includes the utilization of the RAI, a standardized interview instrument, upon patient admission to collect information about a resident. The RAI is used to promote an outcome-oriented resident care plan so as to ensure the quality of care and the resident's quality of life through the early identification of problems and risk factors that can be avoided, managed, or reversed (American Society of Consultant Pharmacists, 1998). This instrument includes three sections: (1) the Minimum Data Set (MDS), a tool used to collect the information needed to evaluate a resident; (2) the Resident Assessment Protocols (RAPs), which address and assess the issues identified from the information on the resident's MDS; and (3) the utilization guidelines.

The MDS data help to identify issues that place a resident at risk for an adverse outcome. These issues or "triggers" are addressed by using the RAP, a protocol that helps to mitigate the trigger. The RAPs are structured, problem-oriented frameworks developed by clinical experts to address the 18 areas that represent the most common problem areas or risks for nursing home residents. Through this process, the RAPs provide a systematic linkage to the resident's care plan (American Society of Consultant Pharmacists, 1997, 1998). As part of these requirements, the medication regimen for each resident must be reviewed monthly by a registered pharmacist (Gooen, 1990; OBRA, 1987).

Another part of OBRA 87 dealt with the use of "unnecessary drugs." Under this section of the legislation, patients' medication regimens must be free from unneeded medications—defined as any medications used in excessive doses (including duplicate therapy), for excessive durations, without adequate monitoring, without indications for use, in the presence of adverse drug reactions that indicate that the dose should be reduced or discontinued, or any combination of these reasons (Gooen, 1990). Several guidelines targeting the use of medications have been developed that will directly affect the consultant pharmacist's practice in long-term care; these can be found in Appendix PP of the SOM. Included are general guidelines for the DRR process performed by the consultant pharmacist and guidance for the use of medications in the elderly. Identification of use of inappropriate medication in this population is primarily based on the Beers criteria, which specifically outline inappropriate medications for elders (Beers, 1997; Fick, Cooper, Wade, Waller, Maclean, and Beers, 2003).

Drug-Regimen Review

The role of pharmacists has evolved since DRR first emerged in 1974 as part of a quality assurance program for the care of Medicaid recipients (Kubacka, 1996). DRR is a systematic process of review to assess a patient's medication therapy and make recommendations to that patient's health care provider regarding optimizing the patient's medication (Kubacka, 1996; Miller, Huey, Hord, and Jackson, 1996). As directed by federal mandate, the guidelines for DRR can be divided into several categories—for example, unnecessary medications/excessive doses, excessive duration of drug therapy, inadequate drug monitoring, absence of documented diagnosis or clinical symptoms, and psychoactive/antipsychotic medication use (Miller et al., 1996). To be efficient in the process of DRR, a pharmacist must develop a systematic approach of identifying actual and potential drug therapy problems. **Exhibit 8-5** provides an organized framework for the pharmacist to utilize when conducting DRR, along with examples for each category.

DRR has been shown to be an effective mechanism to reduce medication use and costs. The DRR that is required in the LTC setting is the heart of the process of monitoring outcomes of medication therapy (Gore, 1994). In a study by Cooper (1985), the use of DRR by a consultant clinical pharmacist in an LTC facility resulted in a 50% decrease in medication use. Miller, Panek, Barger, Cyrek, and Bolles (1994) also reported a decrease in medication use by using DRR in an adult day care facility. An analysis of 23 studies by Kidder (1987) revealed the efficacy of DRR and identified a net cost savings of $220 million to Medicaid and Medicare from such reviews.

Exhibit 8-5   Drug Regimen Review Framework

1. Drug use without indication. The resident is taking a medication for no medically valid indication.
2. Untreated indication. The resident has a medical problem that requires drug therapy but is not receiving a drug for that indication.
3. Improper drug selection. The resident has a drug indication but is taking the wrong drug or is taking a drug that is not the most appropriate for the special needs of the resident.
4. Subtherapeutic dosage. The resident has a medical problem that is being treated with too little of the correct medication.
5. Overdosage. The resident has a medical problem that is being treated with too much of the correct medication.
6. Adverse drug reaction. The resident has a medical problem that is the result of an adverse drug reaction or adverse effect.
7. Drug interaction. The resident has a medical problem that is the result of a drug-drug, drug-food, or drug-laboratory test interaction.
8. Medication errors. A deficiency or weakness of the medication use process of the facility has resulted in an actual or potential medication error.
9. Medication monitoring. Evaluation of medications for effectiveness and toxicity or adverse effects.
10. Medication costs. Intervention is needed to assist the resident with obtaining access to a lower-cost medication or overcoming a barrier to medication access, such as formulary restriction or prior authorization.

Source: From "Revisiting drug regimen review, part III: A systematic approach," *The Consultant Pharmacist,* 18, pp. 656–666, 2003. Reprinted with permission of The American Society of Consultant Pharmacists, Alexandria, VA. All rights reserved.

Drug Utilization Evaluation

Drug utilization evaluation (DUE) entails a sophisticated analysis of medications, their uses, and their contributions to various patient outcomes. Member institutions of the Joint Commission on Accreditation of Healthcare Organizations regularly perform this function. DUE may focus on a particular medication, evaluate the use of an entire class of medications, or monitor the therapy of a medical condition.

DUE is a criteria-based, ongoing, planned, and systematic review of medication. It is often prospective, in that the criteria to be applied are determined first, and then the medication for review is evaluated. Patient data and laboratory data are often included and available for review. DUE is frequently population-based in a specific institution and often part of an institution's quality assessment program. The Joint Commission recommends that a medication's inclusion be based on the following criteria: Is the medication frequently prescribed, known or suspected to present significant risk, known or suspected to be problem-prone, or a critical component of the care provided for a specific diagnosis, condition, or procedure?

As of 1995, the Joint Commission encouraged the use of an interdisciplinary approach to DUE and development of collaborative medication use review. Newer standards continue to support an interdisciplinary approach and focus on how patient care can be improved in LTC facilities as a result of problems identified through the review process (Kubacka, 1996).

Drug Utilization Review

Drug utilization review was established by the 1990 Omnibus Budget Reconciliation Act (OBRA, 1990). Pharmacists performing DURs are required to review past patterns of medication misuse, monitor current medication therapy, and offer patient counseling. By some practitioners' definition, DUR is a subset of DUE. Whereas DUE is prospective, DUR is frequently retrospective. DURs may use large databases and become part of a system's quality assurance program. In the past, use of such reviews has decreased medication costs and the use of inappropriate medications in LTC facilities (Kubacka, 1996).

DRR, DUE, and DUR have comparable functions, and the outcomes they measure can be classified into four categories: (1) therapeutic, (2) functional, (3) quality of life, and (4) economic (Gore, 1994; Kubacka, 1996). Documenting the patient outcomes of pharmacists' recommendations allows the practitioner to chronicle internal quality assurance. Documentation of patient outcomes also provides evidence that the pharmacists themselves are delivering quality patient care (Gore, 1994).

Examples of Consultant Pharmacy Services

Fleetwood Project

In an effort to demonstrate how consultant pharmacists can influence patient care in the nursing home environment, the American Society of Consultant Pharmacists initiated the Fleetwood Project. This project includes three phases: (1) assessment of the baseline costs of medication-related problems in the nursing home setting and the impact pharmacist DRR has on patient outcomes and costs; (2) assessment of prospective interventions utilizing a formal pharmaceutical care planning model for nursing home patients at high risk for medication-related problems (the Fleetwood model); and (3) assessment of the effectiveness of the Fleetwood model in assisted living facilities and nursing homes (Lombardi and Kennicutt, 2001).

In the first phase of the model, researchers conducted a cost-of-illness study to assess medication therapy in nursing homes. This study estimated that consultant pharmacists reduce medication-related morbidity and mortality costs by $3.6 billion annually in the United States (Bootman, Harrison, and Cox, 1997).

The second phase of the project focused on the feasibility of implementing formal pharmaceutical care planning in the nursing home setting. A 6-month pilot program was implemented in six nursing homes in Wisconsin. From the pilot study, it appeared that this approach to care was feasible (Moskowitz, 2003).

The third phase of the Fleetwood Project tested the effectiveness of the Fleetwood model and was conducted in 26 nursing facilities in North Carolina (Cameron, Feinberg, and Lapane, 2002). The investigators developed screening tools to help pharmacists identify patients at high risk for adverse events and treatment algorithms for alternatives to potentially inappropriate medications (Lapane and Hughes, 2004a; Christian, vanHaaren, Cameron, and Lapane, 2004). In addition, Fleetwood Phase III reported high job satisfaction among pharmacists participating in the project (Lapane and Hughes, 2004b).

North Carolina Nursing Home Polypharmacy Initiative

After determining that many nursing home patients covered by Medicaid were taking six or more prescription medications daily, the state of North Carolina initiated a pharmacy case management program. Thirteen nursing homes were selected to participate in this program. The goal was to reduce the total number of prescription medications taken by addressing problems such as therapeutic duplication, inappropriate drug utilization, multiple prescriber issues, and higher-than-normal drug use. In addition, there was an effort to switch brand prescription medications to generics or other therapeutic alternatives. After analysis by pharmacist–physician teams, 37% of patients were identified as needing medication changes. Results from the analysis indicated that the economic benefits outweighed the costs of implementing the program by a ratio of 13 to 1 (Henry, Mendelson, and Fallieras, 2003).

Opportunities for Pharmacists in Long-Term Care

Participation in other quality assurance activities and on the pharmacy and therapeutics committees of LTC institutions offers the pharmacist more chances to expand beyond the traditional dispensing role. The areas of pain control and managing patients with substance abuse problems also offer distinctive practice opportunities (Britton, Lobeck, and Kelly, 1994). At present, both of these areas sorely lack pharmacists' involvement. In addition, pharmacists are teaming up with primary-care providers in disease state management.

The Medicare Modernization Act (MMA) has also provided an opportunity for pharmacists to offer Medication Therapy Management Services (MTMS) to Medicare beneficiaries. The eligible providers, covered services, and reimbursement structures vary among the prescription drug plans (PDPs).

Many training programs are offered for pharmacists who are interested in working with the elderly population. The American Society of Consultant Pharmacists (ASCP) Research and Education Foundation is just one organization that has partnered with industry sponsors to offer advanced training in this area [1321 Duke Street, Alexandria, VA 22314-3563; phone: (703) 739-1300, fax: (703) 739-1500, e-mail: info@ascpfoundation.org]. Programs available from the ASCP Foundation and its partners include Alzheimer's disease/dementia, HIV/AIDS, geriatric psychiatric/behavioral disorders, pain management, and Parkinson's disease. In addition, there are specific disease-related pharmacotherapy programs, such as those dealing with heart failure, osteoporosis, and osteoarthritis.

Some pharmacists may choose to enhance their practices by obtaining certification in geriatric pharmacy. This is an optional process beyond required pharmacy licensure. A Certified Geriatric Pharmacist has met certain educational and experiential requirements and passed an examination designed to test his or her knowledge and skills in geriatric pharmaceutical care. Continuing education guidelines must be met to maintain this certification. For more information, contact the Commission for the Certification of Geriatric Pharmacy [1321 Duke Street, Alexandria, VA 22314-3563; phone: (703) 535-3038, fax: (703) 739-1500, e-mail: info@ccgp.org].

QUESTIONS FOR FURTHER DISCUSSION

1. Given that the elderly population is growing and that health care dollars are finite, how would you guarantee access to LTC facilities to all patients who need them?
2. The role of the pharmacist in the LTC setting is evolving. How would you ensure this role's continued progress? (Suggest curricular, research, and legislative solutions.)
3. Given the current financing mechanisms of LTC, how would you recommend that your parents or grandparents prepare for their potential LTC needs in the future?
4. Because the baby-boomer population will significantly affect the need for health services, how should the health care community and country prepare for 2030?

KEY TOPICS AND TERMS

Community-based health care
Consultant pharmacy
Elderly
Health insurance
Long-term care
Nursing homes

REFERENCES

Administration on Aging. (2005). *A profile of older americans: 2005*. Retrieved July 25, 2006, from http://www.aoa.gov/PROF/Statistics/profile/2005/2005profile.pdf

Administration on Aging. (2006). *Medicare drug coverage under Part A, Part B, and Part D*. Retrieved January 29, 2007 from http://www.aoa.gov/Medicare/resources/PartsBDFeb6finaldraftV6.doc

American Seniors Housing Association. (2004, July 30). *Senior housing construction continues at modest pace* [press release]. http://seniorshousing.org/OutsideOfStore/InteractiveFolders/DynamicDocs/showFile.aspx?Parent=152&File=2004SeniorsHousingConstructionReport.doc

American Society of Consultant Pharmacists. (1997). *RAPS and the consultant pharmacist*. Retrieved January 29, 2007 from www.ascp.com/ public/pubs/tcp/1997/jan/raps.html

American Society of Consultant Pharmacists. (1998). *Policy statement: Statement on the role of the consultant pharmacist in resident assessment and care planning*. Retrieved July 24, 1998 from www.ascp.com/public/pr/policy/resident.shtml

Beers, M. H. (1997). Explicit criteria for determining potentially inappropriate medication use by the elderly. *Archives of Internal Medicine, 157,* 1531–1536.

Bootman, J. L., Harrison, D. L., & Cox, E. (1997). The health care cost of drug-related morbidity and mortality in nursing facilities. *Archives of Internal Medicine, 157*(18), 2089–2096.

Boyd, S. L., & Treas, J. (1989). Family care of the frail elderly: A new look at "women in the middle. " *Women's Studies Quarterly, 1*(2), 66–73.

Britton, M. L., Lobeck, F. G., & Kelly, M. W. (1994). Multidisciplinary committee on the abuse of prescription medications. *American Journal of Health-System Pharmacists, 51,* 85–88.

Brooks, S. (1994). Subacute care. *Contemporary Longterm Care, 17,* 42–50.

Buss, D. B. (1994). Assisted living. *Contemporary Longterm Care, 17,* 60–61.

Cameron, K., Feinberg, J. L., & Lapane, K. (2002). Fleetwood Project phase III moves forward. *The Consultant Pharmacist, 17,* 181–198.

Centers for Medicare and Medicaid Services. (2006a). *Medicare and you*. Retrieved July 25, 2006 from http://www.medicare.gov/publications/pubs/pdf/10050.pdf

Centers for Medicare and Medicaid Services. (2006b). *Medicare coverage of skilled nursing facilty care*. Retrieved December 15, 2006 from http://www.medicare.gov/Publications/Pubs/pdf/10153.pdf.

Centers for Medicare and Medicaid Services. (2006c). *National health care expenditures, 1960–2004*. Retrieved July 25, 2006 from http://www.cms.hhs. gov/NationalHealthExpendData

Christian, J. B., vanHaaren, A., Cameron, K. A., & Lapane, K. L. (2004). Alternatives for potentially inappropriate medications in the elderly population: Treatment algorithms for use in the Fleetwood phase III study. *The Consultant Pharmacist, 19,* 1011–1028.

Connor, S. R., Tecca, M., LundPerson, J., & Teno, J. (2004). Measuring hospice care: The National Hospice and Palliative Care Organization national hospice data set. *Journal of Pain and Symptom Management, 28*(4), 316–328.

Cooper, J. W. (1985). Effect of initiation, termination, and reinitiation of consultant clinical pharmacist services in a geriatric long-term care facility. *Medical Care, 23*(1), 84–88.

Cox, N., Starke, M., & Holmes, C. (2001–2002). *National study of adult day services.* Retrieved January 29, 2007 from www.rwjf.org/news/Special/adultday-ServicesReport.jhtml.

Cubanski, J., & Kline, J. (2002). *In pursuit of long-term care: Ensuring access, coverage, and quality. Issue Brief #536.* New York: The Commonwealth Fund.

Cutchin, M. P. (2003). The process of mediated aging-in-place: A theoretically and empirically based model. *Social Science and Medicine, 57,* 1077–1090.

Dunkle, R. E., & Kart, C. S. (1990). Long-term care. In K. Ferraro (Ed.), *Gerontology: Perspectives and issues* (pp. 225–246). New York: Springer.

Feder, J., Komisar, H. L., & Niefeld, M. (2000). Long-term care in the United States: An overview. *Health Affairs, 19*(3), 40–56.

Federal Interagency Forum on Aging-Related Statistics. (2006). *Older Americans update 2006: Key indicators of well-being.* Washington, DC: U. S. Government Printing Office.

Fick, D. M., Cooper, J. W., Wade, W. E., Waller, J. L., Maclean, J. R., & Beers, M. H. (2003). Updating the Beers criteria for potentially inappropriate medication use in older adults. *Archives of Internal Medicine, 163*(22), 2716–2724.

Gabrel, C. S. (2000). Characteristics of elderly nursing home current residents and discharges. Data from the 1997 National Nursing Home Survey. *Advance Data from Vital and Health Statistics, 312.* Hyattsville, MD: National Center for Health Statistics.

Gooen, L. C. (1990, November). Consultant pharmacy: An evolving practice. *Pharmacy Times, 56,* 47–53.

Gore, M. J. (1994). Embracing pharmaceutical care: Consultant pharmacists lead the way. *The Consultant Pharmacist, 9*(2), 143–156.

Hawes, C., Wildfire, J. B., & Lux, L. J. (1993). *The regulation of board and care homes: Results of a survey in 50 states and the District of Columbia.* Washington, DC: American Association of Retired Persons.

He, W., Sengupta, M., Velkoff, V., & DeBarros, K. (2005). *U. S. Census Bureau, current population reports, P23-209, 65+ in the United States.* Washington, DC: U. S. Government Printing Office.

Hegland, A. (1991). Aging mentally retarded: Are we keeping up? *Contemporary Longterm Care, 14,* 58–84.

Henry, D., Mendelson, D., & Fallieras, A. (2003). *Clinical pharmacy management initiative: Integrating quality into Medicaid cost containment.* Lawrenceville, NJ: Center for Health Care Strategies.

Hetzel, L., & Smith, A. (2001, October). *The 65 years and over population: 2000.* Washington, DC: U. S. Census Bureau.

HHS Press Office. (1995). *HHS releases report on board and care regulation.* Retrieved January 29, 2007 from http://www.hhs.gov/news/press/1995pres/950828.html

Jones, A. (2002). The National Nursing Home Survey: 1999 summary. *Vital Health Statistics, 13,* 152.

Kaiser Family Foundation. (2006). *Medicaid and long-term care services.* Retrieved July 25, 2006 from http://www.kff.org/medicaid/2186.cfm

Kane, R. A. (1995). Expanding the home care concept: Blurring distinctions among home care, institutional care, and other long term care services. *Milbank Quarterly, 73*(2), 161–186.

Kane, R. A., & Kane, R. L. (1987). Long-term care: Principles, programs, and policies. New York: Springer.

Kidder, S. W. (1987). Cost-benefit of pharmacist-conducted drug regimen reviews. *The Consultant Pharmacist, 2*, 394–398.

Kramarow, E., Lentzer, H., Rooks, R., Weeks, J., & Saydah, S. (1999). *Health and aging chartbook. Health, United States, 1999.* Hyattsville, MD: National Center for Health Statistics.

Kubacka, R. T. (1996). A primer on drug utilization review. *Journal of the American Pharmaceutical Association, 36*(4), 257–262, 279.

Lapane, K. L., & Hughes, C. M. (2004a). Identifying nursing home residents at high-risk for preventable adverse drug events: Modifying a tool for use in the Fleetwood phase III study. *The Consultant Pharmacist, 19*, 533–537.

Lapane, K. L., & Hughes, C. M. (2004b). Job satisfaction and stress among workers providing long-term care pharmacy services. *The Consultant Pharmacist, 19*, 1029–1037.

Liu, K. (1994). A data perspective on long-term care. *Gerontologist, 34*(4), 476–480.

Lombardi, T. P., & Kennicutt, J. D. (2001). Promotion of a safe medication environment: Focus on the elderly and residents of long-term care facilities. *Medscape Pharmacists, 2*(1). Retrieved October 6, 2003 from http://www.medscape. com/ viewarticle/421217

Marion Merrell Dow, Inc. (1994). *Managed care digest: Long term care edition.* Kansas City, MO: Marion Merrell Dow, Inc.

Mead, V. (1994). Solving medication problems in board and care facilities. *The Consultant Pharmacist, 9*, 735–744.

MetLife Mature Market Institute. (2005). *The MetLife Market Survey of Nursing Home and Home Health Care Costs.* Westport, CT: MetLife Life Insurance Company.

Miller, R. J., Panek, D., Barger, M., Cyrek, B., & Bolles, N. (1994). Drug-regimen review in an adult care facility. *The Consultant Pharmacist, 9*(4), 437–445.

Miller, S. W., Huey, C. E., Hord, R. S., & Jackson, R. A. (1996). Drug-regimen review in pharmaceutical care: Regulation-versus-resident centered review. *The Consultant Pharmacist, 11*(3), 257–261.

Mollica, R. L. (2003). Coordinating services across the continuum of health, housing, and supportive services. *Journal of Aging and Health, 15*(1), 165–188.

Mollica, R. L., & Johnson-Lamarche, H. (2005). *State residential care and assisted-living policy: 2004.* Retrieved January 29, 2007, from www.nashp.org

Moskowitz, D. B. (2003). The pharmacist as care provider: Three projects support role. *Drug Benefit Trends, 15*(7), 43–46.

National Adult Day Services Association. (2000). *Adult day services fact sheet.* Retrieved October 10, 2000 from http://www.ncoa.org/nadsa/ADS_factsheet. htm

National Alliance for Caregiving and American Association of Retired Persons. (1997, June). *Family caregiving in the U.S.: Findings from a national survey.* Retrieved January 29, 2007 from http://www.caregiving.org/finalreport.pdf

National Alliance for Caregiving and American Association of Retired Persons. (2004, April). *Caregiving in the United States.* Bethesda, MD. Retrieved from http://www.caregiving.org/data/04finalreport.pdf

National Center for Health Statistics. (2005). *Health, United States, 2005 with chartbook on trends in the health of Americans.* Hyattsville, MD: National Center for Health Statistics.

National Hospice and Palliative Care Organization. (2000, August). *Facts and figures on hospice care in America.* Alexandria, VA: Kimberly Plake.

National Hospice and Palliative Care Organization. (2003, January). *NHPCO facts and figures.* Alexandria, VA: NHPCO Research Department.

National Hospice and Palliative Care Organization. (2004). *NHPCO facts and figures.* Alexandria, VA: NHPCO Research Department.

Nielson, J., Henderson, C., Cox, M., Williams, S., & Green, P. (1996, May–June). Characteristics of caregivers and factors contributing to institutionalization. *Geriatric Nursing, 17*(3), 124–127.

OBRA. (1987). *Omnibus Reconciliation Act (1987). Public Law 100–203.*

OBRA. (1990). *Omnibus Reconciliation Act (1990). Public Law 101–108.*

Ouslander, J. (1989). Medical care in the nursing home. *Journal of the American Medical Association, 262*(18), 2582–2590.

Pastor, P. N., Makuc, D. M., Reuben, C., & Xia, H. (2002). *Chartbook on trends in health of Americans. Health, United States, 2002.* Hyattsville, MD: National Center for Health Statistics.

Pierce, C. A. (2002). Program of all-inclusive care for the elderly in 2002. *Geriatric Nursing, 23*(3), 173–174.

Riley, K. Y. (1996). The role of the consultant pharmacist in hospice care. *The Consultant Pharmacist, 11*(12), 1313–1315.

Rosenwaike, I. A. (1985). Demographic portrait of the oldest old. *Milbank Quarterly, 63,* 187–205.

Scanlon, W. J. (2000, September). *Long term care insurance: Better information critical to prospective purchasers. United States General Accounting Office testimony before the Special Committee on Aging.*

Scanlon, W. J. (2001, March). *Long term care: Baby boom generation increases challenge of financing needed services. United States General Accounting Office testimony before the Committee on Finance.*

Schneider A., Fennel, K., & Keenan, P. (1999, May). *Medicaid eligibility for the elderly. Kaiser Commission on Medicaid and the Uninsured.* Washington, DC: Kaiser Family Foundation.

Schneider, E. L., & Guralnik, J. M. (1990). The aging of America: Impact on health care costs. *Journal of the American Medical Association, 263*(17), 2335–2340.

Simonson, W. (Ed.). (1996). *Consultant pharmacy practice.* Nutley, NJ: Hoffmann-La Roche.

Simonson, W. (1997). Pharmacy practice in the long-term care environment. *Journal of Managed Care Pharmacy, 3*(2), 189–194.

Sirroco, A. (1987). The 1986 inventory of long-term care places: An overview of facilities for the mentally retarded. *National Center for Health Statistics Advanced Data,* no. 143.

Somers, A. R. (1993). Lifeline: A viable option for the long-term care of the elderly. *Journal of the American Geriatrics Society, 41,* 188–191.

Storey, P. (1996). *Primer on palliative care.* Gainesville, FL: American Academy of Hospice and Palliative Care.

Stucki, B. R. (2005). *Use your own home to stay at home: Role of reverse mortgages to pay for long-term care at home, a blueprint for action.* Washington, DC: National Council on Aging.

U. S. Census Bureau. (2004a). *Population profile of the United States: Dynamic version.* Retrieved July 21, 2006 from http://www.census.gov/population/www/pop-profile/profiledynamic.html

U. S. Census Bureau. (2004b). *U. S. interim projections by age, sex, race, and Hispanic origin.* Retrieved July 21, 2006 from http://www.census.gov/ipc/www/usinterimproj/

U. S. Senate Special Committee on Aging. (1982). *Developments in aging (vol. 1, Report No. 97-314).* Washington, DC: U. S. Government Printing Office.

Walker, D. M. (2002, March). *Long term care: Aging baby boom generation will increase demand and burden on federal and state budgets. United States General Accounting Office testimony before the Special Committee on Aging.*

Williams, M. E. (1995). *The American Geriatric Society's complete guide to aging and health.* New York: Harmony Books.

Williams, M. P., Doyle, G. C., Feeney, E., Lenihan, P., & Salisbury, S. (1991, January–February). Alzheimer's unit by design. *Geriatric Nursing, 12*(1), 34–36.

Mental Health Services Delivery

Helen Meldrum, Bruce Lubotsky Levin, and Ardis Hanson

Case Scenario

You have just taken a new position as a community pharmacist in a busy chain store in an urban neighborhood. When you interviewed for the position, you met with managers at the regional office, so you never had the opportunity to get a feel for your patient population. After only one week on the job, you are now wondering if you are adequately prepared for some of its special challenges. As it turns out, your store is located in a block that has two psychiatric halfway houses and a large day treatment facility.

Even though you sometimes wonder what to say to some of your patients who have a mental disorder, you know that you are making a sincere effort to treat each person with empathy. Some of the technicians and younger pharmacy interns seem so uncomfortable with certain patients that they do not treat them with the utmost dignity. In fact, immediately after some patients leave the store, you have observed the technicians and interns gathering to gossip about them.

Obviously, at some level, your colleagues feel threatened by the challenge of counseling individuals with mental disorders. To diffuse their fears, they often make jokes and flippant comments. You wonder why pharmacy schools and technician training programs don't make more of an effort to prepare pharmacy professionals to understand the needs of individuals with mental disorders.

LEARNING OBJECTIVES _____

Upon completion of this chapter, the student shall be able to:

- Provide a brief historical overview of mental health services in the United States
- Understand the role of epidemiology and service delivery systems for individuals with mental disorders
- Identify the critical issues facing the treatment of individuals with mental disorders
- Understand the complexity of issues in the provision of mental health services within managed behavioral health care
- Better assess the potential role for pharmacists in caring for the pharmacy needs of individuals with mental disorders

CHAPTER QUESTIONS

1. Which two national laws had the most significant impact on the organization, financing, and delivery of mental health services in the United States?
2. What options are available to prepare for careers in the mental health professions?
3. Why is primary prevention so difficult to implement in the field of mental health services?
4. Why should pharmacists learn to read and interpret the behavior of people with mental illness?
5. What are some of the ongoing controversies regarding managed mental health care?

INTRODUCTION

Alcohol, drug abuse, and mental disorders constitute a complex array of major public health problems. The burden of mental illness on health and productivity in the United States and throughout the world has long been seriously underestimated. According to the Global Burden of Disease Study (Murray and Lopez, 1996), mental disorders accounted for more than 15% of the burden of disease in industrialized countries, such as the United States, and accounted for 4 of the 10 leading causes of disability for individuals five years and older. By this measure, major depression was the leading cause of disability, and suicide was one of the leading preventable causes of death in the United States. Mental disorders ranked second only to cardiovascular disease in the magnitude of disease burden.

Total national expenditures for the treatment of mental disorders and substance disorders were approximately $104 billion in 2001, compared with total national expenditures for all health services of $1.373 trillion (Mark et al., 2005). The mental health spending of $85 billion represented 6.2% of all health care spending in the United States in 2001. In the same year, an estimated $18 billion was devoted to the treatment of substance disorders, representing 1.3% of all health care spending (Mark et al., 2005).

Mark and colleagues (2005) have suggested that the increase in public payments from 57% of total mental health spending in 1991 to 63% in 2001, as well as a 17% increase in mental health prescription drug expenditures from 1991 to 2001, have contributed to the increase in the cost of treating individuals with mental and substance disorders. These expenditures include only direct health care costs, not "indirect" costs stemming from suicide, increased medical morbidity, reduced adherence to outpatient treatment leading to relapse and hospitalization, lost wages caused by missed work, decreased workplace productivity, housing assistance, law enforcement and public safety, and lost productivity (due to injury, illness, or premature death).

Mental disorders and substance disorders account for nearly $450 billion in direct and indirect costs annually. These total costs to society for behavioral disorders far exceed the costs of cancer ($104 billion), respiratory diseases ($99 billion), acquired immune deficiency syndrome (AIDS; $66 billion), or coronary heart disease ($43 billion). And yet, even with the enormous amount of money spent, a recent survey found that the United States falls behind other developed countries in its treatment of serious mental illnesses (Survey finds U.S. has high rate of mental illness, 2003).

In fact, the results of a recent national study suggest that the United States may rank number one globally in terms of prevalence of mental illness. Using a World Health Organization survey, a study of randomly selected Americans estimated that approximately 25% of the individuals met the criteria for having a mental disorder within the past year. The survey (which did not include serious mental disorders such as schizophrenia) also indicated that fewer than half of individuals who need help actually seek treatment. This survey, which was funded by National Institute of Mental Health (NIMH), focused on four categories of mental health disorders: mood disorders, anxiety disorders, impulse control disorders, and substance abuse (Kessler et. al., 2005).

Law enforcement officials have become increasingly concerned with calls to apprehend individuals with mental disorders because many officers lack the appropriate training and resources to deal with individuals who have mental disorders. At the same time, there have been reports of "mercy arrests"—in essence, taking an individual with a mental disorder into custody because he or she was involved in a minor scuffle on the street or similar incident. The same behavior would not warrant an arrest for someone without obvious symptoms of a mental disorder (Earley, 2006).

This chapter presents a brief historical overview of mental health services in the United States, including epidemiologic evidence from national studies on the prevalence of mental disorders in non-institutionalized populations. It reviews the critical issues involved in the treatment of mental disorders, and it examines current issues in managed behavioral health care. In addition, the chapter identifies emerging issues critical to pharmacists who must understand the increasingly complex nature of health and behavioral health care delivery systems in the United States. The chapter is also designed to help pharmacy students develop a better understanding of the needs of individuals with mental disorders, as illustrated in the chapter scenario.

HISTORY OF TREATING MENTAL DISORDERS IN THE UNITED STATES

Historically, the organization, financing, and provision of alcohol, drug abuse, and mental health (also collectively referred to as behavioral health) services in the United States have been complicated by a confusing assortment of uncoordinated public and private delivery systems and multiple funding mechanisms that have been parallel to, rather than integrated with, general (somatic) health services. This lack of integration between health and behavioral health services has contributed to the development of a number of dubious public health policies, including insurance providers' unequal coverage of behavioral health services vis-à-vis somatic health services (Levin, Hanson, Coe, and Kuppin, 2000).

The responsibility for caring for individuals with mental disorders has been shifted among religious, governmental, and health care organizations for many centuries. Throughout European and American history, the treatment of individuals with mental disorders has ranged from neglect or institutional warehousing to more humane treatment in the community. Treatment has often depended on the prevailing societal attitudes. Until the age of science, societies interpreted the etiology of disturbed behavior as supernatural or religious in origin. When the Industrial Revolution began, there were fewer people available in farming communities to care for deviant individuals. Accordingly, individuals with mental illnesses were often warehoused in poorhouses for lack of any practical alternatives.

During the early 19th century, Benjamin Rush, a physician and signer of the Declaration of Independence, called for a more humane approach or "moral treatment" in the care of individuals with mental disorders in the United States. This movement promoted the use of small institutions and community resources, which encouraged close staff–patient interactions. By the mid-19th century, Dorothea Dix, a nurse and well-known social reformer, had convinced state legislatures to establish institutional asylums (or "safe havens") for people with mental disorders. Her devotion to the institutional care and treatment of individuals with mental disorders shaped U.S. mental health policy far into the 20th century.

As Sigmund Freud's ideas became widely accepted in the 20th century, patients without major mental disorders began psychoanalytic treatment to resolve negative patterns established in childhood. Because psychoanalysis was expensive, members of the indigent population residing in mental hospitals were more likely to receive physical interventions such as insulin, lobotomy, or electro-convulsive therapy.

Although asylums sometimes represented modest improvements in the living conditions for people with mental disorders, these state institutions quickly grew in size without sufficient staffing and other needed resources. By 1955, the number of individuals hospitalized in state and county mental hospitals in the United States exceeded 550,000. Even though state mental hospital populations would subsequently decline thereafter, a concurrent increase occurred in the number of admissions of individuals with mental disorders at other health care facilities (often referred to as "trans-institutionalization"), including psychiatric units in general (community) hospitals, jails and prisons, and nursing homes as well as other long-term care facilities (Keisler and Sibulkin, 1987).

Today, the institutions Ms. Dix helped establish are few and far. Instead, we have returned to an era of trans-institutionalization, where an estimated 300,000 individuals with mental disorders are in jails and prisons, and half a million individuals with mental disorders are on probation within the legal system.

Another troubling fact is that the inmates on the psychiatric floors of jails spend six times longer in incarceration than the other prisoners who have committed the exact same crimes. Judges seem hesitant to release prisoners who have mental disorders. Complicating matters further, long-term jailers view these individuals as prisoners, not patients, and treat them accordingly (Earley, 2006).

The post–World War II era fostered more optimism that mental disorders were treatable as well as preventable. Based on the findings of the Joint Commission on Mental Health and Illness (1961), the U.S. Congress made the largest commitment to prevention and treatment of mental disorders in the history of the United States when it passed the Community Mental Health Centers Act of 1963. This initiative culminated in the federally sponsored community mental health center (CMHC) program. This massive program began in 1963 and funded the construction and staffing of CMHCs throughout the United States, one for every 75,000 to 200,000 people (referred to as a "catchment area"). The overall goal of this federal legislative initiative was to reduce state mental hospital populations by 50% within 20 years. At the height of the CMHC movement in 1981, 52% of the U.S. population was living in areas served by a CMHC (U.S. Department of Health and Human Services [DHHS], 1999).

The 1981 Omnibus Reconciliation Act consolidated 57 existing federal aid programs into nine block grants through which states obtained funding that could be used for purposes other than CMHCs (U.S. DHHS, 1999). However, separate community-based mental health organizations were established in selected areas of the United States without legislative or funding links to existing health and mental health care delivery systems (Petrila and Levin, 2004).

Other than the CMHC legislation in 1963, no other federal legislation has affected the financing and delivery of mental health services more than the 1965 passage of Titles XVIII and XIX of the Social Security Act, which established the Medicare and Medicaid programs, respectively (U.S. Congress, 1965). These programs pay for health services provided to the elderly and the poor, two populations who historically have not been covered by private health insurance. Whereas care for the elderly and medically disabled (Medicare) is administered by the federal government, Medicaid is a jointly administered federal–state program that finances long-term care and acute care.

The establishment of these entitlement programs in 1965 enabled states to further "depopulate" state mental hospitals and move a significant number of elderly individuals with mental disorders to long-term care facilities. Although many people believe that the development of new drugs that controlled psychotic symptoms ushered in the era of "deinstitutionalization," the significant reduction in the numbers of patients in state institutions can actually be traced to these financing policy changes. For a further discussion of the mental health benefits provided by the Medicare and Medicaid programs, see Urff (2004) and Frank and McGuire (1996).

The Carter administration proposed the Mental Health Systems Act (U.S. Congress, 1980), which sought to implement an extensive reorganization of mental health services throughout the United States by expanding services provided at CMHCs and offering services to various underserved at-risk populations, including children, adolescents, women, the elderly, and minority populations with severe mental disorders. However, in 1981, the Mental Health Systems Act was repealed (shortly after its enactment) by the Omnibus Budget Reconciliation Act (U.S. Congress, 1981). Since the CMHC legislation, Congress has not passed legislation to establish a national mental health services delivery network.

The 1980s were further characterized by increasing cutbacks in funding for the poor. As a result, the number of homeless people with mental illnesses has increased in the United States. Indeed, an enduring problem with the deinstitutionalization movement is the issue of where individuals with serious mental disorders can live. All too often, assisted living facilities (ALFs) provide a substandard home. For example, in the metro Miami, Florida, area, there are a reported 647 boarding homes operating as ALFs for individuals with serious mental disorders. Only 250 of these ALFs have met state licensing criteria. The others have been issued limited licenses in spite of sometimes appalling conditions. These facilities are often staffed by immigrants who have difficulty reading prescription labels and tracking adherence with medication regimens (Earley, 2006).

This trend has several implications for mental health systems as a whole. For example, a survey conducted by the American College of Emergency Room Physicians indicated that 60% of the physicians believed that the increase in the number of mental health patients seeking care in emergency rooms negatively affects access for all patients. This influx increases wait times and decreases available beds. Almost three fourths of these emergency room physicians believe that this hospitalization trend amounted to default "boarding" of patients with mental disorders, resulting in an overall loss of quality medical care (National Alliance on Mental Illness [NAMI], 2004).

In 1996, the Federal Mental Health Parity Act required insurers to offer the same benefits for mental disorders and substance abuse as they would for physical disorders, including any annual or lifetime limitations and restrictions placed upon such coverage (Levin et al., 2000). Since the 1990s, 39 states have enacted such "parity legislation," which requires equal coverage for mental health and/or substance abuse insurance compared with insurance coverage for somatic or physical disorders (American Psychological Association, 2004; Oregon Statutes, 2006).

In 2000, the General Accounting Office of the United States reported to Congress that almost 90% of employers who complied with the parity law have actually reduced or placed new, more restrictive limits on mental health coverage, such as visits to practitioners and numbers of days for hospitalization. Higher cost-sharing burdens for consumers have also been enacted. Clearly, the "spirit" of parity legislation is being violated on a widespread basis (National Mental Health Association, 2006).

The first Surgeon General's report on mental health, entitled *Mental Health: A Report of the Surgeon General* (U.S DHHS, 1999), examined a number of critical issues in mental health services delivery, including the following topics:

- The definitions and fundamentals of mental health and mental disorders
- Mental health and illness across age-specific populations
- Issues in the organization and financing of mental health services
- Confidentiality of mental health information from legal, ethical, and policy perspectives
- Proposed recommendations for the 21st century in overcoming barriers to mental health treatment and services delivery in the United States

The report recommended the following actions:

• Continuing to build a more thorough scientific knowledge base in mental health
• Overcoming the stigma of mental disorders in the United States
• Improving public awareness of effective treatments for mental disorders
• Ensuring the provision of both mental health providers and services
• Providing current, state-of-the-art mental health care
• Tailoring the treatment for individuals with mental disorders to age, gender, race, and culture
• Assuring access for individuals to seek treatment for their mental disorders
• Reducing fiscal and economic barriers to mental health treatment

The New Freedom Commission on Mental Health (2003) was established to study mental health services delivery in the United States and to suggest ways to overcome the three major barriers to mental health services: (1) the stigma of mental disorders, (2) the insurance and financial limitations placed on individuals with mental disorders vis-à-vis somatic disorders, and (3) the multiple, disjointed, and dysfunctional behavioral health care delivery systems in the United States. The Commission identified six goals as the foundation for transforming mental health care in this country:

• Understanding mental health as a component of overall (somatic) health and well-being
• Viewing mental health care as consumer and family focused
• Eliminating disparities in mental health services
• Implementing early screening, assessment, and referral to mental health services
• Prioritizing mental health services delivery and mental health services research initiatives
• Increasing the utilization of constantly emerging information technology in mental health

THE EPIDEMIOLOGY OF MENTAL DISORDERS

Fundamental to a discussion of mental health services in the United States is an understanding of the epidemiology of mental disorders—that is, the study of the factors that determine the frequency and distribution of mental disorders in human populations.

The most comprehensive mental health epidemiologic study conducted in the United States to date is the *Epidemiologic Catchment Area (ECA) Study,* which began in 1978 (Robins and Regier, 1991). Two elements of the study made it unique: (1) the ECA study was a very large initiative, including more than 20,000 respondents over five catchment areas (New Haven, Durham, Baltimore, Los Angeles, and St. Louis); and (2) the study examined the prevalence and incidence of mental disorders in the community as well as in institutional settings.

The major objective of the ECA study was to obtain prevalence rates of specific mental disorders rather than overall prevalence rates of all mental disorders. In summary, 20% of the people interviewed had a diagnosable mental disorder during a given year, with a lifetime prevalence of 32% for a mental illness or substance disorder. Annually, more than 5% of adults in the United States have a severe mental disorder (schizophrenia, major depression, panic disorder, or manic-depressive disorder) (Kessler, Berglund, et al., 1996). In addition, nearly 6% of adults in the United States have addictive disorders (alcohol and drug problems) (U.S. DHHS, 1999). Approximately 75% of individuals in need of services for alcohol and drug abuse do not receive treatment—a failure that has an enormous impact on the health and stability of individuals, families, and communities alike.

Several studies have examined the frequency and distribution of mental illness based on patients' race and income. For example, one study revealed that people who are uninsured are three times as likely as those who are insured to delay seeking health services due to the expense (Kaiser Commission on Medicaid and the Uninsured, 2003). In a comparative study of white, black, Hispanic, and Asian patients using mental health services in the New York City area, it was shown that a disproportionately high number of black and Hispanic residents use public clinics (including hospital emergency rooms) as primary sources for mental health services rather than seeking care from private providers (Minorities get different mental health care, 2003). This type of disparity in access to care may partially account for the difficulty in tracking the occurrence of mental illness in minority populations.

Another important national study on serious mental illness and co-occurring disorders was the *National Comorbidity Survey (NCS)* (Kessler et al., 1994). The NCS had two goals. First, it sought to improve upon the ECA efforts by incorporating revised nomenclature from the *Diagnostic and Statistical Manual of Mental Disorders* (*DSM*), third edition (American Psychiatric Association, 1987), and by more extensively examining risk factors that affect particular mental disorders. Second, it intended to determine the comorbidity of psychiatric disorders (Blazer, Kessler, McGonagle, and Swartz, 1994). Individuals with comorbid disorders include those diagnosed with more than one physical, mental, or substance disorder. As part of the NCS, more than 8,000 persons between the ages of 15 and 54 who lived in the continental United States were interviewed between 1990 and 1992.

Results from the NCS indicated a higher lifetime prevalence for mental disorders than the ECA study found, particularly for individuals with depression, alcohol dependence, and phobia. The NCS reported a prevalence of 3.2% compared with the ECA report of 2.8% for individuals with severe mental illness. The lifetime prevalence was 48% for any disorder (mental illness or substance abuse), and 29% of the respondents reported at least one mental disorder during the previous 12-month period. Approximately 40% of those who reported at least one mental disorder during their lifetime sought treatment in the mental health specialty sector.

The National Institute of Mental Health estimated that 1.8 million people in the United States have severe mental illness and a co-occurring substance disorder. More than 15% of Americans older than age 18 (25.6 million people out of a total population of 166 million) met the criteria for at least one alcohol, drug, or mental disorder (U.S. DHHS, 1999). People who suffered from a mental disorder were more likely to abuse drugs and alcohol. The NCS and follow-up reports also found that 83.5% of those individuals with lifetime comorbidity said that their first mental disorder preceded their first addictive disorder, and co-occurring disorders tended to be more chronic than mental disorders.

Kessler, Nelson, et al. (1996) used data from the NCS to study the prevalence of co-occurring addictive and mental disorders. These researchers found that the total number of people with co-occurring disorders (anyone with both a substance disorder and any mental disorder as described in the *DSM* classification system) was between 7 million and 9.9 million people, depending on the definition of alcohol abuse. Kessler et al. (2005) updated these findings to suggest that nearly half of people with mental disorders met the criteria for a diagnosis of two or more illnesses.

Kessler and colleagues (2005) also studied the trends in the prevalence and rate of treating individuals with mental disorders based on data from the original NCS study as well as data from the NCS Replication (conducted between 2001 and 2003). They found that while the prevalence of mental disorders did not change from the earlier NCS to the NCS Replication (approximately 29% between 1990 and 1992 versus approximately 30% between 2001 and 2003), what did change was the rate at which individuals with mental disorders received treatment—this percentage increased from approximately 20% in the NCS to nearly 33% in the NCS Replication. Nevertheless, despite an increase in treating individuals with mental disorders from 1990–1992 to 2001–2003, the majority of individuals with mental disorders do not receive treatment.

While space does not permit a more extensive review of the results of epidemiologic studies of mental disorders, Levin, Petrila, and Hennessey (2004) present additional information about the epidemiology of mental disorders in special populations.

TREATING INDIVIDUALS WITH MENTAL DISORDERS

There is no definitive etiology for all mental disorders. Instead, the roots of mental disorders may lie in developmental, biological, environmental, social, or cultural causes. Some severe mental illnesses can be treated but never cured.

The *DSM-IV* (American Psychiatric Association, 1994) originally identified approximately 60 types of mental disorders, including disorders usually first diagnosed in infancy, childhood, or adolescence; cognitive disorders such as delirium, dementia, and amnesia; mental disorders due to a general medical condition; substance-related disorders; psychotic disorders such as schizophrenia; mood disorders such as depression; anxiety disorders; somatoform disorders; dissociative disorders; sexual and gender-identity disorders; eating disorders; sleep disorders; impulse-control disorders; adjustment disorders; personality disorders; and other disorders. The current edition, *DSM-IV-TR* (American Psychiatric Association, 2000), specifies approximately 350 possible diagnoses for mental disorders.

Pharmacists are most likely to come in contact with individuals with cognitive disorders (delirium, dementia, and amnestic disorders); anxiety disorders, including acute stress disorder; depressive disorders (mood disorders); and psychotic disorders (including schizophrenia). Therefore, it is very useful for pharmacists to learn to distinguish among the different conditions associated with mental disorders.

People with various types of mental disorders can be treated with a wide range of pharmacological and/or psychological therapies. New psychopharmacologic therapies have allowed the deinstitutionalization of many patients (particularly individuals with schizophrenia) who previously required hospitalization. However, while these new antipsychotic medicines help control some symptoms, they do not arrest or reverse the progress of the disease itself.

Soon after the introduction of antipsychotics, monoamine oxidase inhibitors and tricyclic antidepressants were introduced to treat depression. In 1988, the first selective serotonin reuptake inhibitor (SSRI) was introduced. Today, these newer drugs for depression, which have fewer side effects, are prescribed more often by internists and general practitioners than by psychiatrists. Additional drug treatments include lithium for bipolar disorder and anxiolytics for anxiety disorder.

Pharmacotherapy is always evaluated in terms of costs and benefits to the patient. Given that no cure exists for individuals with the most severe mental disorders, the goal is to increase the patient's functioning to the highest level possible. It is true that these medications have revolutionized the treatment of individuals with severe mental disorders as well as the atmosphere inside mental hospitals. At the same time, some scholars have questioned the proliferation of direct-to-consumer media advertising, which suggests that pharmacotherapy is an easy answer to complex problems. These critics suggest that the increase in the number of patients seeking treatment (for a variety of conditions) is merely a reaction to these persuasive vehicles rather than a reflection of their efficacy (Karp, 2006).

MENTAL HEALTH PROFESSIONALS

A wide range of mental health professionals serve individuals with mental and emotional disorders in both hospital and ambulatory care settings.

Psychiatrists are licensed physicians with five years of additional specialized training after medical school. In 2000, there were approximately 41,000 clinically trained psychiatrists in the United States (Duffy et al., 2004).

Psychologists are nonmedical professionals who generally hold a doctoral degree in clinical psychology. In 2002, there were more than 88,500 licensed psychologists in the United States (Duffy et al., 2004). Licensed psychologists are generally able to bill third-party payers directly for services provided to clients.

Social workers find themselves in competition with psychologists at times because they also provide psychotherapeutic services at a lower cost. In 2000, there were in excess of 97,000 clinically trained social workers in the United States (Duffy et al., 2004).

Nurses also have the opportunity to specialize in psychiatric nursing. In 2002, more than 8,500 nurses were certified as specialists in psychiatric mental health nursing (Duffy et al., 2004). Particularly in inpatient settings, nurses with psychiatric training are responsible for conducting substantial patient assessment and assisting with the activities of daily living.

Individuals with mental and emotional disorders are also served by a variety of other practitioners, including (but not limited to) counseling psychologists, marriage and family therapists, professional counselors, psychosocial rehabilitation professionals, school psychologists, and pastoral counseling professionals. These mental health professionals work in diverse settings, including private psychiatric hospitals, federally funded medical centers (such as Veterans Affairs hospitals), general hospitals, residential treatment centers for children with severe emotional disorders, free-standing day treatment facilities, psychiatric ambulatory clinics, nursing homes, and community mental health centers.

THE ROLE OF PHARMACISTS

Pharmacists may interact with and counsel individuals with mental disorders as described in the chapter-opening case study. Unfortunately, some feel embarrassed, helpless, frightened, powerless, uncomfortable, or self-protective when working with patients with mental disorders. Furthermore, some pharmacists worry about the stigma associated with interaction with a person who has a mental disorder. Although pharmacists cannot function as psychotherapists, they can acquire the basic knowledge and skills needed to respond more effectively as a member of the health care team that provides services to people with mental disorders.

Although many articles are available about how to select the appropriate drugs to treat particular psychiatric conditions, no written advice has been available on how to recognize and respond to patients who have mental disorders and who present themselves to pharmacists. To learn more about individuals with mental or emotional disorders, pharmacists should consult supplementary resources on mental health and mental disorders (Levin et al., 2004; U.S. DHHS, 1999).

Pharmacists should also familiarize themselves with the Mental Status Exam (MSE), which is a standard procedure that has been used for decades by many members of the health care team to screen and gather information on patients (Ewalt and Farnsworth, 1963). The MSE includes questions about moods, thoughts, perceptions, and memory (Slater, Daniel, and Banks, 2003). Pharmacists need to be aware of this type of assessment so that they can communicate effectively with physicians, social workers, and (the patient's) other health care providers.

Patients with a wide variety of mental, cognitive, and emotional disorders may present in an equally wide variety of ways to pharmacists. For example, dementia may cause individuals to look sleepy or disoriented. Individuals with dementia may have impaired memory, and they may have an attention span deficit. Some pharmacists have experienced the difficult situation of a patient experiencing an anxiety attack in the pharmacy. Patients in such a state often have palpitations, difficulty breathing, hyperventilation, dizziness, faintness, and hot flashes or freezing in place.

Depression ranks as the leading cause of disability worldwide (Murray and Lopez, 1996). While depression is found more often in women than in men, individuals with depression often have co-occurring behavioral disorders (U.S. DHHS, 1999). Such patients often have difficulty concentrating, low physical energy, and a loss of interest in their usual activities, and they may increasingly withdraw from social interactions. Factors that have been associated with suicidal depression have historically included past and ongoing psychiatric treatment, previous suicide attempts, poor health, alcoholism, suicide of a close family member, recent loss of a job, divorce, or death of a loved one.

The patient with a psychotic disorder generally manifests inappropriate behavior and reality testing. They present behavior that is not the norm; for example, they might be too loud, bullying, paranoid, or expressionless. Thought disturbances create delusions and hallucinations that often leave patients appearing preoccupied and unable to clearly perceive the world around them.

To understand how a mental or emotional problem can be situational instead of chronic, consider the issue of grief and bereavement. Often pharmacists find themselves serving elderly couples together for years at a time and then not knowing what to say the first time the widow or widower comes in alone. Patients suffering from grief are likely to express guilt or anger. They may feel worthless and fear that the pain will never lessen. Some people stay in a period of denial, shock, or disbelief for a long time. In addition, people experiencing emotional pain are more likely to experience co-occurring somatic or behavioral disorders.

COMMUNICATION SKILLS

The opening case study suggested that some pharmacists, technicians, and pharmacy interns may be apprehensive or uncomfortable when interacting with individuals who have a mental illness or a substance disorder. However, persons with mental illnesses or substance disorders, parents of children with mental illnesses, and family members who are primary caretakers may have concerns about the use of antipsychotics, antidepressants, and other medications that should be addressed with their local pharmacist (Ewan and Greene, 2001; MacHaffie, 2002; Ranelli, Bartsch, and London, 2000).

Barriers to effective communication between pharmacists and their patients include the pharmacy environment, lack of awareness by patients, and trust in and loyalty to their physician. Confidential consultations are seen as a way for persons with mental illnesses to obtain this information without having to self-disclose their treatment history in a public setting (Schommer, 2000). Common questions for pharmacists revolve around therapy choice and medication side effects.

Although pharmacists are not expected to function as mental health practitioners, they can be caring and thoughtful allies to patients with mental or substance disorders. Pharmacists can do a lot more than simply wait for other health care professionals to treat patients. Specifically, they can play an active role in determining the main problem of an individual with a mental disorder and can gather information that can be given to a physician or emergency medical staff.

MEDICATION ADHERENCE

Pharmaceutical care is "the responsible provision of drug therapy for the purpose of achieving definite outcomes that improve a patient's quality of life" (Hepler and Strand, 1990, p. 539). For persons with mental illnesses, psychopharmacology can dramatically improve not only their own lives, but the lives of their family members as well.

Persons with mental illnesses often have co-occurring disorders (e.g., a mental and a somatic disorder, multiple mental disorders, or a mental disorder with a substance abuse disorder). Although taking multiple prescriptions for multiple disorders is not uncommon, the risk of side effects and adverse drug reactions increases with this practice. To avoid these complications, persons with mental illnesses may choose not to comply with their medication regimens.

Treatment guidelines in the United States suggest 1 year of antipsychotic therapy for patients who are experiencing their first psychotic episode and a minimum of 5 years of maintenance therapy with antipsychotics for patients who have experienced multiple episodes (American Psychiatric Association, 1997). A recent study of adherence with antipsychotics among schizophrenics indicated that 24% were noncompliant with their medication regimens, 16% were partially adherent, and 19% were excess fillers (Gilmer et al., 2004).

Vanelli, Burstein, and Cramer (2001) examined the medication adherence of patients in the community who obtained their initial prescription for an antipsychotic medication at a national retail pharmacy chain. Their study indicated that working with persons with serious mental illnesses requires a heightened accountability on the part of psychiatrists and pharmacists to enhance adherence among patients taking antipsychotic medication. They also suggested that "premature medication discontinuation may be not just a patient issue, but a larger systems issue that may be responsive to processes that improve medication administration and patient tracking" (Vanelli, Burstein, and Cramer, 2001, p. 1250). A recent study of follow-up care of patients with major depression by community pharmacists found that consultation and education by the pharmacists was an effective way to improve depressive primary-care patients' attitudes toward their medications (Brook, van Hout, Nieuwenhuyse, and Heerdink, 2003).

Baker (2001) suggests that nonphysician members of a mental health treatment team, such as pharmacists, can fulfill several essential roles in improving medication adherence. For example, pharmacists can assist in monitoring medication compliance and help shape patients' and families' attitudes toward changes in treatment. Furthermore, they may be able to provide critical feedback to prescribers about a patient's clinical state and treatment response. As pharmacy practice continues to move toward an integrated, holistic model, pharmacists, consumers, and their family members should all be involved in treatment and maintenance discussions, including choosing a therapeutic option and providing feedback about the response to this treatment.

Elderly patients who take antipsychotic medications may present some special concerns in terms of medication adherence. A national survey of the non-institutional adult population in the United States indicated that more than 90% of persons aged 65 years or older used at least 1 medication per week, more than 40% used 5 or more different medications per week, and 12% used 10 or more different medications per week (Kaufman, Kelly, Rosenberg, Anderson, and Mitchell, 2002). Although they account for only 15% of the U.S. population, seniors 65 and older consume 40% of all prescription drugs (Edlin, 2003).

Many elderly patients have a heightened susceptibility to adverse drug events. Misuse of prescription drugs is a significant issue among elderly populations, especially with the use of psychotropics. Atypical antipsychotics, for example, are frequently prescribed as first-line antipsychotics for persons with dementia who are experiencing behavioral problems, despite the poor evidence base for their efficacy and safety in this population (Beck, Paton, Euba, and Goddard, 2001). Under-monitoring of side effects may remain a problem as therapy continues.

Mort and Aparasu (2002) examined causes of errors in medication prescribing for the elderly, but many of the same problems apply equally to persons with serious mental illnesses and substance disorders. These include a basic lack of knowledge of drug effects, confusion or lack of consensus on treatment criteria, and inappropriate medications started by a previous provider. Often multiple prescribers and multiple pharmacies are involved in the care of a single patient, which exacerbates the problem and increases the chance of adverse reactions or noncompliance with a medication regimen. Patients may also demand an inappropriate medication or base their decision to take a drug strictly on its cost, rather than the efficacy of the drug. Patients may also choose to use an over-the-counter medication rather than a prescription drug without understanding the ramifications of such a choice.

While Gurwitz et al. (2003) advocate further development and testing of new approaches to enhance collaborations between those who prescribe drugs and pharmacists to be pursued in the ambulatory setting, collaborations between home health care delivery workers and pharmacists are proving fruitful as well. Home care pharmacy consultation can also reduce medication-related risks. Barriers to this type of intervention include brief enrollment restrictions, heterogeneous care environments, discontinuity of care, scheduling and travel difficulties, and lack of reimbursement polices for pharmacists (Boling, 2002).

PREVENTION

The field of public health has long utilized the concept of prevention—to prevent the initial occurrence of major public health problems (primary prevention), to prevent recurrences or exacerbations of diseases already diagnosed (secondary prevention), and to reduce the amount of disability caused by diseases so that at-risk populations can reach the highest possible level of functioning (tertiary prevention). Initially, efforts in disease prevention were directed toward infectious/tropical diseases through community immunization, water treatment, improved sanitation, use of healthier foods, and other methods focusing on personal and public hygiene. Later, when the community mental health movement was developed, mental health professionals extended the concept and principles of prevention to mental disorders.

Primary prevention has proved challenging to operationalize for individuals with severe mental illnesses because of the complex etiology of mental disorders. Secondary prevention has shown the most promise in the field of children's mental health services (Friedman et al., 2004). Tertiary prevention has been the thrust of most mental health interventions in the United States. Successful initiatives in the delivery of mental health services have been achieved through innovative efforts including the community support programs financed by the National Institute of Mental Health, psychosocial rehabilitation, and assertive community treatment programs (Young and Magnabosco, 2004; Elpers and Levin, 1996).

Nevertheless, an Institute of Medicine (1994) report on preventive intervention research of mental disorders identified significant problems in applying the public health definitions of primary, secondary, and tertiary prevention to mental disorders—namely, difficulty in diagnosing mental disorders (i.e., the notion of "caseness") and changing definitions and diagnostic classifications systems of mental disorders over time. As a consequence of its findings, the Institute of Medicine established a mental health intervention spectrum for mental disorders that defined three core activities: prevention, treatment, and maintenance.

Prevention activities are similar to the concept of primary prevention in public health: interventions that would occur prior to the initial onset of a mental disorder (with the aim of reducing the occurrence of new cases). In addition, preventive measures were categorized into three types: universal, selective, and indicated (Gordon, 1983). Universal preventive interventions for mental disorders target the general public. Selective preventive interventions target individuals or portions of a population with a significantly higher than average risk of developing a specific mental disorder. Indicated preventive interventions target high-risk individuals who are identified as having symptoms of a potential mental disorder, but have not been formally diagnosed with a mental disorder.

Treatment interventions include the identification of individuals with mental disorders and the standard treatment for individuals with those disorders. They also include interventions to reduce the likelihood of future co-occurring disorders. Maintenance refers to interventions that reduce the rates of relapse and recurrence as well as the provision of rehabilitation.

Although these alternative prevention definitions have been important in conceptualizing the nature of the prevention of mental disorders, they have been neither universally accepted nor universally utilized by mental health professionals. In addition, there has been heightened debate in recent years regarding whether to offer mental health services as part of an integrated health care delivery system or as separate, "carved-out" specialty services.

Mental health research has also identified certain risk and protective factors that might potentially function to predispose or protect against the occurrence of mental disorders (Institute of Medicine, 1994). Risk factors are characteristics, variables, or hazards that make it more likely (for a person selected at random from the general population) that an individual would develop a mental disorder. They may reside in an individual, a family, a community, or institutions (i.e., the environment) that surround the individual. Risk factors can be biological or psychosocial in nature. Some risk factors (e.g., gender and family history) are fixed or determined by genetics; others (e.g., lack of social support) can be altered through interventions.

By contrast, protective factors may potentially improve an individual's response to some environmental force or problem. Such factors may assist individuals in adapting, withstanding, and/or becoming resistant to a mental health problem (e.g., stress, divorce, or other traumatic life events). Protective factors can reside in individuals, families, or the community. Obviously, researchers have an appreciable amount of work ahead of them in conducting research into the effects of protective factors on individuals, families, and the community, and across an individual's lifespan.

To date, certain risk factors have been identified as common to a number of mental disorders: chronic physical illness, low socioeconomic status, paternal criminality, maternal mental disorder, difficult temperament, neurophysiologic deficits, severe marital discord, overcrowding or a large family size, and some community factors (e.g., living in a community with inadequate schools). In addition, certain risk factors appear to heighten an individual's vulnerability to multiple risk factors (i.e., an accumulation of risk factors) that may increase the likelihood of disease onset. Nevertheless, the introduction of protective factors can often ease this situation (Institute of Medicine, 1994). Thus community preventive interventions for mental disorders might focus on decreasing risk factors (for a specific mental disorder) and increasing protective factors in an effort to reduce the incidence of mental disorders in the community or specific population subgroup.

One of the most controversial aspects of the mental health intervention spectrum for mental disorders has been the omission of mental health promotion. The Institute of Medicine (1994) suggested that mental health promotion should focus on the enhancement of well-being rather than serve as a preventive intervention for mental disorders. As a result, the focus on mental health versus mental illness has differentiated mental health promotion from the enhancement of protective factors in preventive mental health interventions (Institute of Medicine, 1994).

MENTAL HEALTH PROMOTION

Mental health promotion activities have been developed for individuals, groups, and communities in an effort to enhance individuals' competence, self-esteem, and sense of well-being rather than to intervene in the prevention of emotional problems, social problems, or mental disorders. Mental health promotion initiatives (including those focusing on the enhancement of mental health, positive mental health, mental well-being, and self-esteem maintenance and enhancement) have been introduced by numerous organizations, including schools, health organizations, industry, governmental organizations, and religious institutions. In addition, societies and the multiple cultures they contain offer varying abilities to provide mental health promotion activities.

Regardless of the focus of a particular mental health promotion initiative, social resources are critical elements in all mental health promotion activities (Kulbok, 1985). In particular, supporting and strengthening family functioning is a major component of many mental health promotion programs (Duffy, 1988). Nevertheless, mental health promotion represents a diverse and complex array of activities that have been found to be difficult to validate empirically.

NATIONAL MENTAL HEALTH OBJECTIVES

The overall mental health goal for Americans, as outlined in *Healthy People 2010* (U.S. DHHS, 2000), has been to improve mental health and ensure access to appropriate, quality mental health services. This has not been an easy task in the United States, given the significant prevalence of mental disorders in this country (as discussed earlier in this chapter). In addition, the co-occurrence of mental disorders and substance abuse (as well as the co-occurrence of mental disorders and somatic disorders) is a significant factor in determining the success of any national mental health initiative. According to data from the U.S. Department of Health and Human Services (1999), in the United States, 29% of individuals 18 years and older with a lifetime history of any mental disorder also have an addictive disorder, 37% of adults with an alcohol disorder also have a mental disorder, and 53% of adults with a drug disorder also have a mental disorder.

From a services delivery perspective, the unequal insurance coverage of mental disorders relative to the coverage available for somatic disorders (Levin et al., 2000), combined with the stigma associated with the identification, diagnosis, treatment, and rehabilitation of individuals with mental disorders, has made goals related to mental health quite difficult to attain. Nevertheless, *Healthy People 2010* (U.S. DHHS, 2000) has established 14 mental health objectives for the United States, grouped under three categories: mental health status improvement, treatment expansion, and state activities.

Five objectives were established under mental health status improvement:

1. Reduce the suicide rate
2. Reduce the rate of suicide attempts by adolescents
3. Reduce the proportion of homeless adults who have a severe mental disorder
4. Increase the proportion of individuals with a severe mental disorder who are employed
5. Reduce the relapse rates for individuals with eating disorders

Six objectives were established under treatment expansion for mental disorders:

1. Increase the number of individuals seen in primary health care who receive mental health screening and assessment
2. Increase the proportion of children with mental health problems who receive treatment
3. Increase the proportion of juvenile justice facilities that screen new admissions for mental health problems
4. Increase the proportion of adults with mental disorders who receive treatment
5. Increase the proportion of individuals with co-occurring substance abuse and mental disorders who receive treatment for both disorders
6. Increase the proportion of local governments with community-based jail diversion programs for adults with severe mental disorders

Three objectives were established under state activities for mental health services:

1. Increase the number of states that track consumers' satisfaction with the mental health services

2. Increase the number of states that address cultural competence
3. Increase the number of states that address mental health screening and treatment services for older adults

MANAGED CARE

The concept of "managing" health care can be traced to the early part of the 20th century and the evolution of prepaid health plans in the United States (Levin, 1992). While the growth of managed care has gone through a number of major evolutionary stages over the last half-century, managed care strategies have remained an evolving array of health care review and service coordination mechanisms that ultimately attempt to control (reduce) the utilization and costs of health and behavioral health services. A multitude of hybrid and specialty models of managed care organizations (MCOs) exist, including managed behavioral health care organizations (MBHOs). Nevertheless, the predominant managed care systems remain health maintenance organizations (HMOs), preferred provider organizations (PPOs), and point-of-service plans.

With the proliferation of state-mandated mental health and substance abuse benefits in the 1980s, managed behavioral health care companies were created to manage the behavioral health benefits within health insurance plans as well as to manage mental health and substance abuse benefits that were contracted out (i.e., "carved out") from HMO and PPO benefit plans. Dental health and pharmacy benefits have also been carved out in some managed care benefit packages.

In addition to providing mental health and substance abuse services to employed populations, MCOs have actively expanded into the public sector. In recent years, an increasing number of public mental health systems have shifted their priorities from providing mental health and substance abuse services to purchasing these services, and from maintaining institutions and other services to using a "systems-of-care" approach to the delivery of mental health services (Essock and Goldman, 1995).

During the past 25 years, numerous employers and government programs have carved out or separated mental health service benefits from somatic health care benefits through contractual arrangements with specialized vendors that may assume some level of financial risk. Specialty managed mental health organizations have subsequently emerged under the rubric of MBHOs. MBHOs attempt to reduce the costs of mental health care through the utilization of mental health practitioners at discounted fees, reduction in the length of mental health treatment, decreased use of hospital treatment, and increased use of ambulatory mental health care treatment. While these plans initially focused on contracting with employers in the private sector as well as subcontracting with HMOs and other models of MCOs, recent studies have reported significant declines in the costs of mental health care under these MCOs (Cuffel, Goldman, and Schlesinger, 1999; Goldman, McCulloch, and Sturm, 1998; Grazier, Eselius, Hu, Shore, and G'Sell, 1999; Ma and McGuire, 1998).

Managed care "carve-out" organizations have found it cost-effective to substitute drug treatments for other types of mental health services. Under both private insurance and Medicaid, for example, it has become easier to get a referral for medication management than a referral for therapy. Cultural support for psychoactive agents has also allowed "carve-out" organizations to realize economies of scale. If physicians needed only a few thousand pills to treat depressed patients, the price per pill would be astronomical. In contrast, when millions of Americans either demand these agents (often as a result of aggressive marketing of these drugs) or are willing to try them, the per-unit cost of these medications drops dramatically. Competitive market forces and consumer habits, therefore, coalesce in such a way as to boost the business goals of the managed care industry (Karp, 2006; Frank, Conti, and Goldman, 2005).

MCOs also have the potential to encompass the basic principles of health promotion and disease prevention in their dealings with patients with mental illness. Although MCOs have used periodic health screening, immunizations, nutrition education, prenatal care, and other prevention strategies with other patient populations, preventive initiatives in mental health services have been slower to develop, in part because of the variety of limitations on managed mental health insurance benefits. Nevertheless, with the continuing evolution of managed health care in the 21st century, more attention is likely to be paid to mental health promotion strategies associated with lifestyle behaviors. For example, many health plans already run stress management seminars that focus on reducing "Type A" behavior, which is characterized by an orientation toward competitive achievement, a focus on time urgency, and an ever-present anger and hostility.

JUSTICE SYSTEMS

Traditional mental health delivery systems are not the only settings in which individuals with mental and emotional disorders receive treatment. Increasingly, individuals with mental disorders are being treated in a variety of delivery systems, including general health care delivery systems, long-term care facilities, jails and prisons, social service agencies, and education systems. In addition, the majority of individuals with behavioral disorders are not treated within mental health care delivery systems.

It's hard to imagine a more difficult situation than managing individuals with mental disorders in a homeless shelter, yet Kaplan (2000) has suggested that jails are fast becoming the "mental hospitals of last resort."

Whereas a patient leaving a psychiatric facility would have a discharge plan, a drug regimen, and a referral for medical assistance or an after-care program, jails and prisons have no obligation to help the released person cope with his or her problems of reentering society. In fact, individuals may have an incentive to seek entrance into jails and prisons, because they guarantee food, shelter, and medical care. Furthermore, law enforcement officials have become increasingly frustrated with calls to apprehend individuals with mental disorders because officers often lack appropriate training and resources to deal with these individuals.

CONTROVERSIES IN MANAGED CARE

Managed care has some decided shortcomings for patients with mental health issues. Increasingly, many MCOs cover only acute mental health care. Because people with mental disorders are highly stigmatized, they are at a decided disadvantage when acting as self-advocates within this kind of managed care system. In addition, because many case management programs are linked to workplace employee-assistance programs (EAPs), there is a risk that the employer will learn about an employee's personal problems if he or she seeks mental health care through such a program.

In addition, the systems of mental health care delivery in the United States have not adequately met the needs of individuals with different cultural and socioeconomic backgrounds. A large national study found that individuals with severe mental disorders were disproportionately African American, unmarried, less educated males with lower incomes (McAlpine and Mechanic, 2000). It has been suggested that current psychopharmacological and psychological interventions may be inadequate for multicultural populations because these treatments were designed primarily for Americans of European descent (Dana, 1998).

A major consequence of the growth of managed behavioral health care has been the devastation of the specialized providers and programs that focused on patients with chemical dependency issues. Between 1989 and 1992, one third of the private treatment centers in the United States that specialized in problems with addictions closed. Because many managed mental health plans pay only for chemically dependent patients who have a dual diagnosis with a medical or mental illness, there is an incentive to misdiagnose the secondary symptoms of addiction as a mental disorder so that the patients qualify for health insurance coverage (Gorski, 1994).

States' ability to experiment with large-scale health reform is limited by the Employee Retirement Income Security Act of 1974 (ERISA), which hinders the ability of state governments to regulate self-insured employee benefit plans (Ridgley and Goldman, 1996). Because ERISA was originally designed to regulate employee pension plans, it contains few codes pertaining to health care; with this law's passage, the federal government unwittingly created a "regulatory gap" that has frustrated states' efforts to provide for their citizens' health (Francesconi, 1995). However, this gap may now be narrowing. The Mental Health Parity Act (U.S. Congress, 1996) set a precedent in terms of congressional lawmakers' willingness to impose benefit mandates on ERISA plans. A 2003 court decision, *Rush Prudential HMO v. Moran,* also boosted states' abilities to regulate HMOs and other health care providers that formerly were the sole domain of the federal government (Zelinsky, 2003). However, although 38 states have passed some form of parity provisions, their full impact on the insurance market cannot be assessed, because a majority of the plans are preempted from compliance with many state insurance mandates by ERISA.

At the heart of the debate over managed behavioral health care as well as parity legislation is the difficulty inherent in determining the impact of mental health care benefit changes on services utilization and costs. In other words, how do carve-out mental health services affect service delivery outcomes (Barry, Frank, and McGuire, 2006)? This question remains to be answered.

THE FUTURE OF THERAPEUTIC SERVICES

Because of the complexity involved in determining the etiology, diagnosis, and treatment of mental disorders as well as the high prevalence of co-occurring disorders, insurance providers and MCOs continue to offer unequal coverage for behavioral disorders vis-à-vis somatic disorders. And yet, effective therapy can function as a social service that has a broader impact on health by restoring and improving functioning and preventing dysfunction. In addition, the literature provides evidence that the timely treatment of mental and substance disorders generates a corresponding reduction in the utilization and cost of somatic health services (Fiedler and Wight, 1989).

The National Association of Psychiatric Health Systems (NAPHS) tracks the average length of stay in psychiatric hospitals on an annual basis. As of 2005, the average length of stay in mental hospitals was typically less than 10 days (NAPHS, 2006). The problem is that in the past, the longer stays of patients with high-end indemnity insurance have typically "subsidized" innovative clinical and research programs that generated little income at many hospitals. Managed care companies, however, prefer that patients receive intensive therapy with a focus on pharmacotherapy. Psychiatrists at McLean Psychiatric Hospital (Belmont, Massachusetts), for example, have recounted experiences of conflict with managed care reviewers (many of whom are not licensed medical professionals) regarding what drug to use or what treatment plan to pursue.

The practice of psychotherapy has been an easy target for cost-conscious managed care administrators. HMOs prescribe medication instead of other types of therapy because it is less expensive. Psychotherapists have divided into three groups based on their responses to these managed care trends. The first group embraces the changes and dismisses critics as living in the past. The second group includes providers who do not like the changes but are trying to fit at least part of their practice into the managed care environment. The third group tries to survive in what is left of the fee-for-service system while avoiding any association with managed care. Overall, the changes in the environment for psychotherapy have meant that most therapists have seen a drop in income and fewer clients. Many have also been forced to alter treatment plans for patients, in part because clinicians may be legally at risk for failure to provide care, even when payment for such treatment has been denied by a third party.

If long-term psychodynamic psychotherapy is not seen as a useful skill, it will eventually become obsolete—not because patients would not benefit from it, but simply because no one will pay for it. Ironically, in the case where long-term therapy is authorized, the patient may have to be managed for the additional anxiety brought on by worrying that benefits may be reduced and a trusted therapeutic relationship discontinued. Paradoxically, people in emotional crisis may have to advocate for themselves in the process of obtaining care (Shapiro, 1995).

The managed care industry has even implemented policies that seem to contradict its own goals of cost containment. For example, Glenmullen (2000) described trying to get an MCO to approve payments of a few hundred dollars a year to reimburse a patient who was responding well to St. John's wort. The claim was denied, but the patient was instantly approved for a $4,000 annual supply of Prozac. Glenmullen has also written about a case involving a patient who was a Holocaust survivor (the patient had witnessed her parents' murders). After a 20-minute consultation with a primary-care physician, she was approved for an SSRI but not referred to therapy to work through her traumatic memories (Glenmullen, 2005). According to Glenmullen, these cases demonstrate that there is not sufficient oversight of each individual patient's best interests under managed care plans.

Dworkin (2006) cites an equally stunning story about a woman who lived in New York City during the World Trade Center attacks on September 11, 2001. Immediately after these traumatic events, she complained to her physician about feeling edgy and was offered a prescription, but no forum for talking through the event (Dworkin, 2006).

Clinicians from Harvard Medical School (Ware et al., 2000) worry that providers practicing in managed care organizations are being gradually re-professionalized from "critics" into "proponents" and are losing a moral and ethical vision of good treatment standards. In fact, *The New*

York Times has reported that an increasing number of physicians are ignoring FDA labeling by writing prescriptions for psychoactive drugs for preschool populations. In the Medicaid population alone, the number of children younger than age 5 receiving antidepressants has doubled in recent years, even though the long-term consequences of these drugs on brain development are unclear (Goode, 2000b).

While providers favoring drug therapy and those favoring talk therapy have sometimes been in conflict (Kramer, 2005), a study confirmed that for patients with depression, a combination approach of talk therapy and drug therapy works best. By studying three groups of patients, researchers discovered that those patients given drugs only and those patients given psychotherapy showed improvement rates of approximately 52–55%. By comparison, when patients were given both drug and psychotherapy treatments, approximately 85% showed improvement in their symptoms (Goode, 2000a). Another study showed that such a combination of talk therapy and drug treatment works especially well for low-income, minority women (Psychotherapy, medication most effective, 2003).

A trend that is gathering momentum is the idea of a guild or alliance of independent mental health practitioners, built upon the premise that patients are fed up with managed care and are ready to pay out-of-pocket for mental health care (given reasonable rates). Under this framework, therapists market themselves through membership directories that detail their approaches to treatment. The movement is doing particularly well in affluent communities and in college towns across the United States (Murray, 1999).

ETHICAL AND LEGAL ISSUES

There have long been ethical issues in health care delivery in the United States. The cornerstone principle of health services has been to place the patient's welfare above all cost considerations. As health care costs have continued to escalate, however, resource limitations or the rationing of health and mental health services has played a larger role in health policy decisions in the United States.

MCOs, regardless of their organizational model, have also altered the traditional doctor–patient relationship in a variety of ways. For example, they have limited access to mental health and substance abuse services (through various benefit limitations, copayments, and deductibles), introduced additional levels of decision making into decisions previously made by physicians and other clinical staff (utilization management techniques), and implemented various forms of prospective and capitation payment that may influence the financial status of the clinician through some type of risk assumption. The use of capitation financing within MCOs may create incentives to underserve patients, particularly those seeking specialized care, such as behavioral health services.

A number of ethical issues persist within behavioral health services delivery systems, including questions about the capacity of individuals with mental disorders to decline health care and mental health care (the right to refuse treatment and informed consent), coercion, the sexual or financial exploitation of patients by clinicians (i.e., regulation of the patient–therapist relationship), confidentiality, professional licensing laws (particularly in this era of continuous emerging technology), and the protection of patients from decisions made by clinical self-interest (Petrila, 1997; Petrila and Levin, 2004).

In addition to a basic right to privacy, all patients with mental or emotional disorders have a right to know about their therapists' credentials, procedures, services, and policies regarding access to patient records. In the past, patients could be assured that confidentiality would be maintained unless they specifically requested sharing of information, they brought charges against the mental health therapist, or the mental health professional believed the patient posed a clear danger to self or others (Woodside and McCain, 1996). The Health Insurance Portability and Accountability Act (HIPAA) also provides protection for psychotherapy notes (for example, records must now be kept separate from medical profiles and may not be transferred without consent). Although this is considered an improvement in safeguarding confidentiality, further protection is needed for people being treated for stigmatizing disorders (RightsMarket, 2004).

CONCLUSIONS

A number of studies have reported that the majority of people suffering from mental disorders do not seek or receive treatment for their illnesses, despite the presence of effective treatments that promote remission and, occasionally, recovery from mental disorders (Kessler et al., 2005; U.S. DHHS, 1999). In addition, of those individuals with diagnosable mental disorders who do seek treatment, the majority seek treatment in non-mental health service delivery settings.

Even though a wide variety of mental health professionals work closely with patients, pharmacists must master basic knowledge about how to assess the status of the people they treat so that they can avoid feeling uncomfortable when interacting with a patient who has a mental disorder (see the chapter-opening case scenario). One pharmacist at a Veterans Affairs hospital who provides pharmaceutical care for 400 mental health patients has suggested that direct patient care is very rewarding and challenging because in mental health settings pharmacists are called upon to use all of their skills—from patient assessment to advanced interpersonal communication, such as teaching patients and their family members about the importance of compliance in relation to their disease state (M. Carvalho, personal communication, 1997). He is very conscious of his responsibility when selecting and dosing medications with a high potential for toxicity and interactions. The proliferation of new psychoactive drugs opens up a whole new armamentarium from which to choose customized therapeutic plans (sometimes including "strategic polypharmacy") in an effort to achieve an optimal response.

Pharmacists will always have some contact with individuals who have mental and addictive disorders, perhaps under similar circumstances to those presented in the chapter-opening case study. Managed care, as a national movement, is changing the organization, financing, and delivery of mental health care in the United States. It is critical that pharmacists be familiar with the wide variety of programs and services available for treating individuals with mental and addictive disorders and to recognize how they might affect relationships on both the systems level and an interpersonal level.

For pharmacists to be adequately equipped to fulfill these roles, which may involve advising staff as well as patients, relevant graduate and postgraduate training is essential. For students in existing pharmacy programs, additional courses in mental health services delivery represent one way to address these emerging roles. Key content areas include current knowledge on the types and etiology of mental illnesses, an understanding of mental health services delivery systems, familiarity with referral mechanisms to mental health services, and enhancement of communication and counseling skills. Other key content areas include an understanding of individuals with serious mental disorders and the role of medication in disease management.

As public-sector managed behavioral health care organizations become more prevalent in community settings, engaging and educating all stakeholders (both professionals and community members) can be an effective, consensus-driven mechanism for medication cost-containment strategies, such as formularies, in a community mental health plan (Baker, 2001). Pharmacists can play an important role in these policy and delivery planning processes.

The continuing organizational, financing, insurance, and information system changes in health care systems have brought about many controversies regarding the quality of care as well as ethical and legal issues in mental health. A promising sign in this era is the growing recognition of somatic and behavioral health prevention and integration services delivery strategies—particularly services that focus on the mind–body connection. Another hopeful sign is the focus on evidence-based practice in behavioral health. Baker (2001) suggests that successful implementation of evidence-based practice in behavioral health will require collaboration between policy makers, administrators, providers, and consumers of somatic and behavioral health care.

QUESTIONS FOR FURTHER DISCUSSION

1. Should mental health services be integrated into health care delivery systems?
2. What are some of the ethical issues in mental health services delivery?
3. What can be done to address the needs of homeless individuals with mental disorders?
4. How involved should pharmacists become in caring for individuals with mental illness?

KEY TOPICS AND TERMS

Addiction disorders
Barriers to communication
Health care services
Health personnel attitudes
Managed behavioral health care
Medication compliance
Mental health
Patient–professional relationships
Pharmacotherapy
Psychopharmacology
Psychotherapy
Substance abuse disorders

REFERENCES

American Psychiatric Association. (1987). *Diagnostic and statistical manual of mental disorders* (3rd ed., rev.). Washington, DC: Author.

American Psychiatric Association. (1994). *Diagnostic and statistical manual of mental disorders* (4th ed.). Washington, DC: Author.

American Psychiatric Association. (1997). Practice guidelines for the treatment of patients with schizophrenia. *American Journal of Psychiatry, 154*(suppl 4), 1–63.

American Psychiatric Association. (2000). *Diagnostic and statistical manual of mental disorders* (4th ed., text revision) (*DSM-IV-TR*). Washington, DC: Author.

American Psychological Association. (2004). *Mental health parity.* Retrieved July 15, 2006, from http://www.apahelpcenter.org/articles/article.php?id=26

Baker, J. G. (2001). Engaging community mental health stakeholders in pharmacy cost management. *Psychiatric Services, 52*(5), 650–653.

Barry, C. L., Frank, R. G., & McGuire, T. G. (2006). The costs of mental health parity: Still an impediment? *Health Affairs, 25*(1), 623–634.

Beck, S., Paton, C., Euba, R., & Goddard, C. (2001). Atypical antipsychotics in the elderly. *International Journal of Psychiatry in Clinical Practice, 5*(4), 257–261.

Blazer, D. G., Kessler, R. C., McGonagle, K. A., & Swartz, M. S. (1994). The prevalence and distribution of major depression in a national comorbidity sample: The National Comorbidity Survey. *American Journal of Psychiatry, 151*(7), 979–986.

Boling, P. A. (2002). Strategic use of home care pharmacy consultation may be worthwhile. *Journal of the American Geriatrics Society, 50*(9), 1597–1598.

Brook, O., van Hout, H., Nieuwenhuyse, H., & Heerdink, E. (2003). Impact of coaching by community pharmacists on drug attitude of depressive primary care patients and acceptability to patients: A randomized controlled trial. *European Neuropsychopharmacology, 13*(1), 1–9.

Cuffel, B. J., Goldman, W., & Schlesinger, H. (1999). Does managing behavioral health care services increase the cost of providing medical care? *Journal of Behavioral Health Services and Research, 26*(4), 372–380.

Dana, R. (1998). Problems with managed mental health care for multicultural populations. *Psychological Reports, 83*(1), 283–294.

Duffy, F. F., West, J. C., Wilk, J., Narrow, W. E., Hales, D., Thompson, J., et al. (2004). Mental health practitioners and trainees. In R. W. Manderscheid & M. J. Henderson (Eds.), *Mental health, United States, 2002. (DHHS Pub. No. (SMA) 3938)* (pp. 327-368). Rockville, MD: U.S. Department of Health and Human Services.

Duffy, M. E. (1988). Health promotion in the family: Current findings and directives for nursing research. *Journal of Advanced Nursing, 13*(1), 109–117.

Dworkin, R. W. (2006). *Artificial happiness.* New York: Carroll & Graf.

Earley, P. (2006). *Crazy: A father's search through America's mental health madness.* New York: G. P. Putnam's Sons.

Edlin, M. (2003). Seniors enjoy better health with diligent drug management. *Managed Healthcare Executive, 13*(1), 34–36.

Elpers, J. R., & Levin, B. L. (1996). Mental health services: Epidemiology, prevention, and service delivery systems. In B. L. Levin and J. Petrila (Eds.), *Mental health services: A public health perspective* (pp. 5–22). New York: Oxford University Press.

Essock, S. M., & Goldman, H. H. (1995). States' embrace of managed mental health care. *Health Affairs, 14*(3), 35–44.

Ewalt, J., & Farnsworth, D. (1963). *Textbook of psychiatry.* New York: McGraw-Hill.

Ewan, M. A., & Greene, R. J. (2001). A training course in mental health care for community pharmacists. *Pharmaceutical Journal, 266*(7133), 160–161.

Fiedler, J. L., & Wight, J. B. (1989). *The medical offset effect and public health policy: Mental health industry in transition.* New York: Praeger.

Francesconi, G. A. (1995). ERISA preemption of "any willing provider" laws: An essential step toward national health care reform. *Washington University Law Quarterly, 73,* 227–267.

Frank, R. G., Conti, R. M., & Goldman, H. H. (2005). Mental health policy and psychotropic drugs. *Milbank Memorial Fund Quarterly, 83*(2), 271–298.

Frank, R. G., & McGuire, T. G. (1996). Introduction to the economics of mental health payment systems. In B. L. Levin and J. Petrila (Eds.), *Mental health services: A public health perspective* (pp. 23–37). New York: Oxford University Press.

Friedman, R. M., Best, K. A., Armstrong, M. I., Duchnowski, A. J., Evans, M. E., Hernandez, M., et al. (2004). Child mental health policy. In B. L. Levin, J. Petrila, & K. D. Hennessy (Eds.), *Mental health services: A public health perspective* (2nd ed.) (pp. 129–153). New York: Oxford University Press.

Gilmer, T. P., Dolder, C. R., Lacro, J. P., Folsom, D. P., Lindamer, L., Garcia, P., & Jeste, D. V. (2004). Adherence to treatment with antipsychotic medication and health care costs among Medicaid beneficiaries with schizophrenia. *American Journal of Psychiatry, 161,* 692–699.

Glenmullen, J. (2000). *Prozac backlash.* New York: Simon and Schuster.

Glenmullen, J. (2005). *The antidepressant solution.* New York: Free Press.

Goldman, W., McCulloch, J., & Sturm, R. (1998). Costs and use of mental health services before and after managed care. *Health Affairs, 17*(2), 40–51.

Goode, E. (2000a, May 18). Chronic-depression study backs the pairing of therapy and drugs. *New York Times,* p. 23.

Goode, E. (2000b, February 23). Sharp rise in psychiatric drugs for the very young. *New York Times,* p. 1.

Gordon, R. (1983). An operational classification of disease prevention. *Public Health Reports, 98,* 107–109.

Gorski, T. (1994, January/February). Chemical dependency and mental health: Avoiding a "shotgun merger." *Behavioral Health Management, 14,* 22–24.

Grazier, K. L., Eselius, L. L., Hu, T-W., Shore, K. K., & G'Sell, W. A. (1999). Effects of a mental health carve-out on use, costs, and payers: A four-year study. *Journal of Behavioral Health Services and Research, 26*(4), 381–389.

Gurwitz, J. H., Field, T. S., Harrold, L. R., Rothschild, J., Debellis, K., Seger, A. C., et al. (2003). Incidence and preventability of adverse drug events among older persons in the ambulatory setting. *Journal of the American Medical Association, 289,* 1107–1116.

Hepler, C. D., & Strand, L. M. (1990). Opportunities and responsibilities in pharmaceutical care. *American Journal of Hospital Pharmacy, 47,* 533–549.

Institute of Medicine. (1994). *Reducing risks for mental disorders: Frontiers for preventive intervention research.* Washington, DC: National Academy Press.

Joint Commission on Mental Health and Illness. (1961). *Action for mental health.* New York: Wiley.

Kaiser Commission on Medicaid and the Uninsured. (2003). *The Medicaid Resource Book.* Retrieved July 15, 2006 from http://www.kff.org/medicaid/2236-index.cfm

Kaplan, F. (2000, August 28). For mentally ill, jail means care. *Boston Globe,* p. 1.

Karp, D. A. (2006). *Is it me or my meds?* Cambridge, MA: Harvard University Press.

Kaufman, D. W., Kelly, J. P., Rosenberg, L., Anderson, T. E., & Mitchell, A. A. (2002). Recent patterns of medication use in the ambulatory adult population of the United States: The Slone Survey. *Journal of the American Medical Association, 287*(3), 337–344.

Keisler, C. A., & Sibulkin, A. E. (1987). *Mental hospitalization: Myths and facts about a national crisis.* Newbury Park, CA: Sage.

Kessler, R. C., Berglund, P. A., Zhao, S., Leaf, P. J., Kouzis, A. C., Bruce, M. L., et al. (1996). The 12-month prevalence and correlates of serious mental illness. In R. W. Mandersheid and M. A. Sonnenschein (Eds.), *Mental health, United States 1996. DHHS Publication No. (SMA) 96-3098* (pp. 59–70). Washington, DC: U. S. Government Printing Office.

Kessler, R. C., Demler, O., Frank, R. G., Olfson, M., Pincus, H. A., Walters, E. E., et al. (2005). Prevalence and treatment of mental disorders, 1990 to 2003. *New England Journal of Medicine, 352,* 2515–2523.

Kessler, R. C., McGonagle, K. A., Zhao, S., Nelson, C. B., Hughes, M., Eshleman, S., et al. (1994). Lifetime and 12 month prevalence of *DSM-III-R* psychiatric disorders in the United States: Results from the national comorbidity study. *Archives of General Psychiatry, 51,* 8–19.

Kessler, R. C., Nelson, C. B., McGonagle, K. A., Edlund, M. J., Frank, R. G., & Leaf, P. J. (1996). The epidemiology of co-occurring addictive and mental disorders: Implications for prevention and service utilization. *American Journal of Orthopsychiatry, 66*(10), 17–31.

Kramer, P. (2005). *Against depression.* New York: Viking.

Kulbok, P. P. (1985). Social resources, health resources, and preventive health behavior: Patterns and predictions. *Public Health Nursing, 2*(2), 67–81.

Levin, B. L. (1992). Managed mental health care: A national perspective. In R. W. Manderscheid and M. A. Sonnenschein (Eds.), *Mental health, United States, 1992. DHHS Publication No. (SMA) 92-1942* (pp. 208–217). Rockville, MD: Substance Abuse and Mental Health Services Administration.

Levin, B. L., Hanson, A., Coe, R., & Kuppin, S. A. (2000). *Mental health parity: National and state perspectives.* Tampa, FL: Louis de la Parte Florida Mental Health Institute, University of South Florida.

Levin, B. L., Petrila, J., & Hennessey, K. (2004). *Mental health services: A public health perspective* (2nd ed.). New York: Oxford University Press.

Ma, C. A., & McGuire, T. G. (1998). Costs and incentives in a behavioral health carve-out. *Health Affairs, 17*(2), 63–69.

MacHaffie, S. (2002). Health promotion information: Sources and significance for those with serious and persistent mental illness. *Archives of Psychiatric Nursing, 16*(6), 263–274.

Mark, T., Coffey, R. M., McKusick D. R., Harwood, H., King, E., Bouchery, E., et al. (2005). *National estimates of expenditures for mental health services and substance abuse treatment, 1991–2001. SMA No. 05-3999.* Retrieved July 15, 2006 from http://www.samhsa.gov/spendingestimates/SEPGenRpt013105v2BLX.pdf

McAlpine, D. D., & Mechanic, D. (2000). Utilization of specialty mental health care among persons with severe mental illness: The roles of demographics, need, insurance, and risk. *Health Services Research, 35*(1), 277–306.

Minorities get different mental health care in rich neighborhoods (News RX). (2003, June 9). *Managed Care Weekly.* p. 5.

Mort, J., & Aparasu, R. (2002). Prescribing of psychotropics in the elderly: Why is it so often inappropriate? *CNS Drugs, 16*(2), 99–109.

Murray, C. J. L., & Lopez, A. D. (1996). *The global burden of disease: A comprehensive assessment of mortality and disability from diseases, injuries, and risk factors in 1990 and projected to 2020.* Cambridge, MA: Harvard University Press.

Murray, S. (1999, November 22). With a "guild" therapists flee managed care. *Wall Street Journal,* p. B1.

National Alliance on Mental Illness (NAMI). (2004). *Emergency departments see dramatic increase in people with mental illness seeking care.* Retrieved July 15, 2006 from http://www.nami.org/Content/ContentGroups/Policy/Issues_Spotlights/Emergency_Departments_See_Dramatic_Increase_in_People_with_Mental_Illness_Seeking_Care.htm

National Association of Psychiatric Health Systems (NAPHS). (2006). *New NAPHS annual survey tracks behavioral treatment trends.* Retrieved July 15, 2006 from http://www.naphs.org/documents/Annualsurvey2005.pdf

National Mental Health Association. (2006). *Health insurance crisis affecting millions of Americans suffering from depression, other mental health disorders.* Retrieved July 15, 2006 from http://www.nmha.org/newsroom/system/news.vw. cfm?do=vw&rid=840

New Freedom Commission on Mental Health. (2003). *Achieving the promise: Transforming mental health care in America. Final report. DHHS Pub. No. SMA-03-3832.* Rockville, MD: U. S. Department of Health and Human Services.

Oregon Statutes. (2006). *Mandated benefits for chemical dependency and mental or nervous conditions.* Retrieved July 15, 2006 from http://insurance. oregon. gov/rules/attachments/recently%20proposed/id13-2006_rule. pdf

Petrila, J. (1997). *Ethical issues for behavioral healthcare practitioners and organizations in a managed care environment.* Washington, DC: Center for Substance Abuse Treatment.

Petrila, J., & Levin, B. L. (2004). Mental disability law, policy, and service delivery. In B. L. Levin, J. Petrila, & K. D. Hennessy (Eds.), *Mental health services: A public health perspective* (2nd ed.) (pp. 42–71). New York: Oxford University Press.

Psychotherapy, medication most effective to fight minority women's depression (News RX). (2003, July 25). *Drug Week.* p. 65.

Ranelli, P. L., Bartsch, K., & London, K. (2000). Pharmacists' perceptions of children and families as medicine consumers. *Psychology and Health, 15*(6), 829–840.

Ridgely, M. S., & Goldman, H. H. (1996). Health law symposium: Putting the failure of national health care reform in perspective: Mental health benefits and the "benefit" of incrementalism. *Saint Louis University Law Journal, 40*(2), 407–435.

RightsMarket. (2004). *HIPAA and file security.* Retrieved July 15, 2006 from http:// www.rightsmarket.com/hipaa_file_security.html

Robins, L. N., & Regier, D. A. (Eds.). (1991). *Psychiatric disorders in America: The Epidemiologic Catchment Area Study.* New York: Free Press.

Schommer, J. C. (2000). Pharmacists' new communicative role: Explaining illness and medicine to patients. In B. B. Whaley (Ed.), *Explaining illness research, theory, and strategies. LEA's communication series* (pp. 209–231). Mahwah, NJ: Lawrence Erlbaum Associates.

Shapiro, J. (1995). The downside of managed mental health care. *Clinical Social Work Journal, 23,* 441–451.

Slater, L., Daniel, J. H., & Banks, A. E. (Eds.). (2003). *The complete guide to mental health for women.* Boston: Beacon Press.

Survey finds U. S. has high rate of mental illness, low rate of treatment (News RX). (2003, June 8). *Medical Letter on the CDC and FDA.* p. 15.

Urff, J. (2004). Public mental health systems: Structures, goals, and constraints. In B. L. Levin, J. Petrila, & K. D. Hennessy (Eds.), *Mental health services: A public health perspective* (2nd ed.) (pp. 72–87). New York: Oxford University Press.

U. S. Congress. (1965). *Public Law 89–97. The Social Security Amendments.* Retrieved January 23, 2007 from http://www.socialsecurity.gov/OP_Home/ comp2/F089-097.html.

U. S. Congress. (1980). *Public Law 96–398. Mental Health Systems Act.* Retrieved January 23, 2007 from http://www.uscode.house.gov/downloads/pls/42C102. txt.

U. S. Congress. (1981). *Public Law 97–35. Omnibus Budget Reconciliation Act.* Retrieved January 23, 2007 from http://www.socialsecurity.gov/OP_Home/ comp2/F097-35.html.

U. S. Congress. (1996). *Public Law 104-204. Mental Health Parity Act.* Retrieved January 23, 2007 from http://www.mentalhealth.samhsa.gov/cmhs/ ManagedCare/Parity/ParityAct96.asp.

U. S. Department of Health and Human Services (U. S. DHHS). (1999). *Mental health: A report of the Surgeon General.* Rockville, MD: Substance Abuse and Mental Health Services Administration.

U. S. Department of Health and Human Services. (2000). *Healthy people 2010: Understanding and improving health* (2nd ed.). Washington, DC: U. S. Government Printing Office.

Vanelli, M., Burstein, P., & Cramer, J. (2001). Refill patterns of atypical and conventional antipsychotic medications at a national retail pharmacy chain. *Psychiatric Services, 52*(9), 1248–1250.

Ware, N., Lachicotte, W., Kirschner, S., et al. (2000). Clinician experiences of managed mental health care. *Medical Anthropology Quarterly, 14*(1), 3–27.

Woodside, M., & McCain, T. (1996). *An introduction to human services* (2nd ed.). Belmont, CA: Brooks/Cole.

Young, A. S., & Magnabosco, J. L. (2004). Services for adults with mental illness. In B. L. Levin, J. Petrila, & K. D. Hennessy (Eds.), *Mental health services: A public health perspective* (2nd ed.) (pp. 177–208). New York: Oxford University Press.

Zelinsky, E. A. (2003). Against a federal patients' bill of rights. *Yale Law and Policy Review, 21*(2), 443–472.

Home Care

William W. McCloskey and Robert L. McCarthy

Case Scenario

Mary is a 70-year-old woman with osteomyelitis of the left foot who is referred to your home care service for continuation of intravenous (IV) antibiotic therapy upon discharge from a local hospital. Her physician has prescribed cefazolin 2 g every 8 hours for 4 weeks. Mary received her first three doses of cefazolin before leaving the hospital, although the nurse had a difficult time establishing a peripheral IV line. In addition to her infection, Mary has a history of hypertension, insulin-dependent diabetes, osteoarthritis, and an allergy to oxycodone.

The case manager states that Mary is scheduled to leave the hospital today. She lives alone, but her daughter is willing to help, and she can visit her mother each day after work. Mary's insurance is provided by a health maintenance organization (HMO) that has contracted with your service in the past. This HMO expects the home care provider to service Mary in the least expensive way. Your company sales representative is excited because he has been trying to get business from this case manager for the past month.

LEARNING OBJECTIVES

Upon completion of this chapter, the student shall be able to:

- Explain what home care is
- Describe the various types of home care industries
- Describe the various types of therapies provided by home infusion therapy providers
- Explain the major factors influencing the home care industry
- Explain the role of the pharmacist in providing home care services

CHAPTER QUESTIONS

1. What is home care?
2. What are the primary industries that provide home care?
3. What factors influence the home care industry?
4. What is the role of the pharmacist in home care?

INTRODUCTION

The home health care industry is very broad in scope, encompassing a variety of products and services. Three home care industries—home health services, home infusion therapy, and home medical equipment—provide the majority of these products and services. Each of these industries is influenced by government legislation, regulatory agencies, reimbursement policies, and technological developments. Home care services are generally initiated when a patient is unable to provide for self-care due to illness, and they are intended to restore and maintain the patient's optimal level of well-being in a familiar environment (Council on Scientific Affairs, 1990).

The growth of home care has been made possible by advances in clinical practice, medicine, and technology. The first home care agencies were established more than 120 years ago, and today more than 20,000 home care providers deliver care to nearly 8 million people in the United States (National Association of Home Care, 2001). In 2006, U.S. expenditures for home health care services were estimated to be approximately $54 billion; this amount is projected to exceed $100 billion by 2015. Public payers, especially Medicare, have been primarily responsible for this trend (Centers for Medicare and Medicaid Services, 2005). In contrast, private insurance payers generally limit home care coverage to only a small percentage of their overall budgets (Levine, Boal, and Boling, 2003).

Because of the large role that home care plays in today's health care system, pharmacists must understand the diverse nature of the products and services offered by the home care industry and the factors that influence their provision. Armed with this knowledge, the pharmacist can more effectively work with other health care professionals to manage the clinical and financial needs of a home care patient.

This chapter presents an overview of home care by describing the products and services offered by members of each industry, the factors that affect the delivery of those products and services, and the role of the home care pharmacist.

HOME CARE INDUSTRIES

Home Health Services

Home health services are usually associated with nursing care that is provided through a home health agency. Nursing care, however, is only one type of service offered by these agencies. Additional services may include speech therapy, physical therapy, or other types of rehabilitation therapies; homemaker services; social services; and hospice care. Home health agencies employ specially trained staff who provide a variety of services with multiple levels of complexity. These professionals work with other home care providers to obtain additional products, such as medical equipment, medication, and surgical supplies, needed to care for the patient. Home health providers perform a vital role in home care by coordinating the patient's care with family caregivers and other health care professionals. Effective communication between the home health provider and everyone involved with the patient's care is essential to the success of a patient's therapy. The following are some examples of home health services.

Nursing Services

Nursing services are also referred to as "skilled nursing services." Patients in the home may require the insertion and maintenance of an intravenous (IV) line, the application of dressings for wound care, assistance with disease management, or self-care education. Skilled services need to be performed by a licensed nurse to ensure patient safety and therapy effectiveness. Based on the information in the chapter-opening case scenario, Mary would most likely require a nurse to help maintain and reestablish her IV site as necessary.

With the advent of high-tech home IV therapy, the role of the home care nurse has become more diverse and sophisticated. Consequently, it is desirable for nurses to have experience in critical care nursing, IV therapy, and the administration of blood products. The introduction of new therapies often requires that the nurse undergo training in the use of complex infusion devices and access methods.

Home care nurses may be employed by a variety of organizations, including Visiting Nurse Associations (VNAs). VNAs are nonprofit entities that coordinate and provide a variety of nursing services in the home. In addition, nursing services may be available through home care companies and pharmacies that provide home care products and services. Some nurses may even practice as independent contractors.

Hospice Services

Hospice services help manage the end-of-life process for terminally ill patients and their families. These services address the clinical, emotional, and spiritual needs of the patient. Support is extended to family members to help them cope with the dying and bereavement processes. In 2005, nearly 900,000 patients were serviced by hospice, and it is estimated that this number will more than double by 2020 (National Hospice Foundation, 2006).

The focus of hospice is on maintaining quality of life for terminally ill patients. Hospice care aims to make patients as comfortable as possible. Hospice organizations care for patients using a team approach that usually includes health care professionals, clergy, homemakers, and volunteers, who work together to manage the many different aspects of patient care.

Pharmacists are important members of the hospice team. As therapeutic drug experts, they recommend appropriate medications and dosage regimens, especially concerning pain control, while monitoring for side effects and drug–drug interactions.

Speech and Physical Therapy

Rehabilitative services such as speech therapy and physical therapy are commonly offered by home health care agencies. Speech therapy, for example, may be provided to stroke patients who are suffering from aphasia, a condition resulting in the loss of ability to speak or to understand spoken or written communication. Physical therapy may be provided to postoperative orthopedic patients or accident victims. Given Mary's foot infection and history of osteoarthritis, she may require the services of a physical therapist. The opportunity to have these traditionally hospital-based services provided at home is particularly convenient for patients who have difficulty with transportation issues.

Social Services

Social workers are charged with facilitating the transition of a patient from a hospital or long-term care facility to home and coordinating the provision of required home care services. Social services include support with both economic issues (e.g., dealing with the insurance company and assisting with paperwork) and social issues (e.g., coordinating activities with a senior center) (Gill, 1991). Although Mary's daughter may be willing to be a caregiver, she may need the support of a social worker to deal with the complexities that home care entails, especially for older people.

Homemaker Services

With the growing elderly population in the United States, the need for homemaker services has increased rapidly over the past decade. Employment of home care aides is expected to grow much more rapidly than the average for all occupations over the next decade (U.S. Department of Labor, 2006). Many elderly individuals require assistance with at least one of their activities of daily living (ADLs) or instrumental activities of daily living (IADLs). ADLs include personal care activities such as the provision of meals and bathing. IADLs include house cleaning and grocery shopping. Agencies exist that provide support for the elders like Mary who may be unable to complete one or more of these activities.

One of the most well-known homemaker services is the meals-on-wheels (MOW) program. MOW ensures that low-income elderly individuals receive at least one well-balanced meal a day at minimal or no cost. These meals may be served in a congregate setting (e.g., an adult daycare center or senior center) or in the senior's home.

Home Infusion Therapy

The home infusion therapy market in the United States is estimated to amount to $4.5 billion annually (National Home Infusion Association, 2006). Home infusion therapy refers to the parenteral and enteral administration of drugs, solutions, and nutrition to patients in their homes. In the past, infusion therapies required hospitalization because of their complexity. As health care providers gained more clinical knowledge about infusion therapies, however, they were able to develop clinical policies and procedures to ensure their safe administration in the home setting. Home infusion therapy is generally a more cost-effective alternative to hospitalization and is preferred by most patients. In many cases, caregivers or patients may be taught to administer infusion therapies at home. For example, Mary's daughter could be trained to administer her antibiotic therapy. The acceptance of home infusion therapy has reduced the length of hospitalizations and allowed patients to continue active lives.

The following are the primary types of infusion therapies that are administered in the home.

Nutrition

Parenteral nutrition refers to the IV administration of either all (total parenteral nutrition [TPN]) or some (partial parenteral nutrition [PPN]) of a patient's daily nutritional requirements. Parenteral nutrition may be considered the grandfather of home infusion therapies. Home parenteral nutrition has been used for more than two decades (Howard, Alger, Michalek, Heaphey, Aftahi, and Johnston, 1993) because health care providers quickly recognized that most patients requiring chronic therapy did not need to be hospitalized to receive IV feedings.

Home parenteral nutrition is usually administered to home care patients via a central venous catheter or a peripherally inserted central catheter (PICC line). The choice of venous access is primarily dictated by the concentration of dextrose in the solution to be administered. High concentrations of dextrose (generally greater than 10%) must be administered centrally through a large vein, such as the superior vena cava, to allow for rapid dilution by the blood so as to avoid vascular irritation. In addition to dextrose (as a source of carbohydrates), parenteral nutrition solutions contain amino acids (a source of protein), electrolytes, vitamins, and trace elements. They may also contain fat emulsion (a source of lipids), hydrocortisone, heparin, insulin, or other compatible medications.

Although enteral nutrition is not a parenteral therapy, patients requiring long-term enteral feedings are often serviced by home infusion providers. Many of these patients have special feeding tubes through which enteral feedings are delivered directly into the stomach (G-tube) or jejunum (J-tube). Consequently, home care therapy providers need to have the expertise to maintain these devices.

Anti-infective Therapy

Anti-infective therapy was one of the earliest nonnutritive therapies offered at home (Bennett and Allen, 1990), and it remains the most common home infusion therapy. Anti-infective therapy is generally used to manage infections that require relatively long-term IV administration (two weeks or longer), such as osteomyelitis, cellulitis, and respiratory infections in cystic fibrosis patients. Even some serious infections, including endocarditis, can be treated in the home setting.

Pain Management Therapy

The hospice movement and the desire of many patients with a terminal illness (and their families) not to be hospitalized in the final days of life have led to the need for the home infusion of narcotic analgesics. Morphine, hydromorphone, and (less commonly) other opiates are administered via continuous infusion to provide chronic pain relief while allowing the patient to remain alert. Ambulatory infusion devices can be programmed to enable patients to self-administer bolus doses of medication on demand for breakthrough pain. Pharmacists are often consulted to convert an oral or transdermal dose of analgesic medication to an appropriate infusion dose.

Chemotherapy

The administration of potent antineoplastics in the home setting may be considered for certain patients. Clinician acceptance of this type of home care has increased as the understanding of how to manage the complications of chemotherapy has improved (Bennett and Allen, 1990). Agents that are administered over several days (e.g., 5-fluorouracil) are the antineoplastics most commonly administered at home. Despite the feasibility of this change in the setting for care, some oncologists are reluctant to relinquish the attractive reimbursement they receive for office chemotherapy. Other physicians may not have facilities adequate for the safe preparation (e.g., vertical laminar flow containment hood) of cytotoxic agents, so they may utilize the services of a home infusion therapy provider

Miscellaneous Therapies

Several other infusion therapies have also been delivered in the home: hydration for such conditions as hyperemesis and inflammatory bowel disease; heparin for the treatment of thromboembolic diseases; inotropic therapy for the treatment of refractory congestive heart failure; and blood products for hemotherapy. In addition, a number of home therapies have resulted from the development of biotechnology-based products. Growth hormone (for the treatment of growth hormone deficiency in children), interferons (including alpha, beta, and gamma), interleukins, epoetin, and colony-stimulating factors all require long-term parenteral treatment, and thus lend themselves to administration in the home setting. As more of these products emerge, it is anticipated that they will find roles in the management of patients in their homes.

Home Medical Equipment

The home medical equipment (HME) industry provides medical equipment and disposable supplies to treat patients at home. For example, medical equipment is used to facilitate patients' breathing, improve their mobility, and perform diagnostic testing. Such equipment often requires the use of disposable supplies by the patient. Home health providers also use surgical supplies for wound care dressings and diagnostic strips to check sugar levels in blood.

The following are examples of products and services that are provided by the HME industry.

Durable Medical Equipment

Durable medical equipment (DME) is reusable medical equipment that patients have an option to lease or purchase. Examples include wheelchairs, bathroom safety supplies, hospital beds, and ambulatory aids such as canes, crutches, and walkers. Providing DME was one of the original home care services delivered by pharmacists.

Respiratory Therapy and Supplies

Many patients suffering from chronic pulmonary conditions, who previously required hospitalization, may now receive respiratory therapy at home. Respiratory therapies include oxygen, aerosolized medications, continuous positive airway pressure (CPAP), and ventilators. All of these therapies require special monitoring and patient education by a licensed respiratory therapist.

Oxygen therapy represents the largest portion of the respiratory market. Oxygen can be delivered to a patient via a concentrator, a machine that concentrates room oxygen to a higher level of purity; cylinders; compressed gas in tanks; or a liberator, a vessel that stores liquid oxygen. Providers evaluate the individual needs of the patient to determine the best method of delivery. Providing oxygen therapy is extremely profitable for HME providers.

Many patients are able to treat their respiratory conditions by administering medications via nebulization at home. In addition, some providers have developed specialty programs to treat conditions such as asthma. Once a patient is enrolled in such a program, the provider will deliver bronchodilators on a recurring basis and monitor patient compliance. The outcome of the patient's therapy is then reported to the patient's insurance carrier for review. Anti-infectives such as pentamidine may be administered via nebulization to prevent *Pneumocystis carinii* pneumonia (PCP) in AIDS patients. In addition, aminoglycoside antibiotics such as tobramycin are used to treat patients with cystic fibrosis.

Miscellaneous Supplies

Miscellaneous products provided by HME dealers and pharmacies allow patients to care for themselves at home. Patients with diabetes (such as Mary) can monitor their blood glucose levels using portable monitors. A wide variety of appliances and skin care products are readily available to ostomy patients to care for their condition. The urinary incontinence market has expanded rapidly and provides home care patients, particularly the elderly, with many options. Wound care and surgical supplies are available to treat bedridden and postsurgical patients.

FACTORS THAT INFLUENCE THE HOME CARE INDUSTRY

Financial and regulatory issues present difficult challenges to the home care industry. One of the toughest challenges facing home care providers is the ability to provide patients with high-quality care given payers' reimbursement rates. The cost of caring for patients at home is increasing because home care providers are increasingly treating "sicker" patients with more complex therapies. Home care providers must also satisfy the requirements of statutory laws, regulations, and professional standards. These requirements improve patient care, but they also increase the cost of providing therapy.

Whereas the cost of providing therapy is on the rise, many insurance carriers are reducing reimbursement rates. To do more for less, home care providers will need to take advantage of advances in technology and changes in business practices to survive. The following are some of the significant factors affecting the home care industry.

Reimbursement Issues

Insurance carriers or "third-party payers" exert a strong influence on the home care industry because they reimburse providers for home care products and services that are provided to patients. Many types of third-party payers exist, including government, managed care organizations (MCOs), and private insurance. Each payer determines its own levels of coverage, billing rules, and reimbursement rates. This inconsistency makes it difficult for home care providers to be reimbursed quickly and easily for the services they provide.

Government Insurance

The Centers for Medicare and Medicaid Services (CMS) is the federal agency that oversees the Medicare and Medicaid programs in the United States. This agency was formerly called the Health Care Financing Administration (HCFA). The Medicare and Medicaid programs insure about 87 million lives (Kaiser Family Foundation, 2005; see Chapter 16).

Medicare. Medicare is a national health insurance program for patients with end-stage kidney disease, elderly patients, and selected patients with disabilities. It is divided into four components: A, B, C, and D. Part A refers to hospital insurance, and Part B provides medical (physician) insurance. Medicare Part A covers inpatient hospital services, skilled nursing facilities, home health services, and hospice care; Medicare Part B helps pay for the cost of physician services, outpatient hospital services, medical equipment, and supplies (Centers for Medicare and Medicaid Services, 2005). Beneficiaries were given another option in 1997 under Medicare Part C, called Medicare Advantage (originally called Medicare + Choice). This program allows the patient to choose benefits through risk-based plans such as an HMO or other managed care plan, or a private fee-for-service plan. Under Part C, beneficiaries must pay monthly Part B premiums in addition to those for the private insurance. In January 2006, Medicare Part D was implemented. This program expanded coverage to include prescription drugs.

Mary was eligible for Medicare once she reached the age of 65. She chose a Medicare Advantage HMO option.

Unfortunately, Medicare does not generally cover home infusion therapies. Only a small number of therapies that are administered using an electronic infusion device are covered, such as antiviral therapies, some chemotherapies, and dobutamine. For most other therapies, patients need to have alternative insurance coverage.

Medicaid. Medicaid is a health insurance program for low-income and needy people. Unlike Medicare, which is entirely a federal program, Medicaid is actually administered by the states within federal guidelines. Medicaid is more comprehensive than Medicare, and it provides home care coverage as part of its required benefits. Many Medicaid programs also offer outpatient prescription drug coverage, although they are not required to do so. Even when prescription drugs are covered, however, infusion medications may not be.

Managed Care Organizations

The goal of MCOs is to balance the delivery of high-quality health care with cost controls. MCOs control their expenditures by limiting coverage for health care products and services based on the needs of their patients. An HMO (like the one that covers Mary) is an example of an MCO. HMOs contract with multiple health care providers to meet the needs of individual groups. Employers and patients pay an HMO a set fee to manage their health care needs.

As large numbers of patients joined MCOs, these payers were able to negotiate sharp reductions in reimbursement rates from home care providers. Managed care principles decreased the costs of health care, but made many providers unprofitable. In response, a number of providers closed or merged with other providers. Home care providers now try to negotiate prices with MCOs. If the reimbursement levels are not favorable, providers may not choose to work with the organization. Managed care contracts can be successful only if they are beneficial to both provider and payer (see Chapter 17).

Private Sector

Many private third-party payers exist, and some large corporations may be self-insured. These payers reimburse for many home care services in an effort to reduce their costs. The rationale for this coverage is simple:

By eliminating the cost of a hospitalization, the care is less expensive. As with many other payers, the private sector may use managed care principles to contain the rising costs of health care.

Legal, Regulatory, and Professional Standards

The Balanced Budget Act of 1997

The Balanced Budget Act of 1997 introduced legislation that significantly affected the home care industry. Congress passed this act to control health care spending and reduce fraud within the Medicare system. The act required the institution of a prospective payment system (PPS) for home health services, reductions in reimbursement rates for HME, and implementation of competitive bidding processes. Under a PPS, the home health agency is paid a flat rate to care for a Medicare recipient. This rate reimburses the home health agency for all labor and medical supplies needed to care for the patient during a 60-day episode. Even though it has been in effect for some time, the overall impact of this legislation on the home care industry remains unclear, but it is expected that there will be changes in how home care providers conduct business so that they can remain profitable (see Chapter 16).

The Health Insurance Portability and Accountability Act of 1996

The Health Insurance Portability and Accountability Act (HIPAA) was enacted as a direct result of consumer demand. HIPAA is best known for its mandating confidentiality of protected health information, which affects how pharmacies and other providers handle a patient's health care information. However, HIPAA regulations are complex and two other provisions of this act affect the home care industry: (1) insurance reform and (2) administrative simplification.

The insurance reform provision improves insurance coverage when an individual changes employment or health plan. Exclusion from a health plan for preexisting conditions is now subject to strict limitations, which should expand the number of patients who are eligible for home care services.

The administrative simplification provision of HIPAA requires standardization of electronic claims submission. Such standardization will improve operational efficiency and payment cycles for home care providers.

Regulatory Agencies

Many federal and state agencies regulate the home care industry. It is the responsibility of home care providers to understand the legal and regulatory processes that must be followed where they practice. Home health services may be monitored by the state's Department of Public Health (DPH). Pharmacies are monitored by the Drug Enforcement Administration (DEA) and the Food and Drug Administration (FDA). HME providers may be monitored by the Department of Transportation (DOT). Providers may also be accountable to their state board of professional registration. These boards may license the facility as well as the pharmacists, nurses, respiratory therapists, and other health care professionals who work there.

Accrediting Organizations

Accrediting organizations are not federal or state agencies, but rather independent organizations that develop standards of practice for home care providers. Standards address issues such as clinical care, business management, and staff competency. By winning a "seal of approval" from these organizations, home care providers prove the quality of care that they provide to insurance carriers and patients. Providers are required to achieve accreditation by most third-party payers to be eligible for reimbursement.

The Joint Commission on Accreditation of Healthcare Organizations (JCAHO) is perhaps the best-recognized accrediting agency. Other home care accrediting agencies include the Accreditation Commission for Health Care (ACHC) and the Community Health and Preventative Services Organization (CHAPS).

Advances in Technology

The delivery of many parenteral medications to patients in their homes has been greatly improved by advances in technology. Infusion pumps are a good example of advanced technology that has improved the care delivered by the home care industry. Once heavy and bulky, infusion pumps have evolved to be ambulatory, lightweight, and inconspicuous. The latest ambulatory models have the ability to infuse multiple therapies. Taken collectively, these advances provide both clinical advantages and cost savings.

Advances in Internet and wireless communications have enabled home care providers to readily share patient data with other health care professionals. Using point-of-care devices, palm-sized computers, and voice recognition software, pharmacists, nurses, physicians, and other health care professionals can transfer patient data quickly and securely. For more than a decade, telemedicine (i.e., transmission of medical data from a remote site to a central location) has been employed to help monitor patients with chronic conditions such as congestive heart failure, diabetes, and chronic obstructive lung disease as well as patients with acute infections (Eron, King, Marineau, and Yonehara, 2004). Home care providers can also communicate with insurance carriers to approve benefits and submit claims. The latest drug and health care information is also available online. Important sites include those operated by the Centers for Medicare and Medicaid Services (www.cms.hhs.gov) and the Food and Drug Administration (www.fda.gov). Easy access to information and increased communication can reduce costs and improve patient care.

THE ROLE OF THE HOME CARE PHARMACIST

Pharmacists working in home care may do so through a community pharmacy, home care company, or hospital outpatient setting. In all home care organizations, the pharmacist must act as a vital member of a health care team that cares for the patient. This team may include nurses, physicians, caregivers, and the patient. The team members work to together to develop a plan of care that will achieve the desired outcome for the patient's therapy.

Pharmacists are relied on for their pharmaceutical expertise, but they must also be competent in other areas to fulfill their role as a member of a health care team. A home care pharmacist may be responsible for the following roles when providing home care services.

Selection of Home Care Patients: Criteria Evaluation

Although Mary was discharged home to finish her course of IV antibiotic therapy, not all patients are appropriate candidates for home care. The decision to treat a patient at home is generally made jointly by nursing and pharmacy staff, in conjunction with the patient's physician. Patients must be clinically stable, have adequate support systems (e.g., telephone, family), and must be willing to accept responsibility for their own care. Given the current financial climate, patients must also have the ability to pay for home care either independently or through a third party.

Insurance

With the exception of IV medications, the major public-sector insurance programs (Medicare and Medicaid) provide good coverage for general home care services. Likewise, most private third-party payers provide reasonable coverage for home care. As discussed previously, the incentive to cover home care services is linked to the notion that it is less expensive than hospitalization.

Nevertheless, the patient's ability to pay is a component of the assessment process conducted before his or her discharge. Patients who meet medical and social criteria for home care may not qualify financially. Unlike many nonprofit hospitals, for-profit home care companies are not required to provide free care. Some home care companies accept a percentage of "no-pay" patients if they believe that this action will generate additional business with a specific physician, group practice, or hospital. It is the responsibility of the patient care coordinator or reimbursement specialist to verify a patient's insurance coverage before a patient such as Mary is considered eligible for home care.

Social Factors

Social factors play a crucial role in the decision to treat a patient at home. Patients should have family members who are willing and able to support or administer care, because 24-hour nursing care is not cost-effective. Generally, patients and family members are taught to administer therapy without the assistance of a nurse or another health care professional. Further, patients must be positive about receiving their therapy at home for it to be successful. Some patients are reluctant to be discharged from a hospital for fear that they will lose the support a hospital offers (Bennett and Allen, 1990). Fortunately, the support that Mary's daughter provides and Mary's own willingness to be discharged will help with her transition to home care.

Other social factors are also important. For example, the physical condition of the home, its cleanliness, and the availability of refrigeration, running water, and electricity must be considered before providing complex therapies at home. Less invasive treatments such as rehabilitation services are possible without the presence of these conditions.

Another potential hazard is the presence in the home of a family member or others who may be abusing illicit substances. Home infusion therapy patients are supplied with needles and syringes to administer their treatment. Some may receive narcotic analgesics. A careful evaluation and monitoring of the home environment for substance abuse is therefore important.

Development of a Patient Plan of Care

Once a patient is discharged to the home, clear objectives must be developed as part of the patient's plan of care. These objectives include the selection of therapy, nature and frequency of monitoring parameters, and desired therapeutic outcomes. The development of a care plan that outlines the individual care for a given patient will help reduce the possibility of a drug-related misadventure, including the situation in which the patient does not respond to therapy. Specific patient problems should be identified and associated with goals. Detailed interventions should then be designed to ensure the resolution of the problems. The patient care plan should include all of the patient's medical problems, not just the one requiring immediate attention. For example, in addition to her osteomyelitis, Mary's care plan should address her hypertension, diabetes, arthritis, and drug allergy. Home care accrediting bodies require the development of such a care plan.

Selection of Therapy

The choice of drug therapy is even more critical in the home than in an institutional setting. The usual safeguards (24-hour nursing and physician availability and emergency equipment) that are standard procedure in institutions may be absent in the home. As a result, several safety and convenience factors should be considered when selecting a therapy for the home care patient.

For example, because of the potential risks of allergy associated with some medications (such as antibiotics), the first dose may be administered in a controlled setting such as a hospital or clinic. If the first dose is administered at home, it should be done under medical supervision. Other considerations include frequency and ease of administration. Drugs that can be administered once daily are more suitable for home care. In Mary's case, the pharmacist might recommend an alternative antibiotic that could be dosed less frequently than every 8 hours. Medications that are less likely to cause phlebitis (inflammation of the vein) and that do not require administration of large volumes of fluid are also more appropriate for home delivery.

Compounding Issues

A number of pharmaceutical compounding issues are unique to home care. These include drug/solution stability, packaging, infusion devices, and delivery schedules.

Drug/Solution Stability

In the past, most manufacturer-generated stability data were predicated on patients receiving medications in a hospital setting. As a result, expiration dating has traditionally been limited to 24 hours after product preparation. To deliver medications in a cost-effective manner at home, pharmacists need to extend stability data often for up to a month, depending on the product. Manufacturers realize that if they can demonstrate that their product is stable for more than 24 hours, it is feasible to use in the home setting; thus longer-range stability data are now available.

It is important to distinguish between sterility and stability. Unless strict aseptic technique is adhered to, microbial contamination may potentially compromise the integrity of the product—regardless of its chemical stability. Consequently, all home infusion providers should have specially designed, environmentally controlled areas (such as clean rooms and laminar flow hoods) for preparation of sterile products. Home infusion companies and any organization that compounds sterile products must now be in compliance with new standards described in USP Chapter <797>. These standards define how sterile products should be prepared based on three risk levels: low, medium, and high. Risk level is determined by factors such as how many manipulations are involved in preparing the product and whether the final product is prepared from sterile or nonsterile ingredients (United States Pharmacopeial Convention, 2004).

Packaging

In institutional settings, both glass and plastic IV containers are used. However, because of the risk of breakage and potential for patient injury, plastic is generally used at home. Some products may be available or stable only in glass. In such instances, glass containers are used, but with appropriate cautions to patients and caregivers.

Infusion Devices

Two major changes have occurred in IV infusion devices as a result of the growth of home care. First, the size and weight of infusion devices have decreased dramatically. These changes have allowed some patients to receive their medication while going to work or school. The devices are simply placed in a pouch, which may be concealed under the patient's clothing. Second, manufacturers have introduced disposable infusion devices, which are designed to deliver one or more doses of medication and be discarded after use. Pharmacists must be able to choose the appropriate device based on the drug therapy and the patient's needs. The selection and use of the device should be incorporated into the patient's plan of care.

Delivery Schedules

Frequency of drug administration is an important consideration when selecting parenteral medications to be used in the home. Drugs that may be administered once or twice per day are more suitable than those that must be administered four to six times per day. Pharmacists should advise prescribers who are discharging patients to the home about alternative medications that may be more suitable for home use.

Monitoring Drug Therapy

Because home care patients lack the support systems available to hospital patients, monitoring drug therapy for efficacy and for adverse drug events is critical to successful patient management. The pharmacist plays an important role in establishing and coordinating monitoring parameters such as serum drug levels and blood chemistries. The pharmacist needs to ensure that the proper tests are ordered from the time the patient is accepted for care at home until the time the therapy is completed. The pharmacist also communicates the results of these tests to the prescriber and recommends changes as appropriate.

Communication with Physician, Nurses, Patients, and Others

Good communication among members of the health care team is essential for the successful care of home patients. Because the home lacks institutional safeguards, poor communication can quickly result in an adverse event for the patient. Adverse events may result in rehospitalization, which negates any benefits afforded by an early discharge.

The pharmacist has an even greater opportunity to affect patient care in the home than in an institutional setting. This impact, however, is predicated on the pharmacist's ability to communicate effectively with all members of the patient's health care team. For example, a pharmacist might receive lab data regarding Mary that may require a dosage adjustment in her antibiotic. The pharmacist must first communicate with the prescriber to effect a dosage change and then ensure that the patient's nurse is aware of the modification in therapy and the reasons for it.

Drug Information

Home care pharmacists must have adequate information resources to support the care of the patient. As a result, access to a drug information center—or, at the very least, to drug information services—is vital. The pharmacist must have the information necessary to determine whether a medication typically administered in an institutional setting can be safely delivered at home. Pharmacists should have ready access to stability and compatibility information, administration modalities, and potential complications.

American Society of Health-System Pharmacists Home Care Standards

The American Society of Health-System Pharmacists is a professional organization that has established standards for a number of activities pertaining to pharmacy practice, including home care. These standards establish a minimum level of pharmacy services within a component of pharmacy practice.

The home care standards for pharmacists focus on the following issues:

- Preadmission assessment
- Initial patient database and assessment
- Selection of products, devices, and ancillary supplies
- Development of care plans
- Patient education and counseling
- Clinical monitoring
- Effective communication with prescribers, nurses, and other health care providers
- Communication with the patient and the caregiver
- Coordination of drug preparation, delivery, storage, and administration
- Standard precautions for employee and patient safety

- Documentation in the home care record
- Adverse drug event reporting and performance improvement
- Participation in clinical drug research in the home
- Participation in performance improvement activities
- Policies and procedures
- Licensure
- Training, continuing education, and competence (American Society of Health-System Pharmacists, 2000)

Education/Training

Many pharmacists who practice in home care do not have additional training beyond their entry-level degree (BS or PharmD). Curricula in U.S. colleges of pharmacy typically provide either required or elective coursework in sterile product preparation or parapharmaceuticals such as ostomy supplies and DME, which may help better prepare practitioners for a career in home care. Some colleges of pharmacy may offer a course or component of a course that addresses home care, issues of reimbursement, and business management. It is anticipated that as home care pharmacy practice grows, pharmacy programs will incorporate more home care-related courses into their curricula.

Practice Experiences

A number of colleges of pharmacy, in conjunction with home care companies, are offering experiential training in the form of early and advanced practice experiences in home care. Early practice experiences provide students with opportunities to gain initial exposure to home care as a career option early in the professional pharmacy curriculum. Advanced practice experiences are more extended, with a focus on patient care, and occur during the final year of the curriculum.

Residency Programs

At this time, only a very limited number of postgraduate, practice-based training programs—that is, residencies—exist in home care. These programs are available to pharmacists who wish to gain additional skills in home care practice. Expansion of such programs may remain somewhat restricted given the proprietary nature of home care businesses. In particular, concerns exist about training pharmacists who will eventually work for the competition.

CONCLUSIONS

Home care encompasses the provision of many health care products and services to patients. To care for themselves, home care patients like Mary rely on home health agencies, home infusion providers, and home medical equipment dealers to provide products, service, and training.

The provision of home care is influenced by factors such as reimbursement issues, regulatory requirements, and advances in technology. To ensure proper care, each provider must account for these factors when developing a patient's plan of care.

Pharmacists must maintain their competency to fulfill their role as home care providers. As advances in technology result in new therapies and methods of delivery, the importance of the pharmacist's role in home care will continue to grow.

QUESTIONS FOR FURTHER DISCUSSION

1. Will the expansion of managed care affect the growth and development of home care? How?
2. What opportunities are available for other players (e.g., hospitals) in the health care delivery system in home care?
3. How do you believe the role of the home care pharmacist will change in the future?

KEY TOPICS AND TERMS

Home care
Home infusion therapy
Home health services
Medicare
Medicaid
Managed care
Technology
Balanced Budget Act
Health Insurance Portability and Accountability Act (HIPAA)
Regulatory agencies
Accrediting agencies
Home care standards for pharmacists

REFERENCES

American Society of Health-System Pharmacists. (2000, July). ASHP guidelines on the pharmacist's role in home care. *American Journal of Health-System Pharmacy, 57,* 1252–1257.

Bennett, M. A., & Allen, R. D. (1990). High-technology home pharmacotherapy. I: An overview of antiinfective and antineoplastic therapies. *Journal of Pharmacy Practices, 3*(1), 34–39.

Centers for Medicare and Medicaid Services. (2005). *National health care expenditures projections 2005–20015.* Retrieved February 2, 2007 from www.cms.hhs.gov/NationalHealthExpendData.

Council on Scientific Affairs, American Medical Association. (1990). Home care in the 1990s. *Journal of the American Medical Association, 263*(9), 1241–1244.

Eron, L., King, P., Marineau, M., & Yonehara, C. (2004). Treating acute infections by telemedicine in the home. *Clinical Infectious Diseases, 39,* 1175–1181.

Gill, G. M. (1991). Social work intervention with stroke patients and their families. *Journal of Home Health Care Practice, 4*(1), 57–62.

Howard, L., Alger, S., Michalek, A., Heaphey, L., Aftahi, S., & Johnston, K. R. (1993). Home parenteral nutrition in adults. In J. L. Rombeau & M. D. Caldwell (Eds.), *Clinical nutrition: Parenteral nutrition* (2nd ed., pp. 814–839). Philadelphia: W. B. Saunders.

Kaiser Family Foundation. (2005). *Medicare and Medicaid at 40.* Retrieved February 2, 2007 from http://www.kff.org/medicaid/40years.cfm

Levine, S. A., Boal, J. B., & Boling, P. A. (2003). Home care. *Journal of the American Medical Association, 290*(9): 1203–1207.

National Association for Home Care. (2001, November). *Basic statistics about home care.*

National Home Infusion Association. (2006). *FAQs.*

National Hospice Foundation. (2006). *National Hospice Foundation strategic business plan 2005–2009.*

United States Pharmacopeial Convention. (2004). Pharmaceutical considerations—sterile preparations (general information chapter 797) In *The United States Pharmacopeia* (26th rev.)/*National Formulary* (22nd ed.) (pp. 2350–2370). Rockville, MD: U.S. Pharmacopeial Convention, Inc.

U. S. Department of Labor, Bureau of Labor Statistics. (2006). *Personal and home care aides.*

Informatics in Health Care

Ardis Hanson, Bruce Lubotsky Levin, and David M. Scott

Case Scenario

As a consultant to Sheila, a 35-year-old pharmacist, you have been asked to give her advice on whether she should integrate pharmaceutical care and information technology into her community pharmacy practice. For the past 10 years, Sheila has developed a thriving independent community pharmacy practice in a rural community of 5,000 people in a southwestern state. However, the trend toward third-party prescription payment and the increasing number of prescriptions transferred to Web-based pharmacies are competitive pressures for this pharmacy.

Because of the economic squeeze on her business, Sheila is considering developing a computerized monitoring and education program for patients based on information technology. If she decides to pursue this route, Sheila plans to market the pharmaceutical care program initially to her private-pay patients, and by the second year to managed care organizations. The disease state that is most prevalent in this rural community is hypertension.

What should you advise Sheila to do? In your answer, consider how information technology and pharmaceutical care have affected community pharmacy practice and the additional training that Sheila would need to implement this change in her practice.

LEARNING OBJECTIVES

Upon completion of this chapter, students shall be able to:

- Describe the history and application of information technology on health care delivery and pharmacy practice
- Describe how automation in distribution is affecting pharmacy practice
- Describe why information literacy is important for the pharmacy researcher, educator, practitioner, and student
- Describe the ethical issues facing pharmacists from the three perspectives of personal, professional, and customer concerns
- Describe major information technology trends in pharmacy practice today
- Describe the redesign of pharmacy practice with regard to information technology with a focus on public policy and public safety

CHAPTER QUESTIONS

1. How is information technology affecting health care delivery and pharmacy practice?
2. How will further automation in manufacturing affect pharmacy practice?
3. With the continued development of databases for pharmaceutical research, what are possible scenarios for computer-based research?
4. What information literacy skills are important for the pharmacy researcher, educator, practitioner, and student?
5. As the practice of pharmacy shifts from medication dispensing to a more holistic health model, what are some of the emerging barriers to care and how will they alter practice?

INTRODUCTION

Although telecommunication is playing an increasingly important role in society in knowledge exchange and in commerce, it is in the fields of public health, medical care, and pharmacy practice where the most remarkable opportunities and challenges related to telecommunication have emerged. Telecommunication ("tele") strategies, particularly with the growth in broadband services, continue to broaden access to medical care, health education, and health services delivery for at-risk populations in America (Hanson, Levin, Heron, and Burke, 2003; National Telecommunications and Information Administration, 2004). The development of computer-based patient records, health information systems, and unified electronic claims systems has taken advantage of a variety of technologies to streamline and centralize databases. Recent initiatives, such as the President's New Freedom Commission on Mental Health

(2003) and the national electronic health record, are also encouraging policy makers and health professionals to transform the existing health delivery systems into more efficient and effective health care delivery systems.

This chapter examines some of the major issues related to health care informatics. It includes a general discussion of the history of informatics technology and the categories of health care information systems, with an emphasis on pharmacy applications.

HISTORY OF INFORMATICS TECHNOLOGY

Telecommunication technologies have become integral components of general health care, emergency health care, and community-based health care, particularly in rural areas of the United States (Levin and Hanson, 2001). With the greater availability of communication satellites in the late 1970s, interest in applying new technologies to health care increased dramatically, driven by the transition from analog to digital transmission coupled with rapid increases in computer and communications hardware and software development. These developments provided the essential core infrastructure for the Internet.

The Internet

With the advent of graphically based browsers, adoption of Internet technology accelerated dramatically. The Internet's ability to provide access to updated, full-text resource literature has eliminated the main disadvantage of print resource literature—namely, its significant lag time. Publishers of electronically formatted, fee-based literature, previously available only on CD-ROMs or network servers, have been rapidly moving their products into Internet formats, resulting in the ready accessibility of current information from anywhere in the world. Journals, textbooks, medical/pharmaceutical databases, and media productions, such as video-casts and audio-casts, are now available directly online to researchers, health care professionals, and patients alike.

Telehealth

Telemedicine (also known as telehealth) has been described as the use of telecommunications technologies to provide health care in a cost-efficient manner and to strive to improve health care, particularly when distance separates consumers and providers (Angaran, 1999). Whereas in the past telehealth technologies have included videoconferencing, telephones, computers, the Internet, e-mail, fax, radio, and television, newer technologies are increasingly being introduced and winning converts (Moore, 2003). More programs have been delivering health care using a combination of audio, graphic, store-and-forward, and telemetry technologies (i.e., automatic transmission and measurement of data from remote sources by wire, radio, or other means).

Early initiatives associated with the Telecommunications Act dramatically altered the communication rates and services potentially available to telemedicine providers. Approximately $400 million of funding was provided to health providers, libraries, and schools in rural areas to finance telephone-line charges incurred in connecting to the Internet via the Universal Service Fund (Rohde, 1996). Nearly a decade later, telecommunications "reform" became a top priority for both Congress and the Federal Communications Commission. In 2005, key members of Congress announced that the Telecommunications Act of 1996, including universal service and the electronic rates (e-rate) provision, would be reformed; the reform efforts primarily addressed, in different bills, general Telecommunications Act reform, digital television, universal service reform, and e-rate reform.

Today's Internet is still concerned with broadband access, network neutrality, and funding for public access (Communications Opportunity, Promotion and Enhancement Act of 2006; Communications, Consumers' Choice, and Broadband Deployment Act of 2006). The American Broadband for Communities Act of 2006 amends the Communications Act of 1934 to also promote and expedite wireless broadband deployment in rural and other areas, and for other purposes.

Pharmacoinformatics

Informatics is a field that focuses on the creative use of computers in support of patient care, education, and research. Although pharmacoinformatics focused initially on clinical issues, it is now used widely in the pharmaceutical industry for research, product development, quality assurance, business development, marketing, and sales.

Patient Care and Educational Databases

Knowledge bases, such as *Clinical Pharmacology* and *MDConsult*, analyze a patient's drug-related problems and sort though information to help solve the patient's problems. Offline information applications, such as *Clinical Reference Library*, are also available to support the provision of pharmaceutical care. Traditional academic resources have received major enhancements through the development of databases such as *EMBASE*, the *Excerpta Medica* database, and its companion current-awareness file, *EMBASE Alert*. Approximately 10 years ago, the terms "pharmacoeconomics" and "disease management" were added to EMTREE, *Excerpta Medica*'s thesaurus.

The continued trend toward making more information available on the Internet emphasizes the need to ensure that *accurate* information is provided on the Web. New conceptual frameworks and evaluative measures are critical to ensure that users receive accurate clinical and medical referral information (Eysenbach, Yihune, Lampe, Cross, and Brickley, 2000; Seidman, Steinwachs, and Rubin, 2003a, 2003b). Such tools are proving to be reliable and valid methods for evaluating the quality of Internet health sites and can help consumers distinguish between beneficial and misleading information.

Pharmaceutical Research and Development

A major growth area in pharmacoinformatics has been in the development of pharmaceutical research and development databases. Informatics has transformed these databases from a specialist's tool in the 1930s into an accepted and widely used tool on researchers' desktops in the 21st century.

The first bioinformatic databases were constructed a few years after the first protein sequences became available (Holley et al., 1965; Dayhoff, 1972; Abola, Bernstein, Bryant, Koetzle, and Weng, 1987; Bairoch and Boeckmann, 1991). In the future, the unprecedented volume of data arising from the Human Genome Project and other projects of this magnitude will undoubtedly have a profound effect on the ways in which data are used and experiments performed in drug discovery, product development, clinical diagnosis, and treatment (Ioannidis et al., 2006; Kaiser, 2006). Three critical factors for effective use of R&D databases are improved access to large electronic data sets, reliable and consistent annotation, and effective tools for data mining (Bassett, Eisen, and Boguski, 1999; Braibanti, Rao, Rao, Ramam, and Rao, 2002; Scott, 2004).

The traditional technological advantages that one pharmaceutical company might have enjoyed over another competitor are now a thing of the past. To be successful, all pharmaceutical companies must invest in new technologies that provide a more scalable framework for handling information beyond the traditional informatics domain. These technologies, such as high-throughput computation, combinatorial chemistry, microarrays, and interactive visualization tools, reduce the time needed to execute the specific steps required for a complete analysis using distributed processes and parallelized software (D'Agostino, Aversano, and Chiusano, 2005; Kruglyak, 2005; Desiere et al., 2006; Teufel, Krupp, Weinmann, and Galle, 2006). Newer technologies are developed to run on low-requirement hardware components, with a focus on achieving scalability at affordable costs. These technologies allow for greater specificity in mapping, classification, visualization, and clustering of data, based on user-defined subsets, with user-editable features being available to parse enormous data sets (Shah et al., 2005; Zhu et al., 2006).

Given the exponential growth rates of data and the critical need to integrate and analyze information more effectively, retraining and repositioning pharmaceutical information technology and research teams to support and use information-driven research more effectively is critical (Mooney, 2001). Meeting these challenges will require a significant investment in infrastructure and industry personnel, hardware and software, and storage facilities (Owen, 2005; Henry, Doran, Kerridge, Hill, McNeill, and Day, 2005). Ideally, researchers should work in an environment where all of a pharmaceutical company's information about a specific receptor, drug, patent, or patient sample can readily be accessed, correlated with other data, and used to infer or augment knowledge of a particular molecular system (Torr-Brown, 2005; Tummala, Shabaker, and Leung, 2005).

APPLICATIONS IN HEALTH CARE AND PHARMACY PRACTICE

In addition to pharmaceutical research and development (R&D), pharmacoinformatics spans a broad spectrum of areas—from clinical problem solving to computer-based clinical records—that may assist with diagnosis, treatment, and other aspects of patient care. In the late 1950s, crude computerized patient information systems were introduced in hospitals (Collen, 1995). The earliest use of computation for medicine was for dental projects in the 1950s at the U.S. National Bureau of Standards (Ledley, 1960). Early expert systems were also developed in the 1950s; for example, MYCIN was designed to diagnose infectious blood diseases and recommend antibiotics, with the dosage being adjusted for a patient's body weight (Winston and Prendergast, 1984). These early systems, which were used primarily for medical research, differed dramatically from today's patient information systems.

By the mid-1960s, improved computing and communications technology and federal funding for biomedical applications had made the development of patient information systems more feasible. Use of the Internet and the introduction of "smart" drug management systems have dramatically affected the administration of health care organizations. A prime example may be seen in these technologies' effects on hospital and community pharmacies.

Hospital and Community Pharmacies

Computer applications to facilitate dispensing medications first entered into practice in the late 1960s in a limited number of hospital pharmacies. As the costs of computer hardware continued to decrease, technology applications in pharmacy became more widespread. Although most outpatient prescription labels and inpatient orders were typed in the 1970s, virtually all prescription labels are now computer-generated. Editing of labels, storage of prescription information, and easy retrieval made drug distribution a more efficient process than handling individual paper prescriptions.

Tablet-weighting scales (AccuCount or Baker scale) are typically the first step in automation, followed by the more sophisticated Baker Cell Counting machine. The latter device contains a series of cells, each of which holds tablets or capsules that are automatically counted for a prescription. Many of today's counter systems include a verification feature that eliminates potential errors in prescription filling and provide a detailed receipt of the transactions, such as target and actual weights of the ingredients, user identification, lot number, and a time/date stamp. New models include intranet connections to a central drug database that can update independent scales or all scales should the need arise.

By the early 1970s, many hospital inpatient pharmacies had adopted the unit-dose distribution system (Stolar, 1979). Unit-dose systems, in which doses of medications are individually wrapped, labeled, and identified with a patient, have been shown to reduce medication errors in hospital settings. A requirement of the Joint Commission on Accreditation of Healthcare Organizations (JCAHO), the use of the unit-dose distribution system has created a greater reliance on bar-code point-of-care (BPOC) automated distribution systems (Grotting, Yang, Kelly, Brown, and Trohimovich, 2002).

Two automated approaches are typically used: (1) an automated system that operates at the point of use at the nursing unit or (2) a centralized pharmacy system that automates the unit-dose cart-fill process.

A point-of-use system automates the unit-dose system at the nursing unit level. After the physician medication order is entered and checked by the pharmacist, the drug is immediately available at the nursing unit for administration to the patient. Although not all medications can be stored within these units, commonly used medications can be stored and distributed by each unit. Because most physicians prescribe a limited number of drugs and admit patients to a specific nursing unit, such a system can provide unit-of-use packaging under a controlled situation.

An example of a point-of-use system is Pyxis SAFETYnet (Cardinal Health Company). This integrated system combines document imaging of physician orders from initial write-ups, approval by the pharmacist, a point-of-use automated dispensing system, and bar-code scanning by the nurse at the patient's bedside.

By contrast, an automated system in the central inpatient pharmacy uses robotic technology to automate the unit-dose cart filling of patient medication cassettes that are checked by the use of bar-code technology (Nold and Williams, 1985; Chung, Choi, and Moon, 2003). An example of such an automated unit-dose dispensing system is Robot-Rx (McKesson), which integrates dispensing logic with MedCarousel (medication storage system). Using rotating shelves, bar-code scanning, and workflow software, Robot-Rx reduces picking and restocking errors, speeds up cabinet fill time, and decreases the need for pharmacists to check individual doses in the cassette trays.

A second example of a fully automated robotic prescription dispensing system designed for a hospital outpatient pharmacy or a community pharmacy is ScriptPro®. Advantages of this system are its relatively small size (requiring about 15 square feet of floor space), avoidance of medication cross-contamination, and the universality of the 100 or 200 dispensing cells (they can handle either capsules or tablets of various sizes and shapes and support standard pharmacy vials).

Automation is a complex decision and a significant investment, so the decision to automate is largely dependent upon the need for and payback on the equipment. If the workload in any of these areas (i.e., unit-dose filling, syringe filling, or IV admixtures) is relatively low, then purchase of an automated machine may be difficult to justify. However, in a busy hospital pharmacy, the need for an automated machine is often more obvious. As more patient care shifts from inpatient hospitals to ambulatory care facilities, automation for outpatient and community pharmacies will in turn become a significant issue. Given that outpatient pharmacy workload is composed of prescriptions that are generated from a variety of primary care providers and specialists, automation in this setting may be easier to justify (Skrepnek et al., 2006).

For all systems, it is critical that complete and accurate information be entered into the computerized system so that the correct medications are matched to the appropriate patients. Should an adverse event occur, BPOC systems create a vital audit trail to facilitate follow-up (Grotting et al., 2002).

The tools developed for the pharmaceutical industry and its customers are more sophisticated today than ever before (Kager and Mozeson, 2000). Integrated transaction processing systems allow for more timely and accurate reporting of product shipments around the globe. Constraint-based planning tools allow for realistic scheduling of scarce manufacturing and distribution capacity to allow drug makers to meet accurate forecasts of demand. With few other options left to offset the costs of handling the growing number of third-party prescriptions, the nation's drug chains have turned to computers and pharmacy information systems, with the goal of streamlining the prescription filling and distribution process to make it more efficient. Many retailers use automated systems for activities ranging from collecting voice-mail reorders on prescriptions to the control of pharmaceutical inventory (Brookman, 1998).

Owing to the increased volume of prescriptions and the tight labor market throughout the United States, a shortage of pharmacists exists. One workaround for this problem for independent pharmacies and chain pharmacies is use of a central processing high-volume facility, such as TechRx. Prescriptions from a community pharmacy are electronically transferred to a central processing facility where dispensing, claim adjudication, and physician contact for clarifications are completed. Completed prescriptions are then shipped back to the pharmacy overnight (*America's Pharmacist*, 2003).

Pharmacy Benefit Managers

Some drug store chains have sophisticated computer systems and centralized storage sites for prescriptions. When a pharmacist enters a new prescription or a prescription refill, the prescription claim information is transmitted over the telephone line to a pharmacy benefit manager (PBM) computer system or is processed in the pharmacy-owned computer system. The adjudication of a prescription claim occurs in a few seconds or less.

The high costs of prescription drugs remain a major concern in the United States. PBMs, such as Medco Health Solutions, Caremark, and Express Scripts, administer components of prescription drug programs, including claims processing, formulary management, drug utilization review, pharmacy network management, online claims adjudication, eligibility verification, co-payment verification, contracts with pharmaceutical manufacturers, mail-order pharmacy services, and disease management programs. PBMs manage databases that require integration of clinical information and prescription drug information files. Retail pharmacies have also started their own PBMs, including Walgreen's Health Care Plus and Rite Aid's Health Solutions.

PBMs manage prescription costs using a variety of integrated strategies, such as generic drugs, formularies, multitiered co-payment programs, prior authorization, and step therapy. Although PBMs play a vital role in claim adjudication, their inclusion is associated with many potential conflicts of interest and restraint of trade issues, such as rebates from drug companies, limited choices to mail-order pharmacies, lack of disclosure, and complaints of "favoritism."

Warehouse and Distribution Systems

Manufacturers and distributors of all sizes are faced with the conflicting goals of reducing stock on hand to save inventory (carrying) costs while maintaining adequate stock to meet commitments and maintain customer satisfaction. However, for the pharmaceutical industry, achieving 100% accuracy in inventory tracking is the most critical and important goal to achieve. Lot traceability (from point of consumption back to point of manufacture) must be ensured.

An integrated warehouse system passes inventory information and customer orders through a warehouse management system (WMS). Communicating over a wireless data communication system allows order fulfillment associates in a distribution center to have real-time, online tracking of all products as they enter, move through, and then leave the distribution center, providing the validation process required for pharmaceuticals by the government. In addition to improved inventory management, electronic product code/radio frequency identification (EPC/RFID) adoption creates major benefits in the areas of improved supply chain integrity, improved deduction and claims accuracy, and greater warehouse and inventory efficiency (Kearney, 2004).

Web-Based Pharmacies

Web-based pharmacies, such as drugstore.com and CornerDrugstore.com, first emerged in the late 1990s. The National Community Pharmacists Association's (NCPA) CornerDrugstore.com for independent community pharmacies supports individual pharmacy Web sites and features a health information center, a prescription center, communication with the pharmacist, a drug interaction checker, a store locator, and patient centers for shopping and creating family health records. Capabilities include refill reminders, notification concerning new products, and health information (*America's Pharmacist,* 2003).

Computerization has created some problems for community pharmacists, especially with incorporating technology into work flow and staff training issues. Nevertheless, with increased attention to informatics in pharmacy school curricula and continuing education programs, community pharmacists like Sheila (in the chapter-opening case scenario) will undoubtedly be better prepared to use computer and telecommunication technology in their community pharmacy practices.

Rural Pharmacies

The role of the rural pharmacist, as documented in the case scenario, is increasing in importance. Many rural pharmacists are the first health providers seen by patients. As a consequence, the delivery of medications and information to rural pharmacists and their patients is a critical concern (Murray, Loo, Tu, Eckert, Zhou, and Tierney, 1999; Scott, Miller, and Letcher, 1999; Bearden and Holt, 2005; Triller, Donnelly, and Rugge, 2005). Telepharmacy shares the same basic definition as telehealth, but refers to provision of pharmaceutical services via telecommunication. Telepharmacy is not a new concept—pharmacists have provided care by telephone for years, such as through drug information centers, poison control centers, and information help lines. Today, telephone, fax, Internet, e-mail, and interactive video are among the many technologies used to communicate with customers. Vendors of telepharmacy equipment, such as ScriptPro, use commonly available telehealth equipment (Peterson and Anderson, 2004b).

Lack of pharmacy access is both a rural health care crisis and an increasing problem throughout the United States. For instance, in North Dakota, 26 rural community pharmacies have closed in recent years and another 12 are at risk of closing. To address this problem, North Dakota passed legislation in 2001 that would allow pharmacists (by modifying Board of Pharmacy regulations) at a central hub pharmacy to supervise a technician at a remote site in the dispensing of prescriptions using telepharmacy.

North Dakota also sought federal funding for its Telepharmacy Project through the U.S. Health Resources and Services Administration (HRSA), Office for the Advancement of Telehealth (OAT) (Peterson and Anderson, 2004a). The goals of the North Dakota Telepharmacy Project are two-fold: (1) to provide pharmacists with financial assistance and implement telepharmacy in rural locations; and (2) to assess the effects of these services on the targeted communities (Peterson and Anderson, 2004a). As of 2006, the state had 57 telepharmacy sites in 44 retail sites, 13 hospital sites, and 2 interstate sites.

Development of academic and community partnerships can also benefit rural practitioners and communities. The Telepharmacy Project partners, for example, include the North Dakota State University (NDSU) College of Pharmacy, North Dakota Board of Pharmacy, North Dakota State Pharmaceutical Association, rural community pharmacists, and targeted rural communities.

TRENDS IN PHARMACY PRACTICE

Several trends are changing the practice of pharmacy: (1) increased software integration of dispensing and pharmaceutical care; (2) electronic health records; (3) e-prescribing; (4) use of technology to reduce medication errors; and (5) increased use of distance education in pharmacy education and training.

Integration of Pharmacy Dispensing and Pharmaceutical Care Software

Vendors are moving toward comprehensive, integrated computer systems that support numerous pharmaceutical care activities, including screening for problems, documenting interventions, developing patient care plans, billing for cognitive services, and evaluating outcomes. This integration would eliminate the need to double-enter data (e.g., demographics and medication-related information) and would streamline operations (Chung et al., 2003). As pharmacists integrate medication therapy management (MTM) into their practices, the need to identify, monitor, and manage drug therapy will become paramount. The community pharmacist will need the software and skills to accomplish these tasks.

Today's pharmacist is challenged to deliver better patient care and drug information at the point of care. Instead of saying, "Let me get back to you," when asked a difficult drug information question, the pharmacist can use a personal digital assistant (PDA) to immediately access resources and share up-to-date information on prescription drugs with patients waiting for answers (McCreadie, Stevenson, Sweet, and Kramer, 2002). Both pharmacists and pharmacy students are adopting the PDA technologies so that drug therapy decisions can be made quickly and effectively. For clinicians and pharmacists, a growing array of PDA software on clinical and pharmaceutical information is available (Felkey, Fox, and Thrower, 2006). PDAs are also used at the point of care for patient disease state management (e.g., anticoagulation, asthma, diabetes, cardiovascular, and hypertension) (McCreadie et al., 2002; Raybardhan, Balen, Partovi, Loewen, Liu, and Jewesson, 2005). For instance, HemoSense is a handheld pharmacy information system that provides prothrombin time (PT) and international normalized ratio (INR) results using capillary whole blood.

Other computer-aided devices are currently used in pharmacies. For example, automated blood pressure devices measure blood pressure and heart rate, storing this information on a local computer or server. A pharmacist refers the patient to the physician when the blood pressure is not within a defined range. Patients with diabetes may use similar devices to monitor their blood glucose.

Monitoring of medication compliance is also available for patients who are taking numerous medications (Scolaro, Stamm, and Lloyd, 2005). These devices can provide patient reminders and collect data on compliance, which can then be monitored by the pharmacist and downloaded for the physician's review. Computer-aided monitoring devices are an area of informatics that is expected to significantly develop in the near future (Joseph, 2006).

Electronic Health Records

The federal government has set a goal of developing a national electronic health record (EHR) within the next 10 years as a key component of the National Health Information Infrastructure (NHII). Advocates of EHRs have promoted their use for the past three decades (Poon et al., 2006). The Department of Veterans Affairs, for example, developed the Veteran Health Information Systems and Technology Architecture (VISTA), which is a fully integrated EHR system (Department of Veterans Affairs, 2005). The Kaiser Permanente HealthConnect program integrates a patient's clinical record with appointments, registration, and billing, so that patients can go online to make appointments, view lab tests results, refill prescriptions, view prescription histories, and communicate with physicians and other health providers (Raymond, 2005).

A Rand study has suggested that the U.S. health care system could save more than $81 billion annually and improve the quality of care with widespread adoption of EHRs (Hillestad et al., 2005). Electronic medical records would include clinical information systems; scheduling, billing, and other functionalities for fiscal viability; and evaluation and outcomes measures. Challenges include interconnectivity, financing, human factors (such as ease of data entry), network inequity in provider systems, addressing comorbidity, lack of buy-in by providers and their institutions, adoption of common terminology, and universal computer standards. While individually each of these areas poses a significant financial and organizational challenge, taken as a whole, the list is daunting (Newton, Thompson, Campbell, and Spencer, 2006).

Consumer concerns regarding the potential misuse of EHRs also compel providers and payers to protect the security of personal health care information. Although the HIPAA regulations offer some protection, problems with identity theft persist. Thus, while the need for them certainly exists, many obstacles remain to be overcome before EHRs are adopted across the board.

Electronic Prescribing

A third trend affecting pharmacy practice is the continuing demand for electronic delivery of prescription orders. Although virtually all prescriptions were handwritten in 1998 (Schiff and Rucker, 1998), trends toward greater use of computerized prescribing show no signs of stopping. Most states allow prescription transmissions from a prescriber computer to a pharmacy computer. Current e-prescribing vendors generally charge an up-front fee from physicians and a monthly rate for updates, such as drug warnings and label changes from the Food and Drug Administration (FDA).

In a joint venture, members of the NCPA and the National Association of Chain Drug Stores formed SureScript Systems to facilitate e-prescribing between physicians and community pharmacies (Hollon, 2001). In 2006, SureScript Systems began operate an online drug history service that allows doctors in Massachusetts, Rhode Island, New Jersey, Nevada, Tennessee, and Florida to see the consolidated records of most nearby pharmacies, thereby checking on the drugs, doses, and compliance of a patient (Alpert, 2006).

PBMs are also involved in e-prescribing. In 2001, the joint venture RxHub was created by AdvancePCS (Texas), Express Scripts (Missouri), and Merck-Medco Managed Care (New Jersey—a subsidiary of Merck and Company). In 2006, RxHub played a major role in the development of e-prescribing standards that will be tested in Medicare electronic prescribing pilots (*Managed Care Business Week* staff, 2006).

In addition to network e-prescribing, e-prescribing software is available on wireless pocket personal computers or on tablet computers that allow the physician to engage in point-of-care electronic prescribing. These handheld devices may capture information related to a managed care formulary, drug information, a patient medication profile, or a list of pharmacies with electronic data transmission terminals. Physicians can access the Internet to prescribe, check for drug interactions, access medication histories, review drug reference information, and send prescriptions to the pharmacy from virtually anywhere, using a product such as TouchScript. Healtheon/WebMD, for example, has created Internet interfaces and services for medical group practices that connect physicians, insurers, pharmacies, and patients. Its EHR includes lab results, prescribing drugs, clinical tasks, and point-of-care documentation. Clearly, e-prescribing is a growing market.

E-prescribing also holds promise for reducing medication errors. An Institute of Medicine (IOM) report found that 7,000 people die each year from prescription errors made in hospitals and outpatient settings, such as physician offices and pharmacies (Kohn, Corrigan, and Donaldson, 2000). Contributing to these errors are similar-sounding drug names (e.g., Celexa for depression and Celebrex for arthritis), illegible physician handwriting, and expansion of the drug universe (the increasing number of new drugs and number of prescriptions filled annually). E-prescribing might potentially clear up some of this confusion, leading to fewer medication errors.

Use of Technology to Reduce Medication Errors

Another trend in pharmacy practice is greater use of technology to help pharmacists assess and reduce medication errors. In 2003, medication dispensing errors received national attention following publication of a study conducted by Flynn, Barker, and Carnahan (2003). According to this study, dispensing errors occur at a rate of 4 errors per day in a pharmacy filling 250 prescriptions daily, which extrapolates to 51.5 million errors during the filling of 3 billion prescriptions in the United States each year. As Flynn, Barker, and Carnahan (2003) reported, this figure includes an estimated 3.3 million errors of potential clinical importance.

Pharmacy Quality Commitment (PQC), developed by Pharmacists Mutual Company, is a Web-based dispensing error reporting system and quality improvement system for pharmacists. Within this system, an "error" is defined as a mistake that reaches the patient; a "near-miss" is considered a success story, because pharmacy personnel catch the mistake before the prescription is delivered to the patient. Pharmacists and pharmacy technicians probably catch most errors before they reach the patient. Hence, the number of near-misses appears to greatly outweigh the number of errors. Data on such incidents can be used to determine where in the dispensing process errors are occurring. Then, using the quality improvement processes, this information can be shared with pharmacists and pharmacy technicians, enabling them to improve shortcomings in the dispensing process and reduce medication errors.

In 2003, the FDA required bar codes on all medications (when dispensing as well as on prescription bottles) to ensure that patients receive the right drugs in hospitals and in other treatment facilities (Food and Drug Administration, 2003). Physicians enter prescriptions for hospitalized patients into a computer. Pharmacists then fill the prescriptions and check the prescriptions against patient parameters, such as the patient's age, weight, diagnosis, other drugs taken, drug allergies, and drug interactions. At the patient's bedside, a nurse scans the bar code on the patient's bracelet and the bar code on the medication. The computer checks whether the medication is the same drug and matches the dose ordered by the physician, and sounds an alarm if a mismatch occurs.

Medical safety experts, pharmacists, and drug companies support this system to reduce medication errors (Grotting et al., 2002), but are concerned about the high cost to implement the bar-code system. Estimates of the total costs include $50 million for pharmaceutical companies to put bar codes on every product and $7 billion for hospitals to purchase or update scanners and computers. Other concerns relate to the training and adherence rates of physicians, pharmacists, and nurses with this system.

Pharmacist Education and Training

The Pharmacy Education Aid Act of 2001 provided grants to pharmacy schools to use technology for professional (continuing) education and for academic degree programs for students. As pharmacists continue to engage in nontraditional clinical and management functions in a variety of health care settings, the need for coursework has increased for both students and current practitioners (Knapp, Blalock, and Black, 2001; Pedersen, Schneider, and Scheckelhoff, 2005).

Postgraduate educational programs range from traditional one-hour continuing education (CE) programs to intensive certificate programs aimed at helping a pharmacist develop new expertise. Unlike other medical professionals, most pharmacists do not obtain postgraduate qualifications or specialty certifications (Rouse, 2004). Because continuing professional development, lifelong learning, and quality improvement are important measures of professional knowledge, quality-assured CE and certificate programs are essential components of one's professional development as a pharmacist (Rouse, 2004). With this model in mind, the Accreditation Council for Pharmacy Education's (ACPE) Pharmacists' Learning Network (PLAN) allows pharmacists to access information through more than 3,000 live and home study continuing pharmaceutical education programs offered by ACPE-approved providers.

Information literacy skills are critical for successful educational and practice experiences. Many colleges of pharmacy provide students with an array of services, including Internet access, interactive instructional software, and technical support services (Frederick, 1999). The skills associated with information literacy include fundamental knowledge, basic learning techniques, clinical skills, methods for critical appraisal (particularly with Web-based information), and effective use of the pharmacoinformatics research literature. It will be critical for pharmacists at all levels to gain a more comprehensive view of the "information superhighway" as it relates to a particular pharmaceutical question. Information literacy also spills over into communication skills, another critical area for pharmacists.

E-mail (written communication), telephone training, and videoconferencing have become de rigueur in pharmacy practice. These activities (which take place between the clinician and the patient) are usually short and highly focused sessions (Angaran, 1999). Knowing how to communicate well and to be more efficient and effective are critical patient–practitioner skills. Faculty, students, preceptors, and alumni should also receive training in informatics and information technology so they can better integrate telepharmacy into mainstream patient care and remain professionally viable in the increasingly health care networked environment of pharmacy practice.

FUTURE CHALLENGES

A major challenge for both the health care system and pharmacy practice is the integration of available technology (video, e-mail, telephone, and the Internet) into a coordinated practice that improves the therapeutic relationship between patient and practitioner (Angaran, 1999). As the workplace and workforce have changed, it has become clear that the demand for pharmacists has outpaced the supply. Indeed, a study from the American Association of Colleges of Pharmacy predicted a shortfall of 157,000 pharmacists in the United States by 2020 (Cooksey, Knapp, Walton, and Cultice, 2002). The same report also predicted higher workloads and greater use of pharmacist extenders and technology.

As the profession has moved from a product orientation (dispensing medications) to a patient focus, clinical training requirements have expanded, and new business models have been created to capitalize on the changing pharmacist–patient relationship (Cooksey et al., 2002). These new models generate revenue based on value-added patient services, such as health screenings and face-to-face or Web-based information on health issues (Schroff, 2003).

Furthermore, the move toward the disease management/evidence-based practice model is causing the redesign of the medication-use process. Ideally, the redesigned process will reduce preventable drug therapy-related adverse outcomes, identify and evaluate existing and emerging models, and encourage collaboration across disciplines and professions (Kohn et al., 2000). An important part of this process will be efforts to develop and assess new models of pharmaceutical care that embrace the Institute of Medicine's recommendations for improving the safety of the health care system by optimally engaging pharmacists (Institute of Medicine, 2001; Kohn et al., 2000).

The JCAHO standards focus on organizational leadership, improvement of performance, information management, patient rights, staff training, and care delivery. These standards formalize the collection of patient safety data, require annual safety reports to the institution's governing board, commit organizations to prompt disclosure of errors to patients, and require reengineering of care delivery systems to prevent errors before they occur (Gebhart, 2001). Given that medication usage is a central component of medical care (Pedersen, Schneider, and Scheckelhoff, 2006), research efforts to inform the redesign of the medication-use process should be a priority in health care policy (Cooksey et al., 2002). Such system redesign needs to focus on developing an integrated health care delivery model from the perspectives of both the patient and the pharmacy staff, and minimizing barriers to care through improved communication between medical and pharmacy professionals as well as through the use of multiple-approved formularies (Cooksey et al., 2002; Park, 2006; Mann, Lloyd-Puryear, and Linzer, 2006).

A final challenge for pharmacists is to increase their participation in policy and regulatory planning sessions, particularly in the areas of the National Health Infrastructure and electronic health records. For example, universal adoption of EHRs is supposed to occur by 2014. Pharmacists, particularly those who work in concert with other medical professionals in small and solo practice environments, will be significantly affected by this requirement. Nevertheless, EHR adoption is not expected to reach its maximum market share in the small practice setting until 2024 (Ford, Menachemi, and Phillips, 2006). If this scenario holds true, EHR products are unlikely to achieve full diffusion in this critical market segment within the targeted time frame of 2014. Although pharmacists have many opportunities to become engaged in health care informatics, impressive challenges still remain, even as improvements in research technology continue to be introduced to pharmacy students through curriculum changes and to practicing pharmacists through postgraduate training initiatives.

CONCLUSIONS

Technology has had a dramatic impact on health care delivery and pharmacy practice. Twenty-five years ago, very little automation or computerization was used. Personal computers began to replace typewriters in the early 1980s. Today, computers are found in every pharmacy setting and automated dispensing devices are becoming common. While no one has a crystal ball that can reliably predict the future, the potential applications of technology seem unlimited.

Information literacy skills are critical for successful education, training, and practice experiences in any field. Skills associated with information literacy that are essential for pharmacy students and practitioners to acquire include (1) fundamental knowledge, (2) basic learning techniques, (3) clinical skills, (4) methods for critical appraisal, and (5) effective use of the pharmacoinformatics research literature. Pharmacy faculty and students need to be conversant with the databases used within the health and drug information environment. It is critical for pharmacists at all levels to gain a comprehensive view of the information superhighway as it relates to a particular pharmaceutical question.

In recent years, the focus of pharmacy practice has changed in a number of ways. Emerging business models emphasize an integrated health care delivery model, which takes both provider and patient perspectives into account. Important areas of concern in this model include the reduction of barriers to care, such as use of patient medical information. How can pharmacists gain access to the patient's medical history, which may contain critical information on existing or co-occurring medical conditions that may affect the dispensing of medications, particularly drug interactions that may not be evident to the prescribing physician or physician's assistant?

Another barrier to care is the limited communication between medical and pharmacy professionals. Although access to patient records is a critical component in providing more complete patient care, more "real-time" communication between physicians and pharmacists is needed, especially if the physician has questions about new medications that may be part of a drug company's sample or that are seen briefly in advertising.

QUESTIONS FOR FURTHER DISCUSSION

1. What information technology innovations are adaptable for use in institutional and community pharmacy practice?
2. Several information technology applications to pharmacy practice in drug distribution and telepharmacy have been developed in the past decade. What innovations do you envision appearing in this decade?
3. Contrast the strengths and limitations of information technology applications in rural and urban areas in your state.
4. What aspects of technology are nice to have, yet are currently unnecessary for improving patient care?
5. What are important educational technology components in pharmacy school curriculum from a student's perspective? From a professor's perspective?

KEY TOPICS AND TERMS

Licensure and accreditation
Manufacturing and distribution
Medication delivery
Pharmacoeconomics
Pharmacy education
Pharmacy information services
Pharmacy practice
Public policy
Quality assurance
Technology
Telehealth

REFERENCES

Abola, E. E., Bernstein, F. C., Bryant, S. H., Koetzle, T. F., & Weng, J. (1987). Protein data bank. In F. H. Allen, G. Bergeroff, & R. Sievers (Eds.), *Crystallographic databases: Information content, software systems, scientific applications* (pp. 101–132). Bonn, Germany: Data Commission of the International Union of Crystallography.

Alpert, B. (2006). At last, digital doctors. *Barron's, 86*(7), 43–45.

American Broadband for Communities Act of 2006. (2006). S. 2332, 109th Cong., 2nd Session.

America's Pharmacist. (2003, April). Community pharmacy stands at the dawn of the e-prescribing era. *America's Pharmacist,* 16–21.

Angaran, D. M. (1999). Telemedicine and telepharmacy: Current status and future implications. *American Journal of Health-System Pharmacy, 56*(14), 405–426.

Bairoch, A., & Boeckmann, B. (1991). The SWISS-PROT protein sequence data bank. *Nucleic Acids Research, 19*(suppl), 2247–2249.

Bassett, D. E., Eisen, M. B., & Boguski, M. S. (1999). Gene expression informatics: It's all in your mind. *Nature Genetics, 21*(suppl), 51–55.

Bearden, D. T., & Holt, T. (2005). Statewide impact of pharmacist-delivered adult influenza vaccinations. *American Journal of Preventive Medicine, 29*(5), 450–452.

Braibanti, A., Rao, R. S., Rao, G. N., Ramam, V. A., & Rao, S. V. (2002). Data, knowledge and method bases in chemical sciences. Part IV. Current status in databases. *Annali Di Chimica, 92*(7–8), 689–704.

Brookman, F. (1998). Drug chains turn to automated systems to counter shrinking Rx margins. *Stores, 81*(5), 3628.

Chung, K., Choi, Y. B., & Moon, S. (2003). Toward efficient medication error reduction: Error-reducing information management systems. *Journal of Medical Systems, 27*(6), 553–560.

Collen, M. F. (1995). *A history of medical informatics in the United States, 1950 to 1990.* Indianapolis, IN: American Medical Informatics Association.

Communications, Consumers' Choice, and Broadband Deployment Act of 2006. (2006). S. 2686, 109th Cong., 2nd Session.

Communications Opportunity, Promotion and Enhancement Act of 2006. (2006). H. R. 5252, 109th Cong., 2nd Session.

Cooksey, J., Knapp, K. K., Walton, S. M., & Cultice, J. A. (2002). Challenges to the pharmacist profession from escalating pharmaceutical demand. *Health Affairs, 21*(5), 182.

D'Agostino, N., Aversano, M., & Chiusano, M. L. (2005). ParPEST: A pipeline for EST data analysis based on parallel computing. *BMC Bioinformatics, 6*(suppl 4), S9.

Dayhoff, M. (1972). *Atlas of protein sequences and structure* (Vol. 5, pp. 89–99). Silver Spring, MD: National Biomedical Research Foundation.

Department of Veterans Affairs. (2005). *VistA monograph 2005–2006.* Retrieved July 15, 2006 from http://www.va.gov/vista_monograph/docs/vista_monograph2005_06.doc

Desiere, F., Deutsch, E. W., King, N. L., Nesvizhskii, A. I., Mallick, P., Eng, J., et al. (2006). The PeptideAtlas project. *Nucleic Acids Research, 34*(database issue), D655–D658.

Eysenbach, G., Yihune, G., Lampe, K., Cross, P., & Brickley, D. (2000). MedCERTAIN: Quality management, certification and rating of health information on the Net. *Proceedings of the AMIA Symposia, 230–234.*

Felkey, B. G., Fox, B. I., & Thrower, M. R. (2006). *Health care informatics: A skills-based resource.* Washington, DC: American Pharmacists Association.

Flynn, E. A., Barker, K. N., & Carnahan, B. J. (2003). National observational study of prescription dispensing accuracy and safety in 50 pharmacies. *Journal of the American Pharmaceutical Association, 43*(2), 191–200.

Food and Drug Administration. (2003, March 14). *Secretary Thompson announces steps to reduce medication errors.* Retrieved July 16, 2006 from http://www.hhs.gov/news/press/2003pres/20030313.html

Ford, E. W., Menachemi, N., & Phillips, M. T. (2006). Predicting the adoption of electronic health records by physicians: When will health care be paperless? *Journal of the American Medical Informatics Association, 13*(1), 106–112.

Frederick, J. (1999). Rite Aid donates teaching center. *Drug Store News, 21*(14), 17.

Gebhart, F. (2001). Hospital leaders must advance JCAHO patient safety standards. *Drug Topics, 145*(15), 26.

Grotting, J. B., Yang, M., Kelly, J., Brown, M. M., & Trohimovich, B. (2002). *The effect of barcode-enabled point-of-care technology on patient safety.* Retrieved July 15, 2006 from http://www.bridgemedical.com/pdf/whitepaper_barcode.pdf

Hanson, A., Levin, B. L., Heron, S. J., & Burke, M. (2003). Introduction: Technology, organizational change and virtual libraries. In A. Hanson & B. L. Levin (Eds.), *Building a virtual library* (pp. 1–19). Hershey, PA: IDEA Group Publishing.

Henry, D., Doran, E., Kerridge, I., Hill, S., McNeill, P. M., & Day, R. (2005). Ties that bind: Multiple relationships between clinical researchers and the pharmaceutical industry. *Archives of Internal Medicine, 165*(21), 2493–2496.

Hillestad, R., Bigelow, J., Bower, A., Girosi, F., Meili, R., Scoville, R., et al. (2005). Can electronic medical record systems transform health care? Potential benefits, savings, and costs. *Health Affairs, 24*(5), 1103–1117.

Holley, R. W., Apgar, J., Everett, G. A., Madison, J. T., Marquisee, M., Merrill, S. H., et al. (1965). Structure of a ribonucleic acid. *Science, 147*(3664), 1462–1465.

Hollon, T. (2001). In answer to RxHub, pharmacy associations launch SureScript. *Drug Topics, 145*(17), 20.

Institute of Medicine. (2001). *Crossing the quality chasm: A new health system for the twenty-first century* . Washington, DC: National Academy Press.

Ioannidis, J. P., Gwinn, M., Little, J., Higgins, J. P., Bernstein, J. L., Boffetta, P., et al. (2006). A road map for efficient and reliable human genome epidemiology. *Nature Genetics, 38*(1), 3–5.

Joseph, A. M. (2006). Care coordination and telehealth technology in promoting self-management among chronically ill patients. *Telemedicine Journal and e-Health, 12*(2), 156–159.

Kager, P., & Mozeson, M. (2000). Supply chain: The forgotten factor. *Pharmaceutical Executive, 20*(6), 84–90.

Kaiser, J. (2006). Genomic databases: NIH goes after whole genome in search of disease genes. *Science, 311*(5763), 933.

Kearney, A. T. (2004). *Adopting EPC in healthcare: Costs and benefits.* Reston, VA: Healthcare Distribution Management Association (HDMA) Healthcare Foundation.

Knapp, K. K., Blalock, S. J., & Black, B. L. (2001). ASHP survey of ambulatory care responsibilities of pharmacists in managed care and integrated health systems 2001. *American Journal of Health-System Pharmacy, 58*(22), 2151–2166.

Kohn, L. T., Corrigan, J. M., & Donaldson, M. S. (2000). *To err is human: Building a safer health system.* Washington, DC: National Academy Press.

Kruglyak, L. (2005). Power tools for human genetics. *Nature Genetics, 37*(12), 1299–1300.

Ledley, R. S. (1960). *Report on the use of computers in biology and medicine.* Washington, DC: National Academy of Sciences—National Research Council.

Levin, B. L., & Hanson, A. (2001). Rural mental health services. In S. Loue & B. Quill (Eds.), *Handbook of rural health* (pp. 241–256). New York: Kluwer Academic/Plenum.

Managed Care Business Week staff. (2006, February 21). Medicare: RxHub participates in Medicare electronic prescribing pilots. *Managed Care Business Week,* 94.

Mann, M. Y., Lloyd-Puryear, M. A., & Linzer, D. (2006). Enhancing communication in the 21st century. *Pediatrics, 117*(5 pt 2), S315–S319.

McCreadie, S. R., Stevenson, J. G., Sweet, B. V., & Kramer, M. (2002). Using personal digital assistants to access drug information. *American Journal of Health-System Pharmacy, 59*(14), 1340–1343.

Mooney, K. G. (2001). Challenges faced by the pharmaceutical industry: Training graduates for employment in pharmaceutical R&D. *European Journal of Pharmaceutical Sciences, 12*(4), 353–359.

Moore, A. (2003). Welcome to the digital mainstream. *Emedia, 16*(4), S2–S4.

Murray, M. D., Loo, B., Tu, W., Eckert, G. J., Zhou, X. H., & Tierney, W. M. (1999). Work patterns of ambulatory care pharmacists with access to electronic guideline-based treatment suggestions. *American Journal of Health-System Pharmacy, 56*(3), 225–232.

National Telecommunications and Information Administration. (2004). *A nation online: Entering the broadband age.* Retrieved July 15, 2006 from http://www.ntia. doc.gov/reports/anol/NationOnlineBroadband04.pdf

Newton, W. P., Thompson B. L., Campbell, T. L., & Spencer, D. (2006). *Keeping our eye on the ball: Managing the evolution of electronic health records.* Retrieved July 15, 2006 from http://www.annfammed.org/cgi/content/full/4/2/184

Nold, E. G., & Williams, T. C. (1985). Bar codes and their potential applications in hospital pharmacy. *American Journal of Hospital Pharmacy, 42*(12), 2722–2732.

Owen, J. (2005). The impact of computing technology on pharmaceutical and bio-tech research. *IDrugs: The Investigational Drugs Journal, 8*(10), 834–837.

Park, E. J. (2006). Telehealth technology in case/disease management. *Lippincotts Case Management, 11*(3), 175–182.

Pedersen, C. A., Schneider, P. J., & Scheckelhoff, D. J. (2005). ASHP national survey of pharmacy practice in hospital settings: Prescribing and transcribing—2004. *American Journal of Health-System Pharmacy, 62*(4), 378–390.

Pedersen, C. A., Schneider, P. J., & Scheckelhoff, D. J. (2006). ASHP national survey of pharmacy practice in hospital settings: Dispensing and administration—2005. *American Journal of Health-System Pharmacy, 63*(4), 327–345.

Peterson, C. D., & Anderson, H. C. (2004a). The North Dakota telepharmacy project: Restoring and retaining pharmacy services in rural communities. *Journal of Pharmacy Technology, 20*(part 1), 28–39.

Peterson, C. D., & Anderson, H. C. (2004b). *Telepharmacy.* Retrieved July 15, 2006 from http://telehealth. muhealth. org/geninfo/A%20Guide%20to%20Getting% 20Started%20in%20Telemedicine. pdf

Poon, E. G., Jha, A. K., Christino, M., Honour, M. M., Fernandopulle, R., Middleton, B., et al. (2006). Assessing the level of healthcare information technology adoption in the United States: A snapshot. *BMC Medical Informatics and Decision Making, 6*, 1.

President's New Freedom Commission on Mental Health. (2003). *Achieving the promise: Transforming mental health care in America. Final Report.* (DHHS Pub. No. SMA-03-3832). Rockville, MD: President's New Freedom Commission on Mental Health.

Raybardhan, S., Balen, R. M., Partovi, N., Loewen, P., Liu, G., & Jewesson, P. J. (2005). Documenting drug-related problems with personal digital assistants in a multisite health system. *American Journal of Health System Pharmacy, 62*(17), 1782–1787.

Raymond, B. (2005). The Kaiser Permanente IT transformation. *Healthcare Financial Management, 59*(1), 62–66.

Rohde, D. (1996). Schools could get cut-rate network services. *Network World, 13*(47), 27.

Rouse, M. J. (2004). Continuing professional development in pharmacy. *Journal of the American Pharmaceutical Association, 44*, 517–520.

Schiff, G. D., & Rucker, T. D. (1998). Computerized prescribing: Building the electronic infrastructure for better medication usage. *Journal of the American Medical Association, 279*, 1024–1029.

Schroff, K. (2003). Back to the pharmacist. *Pharmaceutical Executive, 23*(5), 170.

Scolaro, K. L., Stamm, P. L., & Lloyd, K. B. (2005). Devices for ambulatory and home monitoring of blood pressure, lipids, coagulation, and weight management, part 1. *American Journal of Health-System Pharmacy, 62*(17), 1802–1812.

Scott, D. M., Miller, L. G., & Letcher, A. L. (1999). Assessment of desirable pharmaceutical care practice skills by urban and rural Nebraska pharmacists. *American Journal of Pharmaceutical Education, 62*, 243–252.

Scott, R. K. (2004). Exploiting the potential of knowledge management in R&D and drug discovery: Extracting value from information. *Current Opinion in Drug Discovery and Development, 7*(3), 314–317.

Seidman, J. J., Steinwachs, D., & Rubin, H. R. (2003a). Conceptual framework for a new tool for evaluating the quality of diabetes consumer-information Web sites. *Journal of Medical Internet Research, 5*(4), e29.

Seidman, J. J., Steinwachs, D., & Rubin, H. R. (2003b). Design and testing of a tool for evaluating the quality of diabetes consumer-information Web sites. *Journal of Medical Internet Research, 5*(4), e30.

Shah, N., Teplitsky, M. V., Minovitsky, S., Pennacchio, L. A., et al. (2005). SNP-VISTA: An interactive SNP visualization tool. *BMC Bioinformatics, 6*, 292.

Skrepnek, G. H., Armstrong, E. P., Malone, D. C., Abarca, J., Murphy, J. E., Grizzle, A. J., et al. (2006). Workload and availability of technology in metropolitan community pharmacies. *Journal of the American Pharmaceutical Association, 46*(2), 154–160.

Stolar, M. H. (1979). National survey of hospital pharmaceutical services—1978. *American Journal of Hospital Pharmacy, 36*(3), 316–325.

Teufel, A., Krupp, M., Weinmann, A., & Galle, P. R. (2006). Current bioinformatics tools in genomic biomedical research (review). *International Journal of Molecular Medicine, 17*(6), 967–973.

Torr-Brown, S. (2005). Advances in knowledge management for pharmaceutical research and development. *Current Opinion in Drug Discovery and Development, 8*(3), 316–322.

Triller, D. M., Donnelly, J., & Rugge, J. (2005). Travel-related savings through a rural, clinic-based automated drug dispensing system. *Journal of Community Health, 30*(6), 467–476.

Tummala, S., Shabaker, J. W., & Leung, S. S. (2005). Building process knowledge using inline spectroscopy, reaction calorimetry and reaction modeling—the integrated approach. *Current Opinion in Drug Discovery and Development, 8*(6), 789–797.

U. S. Congress. (1996). Public law 104-191. Health insurance portability and accountability act of 1996.

Winston, P. H., & Pendergast, K. A. (1984). *The AI business: The commercial uses of artificial intelligence.* Cambridge, MA: MIT Press.

Zhu, T. , Zhou, J. , An, Y. , Zhou, J. , Li, H. , Xu, G. , et al. (2006). Construction and characterization of a rock-cluster–based EST analysis pipeline. *Computational Biology and Chemistry, 30*(1), 81–86.

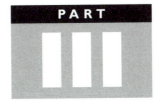

PART III

ECONOMIC ASPECTS OF HEALTH CARE DELIVERY

Basic Economic Principles Affecting Health Care

Kenneth W. Schafermeyer

Case Scenario

Angie Plasty, a recent pharmacy graduate, is trying to determine the reasons for a 15% increase in prescription drug expenditures for a large managed care organization. Angie attributes some of the increased expenditures to manufacturers' price increases. While modest price increases for some commodities can result in large decreases in quantity demanded and, therefore, a decrease in total expenditures, Angie knows that this is not true for most health care services, including prescription drugs. Of even greater concern to Angie, however, is that the prescription drug program experienced a large increase in prescription utilization rates.

Before she can suggest any solutions, Angie must first know the factors that contributed to an increase in demand for prescription drugs. She also needs to know why the quantity of prescription drugs demanded continues to increase even while prices are increasing.

What recommendations could Angie make to try to control the increases in prescription drug expenditures? To answer these questions adequately, one needs to understand some of the basic economic principles affecting health care.

LEARNING OBJECTIVES _____

Upon completion of this chapter, the student shall be able to:

- Define the basic economic concepts of utility, demand, supply, equilibrium price, the price system, price discrimination, and elasticity of demand
- Explain the factors that cause a change in the demand or supply of a product or service
- Determine the impact that a change in demand or supply will have on the equilibrium price and equilibrium quantity of a product or service
- Explain how elasticity of demand influences the effect that a change in price will have on the total revenue earned by a firm

CHAPTER QUESTIONS

1. What factors cause changes in the supply or demand of a product or service?
2. How does a change in the supply or demand of a commodity affect its price and the quantity sold?
3. In what circumstances will an increase in the price of a company's product result in either an increase or a decrease in the total revenue earned by the firm?
4. What factors cause consumers to be more sensitive to changes in price?

INTRODUCTION

Economics is involved in nearly all contemporary issues facing health care, such as the growing demand for health care services, prices for pharmaceuticals, competition among health care organizations, and remuneration for health care professionals. A lack of understanding of basic economic principles contributes to faulty decision making—people form opinions on issues based on emotions and feelings rather than on sound economic principles.

Using real-world examples, this chapter examines the fundamental economic principles that govern how the price system allocates resources in various industries, especially health care. It describes the concepts of utility, demand, supply, and equilibrium price; the causes of shortages and surpluses; the price system; price discrimination; and the effect of elasticity of demand on a firm's pricing decisions and total revenue. Knowledge of basic economic principles will help students and practitioners understand and respond to the economic forces shaping the health care market.

ECONOMIC CONCEPTS IN INDIVIDUAL CONSUMER DECISION MAKING

Consumers' wants may be considered limitless. Our society has never had enough resources to meet the demands of everyone. Because of this scarcity of resources, the science of economics has been developed. Economists have defined economics as "the study of how individuals and societies allocate their limited resources in attempts to satisfy their unlimited wants." The study of economics seeks to answer three important questions:

1. What shall we produce with society's limited resources?
2. How shall they (resources) be used in production?
3. Who shall receive the resulting goods and services?

Utility is the economic term for satisfaction obtained from purchasing a particular good or service. Utility is difficult to measure. For example, if a person eats a pizza, he or she would receive some satisfaction, but the amount of satisfaction could be described only in hypothetical terms. We may conclude with confidence, however, that the pizza provided some utility. The assumption is made in economics that people continually try to maximize their utility, usually within their budget constraints. Generally speaking, if the utility of a good is greater than its cost, people will buy more of that good. Conversely, when the cost exceeds a good's utility, they will not purchase it.

As stated previously, we have an economic system for only one reason: Resources are scarce relative to human wants. Our three basic resources are (1) land, including all natural resources; (2) labor; and (3) capital, including physical resources produced by labor. Economists refer to these resources as factors of production because they are used to produce those things that people desire, which are called commodities. Commodities may be divided into goods and services. Pharmacists provide both goods and services, although when a transaction involves both, they typically receive reimbursement only for the product. However, as pharmacists learn to market cognitive services separately from products, they are beginning to find ways to be reimbursed for these services.

Cost originates from constraints on our resources. With unlimited resources, every good would be free, like air. In reality, we live in a state of economic scarcity. Economic resources, therefore, are allocated according to the price system. Most goods and services are obtained only by those individuals who are willing and able to pay for them.

If no limits existed on resources, goods would have no value because we would use them until totally satisfied. Also, the marginal utility of any good would be zero because the value of any commodity is determined by its marginal utility. Value, then, originates from our personal desires.

Marginal is the economic term for "extra." Thus the value of a good is measured by its marginal utility. For example, the marginal utility of purchasing one pair of tennis shoes may be high if you currently do not have any tennis shoes, but the marginal utility of purchasing a second pair of tennis shoes at the same time would be lower.

When someone decides to make a purchase, he or she is, in a sense, deciding to forgo some other use of that money. This tradeoff is known as an opportunity cost, the value of the best forgone use of a given resource. For example, if a person has enough money for only one pair of shoes, the shoes he or she buys will not only cost the money he or she pays for them, but also the satisfaction (utility) that he or she gives up by not being able to spend that money on something else, such as a new pair of pants. An example that every college student understands is that the true economic cost of going to school full time is more than just the cost of tuition, books, and other direct expenditures; it also includes the loss of the income that could have been earned had the student decided to work rather than go to school. Although this lost income is not a direct expenditure, it certainly is an opportunity cost.

LAW OF DIMINISHING MARGINAL UTILITY

The *law of diminishing marginal utility* states that the value of any additional goods declines as one consumes more of it. In other words, the more we have of a good, the less we desire more of it. A person who likes pizza will receive some utility if he or she eats a piece of pizza for lunch. If the same person eats a second piece, it provides less utility than the first one. A third piece of pizza would provide still less utility. Eventually, the cost of a pizza would exceed its marginal utility, and the person would not purchase more (see **Table 12-1**).

THE LAW OF DEMAND

The two most important economic concepts are demand and supply. The theories of supply and demand explain how millions of individual consumer and supplier decisions interact to determine market prices for available goods and services. Buyers exert a market force on prices by the amount of goods and services they demand, and suppliers exert a market force based on their ability and willingness to supply products for consumption.

A demand schedule shows the various amounts of a commodity consumers are willing and able to purchase at each specific price in a set of possible prices during some specified period of time. Note that demand is not synonymous with "need" or "want." As the term is used in economics, for a person to have a demand, he or she must have both the ability and willingness to pay. Merely wanting a given commodity that he or

Table 12-1 Illustration of the Law of Diminishing Marginal Utility

Quantity Consumed	Total Utility	Marginal Utility
0	0	—
1	3	3
2	5	2
3	6	1
4	6	0

she cannot afford or is not willing to buy does not constitute a demand for that commodity.

Table 12-2 shows a hypothetical demand schedule for pizza. Two variables exist: (1) the price charged (independent variable) and (2) the quantity demanded at each given price (dependent variable). It is assumed, for the sake of simplicity, that all other variables are held constant. According to the table, as the price of pizzas increases, fewer of them are purchased. This illustrates the *law of demand:* As price falls, the corresponding quantity demanded rises; alternatively, as price increases, the corresponding quantity demanded falls. In short, an inverse relationship exists between price and quantity demanded.

The Demand Curve

The law of demand can be illustrated by drawing a demand curve. **Figure 12-1** represents the demand curve for the demand schedule shown in Table 12-2. Readers who have not been exposed to economics before may notice two unusual things about Figure 12-1. First, the relationship between the two variables is often illustrated as a straight line, even though we still call it a "curve." Second, the independent variable (the price charged for the commodity) is plotted on the Y-axis rather than the more conventional way of plotting it on the X-axis. Demand curves slope downward and to the right. This graphic illustration of the data in Table 12-2 shows the inverse relationship between the price of pizzas and the quantity demanded.

Table 12-2 A Demand Schedule for Pizza

Price per Pizza	Pizzas Purchased per Week
$ 6	80
$ 8	64
$10	48
$12	32
$14	16

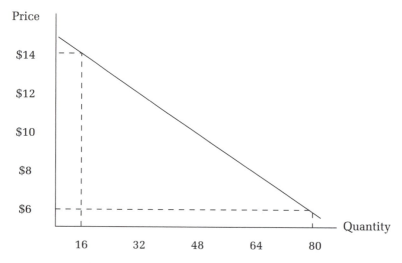

Figure 12-1 A Demand Curve for Pizza

Changes in Demand

It is important to distinguish between the terms "change in quantity demanded" and "change in demand." A change in quantity demanded refers to movement along a given demand curve. In Figure 12-1, for example, a decrease in the price of a pizza from $10 to $8 results in an increase in the quantity demanded, from 48 to 64 pizzas. This increase is referred to as a change in the quantity demanded.

Some factors can result in an entire demand curve shifting; this movement is referred to as a change in demand. **Figure 12-2** shows that demand curve D has moved to the right to demand curve D_1, representing what is meant by a change in demand. Since the demand curve has shifted to the right, the demand has increased. A movement from right to left would mean demand has decreased.

Changes in one or more of five factors can cause consumers to change their demand for a good:

- Prices of related goods
- Money income of the consumer
- Number of consumers in the market
- Attitudes, tastes, and preferences of the consumer
- Consumer expectations with respect to future prices and incomes

Prices of Related Goods

When the price of one good and the demand for another good are directly related, the pair are called substitute goods. An example is the

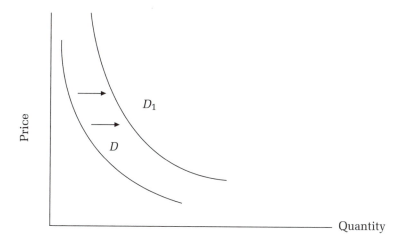

Figure 12-2 Illustration of a Change in Demand

relationship between beef and chicken. As the price of beef increases, the demand for chicken increases (assuming the chicken was reasonably priced), all else being equal. As another example, increases in coffee prices cause the demand for tea to increase. To some degree, many drugs or drug classes may be substitutes for each other (e.g., aspirin, acetaminophen, nonsteroidal anti-inflammatory drugs [NSAIDs], and now COX-2 inhibitors).

When the price of one good and the demand for another good are inversely related, the two products are referred to as complementary goods. In this case, an increase in the price of one good may cause a decrease in the demand for another good. An example would be the relationship between computer printers and printer cartridges. As the price of computer printers decreases, more people will purchase them, thus causing an increase in the demand for printer cartridges. In the prescription market, potassium supplements are often complements of potassium-depleting diuretics. For some patients taking NSAIDs, antacids, H_2 antagonists, or proton pump inhibitors may be complementary products.

Money Income of the Consumer

Commodities whose demand increases with an increase in consumer income are called superior or normal goods. Examples include sirloin steak, new sports cars, and summer homes. Because the demand for health care services increases as consumers' incomes rise, health care is a normal good. (Poor people may have as much need for health care, of course, but their demand—their ability and willingness to pay—is less than that of wealthier individuals. This helps to explain why a higher concentration of hospitals and physicians exists in high-income areas than in the inner city.)

If the demand for a good decreases as income increases, it is known as an inferior good. Examples include used cars and generic liquor or film. An example of an inferior good related to pharmacy could be an over-the-counter (OTC) antacid product that is purchased by a patient who cannot afford to see a physician or purchase a more expensive product such as Pepcid AC.

Number of Consumers in the Market

If a manufacturer is able to attract new customers to a market, demand naturally increases (the demand curve shifts to the right). For example, the U.S. Postal Service discovered that it could increase the number of stamp collectors (and increase its revenue) by creating stamps that are more appealing to children (e.g., cartoon characters rather than historical events or "old dead guys"). Likewise, breweries and cigarette companies have allegedly increased demand for their products by attracting newer, younger customers with advertising featuring cartoon characters.

Manufacturers also use a variety of strategies to increase the number of consumers who are willing to purchase a particular type of pharmaceutical product. That explains why aspirin products are promoted as treatments for minor arthritis, and arthritis products are promoted as treatments for headaches and assorted pains. By finding new indications for prescription drugs, for example, the number of customers (and consequently, demand) for these products will increase. One example is the use of calcium-channel blockers (originally used for treatment of angina) for prevention of migraine headaches. Another example is minoxidil, which was originally marketed as Loniten for treatment of hypertension, but reformulated as Rogaine for hair growth applications.

Attitudes, Tastes, and Preferences of the Consumer

Consumer attitudes, tastes, and preferences are affected greatly by advertising or by fashion changes. The manufacturer of NyQuil liquid cold medicine, for example, created a demand for its product by marketing it as a medication that works while a person is sleeping. This appeal, combined with the distinguishing characteristic that the medication was a liquid rather than a tablet or capsule, resulted in an increased demand for the product, and NyQuil's sales skyrocketed. Conversely, the environmental concerns associated with polystyrene containers for fast food decreased demand for products that use such materials.

Consumer Expectations

A good example of how consumer expectations of future prices and personal incomes affect demand was recently seen in the demand for oranges. Newspapers published articles reporting that Florida's orange crop had been badly damaged by freezing weather, and suggesting this shortage of oranges would cause orange juice prices to rise in the United States. Consumers responded by immediately buying several cans of frozen orange juice concentrate to have on hand when orange juice prices were high. The grocers understood economics and had read the same newspaper articles, so they immediately raised the price of orange juice.

As another example, consider the housing market. Despite tremendous increases in the cost of building a home, the number of houses being built has tended to increase over the years. Two reasons underlie this increase: (1) Economists predicted that housing costs would continue to rise, so people are deciding to build now before costs go any higher; and (2) people anticipated a continual growth in their incomes, so they built homes based on what they expected to earn.

In summary, an increase in the demand for Product X can be caused by any of the following:

- An increase in the price of Product Y if it is a substitute for Product X
- A decrease in the price of Product Y if it is a complement to Product X
- A rise in one's income if Product X is a normal good
- A decrease in one's income if Product X is an inferior good
- An increase in the number of buyers for Product X in the market
- A favorable change in the consumer tastes for Product X
- Consumer expectation that the price of Product X will increase in the future

The case scenario at the beginning of this chapter described an increase in the demand for prescription drugs. This increase in demand could have been due to several factors: (1) an increase in enrollment in health plans, (2) an increase in the average age of enrollees, (3) an increase in the cost of alternative therapies such as surgery, or (4) an increase in physicians' and patients' tastes and preferences in response to the increase in drug advertising aimed directly at consumers. Examples of factors that can affect the demand for health care services are shown in **Table 12-3**.

Exercise 1: Change in Demand

A rightward shift in the demand curve for a commodity means that

a. Consumers' incomes may have fallen.
b. Supply conditions are more favorable.
c. Consumers are willing to buy more of the good at each price than previously.
d. The price of the commodity has decreased.

Answer

Answer "a" is incorrect because a drop in buyers' incomes would decrease their ability and willingness to pay and, therefore, decrease their demand, which would be represented by a leftward shift of the demand curve.

Answer "b" is incorrect because a change in supply does not cause a change in demand. Supply and demand are affected by different sets of factors.

Answer "c" is correct because a rightward shift in the demand curve represents an increase in demand. Because of this increase in demand, consumers are willing to buy more at each given price.

Answer "d" is incorrect because a change in price causes a change in the quantity demanded, not a change in demand. In other words, a given demand curve represents the various quantities that would be demanded by consumers for each of the prices that may be charged by the seller. A change in price simply moves you up and down the curve; it does not change the curve itself.

Exercise 2: Change in Demand

If the price of Product A decreases, what is the effect on Product B (a substitute)?

a. The quantity demanded for Product B increases.
b. The quantity demanded for Product B decreases.
c. The demand increases for Product B.
d. The demand decreases for Product B.
e. The supply increases.
f. The supply decreases.

Answer

Answers "a" and "b" are incorrect because a change in price of a product causes a change in the demand of a substitute product, not a change in quantity demanded. In other words, the demand curve itself is changed; you do not just move up and down the curve.

Answer "c" is incorrect because a decrease in the price of Product A means that more consumers will switch from B to A, thereby decreasing the amount of B that people buy at a given price.

Answer "d" is correct for the same reason.

Answers "e" and "f" are incorrect because a change in the price of Product A changes the demand but has no effect on the supply curves. A change in demand does not cause a change in supply. Supply and demand are affected by independent factors.

Table 12-3 Factors That Affect Demand for Health Care Services

Cause for Change in Demand	Explanation	Examples
Prices of related goods 1) Substitutes 2) Complements	Assuming: A is a substitute for B and X is a complement of Y 1) ↑ price of product A = ↑ demand for B 2) ↑ price of product X = ↓ demand for Y	1) ↑ price of brand-name products = ↑ demand for generics 2) ↑ price of NSAIDs = ↓ demand for antacid
Consumers' incomes	↑ income = ↑ demand	↓ income = ↑ self treatment ↑ income = ↑ demand for physician visits and elective surgery
Number of consumers	↑ population = ↑ demand	New indications for old drugs = ↑ demand Aging of population = ↑ drug use
Attitudes, tastes, and preferences	↑ preferences = ↑ demand	↑ advertising of prescription drugs = ↑ drug use.
Expectations	Expected shortage or price increase in future = ↑ demand	Fear of flu vaccine shortage = ↑ demand for flu vaccine

THE LAW OF SUPPLY

Supply, like demand, can be depicted as a schedule. A supply schedule shows the number of goods or services offered for sale at specific prices during some specified period of time. **Table 12-4** shows a hypothetical supply schedule for a producer of pizzas. Again, only two variables are considered; all others are assumed to be held constant. The independent variable in this case is the price that consumers are willing to pay. Notice

Table 12-4 A Supply Schedule for Pizza

Price per Pizza	Pizzas Produced per Week
$ 6	24
$ 8	36
$10	48
$12	60
$14	72

that there is a subtle difference between this variable and the independent variable for the demand schedule. For the demand schedule, the independent variable is the price charged; for the supply schedule, the independent variable is the price customers are willing to pay.

The dependent variable for the supply schedule is the quantity that sellers are willing to supply at each given price. As shown in Table 12-4, as the price that consumers are willing to pay increases, more pizzas are produced. This illustrates the *law of supply,* which states that as the price that people are willing to pay rises, the corresponding quantity supplied also increases. In short, a direct relationship exists between price and quantity supplied.

The Supply Curve

Just as the law of demand was illustrated by drawing a demand curve, so the law of supply can be illustrated with a supply curve. **Figure 12-3** illustrates the supply curve for the supply schedule given in Table 12-4. Supply curves slope upward to the right, in this case illustrating a direct relationship between the price that people are willing to pay for pizzas and the quantity supplied to consumers.

Changes in Supply

The terms "change in quantity supplied" and "change in supply" are used similarly to those discussed under demand. Whereas changes in the quantity supplied are caused only by changes in prices people are willing to pay, changes in several factors can bring about a change in supply:

- Techniques of production, including technology
- Number of sellers in the market
- Resource costs (materials and wages)
- Prices for related goods
- Sellers' expectations

Techniques of Production

When technology advances, the costs of production usually decrease. At a given price, suppliers will make more profits and, consequently, are willing to produce more. Technological advances could include equipment (e.g., more efficient tractors), supplies (e.g., genetically engineered seeds), methods of production (e.g., crop rotation), or management techniques (e.g., using the advice of agricultural experts).

Number of Sellers in the Market

More producers create more output. Therefore, as the number of sellers in a market increases, supply also increases. This outcome is represented by a rightward shift in the supply curve.

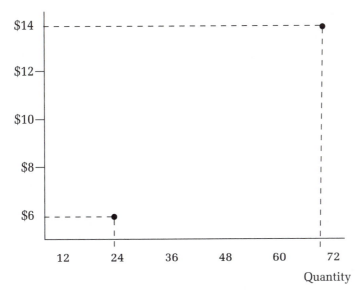

Figure 12-3 A Supply Curve for Pizza

Resource Costs

As the costs of resources (e.g., materials, labor, rents, interest rates) increase, sellers cannot make as much profit at a given price. Companies therefore have less incentive to produce when input costs increase. However, a decrease in resource costs will cause supply to increase. Lower fertilizer prices, for example, can lead to an increase in agricultural production that will encourage farmers to produce more. Some employers have used this same principle to predict that increases in the minimum wage would hurt production levels.

Prices for Related Goods

Producers recognize two types of related goods: (1) substitute products and (2) joint products. Substitute products are those that are produced with the same, or similar, inputs. If the price of one product increases, it will affect the supply of another product. For example, if the price of wheat increases, farmers will start growing less corn and more wheat. Therefore, the price of wheat affects the supply of corn.

Goods that are almost always produced together are known as joint products. Leather and beef, for example, are joint products because they cannot be produced separately. An increase in the price of beef will induce a greater quantity of beef supplied; consequently, the supply of leather will increase even if the price of leather falls.

Seller Expectations

If sellers expect prices to increase in the near future, they may increase production now or withhold some product from the market. This happens in agriculture when farmers try to time their sales to obtain favorable prices. Examples of factors that affect the supply of health care services are shown in **Table 12-5**.

EQUILIBRIUM PRICE

The price system—the interaction of supply and demand—determines how economic resources are allocated. Because buyers in any market always want to demand more units of a good at a lower price and sellers always want to supply more units of that good at a higher price, a market equilibrium price can be achieved that creates economic efficiency by exactly balancing these competing market forces. This market equilibrium price represents the point where the supply and demand curves intersect, as illustrated in **Figure 12-4**.

Table 12-5 Factors That Affect Supply of Health Care Services

Cause for Change in Supply	Explanation	Examples
Prices of related goods 1) Substitutes 2) Joint products	Assuming: A = substitute for B and W = joint product with Z 1) ↑ price of product A = ↓ supply of B 2) ↑ price of product W = ↑ supply for Z	1) ↑ reimbursement for generic substitutes = ↓ brand-name drugs supplied 2) ↑ reimbursement for teaching hospitals = ↑ amount of medical education
Resource costs	↑ production cost = ↓ supply	↑ wages = ↓ personnel hours
Production technology	↑ technology = ↓ production cost = ↑ supply	↑ department automation = ↓ cost to dispense a prescription and ↑ willingness to supply prescriptions
Number of sellers	↑ number of sellers = ↑ supply and ↓ price	↑ number of generic companies = ↑ number of generic products supplied and ↓ price for generic products

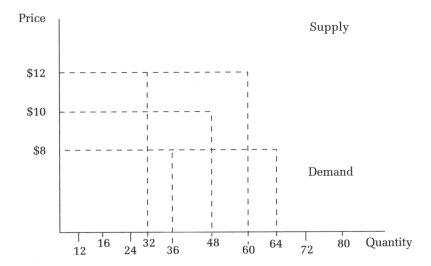

Figure 12-4 Supply and Demand Curve for Pizza

In this case, market equilibrium occurs when pizza is priced at $10. At that price, the quantity demanded equals the quantity supplied. At the equilibrium price of $10, both the seller and the buyer are satisfied with the price. At any price other than $10, economic forces will attempt to change the price. These economic forces can be illustrated with two cases.

Case 1: Price increases to $12. At a price of $12, pizza sellers produce 60 pizzas, whereas consumers want to buy only 32 pizzas. Thus a surplus (excess supply) of pizzas exists. What happens? Consumers buy only 32 pizzas. Eventually, one pizza seller will lower the price to get rid of unsold pizzas, which will increase the quantity demanded for the product. Other sellers also lower their prices until at $10 the demands of the consumers equal what the sellers are willing to produce at that price.

Case 2: Price decreases to $8. At a price of $8, pizza sellers produce 36 pizzas, whereas consumers want to buy 64. Thus a shortage (excess demand) for pizzas exists. What happens? Consumers order a pizza, but the seller is sold out. The seller notices that each day every pizza produced is sold. Consumers might even be calling the seller to say they will pay extra if a pizza is saved for them. This increased demand and the opportunity to increase the price serve as incentives for the seller to produce more pizzas. When the price reaches $10, both the seller and the buyer are satisfied. Everyone who wants to buy a pizza does, and the seller does not have any unsold pizzas remaining.

Exercise 3: Change in Equilibrium Due to an Increase in Supply

When supply increases in a competitive market:

a. Equilibrium price will fall.
b. Demand will fall.
c. Shortages will emerge.
d. Quantities sold will decrease.

Answer

Answer "a" is correct because the new supply curve will shift to the right and intersect with the demand curve at a new point that represents both a decrease in equilibrium price and an increase in equilibrium quantity (see **Figure 12–5**).

Answer "b" is incorrect because a change in supply does not cause a change in demand. Supply and demand are affected by independent factors.

Answer "c" is incorrect because an increase in supply will result in a temporary surplus, which will be corrected when prices drop to a new equilibrium point. At this new equilibrium point, the quantity demanded will equal the quantity supplied.

Answer "d" is incorrect for the same reason given for answer "a."

Note that the equilibrium would also change when there is a change in demand. The increased demand for prescription drugs discussed in the case scenario at the beginning of this chapter, for example, resulted in increases in both the price and the quantity of prescription drugs dispensed.

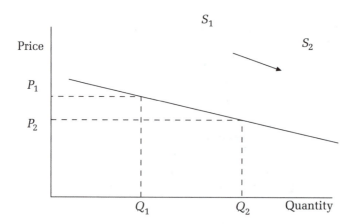

Figure 12-5 Change in Equilibrium for a Product with an Elastic Demand

ELASTICITY OF DEMAND

Elasticity is a widely used economic concept that measures the responsiveness of consumer demands to a change in price. As stated previously, the demand curve slopes downward because as the price of a commodity decreases, the quantity demanded increases. However, the degree (or angle) of this downward slope varies with different types of goods. Depending on the slope, a commodity is said to have an elastic demand, an inelastic demand, or a unitary demand.

The producers (or sellers) of any good typically can charge whatever price they desire. Naturally, they will try to sell the good at a price that maximizes their profits. If they think they can make more money by lowering the price, they will do so. Likewise, if they think they can make more money by raising the price, they will do so. The key factor in such an analysis is not the good's selling price, but rather the total revenue the producer receives. This total revenue equals the selling price multiplied by the quantity sold. Whether a change in the selling price will result in an increase or a decrease in total revenue depends on the elasticity of demand for the particular good.

Elastic Demand

Suppose a producer is faced with the demand schedule shown in **Table 12-6** for one of its goods. As the price of the good increases, the producer's total revenue decreases. This relationship characterizes a good with an elastic demand. Demand is elastic if an increase in price causes the quantity demanded to decrease enough to result in a decrease in total revenue. Conversely, a decrease in price causes the quantity to increase enough to result in an increase in total revenue. Thus, when a good has an elastic demand, the quantity demanded is sensitive to the price.

An example of a good with an elastic demand is a brand of gasoline. If a Shell Oil gas station proprietor lowered his or her price below the competitor's price, sales likely would increase so much that total revenue would increase. The opposite outcome will occur if prices are raised above other brands. That is why gasoline prices are often standardized

Table 12-6 Demand Schedule for an Elastic Good

Price	Expected Number To Be Sold	Total Revenue
$2	56	$112
$3	36	$108
$4	26	$104
$5	20	$100

within a community; the demand for any brand of gasoline is extremely sensitive to price. (Note that gasoline is narrowly and specifically defined here as a particular brand of gasoline at a particular station, and it is understood that this station's gasoline has interchangeable substitutes at many competing stations. When we look at prices for gasoline in general, rather than prices at particular stations, demand is more inelastic.)

Inelastic Demand

Suppose a producer is faced with a demand schedule like the one shown in **Table 12-7** for one of its goods. As the price of the good increases, total revenue increases. This relationship characterizes a good with an inelastic demand. With inelastic demand, an increase in price causes only a slight decrease in the quantity demanded, resulting in an increase in total revenue. Conversely, a decrease in price causes the quantity demanded to increase, but the increase is so small that the result is a decrease in total revenue. Thus, when a good has an inelastic demand, the quantity demanded is relatively insensitive to price.

An example of a good with an inelastic demand is gasoline (when broadly defined as noted in the preceding section). An automobile will not operate without gasoline, so when the price of gasoline increases, people will buy a little less, but they will still buy enough to give the gas station proprietor an increase in total revenue. Thus gasoline has a relatively inelastic demand. Although the quantity of gasoline demanded by consumers does not tend to depend too much on price (inelastic demand), the quantity purchased at a particular station does depend on how prices at that station compare with the competitors' prices (elastic demand).

As described in the case scenario at the beginning of this chapter, studies show that the demand for health care services, including prescription drugs, is inelastic. People with true emergencies (such as a broken arm or a heart attack) will seek treatment without regard to the cost. Nevertheless, high prices may create an elastic demand for emergency treatment of routine problems or minor ailments. This explains the rationale

Table 12-7 Demand Schedule for an Inelastic Good

Price	Expected Number To Be Sold	Total Revenue
$2	45	$ 90
$3	31	$ 93
$4	24	$ 96
$5	20	$100

behind patient cost-sharing mechanisms, which are designed to discourage unnecessary use of services while not inhibiting demand for truly necessary services.

A logical question to ask at this point is this: If total revenue increases every time the price of an inelastic good increases, what keeps the price from rising to infinity? Usually competition keeps prices in check or, in the case where not much competition exists (such as public utilities), government intervention may be needed to regulate prices. Although managed care organizations in the United States have controlled costs by facilitating competition among some pharmaceutical products through generic and therapeutic substitution, government agencies in Canada and Europe control costs by regulating pharmaceutical manufacturers' prices.

Unitary Demand

Suppose a producer is faced with a demand schedule like the one shown in **Table 12-8** for one of its goods. As the price of the good increases or decreases, the producer's total revenue remains the same. This relationship characterizes a good with a unitary demand. Unitary demand is not common in the actual marketplace; instead, products tend to have either an elastic or inelastic demand.

Exercise 4: Elasticity of Demand

If demand is price elastic, an increase in supply will cause a relatively

a. Large decrease in quantity demanded.
b. Large increase in quantity demanded.
c. Small decrease in quantity demanded.
d. Small increase in quantity demanded.

Answer

Answers "a" and "c" are incorrect because an increase in supply will result in an increase in quantity demanded.

Answer "b" is correct because an elastic demand curve, by definition, means that consumers are sensitive to changes in price and any change in price will result in a proportionately greater change in quantity demanded. Therefore, an increase in the supply of a product with an elastic demand curve will result in a large increase in quantity demanded (see Figure 12–5).

Answer "d" is incorrect for the reason explained for answer "c."

Table 12-8 Demand Schedule for a Unitary Good

Price	Expected Number To Be Sold	Total Revenue
$2	50	$100
$2.50	40	$100
$4	25	$100
$5	20	$100

Determinants of Elasticity of Demand

What makes the demand for a particular good or service elastic or inelastic in the short run? To differentiate between the terms "short run" and "long run," consider that a consumer has two resources when shopping: money and time. In other words, a person can purchase a demanded good with money now or wait until a later time when more money is available, when the price of the demanded commodity decreases, or when the consumer's demand may change to favor another commodity. Elasticity of demand for a given commodity changes when one talks about the short run versus the long run because a longer time span allows people to pursue more alternatives (substitutes).

For example, when the price of gasoline increases, automobile owners continue to buy gas in the short run because they need their cars for business or other important purposes. In the long run, alternative means of transportation such as buses, commuter trains, or carpools may be sought as companies continue to work on developing a car that operates on some form of energy other than gasoline. The desired result, of course, is eventually to decrease one's need for—and thus one's demand for—gasoline.

Three determinants of elasticity exist: (1) the availability of substitutes for the commodity, (2) the price of a commodity relative to consumers' incomes, and (3) the number of alternative uses for the commodity.

The Availability of Substitutes

When the price of one good and the demand for another good are directly related, the two products are substitute goods, like beef and chicken. The greater the number of substitute goods available for a particular commodity, the more elastic the demand for that commodity.

The more narrowly and specifically a commodity can be described, the more substitutes it will have. Consequently, the demand for such a commodity will be more elastic. For example, when a person is suffering from athlete's foot, he or she probably has a strong desire for an antifungal. Because no other kinds of OTC drugs will help relieve athlete's foot, the demand for antifungals is inelastic. Because numerous antifungal products are available, however, the demand for any particular brand of antifungal is elastic.

Sellers have found that some customers have more substitutes available than other customers. For example, business travelers are not as flexible in their plans as individuals planning vacations. Therefore, vacation travelers have a more elastic demand for air travel and can obtain less expensive airfares.

Segregating customers and charging prices according to customers' elasticity of demand is known as differential pricing (also known as price discrimination). Because hospitals and managed care organizations use formularies (and consequently have more substitutes available), they can obtain larger discounts or rebates from pharmaceutical manufacturers. Another example of differential pricing is the higher long-distance telephone rates charged during working hours as opposed to weekends and evenings. For price discrimination to work, it must be difficult for buyers to resell to one another. Price differences reflecting actual production cost differences, such as volume discounts, do not represent true price discrimination.

The Price Relative to Consumers' Incomes

The demand for commodities that account for a large portion of a person's income will be more elastic than the demand for purchases that are relatively inexpensive. For example, most managers are more price conscious when they are shopping for a computer than when shopping for envelopes or paper clips. Because envelopes and paper clips account for a negligible fraction of a company's budget, changes in price likely will have little effect on the quantity demanded. Thus the demand for these products is relatively inelastic.

The Number of Alternative Uses

The fewer uses that a commodity has, the more likely that its demand will be inelastic. People tend to become more selective about a commodity's use as its price increases. An example of this occurred several years ago when the price of sugar rose greatly. When the price of sugar increased, people found that they still needed it for some types of foods, but they could reduce the amount they used. Thus consumers were able to change the demand for sugar from elastic to inelastic.

Exercise 5

Elasticity of demand will increase as the

a. Number of available substitutes decreases.
b. Price of the good relative to income decreases.
c. Time horizon increases.

Answer

Answer "a" is incorrect because the greater the number of substitute goods available for a particular commodity, the more elastic the demand for that commodity.

Answer "b" is incorrect because those commodities that account for a large portion of a person's income will have a more elastic demand than those purchases that are relatively inexpensive.

Answer "c" is correct because the longer time frame allows consumers to consider more alternatives and find more substitutes for a product in the long run.

Elasticity of Demand for Prescription Drugs

The three determinants of elasticity can be applied to prescription drugs. First, when a physician writes a prescription order for a specific drug for an ambulatory patient, usually no substitute goods are involved. The patient has the choice of having the prescription filled. If he or she decides to have the prescription filled, the patient often has no choice as to which drug will be dispensed by the pharmacist. (Product selection legislation gives the patient some choices in certain cases, but this description is accurate for drugs protected by patents. This situation is altered to some degree by the adoption of formularies and the practice of therapeutic selection.)

Second, prescription drugs take up a relatively small portion of most people's income.

Third, prescription drugs have few alternative uses. An antibiotic is prescribed for a specific type of infection, but it has no value in treating most other types of physical or mental ailments.

In summary, prescription drugs have few—if any—substitutes; they take a relatively small portion of one's income (particularly if the patient pays only a co-payment); and they have few uses other than the purpose for which they are prescribed. Thus a prescription drug has an inelastic demand. As described in the case scenario at the beginning of this chapter, the quantity demanded is relatively insensitive to changes in price.

Three additional factors unique to the pharmaceutical industry contribute to the inelasticity of demand for prescription drugs. First, the decision maker (the physician) is not the payer (the patient and/or prescription benefit plan); consequently, price is not usually the primary consideration when prescribing a particular drug. Second, the industry promotes product differentiation between drug products, reducing the importance of price in selecting a particular drug to prescribe. Third, having a third-party plan pay all or part of the cost of a person's prescription drugs significantly increases the inelasticity of demand for those drugs.

CONCLUSIONS

This chapter introduced some basic economic concepts, such as supply, demand, equilibrium price, the price system, price discrimination, and elasticity of demand. Chapter 13 discusses how economic forces in the health care marketplace compare with those of other industries and how health care can be influenced by competition.

Health care professionals should understand and use economic principles to work effectively with health care organizations and health benefit programs. By understanding these basic principles, one can begin to appreciate the factors affecting the economics of the health care industry.

QUESTIONS FOR FURTHER DISCUSSION

1. For most products, when substitutes appear in the market, the innovator must usually decrease its price to be competitive. Why don't the prices of brand-name prescription drugs tend to decline when generic substitutes become available?
2. What steps can be taken to control the rapid increase in the quantity demanded for prescription drugs?
3. A demand for a product or service exists only if the potential customers have the ability and willingness to pay for it. What would pharmacists have to do to be reimbursed for nondispensing services?
4. If many health care products and services have inelastic demand, how might companies compete with one another to increase their market shares?
5. Give examples of health care products or services that have an elastic demand. Do competitors compete on price?

KEY TOPICS AND TERMS

Changes in demand
Changes in quantity demanded
Changes in quantity supplied
Changes in supply
Complements
Demand
Demand curve
Demand schedule
Economic resources
Economics
Elastic demand
Elasticity
Equilibrium point
Equilibrium price
Equilibrium quantity
Law of demand
Law of diminishing marginal utility
Law of supply
Marginal utility
Shortage
Substitutes
Supply
Supply curve
Supply schedule
Surplus
Utility

Unique Aspects of Health Economics

Kenneth W. Schafermeyer

Case Scenario

There has been a great deal of controversy and debate over how to control rapidly rising health care costs and expand health care services to the millions of Americans who do not currently have health insurance. Some observers believe that these problems can be resolved by encouraging more competition into the health care system. Others believe that health care is such a unique industry that more competition will not necessarily create efficiencies that will reduce costs and improve access. Some members of the latter group also question the morality of using the price system to allocate health care resources.

Using your knowledge of economics and the health care system, what do you think are some of the arguments that would be used by both sides in this debate?

LEARNING OBJECTIVES _____

Upon completion of this chapter, the student shall be able to:

- Give examples of how basic economic principles apply to contemporary health care issues
- Compare and contrast the various types of market structures: perfect competition, monopolistic competition, oligopoly, and monopoly
- Explain how the economics of health care is different from the economics of other industries
- Describe how economic performance of the health care system could be improved
- Explain the factors that can cause health care costs to increase
- Describe how various forms of reimbursement can create different incentives to control utilization of health care

CHAPTER QUESTIONS

1. To what extent is health care a competitive industry? Does competition always result in decreases in price?
2. How is the economics of health care different from the economics of other industries?
3. What factors can cause health care costs to increase?
4. How do various forms of reimbursement create different incentives to control utilization of health care?

INTRODUCTION

This chapter is designed to help students and practitioners understand and respond to the economic forces shaping the health care market. Chapter 12 presented the basic economic concepts of supply, demand, equilibrium price, the price system, price discrimination, and elasticity of demand. This chapter discusses some of the factors that influence supply and demand for health care services and describes how economic forces in the health care marketplace compare with those of other industries.

In recent years, there has been renewed interest in reforming the health care system through the use of market forces rather than government regulations. One example of such a "market-based policy" is the provision of subsidies to low-income patients for the purchase of health insurance rather than direct payments for health care services. Another example is the increased use of higher cost-sharing levels (Rice, 1997). The critical question, and the one discussed in this chapter, is this: Is the health care market a competitive market?

PERFECTLY COMPETITIVE INDUSTRIES

To describe the unique aspects of the health care market, it is helpful to compare it with the four basic types of market structures: (1) perfect competition, (2) monopolistic competition, (3) monopoly, and (4) oligopoly. First, this chapter describes a market structure known as perfect competition. Next, it contrasts the perfectly competitive market with the other types of market structures and discusses how the health care industry may or may not resemble one or more of these basic structures.

Perfect competition has the following characteristics:

- Many buyers and sellers
- Freedom of entry and exit
- Standardized products
- Full and free information
- No collusion

Many Buyers and Many Sellers

In perfect competition, the number of buyers and sellers has to be large enough so that the entry (or exit) of one firm or one customer into (or out of) the marketplace does not affect market prices. Companies in a perfectly competitive industry do not set prices; instead, prices are set by the market. These firms are referred to as "price takers, not price makers." The demand curve for a company's product is horizontal and referred to as perfectly elastic. In other words, if a single company increased its price, customers would not demand the product from that company—they would just switch to another company.

Freedom of Entry and Exit

Most industries have barriers to entry or exit. Entry barriers may consist of patents, licenses, zoning, environmental regulations, or large investments in technology, training, inventories, or fixed assets such as buildings, specialized equipment, or research and development. Exit barriers exist when a firm's fixed assets cannot be transferred to another use, thereby preventing a company from easily switching to a more profitable industry. Low barriers to entry into and exit from an industry stimulate competition; high barriers inhibit it. In perfect competition, there are no barriers to entry or exit.

Standardized Products

By "standardized products," we mean all products are similar and interchangeable and, therefore, many substitutes exist. Clothing, building materials, gasoline, tires, and many other products have standard sizes or grades, so consumers can easily identify substitutes. In perfect competition, products are perfectly substitutable for each other.

Full and Free Information

In perfect competition, customers have complete information on the prices of goods and services and can compare the prices offered by competing sellers. Equally important, consumers can identify and compare the quality of these goods and services.

No Collusion

In perfect competition, companies in a given industry compete with each other rather than colluding or getting together to set prices. Collusion is more likely to be successful when there are few sellers, because the competitors know each other well and can easily retaliate against each other if the agreement is broken. Because of its anticompetitive nature, collusion is illegal in the United States. Collusion does occur in international trade, where it is referred to as a cartel. The most famous cartel is the Organization of Petroleum Exporting Countries (OPEC).

Although no industries fit the perfectly competitive model exactly, agriculture is usually cited as the industry that most closely matches this description. Although farmers can transfer their resources to producing different crops, they cannot usually do so in the short run. Also, products are fairly standardized, although some differentiation exists by grade and by production method (e.g., organically grown or genetically engineered). Most industries, however, can be categorized into one of the other market structures.

OTHER MARKET STRUCTURES

Monopolistic Competition

The market structure closest to perfect competition is known as monopolistic competition. Despite its somewhat confusing name, monopolistic competition is similar to perfect competition except that it does not have standardized and interchangeable products. In most cases, firms in this industry rely heavily on product differentiation. They minimize price competition by differentiating their products from those of their competitors by promoting perceived or real advantages in style, image, quality, or other attributes. The automobile industry is an example of monopolistic competition.

Monopoly

At the opposite extreme is a market structure known as monopoly, which features only one seller of a product that has no close substitutes. To maximize income, monopolists do not have to produce as much output as possible; they can accomplish this same purpose by producing less and charging higher prices. Some monopolies are formed by controlling the supply source. Barriers that prevent other firms from entering a market, such as legal restrictions (e.g., licenses, government approval, or patents), can also create monopolies. By granting patents, the government allows temporary monopolies to encourage research and innovation. According to Folland, Goodman, and Stano (1997), pharmaceutical firms that control patents for certain drugs that lack close substitutes may be considered monopolists during the life of the patent. With managed care formularies, however, competition can be created between some patented drugs and other therapeutic alternatives.

Other monopolies exist because the required infrastructure for the industry is so expensive that the presence of competing firms would increase—rather than decrease—prices. The prime example of these natural monopolies is utilities. To ensure adequate output at reasonable prices, natural monopolies are usually regulated by government agencies such as public service commissions.

Although a monopoly consists of only one seller, situations exist in which there is only one buyer. In this situation, which is known as a monopsony, the buyer sets the price. The federal government is often a monopsony for military hardware and for health care services for Medicare and Medicaid patients. Unlike private businesses, however, the government is sometimes unable to fully exploit its market power to set prices because it is subject to political pressure and due process.

Oligopoly

Between perfect competition and monopoly is a market structure known as oligopoly, which consists of a few sellers and many buyers. Firms in oligopolies are often interdependent, and a dominant firm can exert influence through price leadership. Although this situation falls short of meeting the definition for collusion, the pricing practices of the oligopolists tend to coincide, with one firm usually taking a leadership role. Oligopolists know that the firms in the industry will not benefit if all of them decrease their prices. However, a single firm that increases its price may lose business if the other firms do not follow suit. This factor usually restricts the ability of smaller companies to change prices unilaterally. If a dominant firm increases prices, however, the other competitors usually follow.

Cereal manufacturers constitute a well-known oligopoly: Four major companies have at least 80% of the market share for cereal. In medium-sized urban areas, hospitals may represent an oligopoly. Certain drug classes with market share concentrated among a few manufacturers may also be oligopolies.

THE HEALTH CARE MARKET

Having just described the characteristics of the various market structures, we now consider whether the health care market fits these characteristics. As pointed out in the case scenario at the beginning of this chapter, this remains a highly debated issue in economic circles. In a survey of health economists, 50% thought the competitive model could apply to the health care industry, whereas 50% did not (Feldman and Morrisey, 1990). Those who did not believe that health care qualifies as a competitive market cited the following factors:

- Numbers of buyers and sellers
- Entry to and exit from the market
- Variation in products, services, and quality
- Full and free information
- Inelastic demand
- Universal demand
- Unpredictability of illness
- Health care as a "right"
- Supplier-induced demand
- Third-party insurance and patient-induced demand

Numbers of Buyers and Sellers

A maldistribution in the supply of health care services exists by geographic and specialty area. Although some health care markets are served by large numbers of sellers (e.g., retail pharmacies), some communities have a shortage of health care providers or health care facilities. In addition, although the United States as a whole has a sufficient supply of physicians, a shortage of primary care physicians (and an oversupply of specialists) exists. In some cases, the shortage exists because the market size is just too small to support enough hospitals or providers in each specialty to create a competitive market (e.g., transplant services).

Further, consolidation among buyers and sellers is occurring. The number of sole practitioners and small group practices is shrinking, while large medical groups are growing larger. Likewise, health maintenance organizations, pharmacy benefit managers, pharmaceutical manufacturers, and drug wholesalers are merging into fewer, but larger organizations. Employer groups have also pooled their purchasing power in many cities by forming employer health coalitions to negotiate better rates for health care services. Retail pharmacies have also participated in this trend through consolidation of chain pharmacies and by independent pharmacies forming volume purchasing alliances and cooperatives.

By consolidating, buyers and sellers find they can lower costs and have more market power to negotiate favorable prices. The concern is that too much consolidation could reduce competition. In some cases, the Federal Trade Commission has intervened to restrict or prevent acquisitions and mergers that it believed would unduly inhibit competition.

Entry to and Exit from the Market

High barriers to entry exist for suppliers of health care, whether they are individual providers or institutions. To pursue a career as a health care provider, one must apply to a limited number of schools and seek out one of a limited number of positions. Becoming a health care professional can require a great deal of education and compulsory licensure. These entry barriers effectively limit the number of new health care professionals who can be added to the labor force at any one time. Health care facilities must also be licensed, certified, and inspected and often require large capital investments. Pharmaceutical manufacturers face extremely large financial barriers to get new drugs approved by the Food and Drug Administration. These same barriers, however, can also inhibit potential competitors.

Because health care resources are not easily transferred to producing other products and services, exit barriers are also formidable. For example, closing a hospital is difficult in part because it is not always possible to convert the building and equipment to other uses.

Variation in Products, Services, and Quality

Instead of producing standardized products and services, health care is usually customized for individual patients. Well-documented variations exist in patterns of medical care. Quality, although hard to measure, also varies; that is why requesting a second opinion is common. For all these reasons, it can be difficult to identify true substitutes for a particular product or service.

Full and Free Information

Most health care services require specialized knowledge. Although patients have more sources of information available today than ever before, they nevertheless may have incomplete information about the prices and quality of health care services. Patients and other health care purchasers often do not know what constitutes good physician care or pharmaceutical care and cannot often tell when they are getting accurate information.

Inelastic Demand

In perfect competition, even small price increases may result in significant loss of quantity demanded and, therefore, losses in revenue; thus demand is relatively elastic. Demand for health care services, however, is relatively inelastic. In other words, patients who need health care services are usually not price sensitive, especially in emergency situations. In part because of this sensitivity, prices for health care services increase more rapidly than the prices for most consumer goods and services. According to the Bureau of Labor Statistics, the Consumer Price Index for Urban Consumers (CPI-U) has increased during the past decade at nearly twice the rate for medical care (49.5%) as it has for all items (28.4%). Demand, however, has not decreased. Per capita prescription utilization for non-Medicaid patients enrolled in health maintenance organizations has increased from 5.7 prescriptions per person per year in 1990 to 8.5 in 2004. Per capita prescription utilization for Medicare beneficiaries enrolled in HMOs increased from 16.5 prescriptions per year in 1994 to 21.3 prescriptions per year in 2004 (Aventis, 2001, 2005).

Universal Demand

Many products and services offered for sale in the United States are used by only part of the potential market (e.g., rollerblades, cordless power tools, high-adventure vacations). Health care products and services, however, are used by nearly everyone. Not only is demand universal, but it is also nearly insatiable. Because of the lack of complete knowledge, many people demand health care services that are of questionable value. Even those services that are usually helpful are sometimes used in inappropriate ways that produce little or no value (e.g., antibiotics for the common cold or heroic efforts to prolong the life of a patient who is in the last stages of a terminal illness). In some cases, too many services may produce net losses in value (e.g., antibiotic resistance, addiction, iatrogenic disease, or unnecessary pain and suffering).

Unpredictability of Illness

Given a large enough group of people, we can predict with some certainty the number of individuals who will need trauma care in the emergency department during a given time. We cannot, however, predict exactly which individuals will need this care. Because consumers are often unable to time their health care purchases, they are typically not in a negotiating position when they need services. An obvious implication of this unpredictability is the need to pool risk through health insurance, especially if done so through a managed care organization that is in a position to negotiate discounts before services are actually needed.

Health Care as a "Right"

Many people view health care as a "right" because it is a prerequisite for individuals to become useful, productive members of society (much like public education). Those who espouse this viewpoint also believe that the allocation of scarce resources should not be determined by people's ability and willingness to pay, as is the case with most goods and services in the United States; instead, some level of health care should be provided to everyone. This position holds, therefore, that the price system should not be the sole determining factor in deciding who will receive health care products and services.

Supplier-Induced Demand

Physicians are in the unique position of controlling both the supply of and the demand for health care services. Although patients do not usually gain financially from illness or injury, their physicians often do. Acting as the patients' agents, physicians can create demand for their services and, at the same time, supply the services. This potential conflict of interest is an inherent element of health care under fee-for-service reimbursement and is difficult to prevent completely. Many managed care organizations, however, have restricted physicians' abilities to create self-referrals for laboratory, radiology, and other health care services.

Chapter 12 illustrated that an increase in the supply of most goods and services will result in an increase in the equilibrium quantity and a decrease in the equilibrium price. This is not necessarily the case in health care, however. Studies conducted in 1959 and 1961 first illustrated the effect of what is now called supplier-induced demand by showing a close correlation between the number of hospital beds per 1,000 people and rates of utilization measured as hospital days per 1,000 people (Roemer, 1961; Shain and Roemer, 1959). This led to an observation known as Roemer's Law: "A bed built is a bed filled."

The effect of supplier-induced demand has also been demonstrated by the increases in utilization that often accompany attempts to impose controls on physician fees (Folland et al., 1997). Other studies have shown that physicians' clinical decisions can be influenced by financial incentives (Hemenway, Killen, Cashman, Parks, and Bicknell, 1990; Hillman, Pauly, and Kerstein, 1989). This may explain, in part, why increases in the supply of physicians during the 1980s and 1990s were accompanied by acceleration—rather than moderation—in the growth of health care costs. However, increases in the supply of health care services may be favorable if they allow more people to access care or if they lead to improvements in quality.

Third-Party Insurance and Patient-Induced Demand

The availability of insurance creates a form of induced demand that is initiated by patients. As discussed in Chapter 12, when the price of a product or service decreases, the quantity demanded tends to increase. By decreasing patients' out-of-pocket expenses, health insurance has encouraged patients to consume more health care services than they would if they had to bear the full cost of the product or service (Torrens and Williams, 1993). One concern with expanding Medicare coverage for outpatient prescription drugs, therefore, is the potential for growth in prescription drug utilization resulting from induced demand. A potential solution is patient cost sharing that—if structured properly—can reduce unnecessary utilization without decreasing the quality of care (Manning et al., 1987).

The open-ended nature of most health insurance coverage leads to a situation that economists call "moral hazard," where people overconsume health care. For health insurance plan enrollees, the out-of-pocket costs for health care services are generally much less than the actual cost for providing those services. At some point, the additional health benefits achieved from consuming additional health services are not really worth their full costs; nevertheless, because the enrollees are paying only a fraction of the costs, they still want to use these services. Overconsumption of health services from moral hazard increases total health expenditures and insurance premiums.

Not all induced demand is undesirable, of course. In some cases, reducing financial barriers to health care may encourage patients to seek health care services earlier, thereby avoiding more expensive health expenditures in the future, particularly for lower-income and more severely ill persons.

IMPROVING ECONOMIC PERFORMANCE OF THE HEALTH CARE SYSTEM

Using Market Forces

From the preceding discussion, it should be clear why many observers feel that the economic aspects of health care are unique. Strategies that successfully reduce costs in most industries (e.g., promoting an increase in supply or an increase in competition) are often not seen as effective in the health care industry. Some individuals and groups, however, believe that health care is more monopolistic than competitive and, consequently, advocate that health care services should be considered a public utility and regulated accordingly. Many industrialized nations have already adopted this stance and regulate both provider fees and manufacturers' prices for pharmaceuticals.

Recognizing that health care is unique, many public policy leaders and payers for health care services advocate instead that the health care industry be managed in a way that allows market forces to work more effectively. Some of the more common approaches are described next.

First, patients can be made aware of and sensitive to health care costs. For example, patients can be given itemized receipts showing the actual costs paid by their insurance programs. They can also be required to pay more through patient cost sharing, especially through tiered co-payments, which allow lower co-payments for preferred products, such as generic drugs, and require higher co-payments for nonpreferred drugs, such as expensive brand-name products.

Second, health care providers can be given feedback about variations in the cost, quantity, and quality of health care services through performance reports and academic detailing.

Third, managed care organizations can design physician and hospital reimbursement so as to create incentives for reducing costs. Because costs are a function of price and quantity, both factors need to be considered. Price (i.e., cost per unit) increases are attributable to inflation and can be controlled to some extent through contracting and competitive bidding. Increased utilization, by contrast, is a function of three separate components (as illustrated in **Table 13-1**): population effects, duration of treatment, and intensity of services.

Creating Incentives

As discussed in Chapter 12, managed health care plans have designed reimbursement methods that seek to reduce unnecessary hospital admissions, decrease hospital length of stay, and decrease the intensity of services provided to hospitalized patients. Similar steps have been implemented to control the cost and utilization of ambulatory services.

Table 13-1 Examples of Utilization Measurements for Various Types of Health Care Services

	Hospital	**Physician**	**Pharmacy**
Population effects	Number of admissions	Number of new patients	Number of new prescriptions
Duration	Length of stay	Episode of care	Number of prescription drug refills
Intensity	Number and types of diagnostic tests	Number and types of treatments ordered	Relative expense of prescription drug or mix of brands versus generics

Health care providers, like everyone else, usually respond to incentives. **Table 13-2** shows the incentives created by each of the various types of hospital reimbursement. Discounted fee-for-service reimbursement (i.e., retrospective reimbursement based on a negotiated fee schedule), for example, creates incentives to increase admissions (population), length of stay (duration), and intensity of services. Per diem reimbursement (i.e., prospective reimbursement of a flat rate per day without regard to actual cost), the most common form of managed care reimbursement for hospitals (Kongstvedt, 1997), creates incentives for hospitals to increase admissions and length of stay but decrease the intensity of services. Prospective reimbursement of a flat rate based on the patient's admission diagnosis, known as diagnosis-related group (DRG) reimbursement, creates incentives to increase admissions but minimize length of stay and intensity of services. Capitation (i.e., prospective reimbursement of a fixed amount each month for each enrolled patient, regardless of the amount of health care services actually provided) creates incentives to minimize all three utilization measures.

Physicians and pharmacies that are paid under discounted fee-for-service systems have the same incentives to increase utilization as do hospitals. Per diems, however, are difficult to apply to outpatient care services. Capitation reimbursement can also be applied to outpatient services in the form of case management (or disease state management). As under DRGs, prospective payments for outpatient services are based on diagnosis but are known as ambulatory patient groups (APGs). Although these programs continue to evolve, they are expected to work best for chronic conditions with a wide range of costs. Again, health care providers in the outpatient setting would have the same types of incentives as would hospitals under prospective (APG) and capitation reimbursement.

Balancing Cost and Value

Another approach to improving the economic performance of the health care system is balancing the cost of health care services with the value received. As described in Chapter 12, most consumers make purchases only when the marginal value of those services meets or exceeds the mar-

Table 13-2 Incentives under Various Forms of Hospital Reimbursement

	Number of Admissions	Length of Stay	Intensity of Services
Discounted fee-for-service	↑	↑	↑
Per diem	↑	↑	↓
DRGs	↑	↓	↓
Capitation	↓	↓	↓

ginal cost. This principle does not always apply in the health care industry, however. To illustrate, assume that the quantity of medical services (*M*) provided to a patient is compared with the patient's resulting health status (*H*) as shown in **Figure 13-1.** The curve in Figure 13-1 illustrates a variation of the law of diminishing marginal utility discussed in Chapter 12—marginal increases in the number of resources consumed result in ever smaller marginal increases in utility. Providing initial medical care services causes health status to improve rapidly at first; as more medical care is provided, however, health status increases more slowly. At some point we will reach the "flat of the curve," where additional health care expenditures produce very little incremental benefit (Jacobs, 1991, 1996).

When patients are isolated from costs, they often demand additional services, even though these services may provide limited or no benefits. It is important to consider the marginal benefit of additional medical services and to determine whether increases in services will produce proportional increases in benefits. If a great deal must be spent to produce a small incremental benefit, this usage may be a waste of limited health care resources.

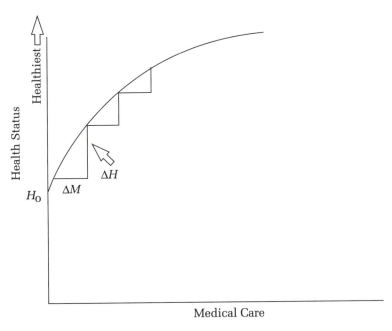

Figure 13-1 Hypothesized Relationship Between Health and Medical Care. In this representation, additional doses of medical care have diminishing impacts on health; eventually, a situation of low medical productivity, termed "flat of the curve medicine," is reached. *Source:* Reprinted from *The Economics of Health and Medical Care*, Fourth Edition, by P. Jacobs, p. 12, 1996, Jones and Bartlett Publishers.

This concept was used by the state of Oregon when it faced a shortage of funds for its Medicaid program and needed to reform its health care system. Use of limited funds for some services meant that opportunities to help other patients had to be forgone. To minimize these opportunity costs, Oregon wanted to allocate resources in a manner that would maximize marginal outcomes. A decision was made to provide coverage for those treatments that provided the greatest benefits compared with the cost of services. By not covering procedures such as removal of benign skin cancer, removal of benign tumors in the gastrointestinal system, and liver transplants for liver cancer patients, the state expanded basic services to approximately 120,000 more uninsured patients (Clewer and Perkins, 1998; for a more detailed discussion of Oregon's Medicaid program, see Chapter 20.)

Although Oregon's experience has not been widely adopted, many other examples exist where this principle is applied to some degree. Managed care organizations are giving more attention to pharmacoeconomic considerations (e.g., cost-effectiveness, cost-benefit, and cost-utility analyses; see Chapter 18). Formulary decisions, step care protocols, and disease management, for example, all consider the incremental costs and outcomes of health care services. More attention will be given in the future to ways in which scarce health care resources can be applied more efficiently and effectively.

CONCLUSIONS

This chapter described some of the unique aspects of health economics and ways to enhance the economic performance of the health care system. Health care practitioners should understand and use these economic principles to work effectively with or for health care institutions and insurance programs. Because of the unique nature of the health care industry, payers are still investigating how they might better control health care costs and improve quality so that patients can receive more benefits from the limited resources available.

QUESTIONS FOR FURTHER DISCUSSION

1. To what extent is health care a monopoly or oligopoly?
2. What can be done to enhance competition in the health care industry? Are there cases where competition will not decrease prices?
3. If pharmacists are able to charge for nondispensing services, how might payers act to prevent or minimize potential supplier-induced demand?
4. In addition to the health care services listed in the text, what other types of health care services might be considered for elimination from health insurance coverage because their marginal cost is likely to exceed their marginal benefits?
5. Which disease states would lend themselves best to pharmacy reimbursement on a capitation basis through ambulatory patient groups (APGs)? Why?

KEY TOPICS AND TERMS

Ambulatory patient groups (APGs)
Capitation
Diagnosis-related groups (DRGs)
Discounted fee-for-service
Duration of treatment
Flat of the curve
Intensity of services
Market structure
Monopolistic competition
Monopoly
Monopsony
Oligopoly
Oligopsony
Patient-induced demand
Per diem
Perfect competition
Population effects
Roemer's Law
Supplier-induced demand
Tiered co-payments

REFERENCES

Aventis. (2001). *Managed care digest series, 2001.* Bridgewater, NJ: Aventis Pharmaceuticals, Inc.

Aventis. (2005). *Managed care digest series, 2005.* Bridgewater, NJ: Aventis Pharmaceuticals, Inc.

Clewer, A., & Perkins, D. (1998). *Economics for health care management.* Hertford-shire, UK: Prentice Hall Europe.

Feldman, R., & Morrisey, M. A. (1990). Health economics: A report on the field. *Journal of Health Politics, Policy and Law, 15,* 627–646.

Folland, S., Goodman, A. C., & Stano, M. (1997). *The economics of health and health care* (2nd ed.). Upper Saddle River, NJ: Prentice Hall.

Hemenway, D., Killen, A., Cashman, S. B., Parks, C. L., & Bicknell, W. J. (1990). Physicians' responses to financial incentives: Evidence from a for-profit ambulatory center. *New England Journal of Medicine, 322,* 1059–1063.

Hillman, A. L., Pauly, M. V., & Kerstein, J. J. (1989). How do financial incentives affect physicians' clinical decisions and the financial performance of health maintenance organizations? *New England Journal of Medicine, 321,* 86–92.

Jacobs, P. (1991). *The economics of health and medical care* (3rd ed.). Gaithers-burg, MD: Aspen.

Jacobs, P. (1996). *The economics of health and medical care* (4th ed.). Sudbury, MA: Jones and Bartlett.

Kongstvedt, P. R. (1997). Negotiating and contracting with hospitals and institu-tions. In P. R. Kongstvedt (Ed.), *Essentials of managed health care* (2nd ed.). Gaithersburg, MD: Aspen.

Manning, W. G., Newhouse, J. P., Duan, N., Keeler, E. B., et al. (1987). Health insurance and the demand for medical care. *American Economic Review, 77,* 251–277.

Rice, T. (1997). Can markets give us the health system we want? *Journal of Health Politics, Policy and Law, 22,* 383–426.

Roemer, M. I. (1961). Bed supply and hospital utilization: A national experiment. *Hospitals, Journal of the American Hospital Association, 35,* 988–993.

Shain, M., & Roemer, M. I. (1959). Hospital costs relate to the supply of beds. *Modern Hospital, 92,* 71–73.

Torrens, P. R., & Williams, S. J. (1993). Understanding the present, planning for the future: The dynamics of health care in the United States in the 1990s. In S. J. Williams and P. R. Torrens (Eds.), *Introduction to health services* (4th ed.) (pp. 421–429). Albany, NY: Delmar.

ACKNOWLEDGMENT

Adapted with permission from the Academy of Managed Care Pharmacy. Copyright 2000. All rights reserved.

CHAPTER 14

Private Health Insurance

Kenneth W. Schafermeyer

Case Scenario

Barb Ital recently graduated from pharmacy school and is considering a job offer from a large pharmacy chain. As part of her benefits package, the company will pay one half of the premium for Barb's health insurance coverage. Barb knows that this is a good deal: Even if she paid 100% of the premium, the group policy would be much less expensive than a policy that she could buy on her own. Barb also knows that if she does not elect to participate in the plan when she begins her employment, she will have to wait until next year before she can join the plan during another open enrollment period. Also, if she joins later, there will be an elimination period; she will have to wait a specified period of months before any preexisting health conditions are covered. Upon reading the policy, Barb discovers that she is required to pay part of the cost for most health care services and that some health care procedures, such as cosmetic surgery, are not covered.

Questions

1. Why are group policies less expensive than individual policies?
2. What is the purpose of the open enrollment period and the elimination period?
3. Why are patients required to pay part of the cost of most health care services?
4. Why are some procedures not covered?

LEARNING OBJECTIVES _____

Upon completion of this chapter, the student shall be able to:

- Identify the factors that determine whether an event is insurable
- Describe the original purpose of health insurance
- List and define the various parties involved in the health insurance industry
- Explain how prepaid prescription programs are inconsistent with the principles of health insurance
- Explain why health insurance plans cover prescriptions despite their incompatibility with some risk management principles
- Outline the advantages and disadvantages of the U.S. practice of offering health insurance as an employee benefit
- Describe the potential risk management problems faced by health insurance programs, and explain how insurance companies try to minimize these risks
- Describe the purpose of pharmacy benefit managers and the types of services they provide to control prescription cost and quality
- Given a third-party plan's reimbursement formula, the pharmacy's actual acquisition cost, and the pharmacy's cost of dispensing the prescription, calculate the pharmacy's earned discount, gross margin, and net profit for that prescription when reimbursed by the third-party plan
- Describe how private health insurance has affected pharmacy practice

CHAPTER QUESTIONS

1. What determines whether an event is insurable or uninsurable?
2. What was the original purpose of health insurance?
3. How are prepaid prescription programs inconsistent with the principles of health insurance?
4. Why do health insurance plans cover prescriptions despite their incompatibility with some risk management principles?
5. Why are most private health insurance policies offered through employers?
6. What can insurance programs do to reduce their risk?

INTRODUCTION

The last half of the 20th century witnessed dramatic changes in the way health care is provided, paralleled by equally profound transformations in the way health care is financed. Although health insurance has preserved financial security and improved access to health care for millions of Americans, it has also ensured payment for health care providers and fueled the growth of hospitals and the development of new health services. Without health insurance, many Americans could not afford the services they need to stay healthy and to continue working as productive members of society.

THE UNINSURED

In 2005, 46.6 million Americans (15.9% of the population) lacked health insurance—1.3 million more people than in 2004 (DeNavas-Walt, Proctor, and Lee, 2006). These uninsured individuals face greater barriers to receiving health care, are generally in poorer health, and have shorter life expectancies than do individuals with health insurance coverage.

Catastrophic medical bills also are a major cause of personal bankruptcies in the United States, accounting for about 40% of these filings in 1999 (Associated Press, 2000). Financial difficulties resulting from such health care expenses affect not only the uninsured, but also individuals with inadequate insurance coverage. The demographic groups most likely to be financially devastated by noncovered medical expenses are the elderly, women, and families headed by single women.

Surprisingly, the individuals most likely to be uninsured are not the groups that were traditionally considered "uninsurable"—the poor, the disabled, and the elderly. These groups are provided some protection by the public sector through Medicare and Medicaid (discussed in Chapter 17). Who, then, are the uninsured? Following are some of the highlights from a U.S. Census Bureau report shown in **Table 14-1** (DeNavas-Walt, Proctor, and Lee, 2006):

- Among adults, the largest group of uninsured comprises the working poor—individuals who are working in low-paying jobs that either do not offer health insurance benefits or require workers to pay premiums that are unaffordable.
- Foreign-born U.S. residents are about 2.5 times as likely as U.S.-born individuals to be uninsured (33.6% versus 13.4%). The highest rate of uninsured status is found among foreign-born Hispanics. This finding has serious public health implications for areas of the country with large numbers of immigrants (Thamer, Richard, Casebeer, and Ray, 1997).
- About one third (30.6%) of young adults between the ages of 18 and 24 are uninsured (about twice the rate of the general population). Young adults who are full-time students fare better because many stay on their parents' health insurance policies through college. A disproportionately large percentage (more than one fourth) of adults between the ages of 25 and 34, however, are also uninsured.
- As might be expected, the proportion of individuals with health insurance increases with household income; only 8.5% of individuals living in households with incomes greater than $75,000 lack health insurance.

Table 14.1   People Without Health Insurance Coverage by Selected Characteristics, 2005

	Percentage
Total Population	15.9
Race	
White, not Hispanic	11.3
Black	19.6
Asian	17.9
Hispanic	32.7
Age	
Under 18 years	11.2
18 to 24 years	30.6
25 to 34 years	26.4
35 to 44 years	18.8
45 to 64 years	14.6
65 years or older	1.3
Nativity	
Native born	13.4
Foreign born	33.6
Region	
Northeast	12.3
Midwest	11.9
South	18.6
West	18.1
Household Income	
Less than $25,000	24.4
$25,000 to $49,999	20.6
$50,000 to $74,999	14.1
$75,000 or more	8.5

Source: U.S. Census Bureau, Current Population Survey, 2005 and 2006 Annual Social and Economic Supplements

Removing financial barriers by providing universal health insurance coverage will not, by itself, eliminate all of the barriers to receiving high-quality health care. For example, insurance coverage was not found to be an independent predictor of vaccination in a study of preschool children (Santoli et al., 2004). An earlier study showed that the barriers to immunization reported by middle/upper-income parents are similar to those reported by lower-income parents: Only about one third identify cost and lack of insurance coverage as problems (Salsberry, Nickel, and Mitch, 1994). Greater health problems faced by poor people are attributable not only to lack of adequate insurance coverage but also to organizational barriers, such as a lack of flexibility in scheduling, long waiting times, and personal barriers such as a lack of reliable transportation, chaotic home environments, and employment conflicts. Other obstacles include lack of knowledge of health care needs and misperceptions about the safety of health care services (Lannon, Brack, Stuart, Caplow, McNeill, Bordley, and Margolis, 1995). Although attempts to reform health care in the United States must focus first on providing adequate insurance coverage, other barriers such as education and transportation must be addressed as well. More discussion about covering the uninsured and reforming the health care system is included in Chapter 20.

Health insurance is a vital component of the U.S. health care system. As important as it is, however, many individuals—including both health care providers and consumers—do not have a clear understanding of how it works. This chapter dispels some of the mystery surrounding health insurance by explaining the evolution of health insurance and some of the basic principles followed by the health insurance industry.

Although health insurance has improved the health status and standard of living in the United States, it also presents some interesting paradoxes:

- Health insurance ensures payment for health care providers, yet it restricts provider reimbursement.
- Health insurance creates patient access to health care services by reducing financial barriers, yet it restricts utilization of those services.
- Health care providers supply services, yet they create the demand for these services—an inherent conflict of interest that can drive up health care costs.
- Health insurance increases access to health care, yet it can encourage unnecessary use of health care services.
- Groups of patients who were once thought of as "uninsurable" (the poor, the disabled, and the elderly) are now covered through Medicaid and Medicare, yet millions of working poor and their families remain uninsured.
- Individuals with chronic or expensive health problems have the greatest need for health insurance, yet they have the most difficulty obtaining it.

Health insurance has been roundly maligned because of these problems, especially by pharmacists and other health care providers who depend on health insurance for payment for services rendered. These paradoxes do make sense, however, when one understands the basic principles of insurance and the needs of the insurance industry. This chapter describes how insurance works and how health care professionals, patients, and insurers can cooperate to accomplish common goals for their mutual benefit. First, it explains the evolution and structure of the health insurance industry, especially as it relates to prescription drug programs. Next, it outlines the basic principles of insurance and highlights the tools that insurers use to manage risk. The impact of health insurance on pharmacy and strategies for working with insurance programs are also discussed.

HISTORY OF HEALTH INSURANCE

Early Health Insurance Programs

Health insurance has a long history in the United States, beginning with the federal Marine Hospital Service, which was first authorized in 1798. Starting in the mid-19th century, accident insurance and life insurance companies began entering the field of health insurance. The Massachusetts Health Insurance Company of Boston was incorporated in 1847, and several health insurance plans were offered for California "Gold Rush" workers in 1849 and for railroad workers in 1860 (Campbell and Newsome, 1995).

Most early health insurance plans were really disability insurance—that is, they did not cover health expenses, but instead protected individuals from the loss of income resulting from illness. At first, only specified diseases such as diabetes, diphtheria, scarlet fever, and typhus were covered. Coverage was later expanded to include more diseases and to reimburse individuals for certain out-of-pocket health expenses. The emphasis, however, remained on protecting income.

Hospital Insurance

In 1929, Baylor University Hospital offered hospital care to a group of Dallas teachers on a prepaid basis. The plan collected premiums of $6 per year for each covered person and then reallocated those funds to the small portion of the group that had hospital expenses.

With fewer financial barriers to hospital care, the demand for hospital services eventually increased. As hospitals experienced empty beds and declining revenues during the Great Depression, the increased revenue and financial stability promised by insurance became increasingly attractive. One problem, however, was that these plans restricted care to a particular hospital. This problem was resolved when the American Hospital Association expanded the prepayment concept by establishing statewide Blue Cross hospital insurance plans allowing free choice of hospitals. These plans did not pay hospitals directly; instead, patients were expected to pay their bills and then were reimbursed by the plan for 80% of the first 21 days of hospital expenses. Although this insurance covered a portion of patients' financial losses, it did not ensure availability of health care services.

Medical Insurance

At the same time that Blue Cross was being created, a medical group practice in Los Angeles organized a similar program to cover medical services. Not only did this plan create insurance for physician services, but it also organized physicians into a large group practice—a unique arrangement at the time that became a model for today's medical foundations and health maintenance organizations (Pharmaceutical Manufacturers Association, 1973). In 1939, the California Medical Association established the first Blue Shield plan to facilitate payment for medical services. Like Blue Cross, Blue Shield focused on reimbursing patients for a portion of their medical expenses, not on organizing or providing health services directly.

Health insurance benefits became an important part of labor negotiations during World War II. Because government wage and price controls prohibited wage increases during the war, companies that wanted to attract workers began offering additional benefits, especially health insurance. Before World War II, health insurance was an occasional employee benefit, covering about 5% of the U.S. population; in just a few years, however, it became commonplace, covering more than 50% of the population (Institute of Medicine, 1993).

Health insurance remains a standard employee benefit today, with 90% of workers in manufacturing jobs covered; it is less common in the service sector (75%) and in agriculture (70%) (Lee, Soffel, and Luft, 1992). Recent evidence suggests, however, that the percentage of workers covered by employment-based health insurance is declining because of decreased unionization, the trend toward using part-time workers, and the decreased percentage of employers sponsoring health insurance plans (Fronstin and Snider, 1996).

Major Medical Insurance

With the merger of Blue Cross and Blue Shield and the formation of several other commercial insurance companies, hospital coverage and medical coverage were combined into comprehensive insurance plans. By the early 1950s, most employee health benefit plans took the form of major medical insurance. These policies were designed to help offset expenses incurred because of catastrophic illness or injury. Until major medical insurance was developed, insurance policies generally limited coverage to a specific dollar amount. Also in the 1950s, the health insurance industry came full circle by reemphasizing income replacement through long-term disability insurance policies.

Indemnity versus Service Benefit Insurance

Blue Cross, Blue Shield, and other health insurers initially reimbursed subscribers—not providers—for a portion (usually 80%) of their medical expenses. These plans, which were known as indemnity insurance, represented the dominant form of health insurance for decades because they were simple and effective in achieving their objectives—to protect both patients and health care providers from financial loss and bankruptcy. Indemnity plans, however, also presented some problems. Patients found it inconvenient to collect receipts and complete claim forms. In turn, insurance companies found the individual claims submitted by thousands of policyholders expensive to process. Premiums for these plans increased rapidly because insurance companies reimbursed on a fee-for-service basis and, consequently, were relatively ineffective at controlling expenditures. Today the term "indemnity" is used loosely to refer to any health insurance program reimbursing on a fee-for-service basis with few cost controls.

Most health insurance programs have discontinued the indemnity approach in favor of service benefit programs, in which health care providers submit claims and are paid directly by the insurance plan. This arrangement allows standardization and automation of claims processing and control of costs through contractual agreements between the insurance plans and health care providers.

Current Trends

Private health insurance has primarily supported and reinforced existing patterns of health services. Those areas that were neglected by the private sector—prevention, control of communicable diseases, and care for segments of society that have the highest incidence of disease and the greatest need for care (persons who are poor, disabled, chronically ill, mentally ill, retarded, and elderly)—have become the responsibility of the public sector (Litman, 1994). This problem was addressed in 1965 when the Social Security Act was amended to provide government-sponsored health insurance coverage for the poor (Medicaid) and for older and disabled persons (Medicare). Medicare and Medicaid are discussed in more detail in Chapter 17 of this book.

Because early health insurance programs, such as Blue Cross and Blue Shield, were controlled by hospitals and physicians, the primary goal was to protect providers—not patients—from financial loss. The form of insurance preferred by these indemnity plans guaranteed that reimbursement would be generous and that little attention would be given to controlling costs (Starr, 1982). Until recently, most health care providers have been reimbursed on a fee-for-service basis—that is, they received a fee for each service performed. This system offered little financial incentive to control utilization, reduce costs, or enhance quality of care.

As health care costs increased rapidly during the 1970s, employer groups that paid for health benefits demanded that health insurance programs control costs and change their governing bodies to reduce the extent of provider control. Health insurance companies responded by restricting reimbursement to providers and by controlling the use of health care services. Until recently, there was little desire or perceived need to improve quality or ensure positive outcomes—ordinary management functions for most businesses. In other words, health care services were not managed.

In the past few decades, traditional health insurance programs have evolved into managed health care plans through the implementation of extensive cost controls and through the use of patient information and claims databases to improve the quality of health care services in an attempt to enhance patient outcomes. Managed care is discussed in more detail in Chapter 16.

Evolution of Prepaid Prescription Drug Programs

Until the early 1970s, most insurance coverage for prescription drugs was offered through major medical insurance programs. The first program to focus primarily on prepayment of prescription drug expenses was the Green Shield plan offered in Ontario, Canada, in the 1950s. Outpatient coverage of prescription drugs through insurance programs other than major medical plans grew only slowly in the United States, however, for several reasons. First, other health care services, such as hospital and medical services, account for a much larger portion of health expenditures; prescription drug coverage, therefore, was a much lower priority. Second, because prescriptions result in a large number of small claims, prescription coverage is not consistent with some of the principles of insurance and risk management. (This point is discussed later in this chapter.) Third, antitrust laws prohibit U.S. pharmacists from doing what Canadian pharmacists had done—working together to negotiate fees.

After the United Auto Workers Union negotiated a prescription drug plan administered by Blue Cross in 1969, labor unions became the major catalyst driving the growth of prepaid prescription plans. In response to this trend, a new industry of fiscal intermediaries was created in the early 1970s to help employer groups provide these prescription benefit programs to their employees. These fiscal intermediaries, which are described in more detail in the next section of this chapter, made it easier for employee benefit plans to include prescription drug coverage.

Although payments to pharmacies through public and private health insurance plans were applied to less than 12% of all retail prescriptions before 1970, more 85% of all prescriptions were subject to such reimbursement by 2004 (West, 2005). About one third of third-party prescriptions dispensed by independent community pharmacies in 2004 were covered directly by Medicaid; the remainder were reimbursed by private-sector plans.

THE HEALTH INSURANCE INDUSTRY

Structure of the Industry

Although the term "third party" implies that only three individuals or companies are involved in a transaction (in this case, the patient, the health care provider, and the payer), the health insurance industry actually includes many different participants, each with its own specific function. To work successfully with third-party programs, health care providers need to understand the structure of the industry and the objectives of each of the participants.

Figure 14-1 outlines the most important participants in employer-sponsored group health insurance. At the top of the diagram is the patient—either an employee of a company that sponsors the health insurance plan or a family member of the covered employee. Sometimes employees are represented by labor unions that negotiate benefits on their behalf. The labor contract may specify the type of health care and prescription coverage that employees and their families receive.

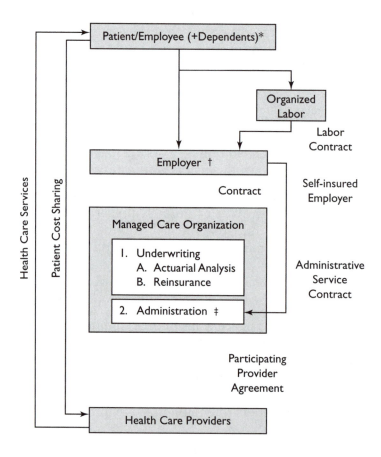

* For public programs = Patient/Qualified Beneficiary
† For public programs = Government Agency (e.g., Medicaid)
‡ Some administrative duties may be assumed by a PBM

Figure 14-1   The Third-Party Prescription Industry.
Source: Schafermeyer, K. W. (1996). Third-party prescription program evaluation. In *Effective pharmacy management,* (8th ed., p. 322). Alexandria, VA: National Community Pharmacists Association.

As shown in Figure 14-1, patients often have to pay a portion of the cost of health services received. This patient cost sharing is designed to control utilization of health services by making patients more cost-conscious. As discussed later in this chapter, patient cost sharing can take one of three forms: a co-payment, a deductible, or co-insurance. Most plans use patient cost sharing as a financial incentive to avoid using unnecessary health care services. To be effective, however, patient cost-sharing provisions should not be so high as to discourage use of truly necessary health services.

Figure 14-1 also shows the sponsor of the insurance program—usually an employer that assumes responsibility for obtaining coverage and pays some or all of the premiums. Because health care costs for small groups (several hundred persons or fewer) can be unpredictable and the payment of claims for health expenditures is complex, most employer groups seek professional help from fiscal intermediaries—companies that provide underwriting and/or administrative services

Underwriting is the process of insuring someone. The underwriter assumes the financial risk for health services in return for premiums paid by the employer group. Because of the unpredictable nature of health insurance coverage, most insurance companies limit their risk by purchasing reinsurance. In essence, the insurance company buys insurance to limit its own risk. Therefore, insurance companies cannot take unreasonable risks because it would make it difficult for them to attract other insurance companies to share the risk with them.

Estimating the amount of risk assumed by an insurance company is known as actuarial analysis. An actuary conducts a statistical analysis of the population served and estimates the income (premiums) that must be earned to cover the estimated expenses, usually expressed as cost per member per month (PMPM). An actuary estimates three expenses: (1) the cost for each type of service; (2) the projected number of services that will be received by the group as a whole (the utilization rate); and (3) the administrative expenses that the fiscal intermediary incurs by insuring and administering the health care benefit program. Actuaries may then adjust their estimates based on the insurance company's overall expenses for a specific geographic area during the previous year (community rating) or adjust the rates for a specific subset of insured individuals—usually an employer group—based on the group's experience for the previous year (experience rating). These adjustments affect premiums for the next year, depending on whether the claims expenses were higher or lower than the actuary's estimate.

Sometimes a large corporation decides that it is unnecessary to use an insurance company to underwrite a health benefit program and decides to self-insure instead. Laws in most states require employers that self-insure health care benefits to put a large sum of money aside into a restricted account that can be used only to pay for employees' health benefits. This restricted account (escrow account) must be large enough to pay any unexpected future health benefit claims. Because self-insurance is a risky strategy and ties up a considerable amount of cash, most employers prefer to use the underwriting services of an insurance company.

Some fiscal intermediaries specialize in providing only underwriting services; others provide only administrative services. A few fiscal intermediaries, such as Blue Cross/Blue Shield, provide both underwriting and administrative services. Because health care providers and administrators are linked through contractual arrangements, administrators are the component of the health care industry that is most visible to health care providers. The elements of this contractual arrangement are discussed later in this chapter.

Viewpoints of the Participants

The various groups involved in the health insurance industry have competing goals. Employees are interested primarily in having convenient access to health care providers, quality services, and reduced out-of-pocket costs. Employers want healthy, satisfied employees but also want to reduce or control the amount they spend on health benefits. Administrators need to satisfy their customers—employer groups—by maintaining an adequate network of participating health care providers and helping employers manage their health benefit programs at a reasonable cost.

Health care providers, however, often see third-party programs as an unnecessary and unwelcome intrusion into the provider–patient relationship and as an unfair market force that controls their practice and limits their earnings. Providers do not like to be viewed as commodities to be purchased at the lowest price. Although providers express concern that cost-containment efforts are imposed at the expense of quality, this concern is difficult to document. Cost control receives more attention because costs are easy to quantify; quality is not. Although aware of providers' concerns, health insurers believe they provide valuable services to policyholders and employer groups and generally conclude that if sufficient numbers of providers agree to their contract terms, then the contract terms must be adequate.

One health economist has pointed out that health care providers want to maximize reimbursement, whereas health care consumers want to maximize health benefits while minimizing personal expenditures. Health insurance may intensify this conflict (Reinhardt, 1994). Given these competing viewpoints, it is often difficult for one party to recognize the needs of the others and, consequently, the various participants can become adversaries. Because the parties also have a common goal—providing services to improve patient outcomes—plenty of room for cooperation exists.

BASIC PRINCIPLES AND STRATEGIES OF HEALTH INSURANCE

Principles of Risk Management

Although insurance seems to be a rather complex subject, the basic principles of insurance are relatively simple. To understand insurance and its effect on the provision of health care in the United States, one must first understand the principle of risk and learn how it can be managed.

The purpose of insurance is to help individuals and businesses manage certain types of unanticipated risk. Death, for example, is inevitable; because it can be sudden or unexpected (unanticipated), however, it is insurable. Most accidents and many other perils are also unanticipated and, therefore, insurable. In contrast, risk that can be anticipated is not insurable (for example, spoilage of products, depreciation of buildings and equipment, or expiration of drugs).

Risk can be described as pure or speculative. Pure risk occurs in situations where a person faces the possibility of loss but no gain. Illness, fires, or storms are unpredictable perils and are often unavoidable. Because these events can cause significant loss but seldom result in any type of gain, they are referred to as pure risk. Speculative risk involves a chance of gain as well as a chance for loss. Gambling is a classic example of speculative risk. Pursuing a business venture also involves speculative risk because an individual accepts the risk of losing money while pursuing the chance of making profits. Speculative risk cannot be insured because risk takers can usually choose the amount of risk they are willing to assume; removing the risk would encourage overspending or careless behavior.

Insurance is designed to help people to reduce pure risk, not speculative risk. Pure risk becomes an insurable hazard when all six of the following elements are present:

1. The probability of a peril occurring in a population can be accurately determined. We can predict with reasonable certainty, for example, the percentage of 60-year-old women who will develop breast cancer in a given year and the percentage of 19-year-old men who will have traffic accidents during a given year.
2. The peril is an irregular event on an individual basis. Although we can predict approximately how many breast cancer cases or traffic accidents will occur in a population, we have no way of knowing to whom these events will occur.
3. The loss must be accidental. For example, arson committed by the insured party is not covered by insurance; neither is murder by a beneficiary of a life insurance policy. The point here is to avoid creating profit-making incentives for purchasing insurance.
4. The event must result in a substantial loss. Insurance is designed to

protect a person's financial security. Although most people can sustain small losses, insurance is needed to cover the large, unexpected losses that can overwhelm an individual's income stream or wipe out a family's accumulated resources.

5. The loss must be measurable. For a loss to be measurable, two conditions must be met: The loss must be attributable to a specific event, and the monetary value of the loss must be relatively easy to determine. For example, normal wear and tear for an automobile does not come from a specific event. In contrast, the loss from a theft or a hailstorm is the result of a specific incident and, therefore, can be insured. Insurance policies state the basis under which the amount of loss will be measured. For personal property, insurance coverage is set at either market value (the amount for which the item could have been sold before it was damaged) or replacement value (the amount it would cost to fix or replace the item). Insurance companies may also establish schedules stipulating the amount they will pay for various services. The intrinsic value of a lost heirloom or a favorite photograph, however, cannot be measured in monetary terms and, therefore, is difficult to insure.

6. The individual must have an insurable interest. Because insurance is designed to compensate for loss, an individual who does not suffer the loss personally usually cannot receive insurance compensation. A person cannot, for example, be reimbursed when a neighbor's house burns down. Likewise, whereas people can purchase life insurance for family members or business partners (with their permission), they cannot purchase insurance on an acquaintance who is a poor driver, thereby speculating that they can cash in when the acquaintance finally has an accident.

Purchasing insurance involves incurring a small, certain loss (prepayment of an annual or monthly premium) in exchange for the possibility of a large, unpredictable loss. Trading uncertainty for certainty reduces risk. Insurance has several other equally valuable benefits: It reduces worry, it makes it easier to borrow money, and it frees up capital for investment.

Insurance does not make risk disappear, but rather transfers risk from individuals to the insurance company for a fee. The insurance company then pools the risk with that assumed from many other insurance policyholders. Transfer of risk and risk pooling are based on the law of large numbers: The larger the number of insured persons, the more accurate the predictions regarding losses. When losses are more predictable, the risk of this loss actually decreases. The insurance company estimates the predicted amount of loss and charges premiums accordingly.

Premiums are based on the claims experience of the policyholders who make up the risk pool. If claims are higher than anticipated, then next year's premiums will increase to make up for this loss. In these experience-rated pools, each insurance subscriber is affected by the aggregate claims experience of the group. A lot of bad risk resulting in a high number of claims results in large premium increases; good risk with fewer claims results in lower premium levels.

Prescription Coverage: An Exception to the Principles of Risk Management

The need for health insurance is obvious. Unexpected injury or hospitalization costing tens of thousands of dollars (or more) can quickly exceed a family's annual income or accumulated savings. Most families consider the financial security provided by health insurance to be a necessity. Insurance coverage for pharmaceuticals, however, is not consistent with all of the requirements of an insurable hazard as described previously. Compared with other health expenditures, the cost of a prescription does not represent a substantial loss. In addition, for some medications, such as oral contraceptives, the prescriptions do not represent an accidental or unpredictable hazard. Because prescriptions represent a large number of small claims, administrative costs are relatively high.

If prescription coverage provides relatively small benefits at a high administrative expense and is inconsistent with some of the basic principles of insurance, why, then, are prescriptions covered by most health insurance programs? A logical explanation is that drug therapy is often preventive in nature and is less expensive than other medical alternatives such as surgery. If medications can keep patients out of the hospital, it is theorized, encouraging proper use of medications may reduce overall health care costs.

Unfortunately, the potential benefits of prescription coverage are not always realized and, consequently, prescription coverage is often viewed as another cost that must be minimized. However, rising prescription expenditures are starting to make prescription drugs more of an insurable risk for some groups of patients, especially older persons.

Potential Risk Management Problems

Theoretically, the law of large numbers allows accurate prediction of losses for insured populations. A number of potential risk management problems, however, can make it difficult to predict losses accurately.

Catastrophic Hazard

One of the most important problems to avoid is catastrophic hazard. Most insurance policies exclude coverage for widespread, catastrophic events that, if covered, would exceed the company's ability to pay. Examples of catastrophic events that are often excluded from property insurance include acts of war and earthquakes. Earthquakes are sometimes covered under special addenda ("riders") to homeowners' policies; acts of war are almost always not eligible for coverage. Companies that provide casualty insurance also limit their exposure to catastrophic events by trying to avoid insuring large numbers of policyholders in the same geographic area.

Adverse Selection

If individuals could predict future losses accurately, they would be more likely to purchase insurance coverage only when they knew they were going to need it and to drop coverage when they did not need it. The situation in which individuals or companies purchase insurance because they expect a loss is known as adverse selection. This practice, of course, makes it difficult for insurers to raise enough premium income from individuals who do not have losses to cover those who do. Adverse selection inevitably results in premium increases for future policyholders.

Flood insurance is notorious for being subject to adverse selection; only policyholders residing in flood plains buy it. Therefore, premiums would be extremely high, and flood insurance probably would not be available, without federal subsidies. Adverse selection is also a problem inherent in health insurance; older or sicker individuals are more likely to use insurance and, therefore, more likely to purchase it. Because large, employer-sponsored groups usually include many healthy individuals, adverse selection is not likely to be a problem and, consequently, premiums for group policies are usually less expensive than individual policies. Dental insurance is also subject to adverse selection because individuals can obtain coverage only when they know they will need it.

For the benefit of insurance companies and policyholders, it is important to avoid adverse selection. Many restrictions in insurance policy contracts (discussed later in this chapter) are aimed at avoiding the problems associated with adverse selection.

Incentives to Create Losses and Supplier-Induced Demand

A third potential risk management problem occurs when an individual actually gains from an apparent loss. For example, insuring a car for more than its value could give the policyholder an incentive to destroy the car. Insurers try to prevent this kind of profiteering by limiting the amount of insurance coverage to the market value of the insured item. For health insurance, however, it is more difficult to avoid incentives to incur losses (i.e., medical claims). Physicians, who serve as the patients' agents, can always create a demand for the same services that they supply. This potential conflict of interest, known as supplier-induced demand, is an inherent element of health care under fee-for-service reimbursement and is difficult to avoid completely. The issue of supplier-induced demand is discussed in more detail in Chapter 13.

Moral Hazard

Health insurance is often subject to a problem know as *moral hazard,* where people overconsume health care. As all consumers know, when the price of a product or service decreases, the quantity demanded tends to increase. This is also true of health care services: By decreasing patients' out-of-pocket expenses for health services, health insurance has encouraged patients to use services that they might not seek out otherwise and has contributed to a dramatic increase in health care expenditures (Torrens and Williams, 1993).

If a person has health insurance coverage, then his or her out-of-pocket costs are generally much less than the true cost of providing the individual's health care. At some point, the benefits of additional health services in terms of improving one's health are not really worth their full costs. Overconsumption of health services can drive up up health expenses and health insurance premiums for everyone. As presented in the case scenario at the beginning of this chapter, insurers often mandate cost sharing (deductibles, co-insurance, or co-payments) as a means to decrease unnecessary demand.

Strategies for Avoiding Risk Management Problems

Insurers must be careful to avoid the problems discussed previously. Failure to do so may result in large increases in premiums or—even worse—make insurance coverage difficult or impossible to obtain. Fortunately, insurance companies have developed a variety of strategies to overcome potential risk management problems and to limit their own risks.

Group Policies

To avoid adverse selection, insurance companies use group policies, which are usually sponsored by employer groups and provided to employees and their dependents. As highlighted in the case scenario at the beginning of this chapter, group policies are usually less expensive than individual policies for two reasons: They are less prone to adverse selection, and they are less expensive to sell and administer. Employer groups assume many of the administrative costs associated with enrolling policyholders and explaining the plan's benefits. Selling costs are lower because the insurance company only has to negotiate a master contract with the employer group; it does not have to sign individual contracts with each insured person. Obviously, for a group policy to be cost-effective for the insurer, enough policyholders must be in the risk pool so that the law of large numbers allows accurate prediction of losses.

Employer-sponsored group health insurance is popular with workers because it reduces their tax liability; if the amount paid in premiums had been given to employees as salary instead, the workers would have paid income tax and Social Security tax on this income first and then purchased premiums out of their own pockets. Employers also bene-fit because their payroll taxes, such as the employers' Social Security matching payments and federal and state unemployment taxes, are not paid on the amount of compensation given as employee benefits.

As introduced in the case scenario at the beginning of this chapter, another contract restriction aimed at avoiding adverse selection is the elimination period (also known as an exclusionary period), in which preexisting health problems are not covered by a new health insurance policy until after the policyholder has been covered for a given period of time. Expenses related to pregnancy and childbirth, for example, may not be covered for the first nine months of a new policy. Elimination periods are often waived during an open enrollment period in which new employees are allowed to join an employer's health insurance plan during a short period of time after they begin their employment. There-after, many policies either impose an elimination period for preexisting health problems or require a health test to demonstrate that the patient does not have preexisting health problems that would result in adverse selection.

Coverage Limitations

Even when a given service is covered, the insurance contract will restrict losses by limiting the amount paid for certain covered expenditures. Health insurance policies commonly limit payments for physician office visits or prescriptions and state that they will not pay the extra cost for a private hospital room unless isolation of the patient is medically neces-sary. When health insurance pays for health care services, usually a limit exists regarding how much the policy will pay.

Insurance companies carefully restrict the perils covered to reduce costs and, more importantly, to avoid adverse selection. This is why health insurance policies, such as the one described in the chapter-opening case scenario, often exclude elective treatments such as cosmetic surgery, fer-tility treatment, abortion, childbirth, and dental care. Mental health and drug and alcohol rehabilitation were commonly excluded until many states adopted laws requiring insurers to cover these services. The perils associated with some injury-prone activities, such as contact sports, avi-ation, and military service, are also commonly excluded from coverage.

Coordination of Benefits

Occasionally individuals have overlapping coverage from two insur-ance policies, and questions may arise about which insurance company should be responsible for payment. This can happen, for example, when a person with health insurance is injured in an auto accident or on the job. In these cases, medical expenses may also be covered by the auto insurance policy or by the employer's workers' compensation policy. To avoid the case in which multiple payments are made for the same care, insurance policies usually include a coordination of benefits provision that limits total reimbursement of all insurance to the amount of loss. An insurance policy's subrogation provision states which company pays first. In the examples cited previously, health insurance policies usually pay after auto, homeowner's, or workers' compensation insurance policies have paid their portion.

Other Strategies

The risk management techniques discussed previously are designed to prevent some of the most common risk management problems and are aimed primarily at policyholders. Reducing risk is extremely important because it is a prerequisite for achieving the basic financial objective of all insurance companies—generating revenues in excess of expenses. (Even nonprofit companies need to avoid losses and build reserves.)

Risk can also be reduced by controlling underwriting—avoiding bad risks by refusing coverage to those individuals who are most likely to incur high costs. In the past, some insurance companies have canceled or refused to renew policies for policyholders who incurred major health care expenses. Most states now prohibit this practice. Insurance companies have also refused new coverage to people with certain preexisting health problems; this practice makes it difficult for some workers to change jobs because they cannot afford to lose their health insurance coverage. Some of these problems were addressed by the Health Insurance Portability and Accountability Act (HIPAA), discussed in Chapter 20.

The facts that health insurance premiums have increased faster than the cost of other goods and services in the United States and that more than 46 million Americans do not have health insurance are evidence that risk management is a complex endeavor and risk management problems are difficult to overcome.

ADMINISTRATION OF PRESCRIPTION DRUG PROGRAMS

Pharmacy Benefits Manager

Given that the administration of prepaid pharmacy programs is complex and requires a large prescription volume to be conducted efficiently, third parties often separate (or "carve out") prescription programs from other health benefits and contract with a type of administrator known as a pharmacy benefits manager (PBM) to manage them. Using a PBM isolates cost centers and concentrates a workforce of prescription benefit experts to manage the prescription program. The administrative services provided by PBMs usually include the following:

- Contracting with health care providers to supply specified services
- Communicating with both patients and providers to explain and update administrative policies
- Providing reports to plan sponsors
- Identifying eligible beneficiaries
- Maintaining formulary systems
- Conducting drug utilization reviews
- Processing claims submitted by providers
- Reimbursing providers
- Auditing providers
- Controlling costs
- Controlling utilization
- Ensuring program quality

Participating Pharmacy Agreement

Even health insurance contracts that are carefully crafted to minimize risk management problems include provisions to control health care expenditures by reducing the costs per claim and the overall number of claims. Many cost-control provisions for prescription drug programs are specified in participating pharmacy agreements—contracts that stipulate the services to be provided by contracting pharmacies in exchange for a specified reimbursement. (These contracting pharmacies are sometimes referred to as "participating pharmacies" or "network pharmacies." If only a selected group of pharmacies is allowed to contract, these entities are known as "preferred pharmacies" or "preferred providers.")

Plan administrators recruit health care providers who are willing to sign participating provider agreements. A clear understanding of the terms of these contracts is important for pharmacy managers and other key employees. Following is a description of some of the most important elements of the participating pharmacy agreement.

Reimbursement

The participating pharmacy agreement specifies the amount and frequency of payment. For pharmacies that dispense large numbers of third-party prescriptions, timely reimbursement is vital. Even more important is the amount of reimbursement. Prescription reimbursement consists of three components: the PBM's cost for the drug ingredients, the dispensing fee, and the amount paid by the patient in the form of co-payments, co-insurance, or deductibles. These factors are shown in **Equation 14-1.**

Rx Payment = Ingredient Cost + Dispensing Fee – Patient Cost Sharing (14-1)

Ingredient Costs

Ingredient costs (also known as the cost of goods sold [COGS]) represents between 75% and 80% of the cost of the average prescription. Pharmacy reimbursement for drug ingredient costs is usually based on the average wholesale price (AWP)—that is, the list price established by the manufacturer. The AWP is higher than the actual acquisition cost (AAC) that pharmacies pay for drug products. As shown in **Equation 14-2,** the difference between the average wholesale price and the pharmacy's actual acquisition cost is known as the earned discount.

$$\text{AWP} - \text{AAC} = \text{Earned Discount} \qquad (14\text{-}2)$$

As shown in **Equation 14-3,** the amount of the pharmacy's earned discount varies depending on the pharmacy's purchasing volume (volume discount), its ability to pay early (cash discount), and special deals and promotions the pharmacy is able to take advantage of (trade discounts).

$$\text{Earned Discount} = \text{Volume Discount} + \text{Cash Discount} + \text{Trade Discount} \quad (14\text{-}3)$$

Earned discounts are very important because they decrease the pharmacy's AAC. A lower AAC, of course, results in a higher gross margin (GM—the difference between the selling price and the cost to the pharmacy for the product that was sold; see **Equation 14-4**). By supplementing low dispensing fees, earned discounts allow pharmacies to participate in managed care plans that would otherwise have been unprofitable.

$$\text{GM} = \text{Reimbursement} - \text{AAC} \qquad (14\text{-}4)$$

Because earned discounts vary among pharmacies and even for the same pharmacy from time to time, managed care plans usually do not reimburse pharmacies for their AAC. Instead, the participating pharmacy agreement usually specifies that reimbursement for drug ingredient costs will be based on an estimated acquisition cost (EAC), which is calculated as a percentage of the average wholesale price (**Equation 14-5**).

$$\text{EAC} = \text{AWP} - (x\% \text{ of AWP}) \qquad (14\text{-}5)$$

When a drug product has generic equivalents, managed care plans usually limit reimbursement to the generic price, referred to as the maximum allowable cost (MAC). Each managed care plan creates its own MAC list. On those occasions when a physician requires the pharmacy to dispense the brand-name product, some managed care plans allow full reimbursement for the higher-cost product if the pharmacist indicates that the prescription was a "dispense as written" (DAW) order.

Dispensing Fees

The second part of the reimbursement for a managed care prescription (Equation 14-1) is the dispensing fee paid to the pharmacy. It is a fixed amount that is paid to the pharmacy for each prescription dispensed. PBMs, of course, try to keep total reimbursement for ingredient costs and dispensing fees as low as possible while still maintaining an adequate provider network.

Patient Cost Sharing

The third component of the reimbursement for a managed care prescription (Equation 14-1) is patient cost sharing. Patient cost sharing effectively decreases managed care organizations' prescription costs by shifting some responsibility for payment directly to the patient. This practice not only decreases prescription costs, but may also decrease the utilization rate. It can take one of three forms: (1) a co-payment, (2) a deductible, or (3) co-insurance. Cost-sharing provisions may also include out-of-pocket limits (i.e., a stop-loss provision) or maximum benefit limits.

Under a co-payment system, patients pay a specified dollar amount every time a service is received (for example, $50 per hospital admission or $5 per prescription). Co-payments are the most common form of patient cost sharing for prescription benefits.

A deductible requires patients to cover their own health care expenses until a specified dollar amount has been paid out-of-pocket during a given period of time, usually a year. (For example, the insurance company might begin paying health expenses once a patient has paid $200 of out-of-pocket health care expenses during the policy year.) Because patients may receive health services from several different providers, in the past it has sometimes been difficult to determine exactly when the deductible requirement has been met. The expansion of online computerized claims processing makes it easier to keep track of expenses, encouraging more plans to use deductibles in their programs.

The third form of patient cost sharing, co-insurance, requires the patient to pay a specified percentage (usually 20%) of the cost of the service; the plan pays the remainder. Although co-payments are the most common type of patient cost sharing, the use of coinsurance has been increasing (*The Takeda Prescription Drug Benefit Cost and Plan Design Survey Report*, 2005). Co-payment levels have been increasing significantly since the mid-1990s; coinsurance levels, by contrast, have not changed because the actual dollar amount paid by patients increases as the price of prescriptions increases.

To encourage patients to ask for generic prescriptions, many prescription plans require patients to pay a tiered co-payment: a relatively low co-payment for generic drugs, a higher co-payment for preferred brand-name drugs, and an even higher co-payment for nonpreferred brand-name products. Some plans have created a fourth tier for certain "lifestyle" drugs (e.g., Viagra) that are subject to very high co-payments or 50% co-insurance. A fifth tier is sometimes reserved for nonformulary products, euphemistically referred to as a "100% co-payment." Multi-tiered cost-sharing levels are often coordinated with formulary systems to encourage patients to request that their physicians prescribe lower-cost medications.

Plans without patient cost sharing offer first-dollar coverage. Although first-dollar coverage once was common, most plans now see patient cost sharing as a financial incentive that encourages enrollees to avoid using unnecessary health care services. To be effective, however, patient cost-sharing provisions should not be so high as to discourage use of truly necessary health services.

Payment

To be adequate, the total reimbursement should cover the cost of drug ingredients dispensed (the COGS or AAC) plus the overhead cost incurred by the pharmacy in dispensing the prescription (the cost of dispensing [COD]) and a reasonable return on the pharmacy's investment (the net profit [NP]); see **Equation 14-6.** If reimbursement covers only the pharmacy's cost without any profit, then it pays at the break-even point (BEP). The gross margin is the portion of the reimbursement that exceeds the pharmacy's actual acquisition cost for drug ingredients.

$$\text{Reimbursement} = \overbrace{\text{AAC} + \text{COD}}^{\text{BEP}} + \underbrace{\text{NP}}_{\text{GM}} \qquad (14\text{-}6)$$

For most plans, total reimbursement for a managed care prescription will not exceed the pharmacy's usual and customary (U&C) price (i.e., the price charged most commonly to private-pay patients). Therefore, pharmacy reimbursement is usually the lower of

1. The specified EAC plus the dispensing fee,
2. The specified MAC plus the dispensing fee, or
3. The pharmacy's usual and customary charge.

Some plans are shifting from paying an estimated acquisition cost for drug ingredients based on a percentage of the AWP to a wholesale acquisition cost (WAC). The WAC is based on surveys of wholesale pricing data rather than manufacturers' list prices. Sometimes reimbursement is specified as the WAC plus X percent, with X being somewhere between zero and 2%–3% (**Equation 14-7**).

$$\text{AAC} = \text{WAC} + X\% \qquad (14\text{-}7)$$

Of course, because the AWP is an artificial price, payers are looking for a better way to estimate actual acquisition costs. Instead of calculating the EAC as a percentage of the AWP, they are considering using a figure known as the average manufacturer's price (AMP). Essentially, this price would be based on actual costs charged by manufacturers rather than the supposed wholesale list price. While public policy experts believe that the AMP may be more accurate, it may also prove to be lower than the EAC currently used.

Other Contract Provisions

The participating pharmacy agreement tells the pharmacy how to determine whether a person is eligible for benefits. Usually, eligible beneficiaries receive some form of identification card. Because cardholders often change jobs or insurance plans, the card itself may not be a guarantee of payment; pharmacies may need to confirm eligibility through a computerized eligibility verification system.

The participating pharmacy contract also specifies how pharmacies are to submit claims for reimbursement. In most cases, this step involves submitting electronic claims through the pharmacy's computer at the time the prescription is dispensed. Such an online adjudication system is a major improvement over the old paper claims system because it is faster and less expensive and tells the pharmacy immediately whether the claim will be accepted, the amount of co-payment that should be collected, and the amount that the plan will reimburse for the prescription.

Not all third-party programs cover the same products. A section of the contract titled "limitations" or "exclusions" specifies what is not covered. Some common exclusions are nonprescription drugs (other than insulin), compounded prescriptions, devices (such as syringes), and products used for cosmetic purposes (such as hair growth or wrinkle removal). There may be a maximum quantity that can be dispensed for some products (for example, a 30-day supply). However, some contracts specify a minimum quantity (such as a 3-month supply) that may be dispensed for certain maintenance medications used for chronic conditions.

Almost all contracts reserve the right to audit the pharmacy's records as a deterrent to fraudulent claims. Preferably, the contract specifies the auditing procedures that will be used.

IMPACT OF HEALTH INSURANCE ON PHARMACY

Health insurance has profoundly affected pharmacy. In the past decade, dispensing fees have declined while inventory costs have increased. This has contributed to a decline in the average pharmacy's gross margin from 32.2% of sales in 1986 to 22.1% of sales in 2004—a drop of 10.1 percentage points (West, 2005). As shown in **Table 14-2,** those pharmacies that have survived have maintained net profits at 3% to 4% of sales. They have done so by becoming more efficient and by decreasing their expenses. These efficiencies have been achieved primarily through automation and increased use of pharmacy technicians.

Table 14-2 Changes in Pharmacy Operations, 1986-2004

	1986 (%)	1996 (%)	2004 (%)	Change 1986-2004 (%)
Sales	100	100	100	0
Cost of goods sold	67.8	74.4	77.9	+10.1
Gross margin	32.2	25.6	22.1	- 10.1
Expenses	29.5	22.5	18.5	-11.0
Net profit	2.7	3.1	3.6	+ 0.9

Source: Dankmyer, T. (Ed.). (1997). *1997 NCPA-Searle Digest.* Alexandria, VA: National Community Pharmacists Association; West, D. S. (Ed.). (2005). *2005 NCPA–Pfizer Digest.* Alexandria, VA: National Community Pharmacists Association.

As shown in **Table 14-3,** there is evidence that pharmacies whose pre-scription volumes are dominated by third-parties and managed care organizations (accounting for 75% or more of their total volume) have significantly lower gross margins and lower proprietor's incomes than do pharmacies with lower third-party prescription volumes (less than 50%) (West, 2005). Lower reimbursement requires higher volume to maintain profits. This shift to an economy-of-scale business requires that pharmacies operate very efficiently and reduce unnecessary costs when-ever possible.

Why do pharmacies participate in third-party plans that offer low reim-bursement? The answer to this question is not simple and varies from pharmacy to pharmacy. Some pharmacies accept third-party plans because

Table 14-3 Effect of Third-Party Prescription Volume on Pharmacy Operations, 2004

	Pharmacies with Low Third-Party Activity (<50%)	Pharmacies with High Third-Party Activity (>75%)
Sales	100	100
Cost of goods sold	77.0	79.9
Gross margin	23.0	20.1
Expenses	18.8	17.4
Proprietor's salary	4.2	3.2
Net profit	4.2	2.7
Total income of self-employed proprietor	8.4	5.9

Source: West, D. S. (Ed.). (2005). *2005 NCPA–Pfizer Digest.* Alexandria, VA: National Community Pharmacists Association.

they are reluctant to lose customers who may be buying over-the-counter products and other goods from the front of the store. For others, as long as reimbursement covers the variable costs of the dispensed prescription, fixed expenses can be spread among the larger percentage of private-pay prescriptions. However, this strategy is effective only as long as third-party prescriptions represent a minority portion of a pharmacy's business. Given that the majority of prescriptions are now paid for by third parties, such cost shifting will not be feasible as a long-term strategy.

To survive or prosper in the managed care environment, pharmacy managers must be more than good clinicians—they must also be good managers. They must know their costs and lower them to the greatest extent possible by managing their operations efficiently. Community pharmacy managers must be familiar with the prescription benefit plans sponsored by major employer groups. They should also be prepared to document the value of their services and market these services to local employer groups, labor unions, or plan administrators.

Most pharmacy managers do not have the time or resources to shoulder all of this burden on their own. Consequently, some have tried to work together through a variety of pharmacy organizations, such as volume purchasing groups and pharmacy associations. (There is a limit, however, to the extent to which pharmacies can work together. Because of antitrust laws, they cannot collectively boycott undesirable plans, nor can they collectively negotiate fees with third parties.) Above all, pharmacy managers must understand the health care marketplace and the roles of the various participants in the health insurance industry. Without this knowledge, even the best manager will be unprepared to work effectively in today's rapidly changing health care environment.

CONCLUSIONS

Health insurance has profoundly changed how health care is financed and delivered in the United States. The health insurance industry has grown rapidly during the past few decades and will continue to evolve toward managed care. Although health insurance presents some formidable challenges for pharmacists and other health care providers, it also presents some promising opportunities. All pharmacists—whether staff or managers, community or institutional—are affected by the problems and opportunities presented by health insurance coverage of prescription drugs. The extent to which pharmacists understand the needs of insurance plan sponsors, underwriters, and administrators and are able to minimize problems while maximizing opportunities will help determine the profession's future success.

QUESTIONS FOR FURTHER DISCUSSION

1. What is the difference between controlling costs and managing care? What are some examples of each?
2. How can experience rating decrease premiums and at the same time increase the number of uninsured?
3. How can health insurance companies reduce or prevent problems associated with adverse selection and moral hazard?
4. What is the traditional role of public insurance programs? How might this role change in the future?

KEY TOPICS AND TERMS

Actual acquisition cost (AAC)
Actuary
Adjudication
Adverse selection
Average manufacturer's price (AMP)
Average wholesale price (AWP)
Catastrophic hazard
Co-insurance
Community rating
Coordination of benefits
Co-payment
Deductible
Dispense as written (DAW)
Earned discount
Elimination period
Estimated acquisition cost (EAC)
Experience rating
First-dollar coverage
Fiscal intermediary
Gross margin (GM)
Group policies
Health Insurance Portability and Accountability Act (HIPAA)
Indemnity
Induced demand
Insurable hazard
Insurable interest
Law of large numbers
Major medical insurance
Maximum allowable cost (MAC)
Moral hazard
Open enrollment period

Participating pharmacy agreement
Patient cost sharing
Pharmacy benefits manager (PBM)
Pure risk
Reinsurance
Risk pooling
Risk transfer
Self-insure
Service benefit
Speculative risk
Subrogation
Underwriting

REFERENCES

Associated Press. (2000, April 25). Massive medical bills accounted for 40 pct. of personal bankruptcies in 1999, study says. *St. Louis Post-Dispatch,* p. A3.

Campbell, W. H., & Newsome, L. A. (1995). The evolution of managed care and practice settings. In S. M. Ito & S. Blackburn (Eds.), *A pharmacist's guide to principles and practices of managed care pharmacy* (pp. 1–14). Alexandria, VA: Foundation for Managed Care Pharmacy.

DeNavas-Walt, C., Proctor, B. D., & Lee, C. H. (2006). *Income, poverty, and health insurance coverage in the United States: 2005. Current population reports* (p60-231). Washington, DC: U. S. Government Printing Office.

Fronstin, P., & Snider, S. C. (1996). An examination of the decline in employment-based health insurance between 1988 and 1993. *Inquiry, 33,* 317–325.

Institute of Medicine. (1993). *Employment and health benefits: A connection at risk.* Washington, DC: National Academy Press.

Lannon, C., Brack, V., Stuart, J., Caplow, M., NcNeill, A., Bordley, W. C., & Margolis, P. (1995). What mothers say about why poor children fall behind on immunizations. A summary of focus groups in North Carolina. *Archives of Pediatric Adolescent Medicine, 149,* 1070–1075.

Lee, P. R., Soffel, D., & Luft, H. S. (1992). Costs and coverage: Pressures toward health care reform. *Western Journal of Medicine, 157,* 576–583.

Litman, T. L. (1994). Government and health: The political aspects of health care—a sociopolitical overview. In P. R. Lee and C. L. Estes (Eds.), *The nation's health* (4th ed., pp. 107–120). Boston, MA: Jones and Bartlett.

Pharmaceutical Manufacturers Association. (1973). *Pharmaceutical payment programs: An overview.* Washington, DC: Pharmaceutical Manufacturers Association.

Reinhardt, U. E. (1994). Providing access to health care and controlling costs: The universal dilemma. In P. R. Lee and C. L. Estes (Eds.), *The nation's health* (4th ed., pp. 263–278). Boston, MA: Jones and Bartlett.

Salsberry, P. J., Nickel, J. T., & Mitch, R. (1994). Immunization status of 2-year-olds in middle/upper- and lower income populations: A community survey. *Public Health Nurse, 11,* 17–23.

Santoli, J. M., Huet, N. J., Sith, P. J., Barker, L. E., Halfon, N., et al, (2004). Insurance status and vaccination coverage among US preschool children. *Pediatrics, 113,* 1959–1964.

Schafermeyer, K. W. (1996). Third-party prescription program evaluation. In *Effective pharmacy management* (8th ed., p. 322). Alexandria, VA: National Community Pharmacists Association.

Starr, P. (1982). *The social transformation of American medicine.* New York: Basic Books.

The Takeda Prescription Drug Benefit Cost and Plan Design Survey Report. (2005).

Thamer, M., Richard, C., Casebeer, A. W., & Ray, N. F. (1997). Health insurance coverage among foreign-born US residents: The impact of race, ethnicity, and length of residence. *American Journal of Public Health, 87,* 96–102.

Torrens, P. R., & Williams, S. J. (1993). Understanding the present, planning for the future: The dynamics of health care in the United States in the 1990s. In S. J. Williams & P. R. Torrens (Eds.), *Introduction to health services* (4th ed., pp. 421–429). Albany, NY: Delmar.

West, D. S. (Ed.). (2005). *2005 NCPA–Pfizer Digest.* Alexandria, VA: National Community Pharmacists Association.

Government Involvement in Health Care

Earlene E. Lipowski

Case Scenario

When the postal facility in Mercer County, New Jersey, was found to be contaminated with anthrax in 2001, the local health department had no physician designated to examine the 1,000 postal workers or advise them about prophylactic treatment with antibiotics. It was a Friday evening when the local mayor asked for help from the state health department. He was told that workers should seek prescriptions for antibiotics from their own physicians. Local pharmacies quickly ran out of the drugs of choice just serving the workers who were able to contact their physicians. Other workers started to panic. The administrator of a private hospital located a supply of the antibiotics and arranged for local police to deliver them to his facility. That hospital treated postal workers for the next three days before federal, state, and local governments were able to coordinate their responses (Kahn, 2003). This incident illustrates the need for the government to be involved in health care and the need for advance preparation to respond to disasters to efficiently mobilize resources from multiple agencies at the local, state, and federal levels.

LEARNING OBJECTIVES

Upon completion of this chapter, the student shall be able to:

- Review the evolution of the government's role in health care during the 20th century
- Explain the system of checks and balances among the three branches of government, and cite the benefits of that system with regard to government involvement in health care
- Identify the three basic functional roles of government in the U.S. health care delivery system
- List the major federal agencies involved in health care delivery, and give examples of the services each provides
- Compare and contrast the roles of the federal, state, and local governments in the U.S. health care system

"We the People of the United State, in Order to form a more perfect Union, establish Justice, insure domestic Tranquility, provide for the common defense and promote the general Welfare . . . do ordain and establish this Constitution." (Preamble to the U.S. Constitution, 1787)

CHAPTER QUESTIONS

1. Give at least one example of a governmental function in health care delivery where the federal government takes primary responsibility. Give at least one example where state and local government agencies have primary responsibility.
2. How does government use its police power in ensuring the health of the population? Propose a definition of police power in the context of health care.
3. What are the advantages and disadvantages of dividing the primary responsibilities for health care among multiple levels of government? How is this division consistent with the philosophy of government in the United States?
4. The U.S. Food and Drug Administration (FDA) must balance concerns for patient safety with the demand for timely access to needed medications. How does the FDA attempt to balance these competing objectives?
5. Cite a recent example from the news that illustrates government involvement in the delivery of health care.

INTRODUCTION

Duty, Authority, and Limits

At the most fundamental level, the role of any government is to provide the foundation for social interaction and mutual security. The founding principles of the U.S. government are affirmed in its Constitution. For the United States, the purpose of the union is to guard the common good, including defense, economic welfare, and social well-being. The Tenth Amendment reserves to the states all powers that are not given to the federal government or prohibited by the Constitution. In exchange for the good of the community, member states agree to subordinate their self-interests to that of the federal government.

Neither the U.S. Constitution nor the Bill of Rights makes specific reference to health care. The government claims authority over health matters at the national and state levels because it is reasonable and consistent with the intent of the Constitution. Because no individual or set of individuals can protect and assure the health of the entire population, promoting the health and well-being of the public is considered to be a common good. An individual may procure some of the necessities of living, including food, shelter, clothing, and even personal medical services. However, it is organized action on behalf of the community that sets limits on individual actions to control infectious diseases and ensure safe and clean water, air, and food. Government, therefore, holds the legal power and duty to provide for the well-being of the people.

The Constitution also is the basis for assigning jurisdiction of power among federal, state, and local governments and for setting limits on that power to protect individual liberties. Limits to government rest on the rights of individuals to autonomy, liberty, privacy, personal expression, property, and economic freedom of contract and uses of property (Gostin, 2001).

Of all the provisions within the Constitution, the power to regulate commerce grants the federal government the greatest authority over the rights of both individuals and the states. The regulation of commerce is the basis for environmental protection, occupational health, food and drug purity, and safe drinking water. The power to tax and spend gives the federal government the means to exercise its duties and responsibilities (Gostin, 2001).

State and local governments retain police power to enforce laws and constrain behavior. In matters of health, the states may curtail proprietary freedoms through inspections of health institutions and licenses for professionals. States control the actions of individuals so as to prevent nuisances that threaten health by regulating smoking, inspecting commercial establishments for fire hazards and environmental contaminants, and checking residential property for unsanitary conditions and vermin. State authority also limits personal freedoms in the interest of public health through mandatory vaccination and diagnostic screening programs. The right to personal privacy is subordinate to state requirements for reporting sexually transmitted diseases and partner notification, and individual liberties may be curtailed through isolation and quarantine.

Evolution of Government Role in the 20th Century

It is not surprising that the Constitution did not make specific references to the role of government in health matters. When the Constitution was written and for the first 150 years after its adoption, citizens did not look to government to get involved in their health care needs. Government intervention was limited to protecting the populace from epidemics and meeting the most basic needs of the poor. That situation changed when the calamity of the Great Depression in the 1930s was felt across all levels of society and dramatically altered public sentiment. Americans turned to government to help deal with their immediate needs and to protect them against future uncertainties. The system of health care delivery in the United States evolved slowly from that point, accompanied by many shifts in the government's role and influence (Litman and Robins, 1997; Turnock, 2001).

The Sixteenth Amendment to the Constitution gave the federal government the authority to levy a tax on income early in the 20th century. The states, however, did not have the authority to raise the sums of money needed to address health problems, so they turned to the federal government for assistance (Turnock, 2001). Federal grants beginning in 1935 made it possible for states to establish maternal and child health care services, public health laboratories, and public health departments. The federal government then gained additional power and influence over health care delivery through a succession of programs, including the establishment of the National Institutes of Health in the 1930s, the Centers for Disease Control and Prevention in 1946, the Hospital Services and Construction Act (Hill-Burton) of 1946, and Medicare and Medicaid in 1965. (For more information, see Chapter 1.)

Political debates over the relative roles of state and federal governments arose in the 1980s and 1990s. The states have enjoyed some measure of flexibility in meeting their own priorities through the distribution of funds provided by the federal government for state health care initiatives (i.e., block grant funds). However, the federal government continues to exert considerable influence over the states through its significant involvement in research, regulation, education and training, and technical assistance in health care delivery.

Responsibilities of the Three Branches of Government

Government power at all levels in the United States is divided among three branches of government in accordance with the Constitution. That is, the responsibilities defined by the Constitution are allocated to the legislative, executive, and judicial branches.

Legislative Branch

The first charge that the Constitution gives to Congress is to provide for the common defense and general welfare of the United States. Congress has the sole authority to decide matters of public policy—that is, to organize, fund, and implement government programs. Members of Congress are accountable to their constituents for securing public health and welfare; their constituents are committed to accepting the responsibility for programs that result from Congressional action (Gostin, 2000a).

Congress serves as the forum for identifying problematic conditions or situations in need of change, debating alternative arrangements, and exhorting others to take action to create change. It is the place where antagonists challenge the diagnosis or the prognosis of alleged problems. Elected representatives pay particular attention to disagreements and the intensity of conflict between or among special-interest groups, or to issues that set the special interests of a group against the larger public interest. Congress attends to public opinion and often learns more about matters by convening public hearings. Secondary problems often come to light in Congress and are placed on the political agenda because they are closely linked to a primary problem that is under examination (Longest, 2002).

The legislative role in the health care system is to enact laws necessary to safeguard the population from harm and to promote health. A member of Congress can propose new legislation or modify existing law by introducing a proposal in the form of a bill. Most general health bills are referred to the House Committee on Energy and Commerce and to the Senate Committee on Health, Education, Labor and Pensions for further investigation and deliberation. Any bills involving taxes and expenditure of public funds must also be referred to the House Committee on Ways and Means and to the Senate Committee on Finance.

The Congressional Budget Office (CBO) plays a role at this point as well (www.cbo.gov). Its purpose is to help Congress formulate budget plans, stay within those plans, assess the effects of federal laws, and estimate the impact of proposals on the federal budget—a process known as "scoring" the bill. The CBO does not offer recommendations on legislative options but merely evaluates their economic impact.

A bill that survives committee deliberation on its merits and economic impact is placed on the calendar for a formal vote by the respective body of Congress. Both the House of Representatives and the Senate must approve identical bills before a bill passes to the President for his signature and adoption into law.

Executive Branch

The executive branch is the administrative arm of government under the direction of the Office of the President of the United States. The President is charged with implementing and enforcing the laws passed by the legislative branch. His advisors make up the Cabinet, which includes the heads of 15 executive departments and the Vice President. President George W. Bush used an Executive Order in 2001 to extend Cabinet rank to the Administrator of the Environmental Protection Agency, the Director of the Office of Management and Budget, the Director of National Drug Control Policy, and the U.S. Trade Representative.

Administrative agencies of the executive branch promulgate the regulations needed to implement laws. Reliance on the regulatory process allows for greater flexibility in the design and subsequent revisions. Administrative agencies issue regulations through the notice-and-comment rule-making process, whose conduct is specified in statutes.

Federal laws leave regulatory agencies with little choice but to include the public in the process. A governmental agency that proposes a new regulation must solicit public commentary and is typically open to any person or any organization (Roth, Dunsby, and Bero, 2003). Administrative agencies are charged with giving each individual comment "full and serious consideration." Officials must incorporate valid comments into the revised rule and explain why they rejected others. At the conclusion of the public commentary period, agency staff review, categorize, and analyze each comment on the proposed rule and publish their findings in the *Federal Register.*

Public comment is an important requirement that allows for public participation in the development of regulations. Even if there is widespread agreement on the scientific evidence, the role of science in health regulation is not independent of politics, law, and the mass media (Abraham and Sheppard, 1999). Comments shape the final version of the proposed regulation, increase its public acceptability, and reduce the risk that special-interest groups will unduly influence the regulatory process. If the regulations are formally challenged, the courts hold an agency's interpretation of a statute in high regard because the regulation has been developed through an open rule-making process. Executive agencies may issue manuals, memos, and guidance to accompany laws and regulations. These documents often specify details, which, in effect, have nearly the same force as regulation (Keough and Greene, 2003).

Federal agencies need the capacity to investigate and impose sanctions for the enforcement of their regulatory policies. To enforce some regulations, government agencies need resources to target beneficiaries, validate eligibility for benefits, manage the supply and quality of goods and services, and deliver the goods, services, and payments. The success of a law depends on whether the executive agency has the necessary resources to enforce it, including the authority, money, personnel, status, prestige, information, expertise, technology, physical facilities, and equipment.

The Office of Management and Budget (OMB; www.whitehouse.gov/omb) is the executive branch's counterpart to the CBO. OMB staff members evaluate the effectiveness of agency programs, analyze competing demands for funding, set funding priorities, and formulate annual budget plans. In accord with the Constitution, the President must report to Congress "from time to time" on the state of the union and recommend for consideration such policies in the form of laws that the President believes to be necessary, useful, or expedient.

Judicial Branch

The role of the judicial branch is to interpret the law and ensure that actions of the legislative and executive branches are in conformance with the Constitution. The courts provide oversight when the effects of one policy infringe on, or conflict with, the desired outcomes of other policies. The courts may make decisions regarding the application of a law in a specific situation and determine whether a specific organization acted appropriately in implementing the law.

Where protection of the public health is concerned, the courts consistently have upheld the right of government to compel adherence to laws and regulations. For example, rulings of the court permit government to collect taxes and expend public resources, and to require members of the community to submit to licensing, inspection, and regulation (Gostin, 2000b). Three general justifications are commonly cited to uphold any intrusion on the rights of a single individual or to force a person to incur economic costs or take other actions that may not be in the individual's self-interest. The courts authorize restraining an individual when (1) there is a risk to the individual, (2) there is a risk to others, or (3) protection is needed for individuals who are judged incompetent or incapable of protecting themselves.

Judicial standards for government actions that affect organizations or groups of individuals require that the government demonstrate (1) a legitimate health threat, (2) compelling reasons for the invasion of personal rights, and (3) the targeted deployment of the least restrictive intervention necessary to substantially reduce the health threat and avoid harm (Gostin, 2001).

Evolution of Government Role in the 21st Century and Beyond

Responsibility for securing the public health and welfare assures widespread government regulatory involvement in modern society. Several historical events at the turn of the 21st century, however, prompted a debate about the appropriate balance between individual liberty, privacy, and paternalism.

First, the emergence of HIV/AIDS and efforts to combat its spread were actually harmed by the traditional practices of disease surveillance and public reporting. HIV-infected persons avoided diagnosis and treatment for fear of being stigmatized. In the meantime, medical practice in general had expanded its regard for individuals' right to refuse treatment, even when they might potentially be life-saving therapies. Public health officials accommodated this higher regard for personal privacy even as it sought to achieve public health ends consistent with the bioethical principles of autonomy and individual rights (Bayer and Fairchild, 2004).

The tension between public health and civil liberties resurfaced with the terrorist attacks carried out on September 11, 2001. Concerns about bioterrorist threats prompted legislative proposals that gave authorities the right to sharply curtail individual freedom and monitor individuals for any conditions that might potentially be related to a sudden outbreak of an infectious disease. The threat of SARS (severe acute respiratory syndrome) and an influenza pandemic generated additional calls for more stringent public health surveillance, isolation, and quarantine. As a result of these events, the tension between the threat of uncertain but potentially catastrophic events and limits to liberty increased.

Although the AIDS crisis and the events of September 11 brought the ever-present balancing act between public and private concerns to the forefront, any resolution of this trade-off will be a long-term process. The leading causes of death in the United States today are, in fact, not acute infectious diseases, but rather chronic illnesses that are related to environmental, social, and behavioral factors such as diet, exercise, smoking, environmental toxins, alcohol and drug abuse, sexual practices, motor vehicle accidents, and firearms. There is broad support for the government's role in restricting individuals when they pose a risk to others. Restrictions imposed on individuals who are at substantial risk to themselves but represent significantly less risk to others smack of paternalism on the part of government, however. Is it an appropriate role of government to mandate motorcycle helmets and seat belts, prohibit smoking outdoors, or regulate fast-food restaurants that allegedly are fueling an epidemic of obesity (Bayer and Fairchild, 2004)? Some view this debate as a matter of moral judgment rather than ethics (Hall, 2003). Other legal scholars argue that it is not a matter of justice if any restrictions on civil liberties are applied equally to all for the good of society as a whole (Epstein, 2003).

The irony is that the current debate has forged strange ideological alliances—for example, libertarians may side with tobacco and other business interests in support of individual rights and be pitted against the social welfare concerns of modern society (Bayer and Colgrove, 2002). Public policy debates of the 21st century will continue to sort out the circumstances in which the rights of the individual must be subordinated to the needs of the community.

GOVERNMENT HEALTH FUNCTIONS AND ORGANIZATION

Functional Roles

The involvement of the U.S. government in the delivery of health care is currently geared toward the identification, formation, and implementation of health policy. Some policies lead to health delivery functions that are funded, organized, and executed by the private sector without direct government intervention. At other times, and in certain circumstances, the government has faced the necessity to fund and organize the delivery of health care itself.

Payer

Government decisions in the financing of health care are meant to satisfy three objectives: (1) ensure adequate funding, while avoiding excessive expenditures; (2) regulate the health insurance market and pool risk when market failure causes uneven distribution of goods and services; and (3) subsidize care for the poor and disadvantaged.

The government is the largest purchaser of health care services in the United States, accounting for nearly half (45%) of all national expenditures related to health (Smith et al., 2006). The major share, representing more than 50% of total federal expenditures, is spent on the Medicare program, which serves 42.1 million elderly and permanently disabled individuals, and the Medicaid program, which serves 44.7 million indigent persons (Smith et al., 2006). The government also is a significant purchaser of health insurance coverage as an employer. Government, including state and local units, school districts, and public utilities, employed 23 million people in 2004, over 15% of the total U.S. workforce (Bureau of Labor Statistics, 2006). Other significant expenditures include the purchase of health care for military personnel and their dependents through the Department of Defense and programs for retired and former members of the military conducted through the Department of Veterans Affairs.

The United States is unique in being the only major developed country that does not provide universal health care coverage for its citizens. In recent years, government financing of health care has moved forward in

incremental steps in response to concerns about the significant proportion of the population without health insurance coverage.

One of the programs that expand the government's role as a payer is the State
Children's Health Insurance Program (SCHIP). Federal funds were made
available to states in 1997 for expansion of Medicaid eligibility to children
younger than 19 years of age who otherwise would not qualify for coverage
because their family income exceeds the Medicaid threshold. SCHIP covers
4.2 million children from families with incomes up to 200% of the federal
poverty level who are not covered under a private insurance plan.

A second, limited example of an expansion program is the Program of
All-inclusive Care for the Elderly (PACE), which was first funded in
1997. PACE provides community-based care for persons aged 55 or older
who would otherwise qualify for placement in a long-term care facility. A PACE team coordinates medical care and social services with the
goal of better coordination of benefits from both Medicare and Medicaid. Medicare also began offering coverage for outpatient prescription
drugs for all Medicare recipients in 2006; this program represents both
an expansion of services and a significant redistribution of prescription
drug expenditures from Medicaid to Medicare.

Provider

Whereas Medicare and Medicaid are financed by the government, the
health care delivered through these programs is purchased from providers in the private sector. For active-duty members of the armed forces
and for veterans, health services are not only financed but also provided
directly by government employees at government-owned facilities. The
Veterans Health Administration (VHA) operates one of the largest integrated health services systems in the United States, which includes
approximately 154 medical centers, 875 outpatient clinics, and 136
nursing homes. More than 5.3 million people received care in Veterans
Administration (VA) health care facilities in 2005 (www1.va.gov).

Originally, the VA health care system was created to treat injuries and
provide rehabilitation services for disabilities resulting from military
service. Although these services remain priorities, the VA has since
extended care to veterans with low incomes or special health care needs
if they can be accommodated using existing resources. As a result, the
VA is supplying increasingly more care for conditions not related to military service. The VA system annually is used by approximately 65% of
all disabled and low-income veterans. In 2005, it treated 587,000 inpatients and registered 57.5 million visits to VA outpatient clinics.

The Department of Defense operates a substantial health care program
that provides medical services to active-duty members and retired personnel of the armed forces, their dependents, and their survivors. The

hospitals and clinics for active-duty members are primarily staffed by military personnel. Dependents of active-duty troops and retirees also can obtain services at military facilities if space is available. Otherwise, they receive medical care under managed care and fee-for-service plans through TriCare. TriCare combines the medical resources of the Army, Navy, and Air Force in the United States, Europe, Latin America, and the Pacific, and then supplements them with networks of civilian health care professionals and facilities.

In addition to directly providing health care services, the government serves an important function as a provider of health care information through agencies at all levels of government and through the public education system (Novick and Mays, 2001). This information ranges from basic scientific research with applications in health care to consumer-friendly health promotion and guidance about self-care practices. Examples of these activities are presented later in this chapter, along with a description of their specific agency sponsors.

Regulator

Laws and regulations are the tools that the government uses to control the public environment and protect it from threats created by the actions of groups and individuals. The government performs surveillance and enforcement functions in addition to carrying out development and implementation of laws and regulations.

When members of the public seek health care, the government regulates the services that are provided and the education and certification of those who provide the services. Government agencies also ensure fair and adequate access to services and basic standards of quality. Finally, the government monitors the health care marketplace to address adverse consequences of market failures that might endanger the availability, cost, or quality of medical care.

A Multilayered, Multifaceted Organizational Structure

Health care delivery rests on many supporting elements, ranging from the discovery, application, and dissemination of scientific research, to the inspection and enforcement of law and regulations, to education of the public and health care professionals, to harnessing and monitoring the impact of changing technology. All three branches of government at the federal, state, and local levels have roles to play in health care delivery, including the roles of payer, provider, and regulator.

Other chapters in this book describe in greater detail how the government carries out many of its most important responsibilities. This chapter provides an overview of the organizational structure that houses the various government functions at the federal, state, and local levels. At the federal level, this chapter can be quite specific in describing the organization and delivery of one or more of an agency's specific functions. Each state and territory, however, is free to organize its own functions in a way that is consistent with the distribution, size, and needs of its population. For this reason, the involvement of government in health delivery at the state level is described here in more general terms. Needs and resources are most closely specified at the level of local governments. By its very nature, health care is delivered to individual persons by individual organizations in specific locales. Consequently, the organizations that deploy health services are highly varied and difficult to characterize in detail.

A policy is rarely implemented by a single organization; instead, when the scope of the policy is broad, a myriad of organizations are involved in turning the policy into reality. The health care system is so complex that many different agencies inevitably come in contact with people. Furthermore, the determinants of health are not confined to the health care sector but require government programs in many areas (Koop, Pearson, and Schwarz, 2002). Overlap is present at the interface between agencies. The flow of goods and services through the health care system generates effects that ripple across organizational charts and geographical divisions. Some degree of overlap is desirable as well as inevitable.

Our brief review focuses on the more particular assignments of responsibilities, rather than the interfaces between government entities. Students of the health care delivery system will inevitably encounter apparent duplications of efforts across organizational and geographical boundaries, just as the roles and responsibilities of various health care professionals overlap to ensure continuity of care.

FEDERAL GOVERNMENT

Department of Health and Human Services

The Department of Health and Human Services (DHHS) is home to many government programs whose functions are related to health care. The Secretary of DHHS is a member of the President's Cabinet and is responsible for nearly 25% of government spending for fiscal year 2007, both discretionary and by entitlement. **Figure 15-1** shows the organization chart for DHHS. This and other chapters in this book describe many offices within DHHS that are engaged in the delivery of health services and directly involved in the formation of health policy. Other offices and agencies provide primarily social services or deliver administrative and support functions within DHHS. DHHS assumes a significant role in the research and development activities of the health care system, by conducting and sponsoring fundamental research, assuring the safety of food and drugs, and monitoring the adoption of information technology.

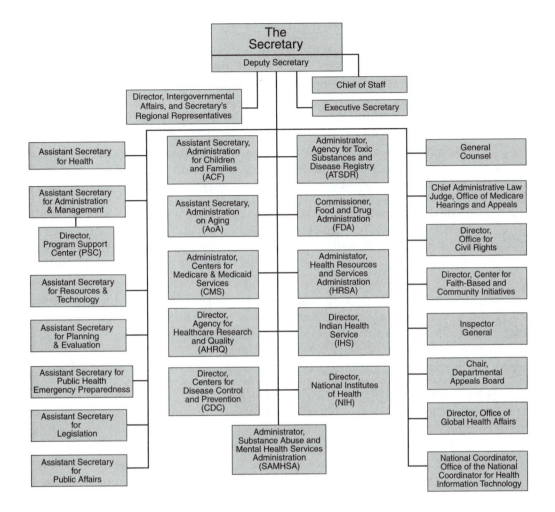

Figure 15-1 Department of Health and Human Services Organizational Chart. *Source:* U.S. Department of Health and Human Services.

Centers for Medicare and Medicaid Services

The Centers for Medicare and Medicaid Services (CMS) is the largest agency within DHHS. Altogether about one fourth of all Americans are covered through health programs operated by CMS. CMS has three operating divisions: the Center for Medicare Management, which oversees the traditional Medicare program; the Center for Beneficiary Choices, which administers Medicare's managed care options; and the Center for Medicaid and State Operations, which has responsibility for state-administered programs including the survey and certification of Medicare providers, operation of the SCHIP, and regulation of self-insured employers. Chapter 17 explains the Medicare and Medicaid programs in more detail.

Health Resources and Services Administration

The Health Resources and Services Administration (HRSA) assures access to health care services for people who have low incomes, are uninsured, or live in rural areas or urban neighborhoods where health resources are scarce. HRSA provides services to people with AIDS under the Ryan White Care Act, works to improve the health of mothers and children, and offers primary care to 14 million people annually through a national network of 3,700 community and migrant health centers or in clinics for the homeless and residents of public housing. HRSA also oversees the U.S. organ transplantation system.

The National Health Service Corps is housed within HRSA. Its goal is to recruit culturally competent clinicians for medically underserved areas in partnership with communities and states, educational institutions, and professional organizations. Under the National Health Service Corps' programs, students in the health professions find career opportunities and professional experiences supported through the Scholarship and Loan Repayment Programs and Student/Resident Experiences and Rotations in Community Health (SEARCH) program.

Indian Health Service

The Indian Health Service (IHS) works with tribes to make health services available to nearly 1.6 million American Indians and Alaska Natives from 557 federally recognized tribes who live on reservations, often in rural and sparsely populated areas. The IHS provides primary and specialized health care services that would otherwise be unavailable, such as dental clinics and residential substance abuse treatment centers. Patients who are covered the IHS and need specialty care are often referred to private facilities for treatment.

Food and Drug Administration

The Food and Drug Administration (FDA) is responsible for assuring the safety of foods and cosmetics and the safety and efficacy of pharmaceuticals, biological products, and medical devices. This agency traces its history to 1906, when Congress passed the Pure Food and Drug Act.

Because drugs have been the fastest-growing cost component of health care in the past decade, and because prescription drugs represent the single most important out-of-pocket medical expense for most Americans, the role of the FDA has come under intense scrutiny. Its role offers a prime example of the tension that exists between government paternalism and individual autonomy. Many citizens misunderstand the function of the FDA and incorrectly believe that the agency itself tests drug products. For all of these reasons, the drug approval process is described here in some detail.

The FDA reviews new molecular entities (NMEs), which are drugs that have never been marketed in the United States. A streamlined application process is in place for generic equivalents of drugs that are already approved for marketing in this country. The FDA issues guidelines for basic research and safety testing in animals before clinical testing may begin. Human testing is conducted in phases, involving progressively larger numbers of people at each phase, as a way to limit exposure to dangerous products. The review process can be halted at any point if findings suggest that the drug lacks efficacy or safety.

In the preclinical (animal testing) phase, scientists study the chemical and physical properties of the molecular entity. Dosage forms are designed and tested, and chemical engineers develop optimal ways to manufacture adequate quantities of the drug product. Patents are filed to protect the intellectual property rights of the inventor.

The approval process begins with the investigational new drug (IND) application, which is filed following toxicology and safety testing of the drug in animals. An IND application includes the results of preclinical tests, research protocols for the initial clinical trials, and a general overview of studies to follow. The applicant also details the manufacturing process—facilities, equipment, and techniques—needed to produce the drug. FDA approval of the IND allows the manufacturer to proceed with clinical trials in humans. At this point, the FDA rates the drug as either "standard" or "priority" to distinguish those chemical entities that will receive priority attention because they may represent a significant therapeutic improvement over existing treatments.

FDA staff members review the procedures and scrutinize data from the trials submitted by the manufacturer. The agency's procedures are intended to ensure that all research participants are well informed of potential benefits and risks and that their decision to participate in a clinical trial is freely given and documented. The first human trials (Phase I) are small, generally including 20–100 healthy volunteers, with the goals of assessing safety, studying drug metabolism and excretion, and documenting pharmacological response. Phase I results are used to calculate the sample size and length of testing needed to establish efficacy in the next phase of clinical studies.

In Phase II trials, the drug is administered to several hundred individuals who are representative of the patients the drug is intended to treat. Response to most new drugs is compared to placebo and less often to existing treatment. Studies are double blind to reduce the likelihood of bias: Neither the patient nor the caregivers know whether the subject receives the experimental drug or the comparison drug or placebo. When the drug is intended for the treatment of chronic diseases, investigators seek data about clinical endpoints including morbidity, mortality, or quality of life in addition to changes in biochemical, physiological, or anatomical attributes. Various doses are compared and additional safety data are gathered. Phase II trials generally last about 2 years.

Phase III trials are controlled clinical studies that are conducted with several hundred to thousands of persons and are intended to demonstrate that the drug has statistically significant safety and effectiveness. Information gathered through these clinical trials determines the content of the product label and package insert required by the FDA. Phase III trials may last as long as 3 years or more so that they can establish the longer-term safety and efficacy of the product.

The drug developer files a new drug application (NDA) after it completes Phase III trials with the drug. The FDA reviews a summary of results from all clinical trials and the procedures planned for the drug's manufacture, formulation, and quality control. The agency may then issue an approval letter, specify conditions under which approval might be granted, or grant no approval. In the latter cases, the sponsor of the NDA may respond to FDA requests for additional information or withdraw the NDA from further consideration. Most NDAs require at least one amendment to the original application and many require several such changes.

FDA approval gives the applicant the right to market the new drug as safe and effective for specific indications supported by evidence. Although individual physicians retain the right to prescribe a drug for "off-label" uses, the manufacturer may promote only the approved uses.

The FDA includes two review centers. The Center for Drug Evaluation and Research (CDER) grants approval to new chemical entities, antibiotics, hormones, and enzyme products pursuant to an NDA. The Center for Biologics Evaluation and Research (CBER) reviews biotechnological drug products and vaccines and grants approval to both a product license application (PLA) to cover the drug and an establishment license application (ELA) to cover safety and quality assurance procedures for facilities where product will be manufactured.

After a drug is marketed to the public, the manufacturer is required to notify FDA about uncommon, yet serious, adverse reactions that were not found in the clinical trial phases but become evident when the drug is used in a broader population. This stage, known as Phase IV or postmarketing surveillance, is especially critical in cases when a priority drug undergoes an accelerated approval process. If the FDA judges a drug to be too hazardous after its original approval, it may request the manufacturer to issue a warning, revise the product label, or withdraw the product from the market.

The FDA regulates all aspects of pharmaceutical marketing. Its regulations aim to assure health professionals and the public that all promotional claims are based on scientific evidence and that the information presented is complete, truthful, and balanced with regard to risks and benefits.

The availability of new drugs has important implications for the nation's overall health status, health expenditures, social equity, and economic growth (Schweitzer, 1997). In 1994, Congress responded to manufacturer complaints about excessive FDA-review times that peaked at 21.2 months. The Prescription Drug User Fee Act authorized the FDA to collect fees from the companies submitting applications and hire more reviewers, improve computer support, and reduce review time. As a result of these measures, review time fell to 12.7 months by 2000 for all new NDAs and 13.4 months for reviews involving NMEs. Congress has continued to reauthorize the collection of user fees.

In the case of the FDA, the role of government involves maintaining a delicate balance between safety and access to potentially beneficial treatments. Criticism of the process is frequent and inevitable from those with competing interests.

National Institutes of Health

The National Institutes of Health (NIH) comprises 27 health institutes and centers that support research on diseases including cancer, diabetes, arthritis, Alzheimer's disease, and investigation of the human genome. NIH funds some 38,000 medical and social science research projects nationwide. In addition, a large research and treatment program is under way at NIH headquarters in Bethesda, Maryland.

Government involvement is particularly critical for the support of health research in cases where economic incentives are lacking or risky. For example, drugs to treat conditions that are poorly understood or that affect small numbers of people have limited appeal to commercial firms. NIH also funds basic research where the commercial application of knowledge to be gained is unclear, uncertain, or unlikely in the short term (Koop et al., 2002).

The National Library of Medicine (NLM) is a part of NIH. NLM is the world's largest medical library. A leader in informatics, it established *Medline* in 1971. Use of NLM's holdings greatly expanded with Internet access and services like *Medline Plus,* which provides worldwide access to full-text, peer-reviewed literature for reference librarians, medical professionals, biomedical researchers, and the general public.

Agency for Health Care Research and Quality

The mission of the Agency for Health Care Research and Quality (AHRQ) is the creation and dissemination of knowledge that enhances the quality, appropriateness, and effectiveness of health services and access to services. AHRQ supports researchers who study the organization, financing, delivery, quality assessment, and improvement of the health delivery system through basic research, evaluation studies, and demonstration projects. In addition, this agency conducts the Medical Expenditure Panel Survey, which produces national estimates related to health status, health insurance coverage, and health care use, expenditures, and sources of payment.

Centers for Disease Control and Prevention

The Centers for Disease Control and Prevention (CDC) works to prevent and control infectious and chronic diseases, injuries, workplace hazards, disabilities, and environmental health threats. It sets national health status goals through its Healthy People program and maintains the National Center for Health Statistics from its headquarters in Atlanta, Georgia. CDC personnel are stationed in more than 25 foreign countries to guard against transmission of disease and respond to health emergencies internationally.

The Agency for Toxic Substances and Disease Registry (ASTDR) is closely affiliated with the CDC. ASTDR coordinates programs that aim to prevent exposure to hazardous substances and conducts public health assessments, studies, and surveillance for persons who are exposed to hazardous materials. The agency maintains exposure and disease registries for study and long-term follow-up.

Assistant Secretary for Planning and Evaluation

The Assistant Secretary for Planning and Evaluation (ASPE) has an important role in health policy formation within DHHS. This office advises the department on policy needs in health, disability, human services, and science. ASPE coordinates the evaluation, research, and demonstration activities of DHHS; it also directly performs some studies and leads other demonstration projects. ASPE staff manages strategic planning, legislative planning, and review of regulations, including policy analyses and cost-benefit evaluations of policy options.

Substance Abuse and Mental Health Services Administration

The Substance Abuse and Mental Health Services Administration (SAMHSA) gathers and disseminates information on health problems related to the use and abuse of drugs and alcohol and the mental health condition of the U.S. population. SAMHSA's work is conducted primarily through block grants to states, which then direct the distribution of funds for substance abuse and mental health services at the local level.

Administration on Aging

The Administration on Aging (AoA) works through a nationwide network to provide services designed to maintain elders in independent living sites—especially those who are disadvantaged by disparities in the financial, social, or health resources available to them. The AoA network provides home-delivered meals, preventive health care services, transportation to medical appointments and shopping, personal care services, adult day care, and caregiver support. In addition, AoA provides health insurance and pension counselors and ombudsmen to serve older persons in long-term care institutions.

Other Executive Agencies

DHHS is, by far, the largest of the federal agencies concerned with the U.S. health care system. Although the remaining Cabinet-level agencies have policy areas that are tangential to health care delivery, they nevertheless play a role in the provision of health care and protect national resources that are essential to the health and welfare of the nation. The well-being of Americans goes well beyond medical care and, because health matters are so pervasive, there is inevitably some degree of overlap and interdependence among all government functions.

Oversight and Advisory Bodies

Congressional Committees

After Congress enacts a law, one of the executive agencies promulgates regulations to implement the law and then enforces the law and its corresponding regulations. However, Congress has the ultimate responsibility for oversight of the implementation of laws it enacts. The objectives of the oversight activities are to ensure that

- The implementation of the law is consistent with congressional intent.
- Programs operate effectively and efficiently.
- Organizations and activities of individuals are managed against fraudulent, dishonest, inept, or capricious behavior.
- The laws and regulations serve the public interest.

Responsibility is assigned to the committee that has jurisdiction over the policy area and to specific oversight committees or subcommittees. Congressional staff members may undertake investigations, subpoena witnesses, and conduct hearings to document these activities.

Government Accountability Office

The Government Accountability Office (GAO) is the investigative arm of Congress. It exists to improve the performance and accountability of the government by supporting the responsibilities of Congress for legislative oversight, policy formation, and funding. GAO staff evaluate federal programs and activities, examine the use of public funds, and provide the office's analyses, options, and recommendations to Congress. Although any member of Congress may make a GAO request, priority is given to work requested by committee chairs and ranking minority members. GAO staff issue public reports of their investigations and frequently testify before Congressional committees.

Office of the Inspector General

The mission of the Office of Inspector General (OIG) is to protect the integrity of executive departments and programs and the health and welfare of the beneficiaries of its programs. The OIG reports both to the Secretary of the Department of Health and Human Services and to the Congress about program and management problems and makes recommendations to correct those problems. OIG staff carry out these duties through nationwide audits, investigations, inspections, and other project-specific strategies.

National Academy of Sciences and Institute of Medicine

The National Academies are nonprofit, honorary societies that were originally established by Congress at the time of the Civil War. The Institute of Medicine (IOM) is one of its component organizations. NAS, including IOM, works independently of the government by convening volunteer committees of experts to seek their advice about science, technology, and medicine. They sponsor symposia, roundtables, and forums on national issues; publish proceedings from conferences and workshops; and issue white papers that take stands on pressing scientific concerns. Recommendations of IOM dealing with health care delivery carry significant weight with members of the public and Congress. Its reports generate some of the nation's most important initiatives to improve health, education, and public welfare.

STATE GOVERNMENTS

Although the federal government is the primary payer for health care of poor and uninsured people through Medicaid, states are responsible for a share of those costs and the administration of the program. Medicaid represents a substantial and ever-increasing portion of individual state budgets (see Chapter 17). In addition to Medicaid, state and local governments administer a small number of programs that provide direct care for persons who do not qualify for any of the federal health care programs. State services frequently include hospitals for the mentally ill and developmentally disabled, general hospitals operated by county and municipal governments, community health centers, and health departments. In recent years, states have taken on an important role in experimenting with innovative health reform strategies in an effort to provide the necessary services with the limited funds available to them.

Each state establishes its own organizational structure for carrying out its responsibilities within the health care delivery system. However, the overall programs and services are similar across states. Two important functions common to state governments are: (1) professional regulation and licensure, and (2) regulation of the health insurance industry.

Professional Regulation and Licensure

Each state has boards that administer a licensure system responsible for controlling entry into the medical professions. Licensure statutes date back to the late 19th century, when allopathic physicians established their control over medical practice. Most state boards of pharmacy were instituted a few years later. Many other health professions achieved license status during the 20th century. Initially the boards were constituted solely of members of the regulated profession, but today many state boards include a number of consumer members. State boards are also subject to legislative oversight.

Licensure assures that applicants to a profession have completed basic educational requirements and demonstrated knowledge by examination. Licensure boards do little at present to assure continuing competency. Instead, they act in response to complaints of incompetence or unprofessional or unethical conduct. The boards take disciplinary action when such allegations are substantiated. The most common disciplinary powers are the power to revoke or suspend licenses (Jost, 2003).

Most states also license health care institutions. However, institutions may be exempt from further state inspection if they are accorded accreditation status from a private agency. Because many hospitals are accredited by a private, nonprofit agency (i.e., the Joint Commission on Accreditation of Health Organizations), state licensure plays a secondary role in this area (Pawlson and O'Kane, 2002).

Health Insurance

Employers provide health insurance benefits for the majority of Americans. The federal Employee Benefits Security Administration within the Department of Labor is charged with protecting the integrity of health plans, pensions, and other employee benefits by assisting employers in understanding and meeting their legal responsibilities and by providing workers with information about their benefit rights. State governments also operate offices that remain on the alert for actions that may have an adverse effect on workers' benefits and introduce initiatives intended to encourage sound benefits programs.

Through a Commissioner of Insurance (or similar agency), states oversee health insurance companies, their organizations, marketing practices, and the products they sell, including the products' content, and price.

States require insurance companies to establish capitalization and financial reserves so that these firms will be able to meet their obligations
to the insured. In addition, state regulations control the marketing and
enrollment activities of insurance companies and the establishment of
insurance rates. States often mandate that health insurance plans cover
specific medical services, such as treatment for alcohol abuse, mental
health services, preventive care, and diagnostic services. Finally, states
support the rights of consumers to file malpractice claims or other actions
that hold insurers and contracted providers accountable for quality care.

Workers' Compensation

Although U.S. workers generally rely on their employers as a source of
health care insurance, injuries and illnesses that occur in the workplace
or are related to workers' employment or occupation are traditionally considered a separate responsibility of industry. That is, an employer is held
financially responsible for treatment of the injury or illness regardless of
how fault is assigned. Workers' compensation was established separately
from health insurance benefits to cover work-related health care. These
funds are used primarily as payment for medical treatment. There are
also provisions for cash payments to replace lost wages, provide benefits
to survivors in the event of an employee's death, and compensate workers who are disabled and unable to resume their former occupation.

Employers are required by law to fully fund workers' compensation
insurance. Employees have no responsibilities for sharing the costs.
The federal government operates separate compensation programs for
coal miners and for railroad workers who suffer injuries linked to these
particular occupations. All other workers' compensation programs are
operated by the states and vary considerably in terms of the financing
mechanisms and levels of benefits they deliver. Depending on the state,
the employer may self-insure by creating its own workers' compensation
fund, purchase private insurance to cover workers' claims, contribute to
a fund established and maintained by the state for this purpose, or participate in some combination of these mechanisms.

Other State Programs

Other activities under state control ensure the public health by taking
the following steps:

- Monitoring the environment, the workplace, and establishments that
  provide food services
- Disease prevention activities that include nutritional services, school
  health, and campaigns to promote healthy behavior regarding tobacco
  use and traffic safety, and communicable disease control
- Public health nursing services, including family planning and prenatal care

Although a state may organize and coordinate these services, their delivery is most often the responsibility of the local government.

LOCAL GOVERNMENTS

National health policy identifies the range of health, morbidity, disability, and mortality issues it intends to address as well as the relevant settings covered by the policy and the framework for implementing the policy in the relevant settings—for example, health services, social services, the education sector, and the workplace. The individual states create political subunits to make those services available to the residents of a particular jurisdiction. Good public policy at the national level specifies the desired goals and the adverse events it intends to minimize, but this merely sets the agenda for planning and delivery of care at a local level (Jenkins, 2001).

The most significant role for local government in the past century centered on three activities: (1) assessing the health needs of the community; (2) devising policies to address those needs; and (3) providing primary and preventive care to all persons without alternative resources. Local emergency situations, including both natural and human-made disasters, also rely on properly trained health care personnel and readily available health care services to meet the immediate needs of citizens. In addition, many localities provide emergency transportation by ambulance as a complement to local fire and rescue services.

Health Department officials are responsible for collecting data on the frequency, trends, and patterns of disease and for maintaining general public health functions such as testing and regulating water quality. They enforce local health codes for sanitation and food safety, implement health education campaigns, and supply population-based preventive care through immunization campaigns, mosquito control programs, and routine health care services for children.

EMERGING ISSUES FOR GOVERNMENT INVOLVEMENT

Health care policy makers continually grapple with a never-ending series of difficult issues. This section presents some issues that currently are demanding government attention.

Privacy and Electronic Medical Records

Concerns for the protection of patient privacy have been a hot topic in discussions about the widespread adoption of electronic medical record systems. Patient advocates fear that a system that maintains sensitive information in an electronic format could be readily accessed and widely distributed. There is a real risk of harm to individuals from disclosure of health information through the health insurance market, particularly when employers purchase that insurance for their workers (Buchanan, Califano, Kahn, McPherson, Robertson, and Brody, 2002).

Although regulations pursuant to the Health Insurance Portability and Accountability Act (HIPAA) are now in place, the unforeseen and unintended consequences of this complex issue—balancing public welfare with individual rights—will continue to demand the attention of the legislative, regulatory, and judicial branches of government. While electronic records offer a clear opportunity for increased efficiency, their adoption remains stymied by concerns about the risk to individual rights as well as technical details and cost constraints related to their implementation.

Consumer-Directed Health Care

The U.S. government is less involved in its citizens' health care delivery than governments in other developed nations. This disengagement in direct care is the result of a strong and persistent belief in the market system as the most appropriate way to organize and deliver health care. The neoconservative view among current elected officials supports the argument that the market can respond better to social and economic problems if there is less interference from government (Williams and Torrens, 2002). As a consequence, there is a growing trend to place more responsibility on the individual to make decisions about the source and mix of health care services to be purchased from a fixed pool of employer or government funding.

If market incentives are favored as the guiding principles of the U.S. health care system, there will continue to be a role for government in assuring that the needs of vulnerable populations are met. Individuals lacking in social status, social capital, or human capital will remain susceptible to harm or neglect. Government intervention will be needed to provide for the health care needs of infants and children, the developmentally disabled and mentally ill, victims of alcohol and substance abuse, immigrants, the homeless, and those disadvantaged by low income or health illiteracy. The extent of government responsibility and the appropriate action will remain a matter of public policy in the United States, just as it has in the past.

The Uninsured

Between 2000 and 2004, the number of uninsured persons in the United States grew by 5 million to reach a total of 45.5 million people (kff.org, 2006). Numerous studies have shown that the uninsured receive less preventive care, are diagnosed at more advanced stages of disease, and once diagnosed receive fewer prescription drugs and other treatment modalities such as surgical procedures (Hadley, 2002). Many of the uninsured seek care that ultimately goes uncompensated—primarily from hospitals, but to some extent from clinics, community health centers, and private physicians. Medicare and Medicaid programs offset a share of the expenses that institutions must shoulder when they render a disproportionate share of charity care. Increasingly, however, a case is being made for establishing a formal direct system of coverage. Incremental programs, such as the expansion of Medicaid benefits to pregnant women and SCHIP programs for uninsured children, may continue to appear in the absence of a coordinated national program to provide a universal health insurance benefit. (See Chapter 20 on health care reform for more details.)

While public awareness about the plight of the uninsured is growing, difficult policy decisions stand in the way of providing a comprehensive approach to the problem. While some factions argue for the expansion of public insurance, opponents point to the large number of persons eligible for existing programs who do not enroll. Some parties favor direct cash payments, others advocate for a tax credit to provide incentives for individuals and small employers to purchase health insurance in the private sector, and still others favor expanding eligibility for existing public programs such as Medicaid, SCHIP, and Medicare (Kovner and Jonas, 2002).

CONCLUSIONS

The government's role in health care in the United States is very different from that of other developed nations; nevertheless, it is extensive. Federal, state, and local governments in the United States serve as providers, financers, and regulators of health care services, information, and research. While the federal government's role as a provider of health care is much more limited than that of national governments in other countries, it does provide health care services through the Department of Defense, Department of Veterans' Affairs, and the Indian Health Service.

Rather than providing direct services, the U.S. federal government is more involved in financing health care services through programs such as Medicare and Medicaid and research and information services through NIH, AHQR, HRSA, and other programs. The federal government, through agencies such as FDA, CDC, and CMS, also provides regulation and oversight of health care.

State and local governments also fulfill important roles, sometimes in collaboration with the federal government and sometimes independently. States collaborate with the federal government by administering and partially funding Medicaid. Independent functions include licensure of health care professionals and institutions, regulation of the health insurance industry, protection of public health, and other programs. State governments directly provide health care services through state hospitals for specific purposes such as mental illness and mental retardation. Local governments provide care through county and city hospitals and health clinics.

The extent of the government's role in health care has always been a matter of controversy. Government success in matters of public policy depends on having a well-defined problem, workable solutions, and a clear direction for developing effective interventions. All three criteria for success require a succinctly articulated consensus. Even when there is a clear mandate and correct decisions are made, circumstances may change over time. Changes that are biological, cultural, demographic, ecological, economic, ethical, legal, psychological, social, and technological in nature make laws and regulations outdated. There is an unrelenting pressure to modify policies and programs.

QUESTIONS FOR FURTHER DISCUSSION

1. Does form follow function in the government's organization of its health care activities? That is, are U.S. government agencies organized around health care activities that have similar functions, similar resource needs, or overlapping jurisdictions? What are the advantages and disadvantages of this organizational structure?
2. Imagine that scientists discover a vaccine for HIV.
   a. What issues might the government face in an effort to establish public policy in this area? Which stakeholders and special-interest groups are apt to be involved in the debate?
   b. What government activities do you think would be involved in public immunization programs?
3. Should the federal government regulate the prices of drugs? If the government were to set prices for drugs, what changes could occur in the market for pharmaceuticals in the United States?
4. What are the advantages and disadvantages of having different roles and responsibilities for federal, state, and local governments with regard to health care?

KEY TOPICS AND TERMS

Administration on Aging (AoA)
Administrative agencies
Agency for Health Care Research and Quality (AHRQ)
Agency for Toxic Substances and Disease Registry (ATSDR)

Assistant Secretary for Planning and Evaluation (ASPE)
Centers for Disease Control and Prevention (CDC)
Centers for Medicare and Medicaid Services (CMS)
Commissioner of Insurance
Congressional Budget Office (CBO)
Department of Health and Human Services (DHHS)
Food and Drug Administration (FDA)
Government Accountability Office (GAO)
Health Insurance Portability and Accountability Act (HIPAA)
Health Resources and Services Administration (HRSA)
Human trials—Phases I, II, III, and IV
Indian Health Service (IHS)
Institute of Medicine (IOM)
Investigational new drug (IND)
Local health departments
Medicaid
Medicare
National Institutes of Health (NIH)
National Library of Medicine (NLM)
New drug application (NDA)
New molecular entity (NME)
Office of the Inspector General (OIG)
Office of Management and Budget (OMB)
Preclinical tests
Program of All-Inclusive Care for the Elderly (PACE)
State Children's Health Insurance Program (SCHIP)
Substance Abuse and Mental Health Services Administration
    (SAMHSA)
TriCare
Veterans Administration
Workers' compensation

REFERENCES

Abraham, J., & Sheppard, J. (1999). Complacent and conflicting scientific expertise in British and American drug regulation: Clinical risk assessment of triazolam. *Social Studies of Science, 29*(6), 803–843.

Bayer, R., & Colgrove J. (2002). Bioterrorism, public health, and the law. *Health Affairs, 21*(6), 98–101.

Bayer, R., & Fairchild, A. L. (2004). The genesis of public health ethics. *Bioethics, 18*(6), 473–492.

Buchanan, A., Califano, A., Kahn, J., McPherson, E., Robertson, J., & Brody, B. (2002). Pharmacogenomics: Ethical issues and policy options. *Kennedy Institute of Ethics Journal, 12*(1), 1–15.

Bureau of Labor Statistics. (2006). U.S. *Career Guide to Industries, 2006-07 Edition.* Retrieved January 24, 2007 from http://www.bls.gov/oco/cg/cg10010.htm

Epstein, R. A. (2003). Let the shoemaker stick to his last: A defense of the "old" public health. *Perspectives in Biology and Medicine, 46*(3 suppl), S138–S159.

Gostin, L. O. (2000a). Public health law in a new century. Part I: Law as a tool to advance the community's health. *Journal of the American Medical Association, 283*, 2837–2841.

Gostin, L. O. (2000b). Public health law in a new century. Part III: Public health regulation: A systematic evaluation. *Journal of the American Medical Association, 283*, 3118–3122.

Gostin, L. O. (2001). Public health theory and practice in the constitutional design. *Health Matrix, 11*(2), 265–326.

Hadley J. (2002, May). Sicker and poorer: The consequences of being uninsured. Menlo Park, CA: Kaiser Family Foundation.

Hall, M. A. (2003). The scope and limits of public health law. *Perspectives in Biology and Medicine, 46*(3 suppl), S199–S209.

Jenkins, R. (2001). Making psychiatric epidemiology useful: The contribution of epidemiology to government policy. *Acta Psychiatrica Scandanavica, 103*, 2–14.

Jost, T. S. (2003). Legal issues in quality of care oversight in the United States: Recent developments. *European Journal of Health Law, 10*, 11–25.

Kahn, L. H. (2003). A prescription for change: The need for qualified physician leadership in public health. *Health Affairs, 22*(4), 241-248.

Keough, C. L., & Greene, A. (2003). Judicial review of CMS policies: An evolving doctrine. *Healthcare Financial Management, 57*(2), 76–80.

Koop, C. E., Pearson, C. E., & Schwarz, M. R. (2002). *Critical issues in global health.* San Francisco: Jossey-Bass.

Kovner, A. R., & Jonas, S. (2002). *Health care delivery in the United States* (7th ed.). New York: Springer.

Litman, T. J., & Robins L. S. (1997). *Health politics and policy* (3rd ed.). Albany, NY: Delmar.

Longest, B. B., Jr. (2002). *Health policymaking in the United States* (3rd ed.). Chicago, IL: Health Administration Press.

Novick, L. E., & Mays, G. P. (2001). *Public health administration: Principles for population-based management.* Gaithersburg, MD: Aspen.

Pawlson, L. G., & O'Kane, M. E. (2002). Professionalism, regulation, and the market: Impact on accountability for quality of care. *Health Affairs, 21*(3), 200–207.

Roth, A. L., Dunsby, J., & Bero, L. A. (2003). Framing processes in public commentary on U.S. federal tobacco control regulation. *Social Studies of Science, 33*(1), 7–44.

Schweitzer, S. O. (1997). *Pharmaceutical economics and policy.* New York, NY: Oxford University Press.

Smith, C., Cowan C., Heffler, S., Catlin, A., et al. (2006). Trends: National health spending in 2004: Recent slowdown led by prescription drugs. *Health Affairs, 25*(1), 186–196.

Turnock, B. J. (2001). *Public health: What it is and how it works* (2nd ed.). Gaithersburg, MD: Aspen.

Williams, S. J., & Torrens, P. R. (2002). *Introduction to health services* (6th ed.). Albany, NY: Delmar.

CHAPTER 16

Managed Health Care

Kenneth W. Schafermeyer

Case Scenario

Viagra, which was approved by the Food and Drug Administration (FDA) in early 1998, is indicated for the treatment of erectile dysfunction but may also improve healthy men's sexual performance. Initial sales of this drug were staggering, with doctors writing as many as 40,000 prescriptions per day (Gillis, 1998b). With such prescription volume, Viagra was on pace to become the best-selling drug in history. Urologists established waiting lists for men seeking appointments that would lead to prescriptions. At a Georgetown University clinic, the phone system was modified to "press 3 for Viagra," creating a waiting list of more than 300 (Gillis, 1998a).

The controversy surrounding insurance coverage of Viagra transcends private and public health care institutions. In July 1998, the U.S. Department of Health and Human Services notified state Medicaid agencies that they had to cover Viagra if their Medicaid programs covered prescription medications. The Director of the American Public Welfare Association argued that Viagra, at $10 per tablet, would add $100 million to $200 million to Medicaid expenses across the country and that to insist on coverage without consultation with the states was "unacceptable" (Goldstein, 1998). The head of the Health Care Financing Administration responded that a 1990 law mandates coverage of any prescription drug that has been approved by the FDA with few exceptions, which include diet pills, smoking cessation products, and fertility treatments.

You work for a pharmacy benefits manager, and clients are asking about your company's stance concerning Viagra coverage. What are the key ethical, political, clinical, financial, and equity issues to consider in deciding whether to cover Viagra? What is your recommendation, and why?

How would your recommendation change, if at all, if the client already covers other impotence medications? What if the client currently does not cover oral contraceptives or infertility medications?

One client has decided to cover Viagra but has indicated that it does not want the drug's utilization, and hence its costs, to skyrocket out of control. What are your recommendations in regard to plan design for Viagra (e.g., prior authorization, quantity limits, and cost-sharing levels)?

LEARNING OBJECTIVES

Upon completion of this chapter, the student shall be able to:

- Describe the objectives of managed health care (i.e., access, quality, and cost)
- Differentiate between insuring health and managing health care
- Differentiate between retrospective and prospective payment for services
- Compare and contrast fee-for-service and capitation reimbursement
- Describe and differentiate among the major types of managed care organizations (MCOs)
- Describe the market power of managed care organizations
- List the functions of a pharmacy benefit manager
- Describe MCO tools used to control costs and enhance quality
- Describe the impact of managed care on pharmacy
- Suggest approaches for pharmacists to work successfully with MCOs
- Define third-party and managed care terminology
- Define the organization and method used to accredit MCOs

CHAPTER QUESTIONS

1. What factors have encouraged or hindered the growth of managed care?
2. How do staff-, group-, network-, and IPA-model HMOs differ?
3. Since 1980, what have the enrollment trends been for the four basic types of HMOs?
4. What are the characteristics of the four major tools used to manage the pharmacy benefit?
5. What measures are considered in NCQA accreditation?

INTRODUCTION

Managed care has profoundly affected the way in which medical care is delivered, consumed, and perceived. While there is no universally accepted definition of managed care, most would agree that any movement away from strict payment of services and toward governing of the provision of medical services is a form of managed care. Managed care organizations (MCOs) provide health care services, including prescriptions, to defined populations such as employer groups on a prepaid basis. Because MCOs assume financial risk for expenditures, they have strong incentives to control costs and utilization of health care services. A major challenge facing MCOs has been the need to balance advocacy for patient care against the efficient allocation of scarce resources.

THE HISTORY OF MANAGED CARE

Managed care's roots can be traced to the lodges, fraternal orders, and benevolent societies established in the 1800s by European immigrants to care for their sick and disabled. The first organized health delivery services were offered to recruit employees to work in isolated areas such as pineapple plantations in Hawaii, lumber camps in Michigan, iron ranges in northern Minnesota, and railroads in isolated pockets across the country. Physicians were usually on contract or salary because the best way to recruit physicians was to provide them with a guaranteed income. Hospital beds were either owned or under contract (Friedman, 1996).

The American Medical Association (AMA) did not object to these plans in the rural areas, considering them "an economic necessity." However, the AMA continued to object to any other form of organized medicine that involved a third-party intermediary (Jecker, 1994). By the 1920s, the AMA had established the solo practitioner with a fee-for-service (FFS) reimbursement (where a fee was paid for each service performed) as the predominant model of medical practice (Miller and Luft, 1994). Despite the AMA's opposition, numerous state courts ruled that medical societies could not take actions against physicians who participated in prepaid plans (plans in which patients paid in advance of receiving service for the cost of predetermined benefits) (Jecker, 1994).

The availability of prepaid plans expanded during World War II. Many of the plans formed during that era still exist today (such as Group Health Cooperative of Puget Sound and Kaiser Permanente), but in the early years they generally had some advantage that allowed them to survive in the anti-managed care environment that prevailed at the time (Miller and Luft, 1994).

Perhaps the most famous MCO was, and is, Kaiser Permanente. Henry J. Kaiser, an industrial contractor, called upon Dr. Sidney Garfield to develop a system for providing medical care to his 15,000 workers and dependents, who were building the Grand Coulee Dam in Washington. The Kaiser Company financed everything from hospital equipment to nurses and staff for outpatient clinics, thereby creating an entire medical delivery system. Kaiser covered workers' industrial injuries and illnesses, and employees had the option of contributing 50 cents per week for themselves, 50 cents per week for each adult dependent, and 25 cents per week for each child to cover nonindustrial injuries and illnesses (Campbell and Newsome, 1995).

Eventually, professional organizations came to accept the insurance company as an intermediary because it did not jeopardize the FFS system, maintained the sanctity of the physician–patient relationship, and enhanced physicians' salaries (Miller and Luft, 1994). The passage in 1973 of the Health Maintenance Organization Act was a major catalyst in the growth of managed care (Davis, Collins, and Morris, 1994). The legislation supported start-up grants and loans for health maintenance organizations (HMOs), a type of MCO, and required employers with 25 or more employees to provide HMO enrollment as an alternative to traditional indemnity insurance for their employees where it was available (see Chapter 14 for a description of indemnity insurance). These factors, taken collectively, had a tremendous effect on the growth of managed care. In 1970, there were 3 million enrollees in HMOs; in 1980, there were 9 million HMO members (Miller and Luft, 1994). In 1989, HMO enrollment grew to 35 million enrollees; by 1998, the number had tripled to 105.3 million participants (Hoechst Marion Roussel, 1999).

Perspectives

While we often think managed care is unique to the health care market, Lynn (1991) has compared the evolution of managed care to the events that shaped America's manufacturing sector. Manufacturing began as a cottage industry characterized by inconsistency in products and few standards. By the 1900s, this sector was populated by unrefined mass producers that employed some inspection techniques. The 1920s saw the development of more sophisticated quality assurance (QA) techniques that have resulted in high aggregate quality standards. Medical care was historically a cottage industry as well. It has only recently incorporated some crude QA techniques. Eventually, as information systems and political forces allowed, more sophisticated QA techniques were implemented that incorporated the use of practice guidelines and statistical analyses (Lynn, 1991). As MacLeod (1996) has pointed out, medical care is no different from other segments of U.S. society that were entrusted to big organizations (the so-called corporatization of America).

Since the early 1980s, employers have pushed the growth in managed care, acting in response to continually rising medical costs and diminished profits (Miller and Luft, 1994). These employers and the federal government (through Medicare and Medicaid) have found that managed care can reduce the costs of health care without reducing quality or limiting access. The question, therefore, is not whether managed care works and should be adopted; clearly, the United States has adopted managed care as the predominant form of health care delivery. Rather, the important issue is the need to study available evidence to determine which cost and quality controls are most effective.

TYPES OF MANAGED CARE ORGANIZATIONS

While the term "managed care" can be defined in many ways and is constantly evolving to meet the demands of the health care market, the differentiating feature of managed care relative to FFS plans is the use of provider networks (Miller and Luft, 1994). A network is a defined group of providers, typically linked through contractual arrangements, who supply a full range of primary and acute health care services (Medicome International, n.d.). Managed care enrollees who use providers outside the network may receive reduced coverage or even no coverage. Four characteristics differentiate the various managed care plans (see **Table 16-1**):

- *Risk-bearing* refers to the amount of risk borne by the providers, which can range from full risk to no risk.
- *Physician type* refers to the relationship between the MCO and the physician(s).
- *Relationship exclusivity* addresses whether the physician provides care to patients from one MCO only or to patients from multiple MCOs.
- *Out-of-network coverage* identifies whether care received from a provider who is not in the MCO's network is a covered benefit. Types of MCOs are discussed below in terms of these distinguishing characteristics (see Miller and Luft, 1994, for a thorough discussion).

Table 16-1 Characteristics of Managed Care Plans

Type	Physician Risk Bearing	Physician Type	Exclusivity of Relationship with Physician	Out-of-Network Coverage
HMO				
Staff	No	Staff	Yes	No
Group	Yes	Large group	Yes	No
Network	Yes	Large group	No	No
IPA	Yes	Solo/small group	No	No
PPO	No	Solo or group	No	Yes
EPO	No	Solo or group	No	No
POS	Varies	Varies	Varies	Yes

HMO—health maintenance organization
IPA—independent practice association
PPO—preferred provider organization
EPO—exclusive provider organization
POS—point of service

Source: Adapted and reprinted with permission from the *Annual Review of Public Health,* Volume 15, copyright 1994, by Annual Reviews, Inc., www.annualreviews.org.

Health Maintenance Organizations

The distinguishing characteristics of HMOs are that they place providers at risk, either directly or indirectly, and generally do not provide coverage for medical care that is received out of network. The risk arrangement can take many forms. In capitation, costs of care for a given population are estimated for some time span (typically one year), and physicians are prospectively paid this set amount of money to provide agreed-upon services (Rognehaugh, 1996). The provider keeps the capitation payment, regardless of whether a patient actually receives any services during the year. The provider is, however, obligated to provide any services—no matter how many—needed by the patient. Thus the physician is taking the risk that the capitation rate will be sufficient to cover all the costs of care for the population. In this way, the provider assumes risk that traditionally was underwritten by the insurance company.

Risk pools, in which a portion of payments for services rendered (i.e., a "withhold") is placed in a pool as a source for any subsequent claims that exceed projections (Rognehaugh, 1996), have been implemented for hospitals and other high-risk services. In these schemes, the physician and the HMO share the surplus or loss from the risk pool at the end of the year (Mack, 1993). The use of this strategy, however, has decreased in recent years; less than one-third of HMOs reported that they used withholds or risk pools in 2004 (Aventis, 2005).

The gatekeeper is a central component of most HMOs. Gatekeepers, who are typically primary-care physicians, must coordinate and authorize all medical services, including laboratory services, specialty referrals, and hospitalizations (Medicome International, n.d.). In many gatekeeper systems, a patient must receive a referral from his or her primary-care physician to receive coverage for a specialist's care. The rationale behind this approach is that it avoids unnecessary and often expensive referrals to specialists. The gatekeeper may be financially at risk—not only for the services that he or she provides, but also for the medical services provided by specialists to whom a patient is referred.

Traditionally, HMOs were classified into four major types:

- *Staff-model HMO:* a type of HMO characterized by direct ownership of health care facilities and direct employment physicians. Physicians in a staff-model HMO typically bear no direct risk, but the HMO can influence the care given by the physicians through utilization review (the review of the necessity and efficiency of patients' utilization patterns). In addition, because the HMO pays most or all of the physicians' salaries, these providers risk termination of their contracts if their treatment patterns do not meet administrators' expectations.

- *Group-model HMO:* a type of HMO characterized by contracts with large, multispecialty medical groups offering services exclusively to the HMO on a capitated basis.
- *Network-model HMO:* a type of HMO characterized by nonexclusive contracts with large medical groups. While networks typically bear risk, the nonexclusivity of the arrangement reduces the influence of the risk on the physician's behavior.
- *Independent practice association (IPA)-model HMO:* a type of HMO in which physicians form a separate legal entity, usually a corporation or partnership, that then contracts with the MCO. The IPA usually shares risk with the MCO, and then individual providers are paid by the IPA for services provided to enrolled patients for a negotiated fee. The IPA may reimburse physicians on a discounted FFS basis or may share some risk with them. These physicians typically maintain their own private practices and are allowed to provide services to patients enrolled in other MCOs.

While these four models represent the traditional categories into which HMOs are classified, recent innovations in plan designs have blurred the distinctions among these models. Plans can have elements of two or more of these categories and, therefore, be difficult to classify as fitting into any single model.

Preferred Provider Organizations

Preferred provider organizations (PPOs) are affiliations of providers that seek contracts with insurance plans. The physicians are usually from solo or small-group practices and have nonexclusive arrangements with the PPO. Under a PPO plan, individuals are free to see any provider they choose but have a financial incentive (i.e., lower out-of-pocket expenses) to receive care from providers in the preferred network. PPOs generally do not capitate physicians who are members of their network. Rather, physicians accept discounted FFS payment in exchange for increased patient volume and a quick turnaround on claims payment. Because physicians bear no risk, plan administrators emphasize fee reduction and case-by-case utilization management to control costs. PPOs have proved more popular than HMOs with sponsors, providers, and patients because they are perceived to be less restrictive. Nevertheless, the number of operating PPO plans has decreased each year since 1998 (Aventis, 2005).

Exclusive provider organizations (EPOs) are a form of a PPO in which no coverage is provided for care received outside the provider network. While some plans require participants to enroll in an EPO, most EPOs are offered to enrollees as one of several options from which they may choose. The number of plans offering EPOs as a choice is increasing, while the number of mandatory EPOs is declining (Aventis, 2005).

Hybrid Plans and Categorical Limitations

Many plans combine two or more of the previously described organizational models and, accordingly, are referred to as hybrid plans. An example of a hybrid plan is a point-of-service (POS) plan. POS plans allow patients to select providers at the time a service is needed rather than when they join the plan. As with PPOs, when care is received from a provider outside the network, partial coverage is provided. As with HMOs, physicians may be at risk or contract exclusively with the plan.

With the rapidly changing health care market, the categorization of the various types of MCOs can become quickly outdated. As HMOs provide more diversified products, the lines of distinction become blurred. For example, mixed-model HMOs, which contract with more than one type of physician organization, are becoming more prevalent as the arrangements among the organizations grow increasingly complex (Miller and Luft, 1994).

Growth and Composition of Managed Care Plans

Early on, managed care plans were predominantly not-for-profit, operating as either staff- or group-model HMOs. IPAs and network-model HMOs appeared in the 1950s in response to physicians' feeling threatened by the staff and group models (Davis et al., 1994). Since then, growth in this market has been greatest in IPA models and slowest in staff and group models. In recent years, however, both the number of HMOs and HMO enrollment have declined. For example, in 1998, there were 902 HMOs licensed in the United States; by 2004, the number dropped to 465. Although IPAs are still the predominant HMO model—accounting for 56% of all HMOs in 2004—the number of plans declined from 606 in 1998 to 261 in 2004 (Aventis, 2002, 2005). Group and staff models remain the least popular options, accounting for 9% and 3% of all HMOs in 2004, respectively (Aventis, 2005).

In 2001, 31.7% of the U.S. population was enrolled in some kind of HMO; by 2004, that percentage had dropped to 26.8%. There were, however, some significant regional differences in acceptance of HMOs. The highest enrollment is in California and Pennsylvania; in both states, slightly more than 40% of patients belong to an HMO. By contrast, eight states posted HMO penetration rates of less than 10%: Alabama, Alaska, Idaho, Mississippi, Montana, North Dakota, South Dakota, and Wyoming (Aventis, 2002, 2005).

Managed health care continues to evolve rapidly. While HMO enrollment has declined in recent years, enrollment in other types of MCOs has increased. Managed health care has also shifted from being predominantly a not-for-profit industry to a for-profit sector (Davis et al., 1994). Concurrently, there has been a marked expansion of managed care to the Medicaid and Medicare populations.

MANAGING THE PHARMACY BENEFIT

Much emphasis is placed on managing the pharmacy benefit in MCOs, despite its relatively small share of the overall health care budget. Companies that manage the pharmacy benefit may offer performance guarantees: If they do not achieve a certain level of performance, they are subject to financial penalties. Performance guarantees can relate to cost savings (e.g., generic substitution rates), customer service (e.g., wait time on calls to customer service), or client reporting (Lipton, Kreling, Collins, and Hertz, 1999).

Pharmacies are rarely reimbursed on a capitation basis because it is physicians—not pharmacists—who have the greatest influence over prescription utilization and costs. Physicians, therefore, are more likely to be held responsible for prescription costs. An effective way to influence prescribing practices is to give physicians financial incentives to control drug costs. These incentives may take the form of performance bonuses or withholds and risk pools. Performance bonuses are becoming more common, whereas the use of withholds and risk pools is declining (Aventis, 2005).

Because managed care prescription programs are reimbursed on an FFS basis, health plans' cost-containment efforts are directed to three types of costs incurred whenever a prescription is dispensed:

- *Unit cost* refers to the amount paid for each prescription, which consists of reimbursement for drug ingredient costs and a dispensing fee.
- *Utilization rate* refers to the number of prescriptions dispensed per patient.
- *Administrative costs* are the charges for processing a claim and managing the prescription benefit program. They are greatly reduced by having pharmacies submit claims for reimbursement electronically, thereby eliminating most, if not all, paperwork. While administrative costs are commonly paid on a per-claim-processed basis, some are paid on a per-enrollee basis.

Pharmacy Benefit Managers

In 2004, approximately 85% of retail prescription claims were paid for by a third party rather than by individual patients (West, 2005). Most often, the payer was a specialized organization known as a pharmacy benefit manager (PBM). As explained in Chapter 14, PBMs administer the prescription drug part of health insurance plans on behalf of plan sponsors, which could be HMOs, self-insured employers, PPOs, or indemnity insurers.

While not always considered a type of MCO, PBMs have many of the characteristics of managed care, including having a provider network. Typically, PBMs contract with existing community pharmacies to create a network of pharmacies from which patients can receive prescriptions at the rate established by the plan sponsor. PBMs negotiate with network pharmacies for decreased product reimbursement prices in exchange for an increased volume of prescriptions to be dispensed.

Because the administration of pharmacy programs is rather complex and requires a claims-processing system and large prescription volume to be handled efficiently, PBMs typically can offer lower costs and patient access to a greater number of pharmacies than can a plan sponsor. Services offered by most PBMs include pharmacy network development, claims processing, eligibility maintenance, client reporting, rebate contracting, generic use programs, formulary management (as described in the case scenario at the beginning of this chapter), therapeutic interchange, mail service, drug utilization review (DUR), patient and provider education, step therapy, and disease management. Following is a description of each of these tools.

Limited Networks

As previously mentioned, PBMs contract with community pharmacies to create a network of pharmacies from which patients can receive prescriptions. In selecting a network, considerations include location, cost, and quality, which are interrelated (Sterler and Stephens, 1999). For example, plans can simultaneously reduce administrative expenses and negotiate greater fee reductions by contracting with fewer pharmacies in return for increased prescription volume. When developing a network, the PBM will model the average distance between pharmacies and patients in the area using geographic information systems based on the pharmacies' and the patients' ZIP codes. An example of a common target is that a pharmacy provider be located within 1 to 5 miles of each enrollee's home in metropolitan areas, within 5 miles in suburban areas, and within 10 miles in rural areas (Sterler and Stephens, 1999).

Once a network has been established, ongoing network communication and provider performance are key issues. The PBM can use a variety of methods to communicate with network providers, including newsletters, online communications, and Internet Web sites (Sterler and Stephens, 1999). When measuring performance, both clinical and economic factors may be considered. Examples of economic measures include average discount off the average wholesale price (AWP) and generic conversation rates: (number of generic claims) ÷ (number of generic claims + number of brand claims for which generics are available). The number and type of responses to DUR alerts is another performance measure (Sterler and Stephens, 1999). By comparing pharmacy providers, PBMs can prepare "report cards" showing how pharmacies adhere to preselected performance criteria, such as customer satisfaction or availability of 24-hour emergency service (Marcille, 1996).

While online adjudication systems help minimize fraud and abuse problems, audits serve as an additional quality control technique. An on-site audit, in which the auditor visits the pharmacy and examines its prescription records, is a commonly used strategy (Sterler and Stephens, 1999). On-site audits may result in no action, termination from the network, a request for reimbursement for select claims, or other actions.

Mail Service

Most PBMs offer mail service pharmacies—either through their own mail-order facility or by contracting with one. As a result of their huge prescription volumes, these mail service pharmacies are able to negotiate discounts on product costs and try to achieve economies of scale that reduce their dispensing costs. PBMs may require members to use only a mail service pharmacy for certain prescriptions (usually refills of maintenance medications for chronic conditions), or they may give incentives, such as discounted co-payments, to encourage patients to use the mail service pharmacy.

Negotiated Discounts, Generic Substitution, and Rebates

Managers of the pharmacy benefit attempt to control product ingredient cost by obtaining significant discounts off AWP from the network pharmacies. Network reimbursement for pharmacy providers is typically based on AWP for brands. AWP is the manufacturer's price to wholesalers and pharmacies before any discounts are taken. The mean payment for brand-name drugs is typically 86% of AWP or less. It is expected that use of AWP as a basis for reimbursing drug ingredient costs will decline in the near future in favor of a new cost estimate known as average manufacturer's price (AMP). AMP promises to provide a more accurate estimate of pharmacies' actual acquisition costs but is also expected to result in lower reimbursement and lower gross margins for pharmacies.

The vast majority of plans use maximum allowable cost (MAC) in setting generic prices. MAC is a maximum ingredient cost that will be paid for a drug, independent of the manufacturer's AWP. Regardless of the discount that is stipulated for brands and generics, most contracts require that the payment be the lowest of three measures:

- The contract rate—usually stated as a percentage of AWP plus a dispensing fee, or
- The MAC plus a dispensing fee, or
- The usual and customary (U&C) price charged to a cash-paying customer.

Thus, in those cases where the pharmacy's U&C is less than the contract rate, the pharmacy is paid the lower U&C price.

PBMs generate significant revenues from the rebates received from pharmaceutical manufacturers in return for putting specific drugs on the formulary or giving these drugs preferred status. The amount of these rebates may be based on performance (i.e., a certain level of prescribing) or market share (i.e., the percentage of all prescriptions within a given therapeutic class that are dispensed for the company's product). The specific amounts of these rebates are difficult to find out because such information is proprietary (Lipton et al., 1999). When a PBM is administering the plan sponsor's pharmacy benefit, the rebate may be shared between the PBM and the plan sponsor or may be awarded solely to one party, depending on the contract between the plan sponsor and the PBM.

Claims Adjudication

PBMs use online electronic claims submission systems to adjudicate claims for prescriptions dispensed by network pharmacies. This electronic data interchange has been standardized and is maintained by the National Council for Prescription Drug Programs (NCPDP). Electronic claims systems can carry out distinct administrative functions, including eligibility verification and claims adjudication. The pharmacy is notified of the formulary status of the prescribed medication, and any limits on medication quantities or refills are addressed. The amount to be remitted to the pharmacy and the patient's co-payment are also determined.

In addition, electronic claims systems can review the prescribing, dispensing, and usage patterns for given patients or drug products and suggest improvements (see the discussion on drug utilization review later). They may also suggest therapeutic alternatives and provide information regarding physician network status and various patient and provider characteristics.

A transaction can be rejected by the PBM during adjudication if the pharmacy violates a clinical or administrative mandate. An online dispensing message that can be overridden by the pharmacist is known as a soft-edit message; a hard-edit message cannot be overridden without approval of the plan or an appropriate change to one or more components of the submitted claim. Under the latest NCPDP guidelines, intervention/outcome codes allow pharmacists to override certain edits by indicating which intervention took place to address the identified issue (e.g., the pharmacist called the doctor to notify him or her about a potentially serious drug–drug interaction).

Formularies

As described in the case scenario at the beginning of this chapter, formulary development and management is a core function of PBMs. Formularies can be described as open, closed, or incented. In an open formulary, all drugs are covered, regardless of their formulary status. In a closed formulary, drugs not on the formulary are not covered by the health plan. In an incented formulary, patients are provided with financial incentives (i.e., lower co-payments) to use preferred drugs; coverage is also provided for nonpreferred products, albeit at higher co-payments. Incented formularies are often referred to as "multiple-tiered formularies" or described as having "tiered co-payments." (Tiered co-payments are discussed in more detail in the "Cost Sharing" section of this chapter.) In recent years, traditional open or closed formularies have been replaced for the most part by incented formularies.

As in the Viagra case scenario at the beginning of this chapter, plans have debated whether they should cover "lifestyle" drugs and, if so, whether they should be subject to higher co-payments or require approval from the PBM. PBMs often exclude specific classes of drugs, such as the following:

- Nonprescription drugs (other than insulin)
- Parenteral products (other than insulin)
- Compounded prescriptions
- Devices (e.g., syringes, blood glucose monitors, blood pressure machines, and glucose test strips)
- Appetite suppressants
- Products for smoking cessation
- Oral contraceptives
- Fertility agents
- Products used for cosmetic purposes (such as hair growth or wrinkle removal) (Takeda Pharmaceuticals of North America, Inc., 2003)

In addition to benefit exclusions, PBMs may limit the size of a particular prescription or the number of refills. Size may be limited to a specified number of dosage units or, more commonly, to a specified day's supply. Usually the day's supply is limited to 30 days. Early refills may not be allowed unless the PBM gives authorization to do so (e.g., the patient is going on vacation). Some PBMs, however, specify a minimum quantity (such as a three-month supply) that may be dispensed for certain maintenance medications used for chronic conditions.

Some plans incorporate a prior authorization (PA) program into their pharmacy benefit. A PA program, which allows a patient's physician to request coverage of nonpreferred or noncovered medications, provides access to certain drugs when they are needed without covering the drug for the general population. A variation on the formulary and prior authorization is step therapy. With step therapy, the use of the more expensive agent is reserved for second-line treatment if treatment with the less expensive agent proves unsuccessful. For example, a patient with arthritis might be required to try aspirin or a generic nonsteroidal anti-inflammatory drug (NSAID) before coverage of a brand-name NSAID or COX-2 inhibitor will be authorized.

Some staff- and group-model HMOs authorize pharmacists to dispense therapeutic alternatives in accordance with previously established formulary guidelines. This practice, known as therapeutic interchange, is used by some PBMs for two reasons: (1) Therapeutic categories are becoming more crowded with very similar drugs, and (2) there is growing pressure to increase the market share of particular products so that the payer can receive manufacturer rebates.

Outside of these tightly managed environments, the term "therapeutic interchange" takes on a somewhat different meaning because the pharmacist contacts the physician to request approval for a switch in medication, typically from a nonformulary medication to a formulary medication. Depending on the particular plan, the pharmacist may also contact the patient to get his or her permission before making the switch. Such programs, which are also called therapeutic conversion, therapeutic substitution, or switch programs, have been more commonly administered in mail service pharmacies than in the retail networks because of the efficiencies that can be achieved in the mail-order setting (Kreling, Lipton, Collins, and Hertz, 1996). Controversy surrounds these therapeutic conversion programs, however. Opponents argue that these programs have negative effects on patients' health and are motivated by rebate revenues; proponents advocate their use as a way to control the growth in drug costs without compromising quality of care.

Drug Utilization Review

The review of physician prescribing, pharmacist dispensing, and patient use of drugs is known as drug utilization review (Palumbo and Ober, 1995). The goal of DUR is to ensure that drugs are used appropriately, safely, and effectively.

Reviews based on claims data for prescriptions that have already been dispensed are known as retrospective DUR. The primary goal of retrospective DUR is educational—to find ways in which drug therapy can be improved and inform prescribers and dispensers about these findings. Retrospective DUR may focus on physicians' prescribing patterns, individual patients' patterns, or patterns of use for certain therapeutic categories—especially for drugs that may be subject to abuse.

Prospective DUR is conducted at the time the prescription is dispensed via the electronic claims adjudication system. Patients' medication records are reviewed during the dispensing process to determine whether the prescriptions are appropriate. If a problem is identified, a message describing the problem is returned to the pharmacy through the computer system before the prescription is dispensed. Examples of reviews performed by these systems include appropriateness of dose, drug interactions, duplication of therapy, and drug–allergy interactions. Online prospective DUR programs may duplicate pharmacists' reviews of their own records but has the added benefit of screening prescription claims from other pharmacies that may have filled prescriptions for the same patient.

Cost Sharing

Cost sharing requires the patient to share in the cost of a medication based on some predetermined rate schedule. It tries to optimize utilization by requiring patients to consider the cost of the medication (at least part of the cost), just as they would in any other purchasing transaction. Cost sharing can take many forms, including co-payments, coinsurance, deductibles, out-of-pocket limits, or maximum benefits. Many health plans use a combination of deductibles and co-payments or co-insurance when designing their pharmacy benefits. These techniques are fully described in Chapter 14.

PBMs commonly use tiered co-payments to drive drug utilization away from high-cost brand-name medications to lower-cost alternatives. In many three-tiered pharmacy benefits, generic drugs are placed on the first tier of the formulary and have the lowest co-payment; preferred brand-name drugs are placed on the second tier with a higher co-payment; and nonpreferred brand-name drugs are placed on the third tier and have the highest co-payment. Some plans specify four-tier co-payments, with certain "lifestyle" drugs (e.g., Viagra) or nonformulary drugs appearing on the fourth tier. This fourth tier often has a co-insurance requirement ranging from 50% to 100%.

Provider and Patient Education

Physician profiling is a tool for comparing the practice patterns of providers on cost and quality dimensions. Measures are generally expressed as a rate over a specific period of time within the physician's patient population (e.g., the average dollars spent per patient per month). These "report cards" are then provided to individual physicians. These reports show not only the specific physician's practice patterns but also the average practice patterns of their physician counterparts, thereby providing a benchmark for comparison. The information on a report card typically includes health care and prescription costs per patient per month, number of prescriptions per patient per month, percentage of brand-name versus generic prescriptions, compliance with formulary guidelines, and prescribing patterns for selected prescription drugs.

As a follow-up to physician profiling, some health plans provide counter-detailing (also known as academic detailing). Plans monitor physicians' prescribing patterns to identify those physicians who are prescribing inappropriately, as viewed by the health plan. A health plan representative (or the contracting PBM) then visits targeted physicians to provide information regarding the most cost-effective use of selected drugs and to encourage physicians to prescribe in ways that will reduce overall costs while maintaining program quality. The targeted physicians are usually identified by the practice profiling program as ones with higher than average costs or unusual prescribing patterns. As discussed previously, the ability to influence providers' behavior depends greatly on how much of the contracted provider's business that the organization controls.

Patient education is becoming more prevalent in health plans. The goal of these programs is to produce voluntary changes in patients' behavior that will improve their health. Such efforts take a variety of forms, from passive educational mailing to more active educational efforts through telephone call centers. More-encompassing patient education programs are sometimes referred to as disease management programs. The idea behind disease management is to take a broad view of a disease, focusing on how it is treated across the continuum of care. Often disease management programs target high-cost or high-prevalence diseases for which pharmaceutical therapy plays a central role, with the goal of improving how patients and physicians manage the disease. Examples include asthma, diabetes, heart disease, acid reflux disorders, and depression.

ETHICAL ISSUES IN MANAGED CARE

Managed care takes an active approach to managing health, and this approach frequently intervenes in the physician–patient relationship. Considering the historical perspective discussed at the beginning of the chapter, it should not be surprising that the growth of managed care has fueled many ethics debates almost since its inception (Jecker, 1994). Ethical concerns related to managed care revolve around four central themes: the sanctity of the physician–patient relationship, the ethics of medicine, the quality of care, and freedom of choice for patients and providers (see **Table 16-2**). The challenge for managed care is to balance these concerns against the limited amount of resources that can be devoted to medical care spending.

QUALITY IN MANAGED CARE

Background

While much of the interest in managed care has traditionally focused on controlling costs, today there is a growing emphasis on ensuring the quality of care. A major difficulty facing those who attempt to measure quality is that there is no universally agreed-upon definition of quality. Which variables should be measured, and how should they be weighed? Donabedian (1978) identified three measures for the assessment of quality that are still used today: structure, process, and outcomes.

Table 16-2 Summary of the Ethical Issues in Managed Care

Anti-Managed Care Position	Pro-Managed Care Position
The financial incentives of managed care threaten the role of physician as the patient advocate, undermining the patient's trust and jeopardizing the oath of doing good while avoiding harm.	The financial incentives of FFS resulted in overtreatment of patients, which can also be detrimental to the patient.
The ethics of medicine will be replaced with the ethics of business.	The ethics of medicine are not as superior as perhaps believed. Physicians do not take vows of poverty. In addition, businesses are increasingly being held to ethical standards. By considering medicine to be both a profession and a business, society will not overlook the ethical issues that can arise as a result of these conflicting agendas.
Physicians' autonomy is removed, which will eventually harm patients.	Physicians did not have complete autonomy under FFS. Nonetheless, reducing physician autonomy is not necessarily a bad thing. Who is to say that physicians are the experts or have special authority about the ethical values that should be considered in making resource allocation decisions? Further, empirical evidence does not show that managed care results in a lower quality of care. Rather, it can provide numerous benefits, such as an emphasis on preventive care.
Patients' freedom to choose providers and obtain medical services is limited, resulting in decreased patient satisfaction.	Patients have limits under FFS. Further, as managed care grows, a greater number of providers will be included in managed care, increasing patients' choice of providers.

Source: Reprinted from *Clinics in Geriatric Medicine*, Vol 10(3), N.S. Jecker, "Managed Competition and Managed Care: What are the Ethical Issues?", pp. 527–540, ©1994 with permission from Elsevier

Structure refers to the personnel and other resources used to provide care as well as the policies and procedures that govern the use of resources and providers' decision making. Examples include availability of X-ray equipment, the type of information system used, the number of physicians and their credentials, and the policy for receiving prior authorization for noncovered services. Structural criteria are generally easy to measure and document, but their relationship to other measures of quality is not always clear.

Process refers to the interactions that occur between practitioners and patients or what was done to the patient. Examples in a community pharmacy include the percentage of patients counseled per day and the number of dispensing errors as a percentage of prescriptions dispensed. For a PBM, a process measure may include the number of patients switched to a preferred medication.

Outcomes are the end results of medical care—that is, what happened to the patient. Examples of outcomes include stroke, death, quality of life, and patient satisfaction. While most would agree that outcomes are the best indicators of quality, quality assessment efforts often focus on the structure and process of care because they are much easier to measure and interpret.

Oversight and Accreditation

Oversight is the process of reviewing and monitoring managed care organizations to determine whether they meet specified criteria. Government agencies, such as state insurance departments, are responsible for ensuring compliance with state laws and regulations regarding issues such as financial solvency, enrollment procedures, and patient rights. Accreditation, by contrast, is a voluntary form of oversight involving independent, nonprofit, nongovernment entities. Accreditation goes beyond oversight in that it evaluates and reports on the quality and performance of MCOs, thereby enabling purchasers and consumers of managed health care to make comparisons and more informed health care purchasing decisions. Accreditation, therefore, serves as a "seal of approval" that is relied upon by employers, patients, and, sometimes, government agencies (Kongstvedt, 2002).

There are three major accreditation agencies in the United States:

- The National Committee for Quality Assurance (NCQA)
- The Joint Commission for the Accreditation of Healthcare Organizations (Joint Commission)
- The Utilization Review Accreditation Commission (URAC)

The majority of HMOs voluntarily submit to accreditation—more than any other type of MCO. NCQA is the dominant accreditation agency for HMOs, but the Joint Commission and URAC are also used. Accreditation of PPOs is increasing but still is not as common as for HMOs. URAC is the main accreditation agency for PPOs, but NCQA and the Joint Commission also accredit PPOs. The accreditation process looks at utilization management, patient satisfaction, access, financial performance, provider credentialing, treatment of specific diseases and outcomes achieved, and other measures (Kongstvedt, 2002). The accreditation survey process involves both on- and off-site components that are assessed by a team of reviewers.

In addition to accrediting HMOs, NCQA promotes performance standards, quality assurance, and review standards. It has also developed the Health Plan Employer Data and Information Set (HEDIS), a group of measures that gives plan sponsors objective information that they can use to evaluate MCOs. **Table 16-3** gives examples of the seven major types of HEDIS standards.

IMPACT OF MANAGED CARE ON PHARMACISTS

As discussed in Chapter 14, the growth of health insurance coverage for prescription drugs has resulted in extra work (e.g., prior authorization, online prospective DUR, and formulary restrictions) and reduced reimbursement for pharmacists. Nevertheless, the concept of pharmaceutical care is consistent with the goals of managed care. Indeed, the growth of pharmaceutical care occurred simultaneously with the growth of managed care. Changes in pharmacy education are preparing pharmacists to manage care and affect positive patient outcomes. It is expected that pharmaceutical care services will ultimately be recognized as a valuable part of managed care and not just a cost to be controlled. Taking a broader perspective, greater focus on patient outcomes and cost-effec-

Table 16-3 Major Categories of HEDIS Measures

Area Measured	Examples
Effectiveness of care	Childhood immunization rates Mammography rates Response to those who are ill
Access	Availability of care when needed
Member satisfaction	Average office wait times Difficulty receiving care Satisfaction with choice of provider Overall satisfaction
Use of services	Mental health utilization Maternity length of stay Well-child visits Cesarean section rates Frequency of selected procedures
Cost of care	Frequency of high-cost procedures Cost trends
Informed health choices	Future measures will be developed to help patients become actively involved in making informed choices among treatment options
Health plan descriptive information	General questions about patient perceptions of the health plan

tiveness will encourage pharmacists, physicians, and other health care providers to collaborate for the benefit of the patient to realize the goal of optimally managed health care.

Managed care has also expanded the roles played by pharmacists. New opportunities include roles as formulary managers, drug utilization reviewers, outcomes researchers, and numerous other positions that combine the clinical and business aspects of pharmacy benefit management.

CONCLUSIONS

Clearly, managed care continues to have a major impact on the U.S. health care system as well as the quality of care and patient outcomes. To see how much managed care has evolved, one needs merely to review the following set of predictions made in 1994:

- Patients will be given financial incentives to use network providers.
- Treatment protocols/clinical guidelines will determine which services are provided, when, and by whom.
- Performance of physicians, hospitals, and other providers will be measured and reported.
- Primary care physicians will serve as gatekeepers to other forms of care.
- Patient education and preventive care will be emphasized.
- QA activities will be emphasized.
- There will be a seamless continuum of care.
- Health care financing will be integrated with delivery (Simpson, 1994).

Many of these predictions are now reality, and the others are currently being addressed. The changes in the delivery and financing of health care over the past several decades offer promise for both patients and providers. Many patients are now more sensitive to the costs of care and are better able to judge the quality of care they receive. MCOs are investing in the information systems needed to truly manage care, and providers are increasingly relying on best practices guidelines. These trends should lead to a more efficient and effective system of health care delivery.

ACKNOWLEDGEMENT

The author wishes to express appreciation to Brenda R. Motheral, PhD, for her contributions on managed health care initially published in the second edition of this text.

QUESTIONS FOR FURTHER DISCUSSION

1. Bad publicity continues to plague managed care. To what extent is the current trashing of managed care an unavoidable cost of bringing change to the U.S. medical system? How much, if any, are the media to blame?
2. What are the strengths and limitations of prospective DUR systems from the perspectives of the PBM and the retail pharmacist? Given your explanation, what could be done to improve prospective DUR?
3. Describe some of the new and innovative career opportunities that have developed for pharmacists as managed care enrollment has grown.

KEY TOPICS AND TERMS

Academic detailing (counterdetailing)
Capitation
Cost sharing
Exclusive provider organization (EPO)
Fee-for-service (FFS)
Gatekeeper
Group-model HMO
Health maintenance organization (HMO)
HEDIS
Independent practice association-model HMO (IPA)
Managed care organization (MCO)
NCQA
Network
Network-model HMO
Pharmacy benefit manager (PBM)
Point of service plan (POS)
Practice profiling
Preferred provider organization (PPO)
Prospective DUR
Rebates
Report cards
Retrospective DUR
Risk-bearing
Risk pool
Staff-model HMO
Tiered co-payments
Utilization review

REFERENCES

Aventis. (2002). *Managed care digest series.* Bridgewater, NJ: Aventis Pharmaceuticals.

Aventis. (2005). *Managed care digest series.* Bridgewater, NJ: Aventis Pharmaceuticals.

Campbell, W. H., & Newsome, L. A. (1995). The evolution of managed care and practice settings. In S. M. Ito & S. Blackburn (Eds.), *A pharmacist's guide to principles and practices of managed care pharmacy* (pp. 1–14). Alexandria, VA: Foundation for Managed Care Pharmacy.

Davis, K., Collins, K. S., & Morris, C. (1994, Fall). Managed care: Promise and concerns. *Health Affairs, 13*(4), 178–185.

Donabedian, A. (1978). The quality of medical care. *Science, 200*(4344), 856–864.

Friedman, E. (1996). Capitation, integration, and managed care lessons from early experiments. *Journal of the American Medical Association, 275*(12), 957–962.

Gillis, J. (1998a, April 22). The impotence pill: Who will pay? *The Washington Post,* p. A1.

Gillis, J. (1998b, April 26). Prescriptions for a better life. *The Washington Post,* p. AO1.

Goldstein, A. (1998, July 3). U.S.: Medicaid must cover Viagra. *The Washington Post.*

Hoechst Marion Roussel. (1999). *HMO-PPO/Medicare–Medicaid digest.* Kansas City, MO: Hoechst Marion Roussel.

Jecker, N. S. (1994). Managed competition and managed care: What are the ethical issues? *Clinics in Geriatric Medicine, 10*(3), 527–540.

Kongstvedt, P. R. (2002). *Managed care: What it is and how it works* (2nd ed.). Sudbury, MA: Jones and Bartlett.

Kreling, D. H., Lipton, H. L., Collins, T. C., & Hertz, K. C. (1996). *Assessment of the impact of pharmacy benefit managers: Final report to the Health Care Financing Administration* (Pub. no. PB97-103683). Springfield, VA: National Technical Information Service.

Lipton, H. L., Kreling, D. H., Collins, T., & Hertz, K. C. (1999). Pharmacy benefit management companies: Dimensions of performance. *Annual Review of Public Health, 20,* 361–401.

Lynn, J. T. (1991). The promise of managed care: An insurer's perspective. *Health Affairs, 10*(4), 185–188.

Mack, J. M. (1993). Managed care relationships from the physician's perspective. *Topics in Health Care Financing, 20*(2), 38–52.

MacLeod, G. K. (1996). An overview of managed health care. In P. R. Kongstvedt (Ed.), *Essentials of managed health care* (pp. 1–9). Gaithersburg, MD: Aspen.

Marcille, J. A. (1996). Contracting: How will you measure up? *Managed Care Pharmacy Practice, 116*(6), 65.

Medicome International. (n.d.). *Medical interface. A thru Z. Managed care terms.* Bronxville, NY: Medicome International.

Miller, R. H., & Luft, H. S. (1994). Managed care plans: Characteristics, growth, and premium performance. *Annual Review of Public Health, 15,* 437–459.

Palumbo, F. B., & Ober, J. (1995). Drug use evaluation. In S. M. Ito & S. Blackburn (Eds.), *A pharmacist's guide to principles and practices of managed care pharmacy* (pp. 51–59). Arlington, VA: Foundation for Managed Care Pharmacy.

Rognehaugh, R. (1996). *The managed health care dictionary.* Gaithersburg, MD: Aspen.

Simpson, R. L. (1994). The role of technology in a managed care environment. *Nursing Management, 25*(2), 26, 28.

Sterler, L. T., & Stephens, D. (1999). Pharmacy distribution systems and network management. In R. P. Navarro (Ed.), *Managed care pharmacy practice* (pp. 89–123). Sudbury, MA: Jones and Bartlett.

Takeda Pharmaceuticals of North America, Inc. (2003). *The prescription drug benefit cost and plan design survey report.* Albuquerque, NM: Wellman.

West, D. S. (2005). *NCPA–Pharmacia digest.* Alexandria, VA: National Community Pharmacists Association.

CHAPTER 17

Medicare and Medicaid

Alan P. Wolfgang

Case Scenario: Medicare

Helen is a retired bank teller, 67 years of age, who was recently afflicted with a serious illness. After spending 10 days in the hospital, she spent 4 weeks in a skilled nursing facility before being discharged to her home. During her recuperation, Helen often reflected on how lucky she was to be enrolled in Medicare. Because of her limited income, it was reassuring to know that Medicare would take care of her substantial health care expenses. Helen was shocked, however, when she began receiving bills that Medicare did not pay. Adding up the bills from the hospital, skilled nursing facility, pharmacy, and her physician, she owed more than $2,000! Helen could not understand how she could owe so much money when she had health insurance through Medicare.

LEARNING OBJECTIVES

Upon completion of this chapter, the student shall be able to:

- Explain the eligibility requirements of the Medicare program
- Describe the sources of funding for Medicare
- Describe the benefits provided under Medicare Parts A and B
- Describes the types of cost sharing imposed on Medicare patients
- Explain the concepts of approved charges and assignment
- Explain the benefits provided under Medicare Part C
- Describe the major provisions of the Medicare Part D prescription drug benefit
- Describe the magnitude of Medicare enrollment and spending
- Explain the need for and types of Medicare supplement policies
- Describe the three broad groups of people who may be eligible for Medicaid
- Describe the roles of state and federal governments in financing and administering Medicaid
- Describe the mandatory and optional benefits provided under Medicaid
- Describe the types of cost sharing imposed on Medicaid patients
- Describe the magnitude of Medicaid enrollment and spending
- Explain the role of waivers in encouraging innovation in Medicaid programs

CHAPTER QUESTIONS: MEDICARE

1. Which groups of people are eligible to be covered by Medicare?
2. How is Medicare financed?
3. What services are covered by Parts A and B of Medicare?
4. What types of cost sharing are imposed on Medicare beneficiaries?
5. What is "assignment," and why is it important to Medicare beneficiaries?
6. What is a Medicare supplement insurance policy?
7. What are some of the future challenges facing Medicare?

CHAPTER QUESTIONS: MEDICAID

1. What are the characteristics of the persons considered mandated categorically needy, optionally eligible, and medically needy?
2. What are the roles of federal and state governments in financing and administering Medicaid?
3. Which services must be covered by state Medicaid programs?
4. What are examples of optional services in Medicaid programs?
5. What types of cost sharing are imposed on Medicaid beneficiaries?
6. How have waivers been used by states to test innovative Medicaid programs?
7. What are some of the future challenges facing Medicaid?

MEDICARE: LEGISLATIVE HISTORY

The development of the Medicare program can be traced back to the 1935 Social Security Act (SSA). Although Medicare was not enacted at that time, this landmark legislation marked the beginning of the federal government's central role in the area of social insurance (Longest, 1994). Passed by Congress during President Franklin Roosevelt's first term, the SSA was designed to provide for the material needs of Americans (Hellman and Hellman, 1991). Title XVIII of the SSA, "Health Insurance for the Aged and Disabled," was established as part of the Social Security Amendments of 1965. More commonly known as Medicare, Title XVIII launched a health insurance program that complemented the SSA's retirement, survivors, and disability insurance benefits (Medicare and Medicaid Statistical Supplement, 1995).

The concept of Medicare was introduced early in 1952, during the Harry Truman administration. Abandoning his advocacy of a universal health program, President Truman suggested a more limited health insurance plan that would cover all Social Security beneficiaries (Ball, 1995). However, Truman's plan received little serious consideration. Fein (1989) believes that the introduction of a bill by Representative Aimee Forand of Rhode Island in August 1957 initiated the legislative activity that led to the enactment of Medicare. This bill, which proposed a social insurance program of health insurance for the aged, and its legislative successors received sustained attention in Congress for the next 8 years. Hearings on the bill held in 1959 helped build a consensus for the belief that many aged Americans faced severe difficulties in obtaining health insurance and that federal action in this arena was necessary.

Health insurance for the elderly was at the top of the federal legislative agenda in 1965 following the election of Lyndon Johnson as President in November 1964. During the early months of 1965, Representative Wilbur Mills of Arkansas, chairman of the House Ways and Means Committee, designed a compromise that encompassed three major proposals that were under consideration at that time: (1) a compulsory health insurance program for the elderly, which was to be financed by payroll taxes; (2) a voluntary insurance program for physician services, which was to be subsidized with general tax revenues; and (3) a means-tested health insurance program for the poor, which was to be administered by the states (Ginsburg, 1988). The first two proposals were combined in the Mills compromise to form the Medicare program; the third proposal was addressed through development of the Medicaid program.

After many years of often acrimonious debate about the government's responsibility for ensuring Americans' access to health services, passage of the 1965 SSA amendments was made possible by Johnson's landslide victory in the 1964 election and the accompanying large Democratic majority in Congress (Longest, 1994). If not for these unique circumstances that existed in 1965, it is unlikely that Medicare could have mustered the votes necessary for passage (Ball, 1995). In fact, some have argued that this comprehensive program could not have been enacted at any time except in 1965. The legislation was signed into law by President Johnson on July 30, 1965, with Medicare's implementation set for July 1, 1966 (Fein, 1989).

PROGRAM STRUCTURE

Medicare was traditionally a two-part insurance program. Part A, also known as Hospital Insurance (HI), pays for care provided to patients in hospitals, skilled nursing facilities, hospices, and home health care programs. Part B, or Supplementary Medical Insurance (SMI), provides coverage for physicians' services, outpatient hospital care, and a variety of other medical services not covered under Part A (Health Care Financing Administration, 1996). Part C, which was added in 1997, was originally known as the Medicare + Choice program, but now is called Medicare Advantage. It expanded beneficiaries' ability to participate in a wide variety of private health plans, including HMOs and PPOs. The Medicare Prescription Drug, Improvement, and Modernization Act of 2003 established a new prescription drug benefit, also known as Part D (Henry J. Kaiser Family Foundation, 2003; Centers for Medicare and Medicaid Services, 2005a).

ELIGIBILITY

Part A

In 2006, approximately 43 million people were enrolled in Medicare (Henry J. Kaiser Family Foundation, 2006a). Most of these people qualify for Medicare by virtue of the fact that they or their spouse worked for at least 10 years in Medicare-covered employment, they are citizens or permanent residents of the United States, and they are at least 65 years old. Persons who are 65 or older are entitled to receive Part A automatically without paying any premium if they (1) are receiving or are eligible to receive retirement benefits from either Social Security or the Railroad Retirement Board, or (2) had Medicare-covered government employment. People age 65 or older who do not meet these criteria can purchase Part A by paying a monthly premium (Health Care Financing Administration, 1996, 1998, 2000c; Medicare and Medicaid Statistical Supplement, 1995). This premium, which varies based on an individual's length of Medicare-covered employment, ranged between $216 and $393 per month in 2006 (Centers for Medicare and Medicaid Services, 2005a).

Two groups of people younger than age 65 can receive Part A without paying a monthly premium: (1) individuals who have received disability benefits from Social Security or the Railroad Retirement Board for at least

24 months, and (2) patients with end-stage renal disease (ESRD) who require dialysis or a kidney transplant (Health Care Financing Administration, 1996; Medicare and Medicaid Statistical Supplement, 1995). Legislation enacted in 2000 allows persons with amyotrophic lateral sclerosis (ALS, also known as Lou Gehrig's disease) to waive the 24-month waiting period for Part A coverage (Centers for Medicare and Medicaid Services, 2005a). Overall, the elderly account for 86.1% of the Medicare population, while disabled and ESRD patients account for 13.6% and 0.3%, respectively (Centers for Medicare and Medicaid Services, 2003c).

Part B

Although most Medicare patients do not pay a premium for Part A coverage, everyone who wishes to be covered by Part B is charged a monthly premium. For Social Security recipients enrolled in Part B, this premium ($88.50 per month in 2006) is deducted from their monthly benefit checks (Centers for Medicare and Medicaid Services, 2005a). Beginning in 2007, higher-income Medicare beneficiaries will begin paying a higher, income-related Part B premium (Henry J. Kaiser Family Foundation, 2005a). Approximately 94% of the Medicare population voluntarily enrolls in Part B (Centers for Medicare and Medicaid Services, 2004). Individuals who would have to pay a premium for Medicare Part A can purchase Part B even if they do not enroll in Part A.

FINANCING

The expenses of providing the benefits and administration of Parts A and B are paid from separate trust funds. Part A expenses are paid from the HI trust fund, which is financed primarily through payroll taxes paid by employees, employers, and self-employed individuals. At present, employees and employers each contribute 1.45% of earnings to the trust fund; self-employed individuals pay 2.9% of earnings. Additional funding is provided by beneficiary cost-sharing mechanisms (such as premiums, deductibles, and co-insurance) that are required for most Part A and B services (Davis and Burner, 1995; Medicare and Medicaid Statistical Supplement, 1995; Social Security Administration, 2003). Approximately 25% of the contributions to the HI fund come from beneficiary cost sharing. Most of the income for the SMI trust fund is provided from general revenues of the federal government (Davis and Burner, 1995; Zarabozo, Taylor, and Hicks, 1996).

ADMINISTRATION

Administration of the Medicare program is the responsibility of the U.S. Department of Health and Human Services (DHHS). Within DHHS, Medicare eligibility and enrollment are the responsibility of the Social Security Administration. The Centers for Medicare and Medicaid Services (CMS), formerly the Health Care Financing Administration (HCFA), is charged with carrying out most other duties pertaining to Medicare, including developing operational policies and guidelines, formulating conditions of participation for providers, maintaining and reviewing utilization records, and overseeing general financing of the program. The U.S. Department of the Treasury manages the HI and SMI trust funds (Medicare and Medicaid Statistical Supplement, 1992, 1995).

To be reimbursed for providing services to Medicare patients, health care providers must comply with the program's conditions of participation, which are requirements relating to the health and safety of Medicare beneficiaries. Agencies of state governments assist CMS in the certification process by surveying and inspecting potential providers (Medicare and Medicaid Statistical Supplement, 1995).

Providers are paid for services delivered to Medicare patients after they file claims with designated administrators (such as Blue Cross/Blue Shield associations and commercial insurers), which are organizations that contract with CMS to administer Part A and B claims. These administrators determine reasonable charges for covered services, make payments to providers, and guard against unnecessary utilization of services. Providers are required to file claims with the administrators on patients' behalf (Medicare and Medicaid Statistical Supplement, 1995).

MEDICARE SERVICES AND COST SHARING

Part A

Inpatient Hospital Care

Services for inpatient hospital care are based on the concept of a benefit period. A benefit period begins on the day an individual enters the hospital and ends when that person has not been a patient in either a hospital or skilled nursing facility for 60 consecutive days. It also ends if the person resides in a nursing home for 60 consecutive days without receiving skilled care. A Medicare beneficiary can have several benefit periods during a given year, and there is no lifetime limit on the number of benefit periods available to individuals (Centers for Medicare and Medicaid Services, 2003d).

Part A covers 90 days of medically necessary inpatient hospital care per benefit period. Each patient also has a lifetime reserve of 60 days that can be used if he or she needs to be hospitalized for more than 90 days in one benefit period. This lifetime reserve is not renewed at the beginning of each benefit period. The services that Medicare covers for hospital inpatients include a semiprivate room, meals, nursing care, operating and recovery room, drugs, laboratory tests, and X-rays. Medicare does not cover extra charges such as those for a private room or the cost of amenities such as a television or telephone.

A separate limit applies to inpatient services received in psychiatric hospitals; each Medicare beneficiary is entitled to just 190 days of inpatient psychiatric care during his or her lifetime. Psychiatric care provided in a general hospital does not count toward this 190-day limit (Centers for Medicare and Medicaid Services, 2003d).

Hospitalized Medicare patients are subject to a schedule of deductibles and co-payments, the amount of which changes each year. For days 1 through 60 of hospitalization during a benefit period, the patient is responsible for paying a deductible ($952 in 2006). Regardless of how many times a person might be admitted to the hospital, as long as he or she has not received more than 60 days of care within the benefit period, he or she pays only this deductible. The patient is not required to pay for any other portion of the costs of covered services during that time period. If, however, a patient is hospitalized for more than 60 days in a benefit period, further cost sharing is required in the form of daily co-payments. For days 61 through 90 of a benefit period, the co-payment amount ($238 per day in 2006) equals one fourth of the inpatient hospital deductible; for the lifetime reserve days, the co-payment ($476 per day in 2006) is one half of that deductible (Centers for Medicare and Medicaid Services, 2005a).

The other form of cost sharing that may be imposed on hospitalized Medicare patients is the blood deductible. Patients are required to pay for or replace (either by themselves or another person on their behalf) the first three pints of blood used each year. Both Parts A and B cover blood. Thus, to the extent that the blood deductible is met under one part of Medicare, it does not have to be met under the other part (Centers for Medicare and Medicaid Services, 2003d).

Skilled Nursing Facility Care

Medicare patients are entitled to 100 days of care in a skilled nursing facility (SNF) per benefit period. During stays in such facilities, covered services include a semiprivate room, nursing care, meals, drugs, medical supplies and equipment, and rehabilitation services (such as physical therapy and speech therapy). A number of criteria must be met before a Medicare patient can qualify for these services. Perhaps most important is the requirement that the patient require daily skilled nursing or rehabilitation services that can be provided only in a skilled nursing facility. Because this benefit is intended to serve acutely ill patients who can be cured or improved by short-term, daily, skilled services, SNF care for patients who need only custodial care (such as assistance with eating, toileting, or taking medication) will not be covered by Medicare. In addition to the requirement regarding level of care, admission to a SNF must be preceded by a hospital stay of at least 3 days, and it typically must occur within 30 days of hospital discharge (Centers for Medicare and Medicaid Services, 2003d; Hellman and Hellman, 1991).

There is no charge to the patient for the first 20 days of care in a SNF. For days 21 through 100 of care within a benefit period, however, Medicare patients are responsible for a daily co-payment. This co-payment ($119 per day in 2006) is set at one eighth of the inpatient hospital deductible (Centers for Medicare and Medicaid Services, 2005a).

Home Health Care

Like the skilled nursing care benefit, Medicare's home health care coverage is designed to help people recover from illnesses through the provision of skilled services—not to provide long-term, unskilled care. Part A and Part B actually share responsibility for home health care services. Part A covers a maximum of 100 home health visits following a hospital or SNF stay of at least 3 days. Thereafter, visits are covered by Part B, as is home health care not associated with a hospital or SNF stay. Home-bound patients may continue to receive home health care benefits so long as they require intermittent skilled nursing care, physical therapy, occupational therapy, or speech therapy. If a patient receives any of those services, he or she is entitled to a variety of other services, including home health aide services, medical social services, medical supplies (such as bandages or incontinence pads), and durable medical equipment (such as wheelchairs and walkers). Services not covered include meal preparation and delivery and full-time nursing care.

Medicare Part A pays the entire bill for most covered services provided by approved home health agencies without requiring any patient cost sharing. The one exception concerns durable medical equipment, for which the patient must pay a 20% co-insurance (Centers for Medicare and Medicaid Services, 2003d, 2005a; Hellman and Hellman, 1991).

Hospice Care

The hospice benefit provides care to patients who have life expectancies of 6 months or less (as certified by a physician) and who voluntarily waive their right to traditional treatment of their terminal illnesses (such as cancer chemotherapy). Hospice services, which primarily are delivered in a home setting, can include relief of pain and other symptoms (such as nausea, diarrhea), physician services, nursing care, counseling, and homemaker services. Short-term respite care in a nursing home or hospital, which provides temporary relief for the family members who regularly assist with home care, is also covered for a maximum of 5 consecutive days. If a hospice patient requires care for conditions not related to his or her terminal illness, these services are covered under the standard Medicare plan (Centers for Medicare and Medicaid Services, 2003d; Hellman and Hellman, 1991).

Very little patient cost sharing is required for covered services provided under the hospice benefit. Patients pay small co-insurance amounts for outpatient prescription drugs and inpatient respite care (Centers for Medicare and Medicaid Services, 2005a).

Other Services

Medicare Part A covers emergency services received in all hospitals, even those that do not participate in the Medicare program, including hospitals in Canada and Mexico under some circumstances. In general, Medicare does not pay for health care services received outside the United States and its territories (Centers for Medicare and Medicaid Services, 2003d). Therefore, elderly patients are advised to obtain other health insurance when they travel outside the country.

Part B

Services Covered

Part B covers services provided by physicians in a wide variety of settings, including hospitals, physicians' offices, nursing homes, and patients' homes. Thus, when a Medicare patient undergoes an inpatient surgical procedure, Part A pays the hospital charges and Part B pays for the surgeon's services. Other services covered under Part B include outpatient hospital services, X-rays and laboratory tests, physical and occupational therapy, home health care (if not associated with a hospital or skilled nursing facility stay), drugs and biologicals that cannot be self-administered (such as flu, pneumonia, and hepatitis B vaccinations), kidney dialysis, durable medical equipment, and ambulance transportation. A variety of other preventive services are covered under Part B, including bone mass measurements, colorectal cancer screenings, diabetes monitoring, mammograms, Pap smears, and prostate cancer screenings. Limited coverage is available for services provided by chiropractors, podiatrists, optometrists, and dental surgeons (Centers for Medicare and Medicaid Services, 2003d; Hellman and Hellman, 1991).

Although a wide variety of physician and outpatient services are covered by Part B, many services are not covered. Services not covered by Medicare Part B include routine physical examinations, routine vision and hearing tests, hearing aids, routine dental care, homemaker services, and most health care services received while traveling outside the United States (Centers for Medicare and Medicaid Services, 2003d; Hellman and Hellman, 1991).

Cost Sharing

Each calendar year, Medicare patients pay a deductible ($124 in 2006) for Part B services. After that deductible has been met, Medicare typically pays 80% of the approved charge for most services; this approved charge may be lower than the amount actually billed by the health care provider. The patient is responsible for paying the other 20% of approved charges and may be financially responsible for the difference between Medicare's approved charge and the provider's actual charge, depending on whether the provider accepts assignment (Centers for Medicare and Medicaid Services, 2003d, 2005a).

When a provider accepts assignment, it means that his or her actual charge will equal Medicare's approved charge. In such cases, Medicare patients are assured that they will be billed only for 20% of the approved charge. However, when patients receive services from providers who do not accept assignment, they can also be billed for the difference between actual and approved charges (see **Table 17-1**). The amount of this balance billing is limited, as federal law prevents providers who do not accept assignment from charging Medicare patients more than 115% of Medicare's approved charges (Centers for Medicare and Medicaid Services, 2003d). States may place even further restrictions on providers' ability to balance bill.

Physicians can agree on an annual basis to accept assignment for all services provided to Medicare beneficiaries; they are then referred to as "Medicare participating physicians." To encourage physicians to sign up for this program, payments for participating physicians are set approximately 5% higher than payments for nonparticipating physicians (Coleman, 1990). In 2001, assignment accounted for 99% of Medicare payments for physician services (Centers for Medicare and Medicaid Services, 2003a).

Table 17-1 Impact of Assignment on Total Payment by Medicare Patients

Assignment Accepted		Assignment Not Accepted
$200	Approved charge	$190
$215	Actual charge	$215
$160	80% of approved charge, paid by Medicare	$152
$ 40	20% of approved charge, paid by patient	$ 38
$ 0	Balance billing (actual charge minus approved charge)	$ 25
$ 40	Total payment due from patient (20% of approved charge plus balance billing)	$ 63

Part C

One solution to controlling Medicare spending might be to implement the types of managed care innovations that appear to have been successful in constraining health care costs in the private sector. Encouraging more Medicare enrollees to obtain their health care services through managed care organizations (MCOs) might allow the federal government to maintain—if not improve—the level of service provided to older Americans while assisting in its efforts to control expenditures. Even though Medicare does not require its beneficiaries to enroll in managed care plans, Medicare managed care enrollment nevertheless increased tremendously in the latter half of the 1990s. The number of Medicare beneficiaries in HMOs increased from fewer than 2 million in 1995 to a peak of 6.3 million (16% of all Medicare beneficiaries) in 1999 (Henry J. Kaiser Family Foundation, 1999a, 2005a).

Enrollment in traditional HMOs was the only managed care option available to Medicare beneficiaries from 1985 until implementation of the Balanced Budget Act of 1997 (BBA). Under the new Part C (Medicare Advantage) program, an expanded set of options for the delivery of health care services became available to Medicare beneficiaries, including PPOs and other types of managed care plans. The addition of these new managed care options made the variety of plans available under Medicare more similar to those available to non-Medicare patients.

Most Medicare Advantage plans are required to provide the traditional Medicare benefit package, excluding hospice care, without imposing additional out-of-pocket costs. If plan costs are lower than Medicare payments, plans are required either to pass those savings along to beneficiaries in the form of lower premiums, cost sharing, or additional benefits (e.g., outpatient prescription drugs, additional preventive care), or to return the excess payments to Medicare. While they may still be responsible for the Part B premium, most Medicare managed care patients receive additional benefits while paying either no additional premium or a premium substantially lower than premiums for supplemental insurance plans (Centers for Medicare and Medicaid Services, 2005a; Health Care Financing Administration, 1998, 2000c; Henry J. Kaiser Family Foundation, 1999a). It has been estimated that Medicare Advantage plans can save beneficiaries $100 per month, on average, compared to traditional fee-for-service (FFS) Medicare (Center for Medicare and Medicaid Services, 2006).

The growth in enrollment in Medicare managed care in the 1980s and 1990s, however, has been reversed in recent years. Between 2000 and 2005, enrollment dropped 22% to 4.9 million persons, representing just 12% of Medicare beneficiaries. The number of plans participating in Medicare Advantage, which had grown to 346 plans in 1998, fell to 143 plans by 2004 (Henry J. Kaiser Family Foundation, 2005a).

Limits on increases in payments from Medicare, increased administrative responsibilities, provider turnover within managed care networks, and other business concerns have been cited as reasons for this decline in plan participation (Henry J. Kaiser Family Foundation, 2005b). For Medicare managed care to succeed, a balance must be found between controlling spending, setting fair payment rates, and providing a stable source of health care for beneficiaries (Henry J. Kaiser Family Foundation, 2003).

Part D

Since January 1, 2006, prescription drug coverage has been available to Medicare beneficiaries through voluntary enrollment in Part D. Individuals obtain this coverage in one of two ways: (1) by enrolling in a free-standing prescription drug plan (PDP) while getting other Medicare benefits through the traditional FFS program or (2) by joining a Medicare Advantage plan that covers all Medicare benefits, including prescription drugs. Beneficiaries will pay an additional premium for Part D benefits. This premium, which is designed to cover approximately 25% of the cost of the standard drug benefit, is estimated to have averaged $32.20 per month in 2006; it may vary considerably between plans. By 2014, this premium is expected to approach $64 per month. Other sources of funding for Part D include contributions from the general fund of the U.S. Treasury and payments from states, which must offset some of the cost of prescription drugs for Medicaid beneficiaries who also are enrolled in Medicare (Centers for Medicare and Medicaid Services, 2005a; Henry J. Kaiser Family Foundation, 2005b).

Under Part D, beneficiaries pay a $250 deductible for prescription drugs in 2006, after which they will pay 25% of the next $2,000 of drug costs. Thus, in total, patients pay $750 of the first $2,250 in prescription drug costs. At that point, there is a gap in Medicare coverage that requires Medicare patients to pay 100% of the next $2,850 in prescription drug costs out of their own pockets. After beneficiaries have reached a catastrophic threshold by spending some $3,600 out-of-pocket, Medicare's catastrophic coverage kicks in; beneficiaries then pay either a 5% co-insurance charge or co-payments of $2 for generic drugs and $5 for brand-name drugs, whichever is greater. The annual deductible, benefit limits, and catastrophic threshold are indexed to rise as Part D spending increases. It has been estimated that the annual deductible may exceed $430 by 2014 (AARP, 2003; Henry J. Kaiser Family Foundation, 2005c). Because free-standing PDPs are free to offer lower premiums and lower patient cost-sharing requirements, patients' actual out-of-pocket expenses can vary considerably from the federal guidelines.

Medicare provides a variety of subsidies for low-income beneficiaries who enroll in Part D. For example, individuals with incomes below the poverty level who are eligible for both Medicare and Medicaid pay no monthly premium or deductible, and their co-payments are $1 for generic drugs and $3 for brand-name drugs. Numerous other groups of Medicare beneficiaries with limited incomes and resources also qualify for some type of assistance with Part D premiums, deductibles, and co-payments (Henry J. Kaiser Family Foundation, 2005c).

Part D coverage includes most FDA-approved prescription drugs and biologicals (drugs currently covered under Parts A and B will still be covered by these Medicare components). However, although they are expected to provide a broad range of drugs, drug plans are allowed to have formularies under Part D. Likewise, plans can use tiered cost-sharing, prior authorization, and other cost-containment tools, so long as they are not deemed unduly restrictive. While the law that created Part D prevents Medicare from negotiating drug prices with manufacturers, individual drug plans will undoubtedly use such tactics to produce savings in their drug expenditures (Centers for Medicare and Medicaid Services, 2005a; Henry J. Kaiser Family Foundation, 2005c).

Part D was not launched without its share of problems. Most notably, widespread eligibility verification problems frustrated both Medicare patients and the community pharmacists who serve them (Pharmacy Times, 2006; Ukens, 2006). As of April 2006, almost 20 million Medicare beneficiaries were enrolled in either a stand-alone PDP or a Medicare Advantage plan with prescription drug coverage; another 10 million individuals had drug coverage through a retiree health plan. Thus more than two-thirds of Medicare beneficiaries had some form of prescription drug coverage (Henry J. Kaiser Family Foundation, 2006a).

EXPENDITURES

Growth in Medicare Spending

Medicare has witnessed tremendous growth since its inception. When this program was first implemented, Medicare served some 19 million enrollees; by 2006, however, more than 43 million Americans were enrolled in Medicare (Centers for Medicare and Medicaid Services, 2005c; Henry J. Kaiser Family Foundation, 2006a).

Accompanying this expansion in the Medicare population has been rapid growth in Medicare program spending. Between 1967 and 2002, expenditures increased from $4.2 billion to approximately $325 billion (Centers for Medicare and Medicaid Services, 2003a; Henry J. Kaiser Family Foundation, 2005).

Spending by Type of Service

Inpatient hospital services and physician services are the largest individual components of total Medicare payments (see **Figure 17-1**). The proportion of Medicare spending attributable to these two types of services has decreased over time due to various payment reforms and cost-containment efforts. While inpatient hospital services and physician services accounted for more than 90% of Medicare payments in 1967, they accounted for just 62% of such payments in 2005. Conversely, the proportion of payments attributable to home health care and other outpatient benefits has increased substantially since 1967, and managed care, which was virtually nonexistent in 1967, now accounts for 15% of Medicare payments (Henry J. Kaiser Family Foundation, 2005a; Medicare and Medicaid Statistical Supplement, 2001).

Medicare is a program in which relatively small groups of patients with serious health problems consume a disproportionate share of benefits. The highest-cost group in the Medicare program is individuals with end-stage renal disease. In 2001, the average payment per ESRD patient was $43,633, compared to $6,061 for non-ESRD patients. Other high-cost groups of Medicare patients include those who died and those were hospitalized during a given year (Centers for Medicare and Medicaid Services, 2003a).

MEDICARE SUPPLEMENT (MEDIGAP) INSURANCE

Need for Supplemental Insurance

Although some Medicare beneficiaries, such as Helen in the case scenario at the beginning of this chapter, may be under the impression that Medicare will pay for all of their health care bills, it does not. Medicare pays for only 45% of the average elderly person's health care charges. Substantial patient cost sharing is required in the form of deductibles, co-payments, co-insurance, and Part B premiums. As an extreme example, a seriously ill Medicare patient who stayed 150 consecutive days in the hospital during 2006 would have been responsible for $36,652 in hospital deductibles and co-payments. But even relatively healthy Medicare enrollees who visit their physicians a few times per year will be liable for the premiums, deductibles, and co-insurance associated with Part B, as well as the full cost of services that are not covered by Medicare. Medicare beneficiaries paid, on average, more than $2,200 out-of-pocket for health care expenses in 2002 (Henry J. Kaiser Family Foundation, 2005b).

Several options are available to help Medicare beneficiaries meet these cost-sharing requirements, aside from paying these expenses out of their

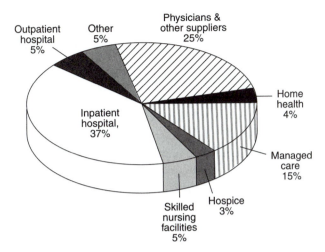

Figure 17-1 Distribution of Medicare Payments by Type of Service, 2005. *Source:* Congressional Budget Office.

own pockets. First, some patients might have additional retiree health insurance through a former employer or union. Second, they might be poor enough to qualify for assistance from Medicaid, which would help pay for their care. Third, they might enroll in a managed care plan that covers more services than does traditional Medicare. Lastly, Medicare beneficiaries can purchase additional private insurance, known as Medicare supplement or "Medigap" insurance, which is designed to pay for many of the charges for Medicare-covered services for which the beneficiary is responsible (Centers for Medicare and Medicaid Services, 2003a).

Types of Medigap Policies

Most states have adopted regulations designed to make it easier for consumers to comparison shop for a Medigap policy. These regulations allow no more than 10 different Medigap policies to be sold. These 10 policies, which were developed by the National Association of Insurance Commissioners and incorporated into state and federal laws, are assigned letter designations from A through J. To further enhance comparison shopping, insurers must use the same format, language, and definitions in describing their plans. In accordance with federal regulations, each state must allow the sale of Plan A, and all Medigap insurers must offer Plan A. Beyond this requirement, states may restrict the number of other plans that may be sold, and insurers are not obligated to sell any of the other nine types of Medigap plans (Center for the Study of Services, 1995).

The most basic type of Medigap policy, Plan A, consists of five basic benefits:

1. Coverage of the co-payment for days 61 through 90 of inpatient hospitalization
2. Coverage of the co-payment for lifetime hospital inpatient reserve days
3. Coverage of 100% of Medicare-eligible hospital expenses after all Medicare hospital benefits are exhausted
4. Coverage of the three-pint blood deductible
5. Coverage of the Medicare Part B co-insurance

Plans B through J offer combinations of other benefits in addition to those provided in Plan A. These additional benefits can include coverage of the SNF co-payment, the Part A hospital deductible, the Part B deductible, and preventive medical care. Three plans (H, I, and J) provide a prescription drug benefit with a $250 annual deductible. After meeting that deductible, Plans H and I cover 50% of prescription drug costs up to a maximum of $1,250 per year, while Plan J covers 50% of these costs up to a maximum of $3,000 per year (Health Care Financing Administration, 2000c). As of January 2006, insurers may no longer issue new Medigap policies that include drug coverage, and two new benefit packages (Plans K and L) became available that offer coverage for catastrophic medical expenses (Henry J. Kaiser Family Foundation, 2005b).

Case Scenario: Medicaid

Charlotte is a single parent of two children younger than age 6, and her annual income is about 10% above the federal poverty level for a family of three. She and her children receive health insurance through her state's Medicaid program.

In a nearby state, Ed and Teresa are married and have an infant daughter. They both work at low-wage jobs, providing a family income equal to the federal poverty level, but neither of their employers offers a health insurance benefit. While their daughter is covered by the state's Medicaid program, Ed and Teresa have no health insurance.

In yet another state, Jack is an agricultural worker with an annual income that is less than half the federal poverty level. Despite his extremely low income, Jack does not qualify for health insurance through his state's Medicaid program.

How can some, but not all, of these people be covered by Medicaid? Why is Medicaid eligibility not uniform across the United States?

MEDICAID: LEGISLATIVE HISTORY

In addition to initiating the Medicare program, the 1965 amendments to the Social Security Act (SSA) established a program popularly known as Medicaid. Officially designated as Title XIX of the SSA, "Grants to the States for Medical Assistance Programs," Medicaid was designed to provide medical assistance to eligible needy Americans and is now the largest source of funding for the provision of health-related services to the United States' poorest people (Medicare and Medicaid Statistical Supplement, 1995).

Medicaid remained a rider on the Medicare bill until late in the 1965 legislative debate, when it became a separate title at the last minute. For this reason, Medicaid has been referred to as Medicare's "kid brother." Some have suggested that no one knew enough in 1965 to predict accurately how large the Medicaid program would become. Of course, Medicaid proponents may have also provided unrealistically low estimates of the program's cost and eligibility to ensure its passage in Congress (Friedman, 1987). Many people viewed the legislation that created Medicaid and Medicare as a stopgap or temporary measure. Democrats assumed that either Lyndon Johnson or Hubert Humphrey would be elected president in 1968 and that a universal health plan for all Americans would become a reality soon thereafter. After Richard Nixon's election, however, movement toward a universal health plan stalled and these temporary measures became permanent fixtures in the U.S. health care market (Friedman, 1990).

ELIGIBILITY

Three broad groups of people may be covered by a state's Medicaid program: the mandated categorically needy, the optionally categorically needy, and the medically needy (Oberg and Polich, 1988). Because Medicaid is a joint state–federal program, states have some flexibility in determining criteria for Medicaid eligibility. States establish their own criteria within federal guidelines, so eligibility for each of these groups varies considerably from state to state.

Mandated Categorically Needy

If a state has a Medicaid program and wishes to receive matching federal funding, it must provide coverage for several groups of people. Federal welfare reform legislation enacted in the latter half of the 1990s made a major change with respect to individuals who must be provided Medicaid coverage. Prior to enactment of the Personal Responsibility and Work Opportunities Act of 1996, individuals who received cash assistance (welfare) through Aid to Families with Dependent Children (AFDC) were automatically eligible for Medicaid. The 1996 welfare reform act, however, cut the link between Medicaid and cash welfare by replacing the AFDC program with the Temporary Assistance for Needy Families (TANF) program, which provides block grants to states to be used for time-limited cash assistance. TANF generally allows a family to receive cash welfare benefits for no more than 5 years and allows states to impose other requirements related to employment.

Even if they are not receiving welfare, families are still eligible for Medicaid if they meet the AFDC eligibility criteria that were put in place in July 1996 (FamiliesUSA, 2000; Health Care Financing Administration, 2000a, 2000b). Such eligibility has two basic requirements:

- A maximum limit is placed on family income and resources. States establish these income and resource limits that determine access to Medicaid services (Health Care Financing Administration, 2000a). In 2005, for example, the maximum annual income limit for working parents to be eligible for Medicaid ranged from 19% of the federal poverty level (FPL) in two states to 275% of the FPL in a single state (Henry J. Kaiser Family Foundation, 2006b).
- A child typically must be living with a parent or other relative while being deprived of parental support or care due to death, absence, incapacity, or unemployment (Health Care Financing Administration, 2000a).

A second mandatory group of individuals qualifies for Medicaid because they receive government cash assistance through the Supplemental Security Income (SSI) program (Health Care Financing Administration, 2000a). This program provides assistance to persons who are poor and either elderly, blind, or disabled. As with TANF, eligibility for the SSI program is based on income and asset limits. The 2006 federal maximum monthly income for individuals in the SSI program, the standard used by most states, ranged from $623 for an individual whose income comes not only from wages to $1,893 for couples whose income does come only from wages (Social Security Administration, 2006).

Several other mandated categorically needy groups of low-income individuals do not meet the SSI or previous AFDC requirements. For example, Medicaid programs must cover pregnant women (for pregnancy-related services) and children younger than 6 years of age in families with incomes up to 133% of the FPL. In families with incomes at or below the FPL, Medicaid must cover all children younger than 19 years of age (Centers for Medicare and Medicaid Services, 2002a).

States must also provide limited Medicaid coverage to certain groups of low-income Medicare enrollees. Medicare-eligible individuals with incomes below the FPL and limited assets are known as Qualified Medicare Beneficiaries (QMBs). Medicaid must pay the premiums and other cost-sharing expenses (such as deductibles and co-insurance) incurred with Part A and Part B of Medicare for QMBs. For low-income Medicare beneficiaries with incomes between 100% and 120% of the FPL, Medicaid must pay only the Part B premiums. Individuals who have lost their Medicare disability benefits because they returned to work but are allowed to purchase Medicare coverage (called Qualified Disabled and Working Individuals) can qualify to have Medicaid pay their Medicare Part A premiums if their incomes are less than twice the FPL (Centers for Medicare and Medicaid Services, 2002a).

Optional Eligibility Groups

States have the option of providing coverage for other groups of needy individuals who do not meet the requirements for mandated coverage, although they may share certain characteristics with people in the aforementioned categories. Many of those considered optionally eligible are children or pregnant women. For example, states may cover infants up to 1 year of age and pregnant women in families not qualifying for mandated coverage but with incomes below 185% of the FPL. Likewise, children younger than age 21 who meet the income and asset requirements for TANF, but not the family status requirements, can be covered by state Medicaid programs (Centers for Medicare and Medicaid Services, 2005a). If a state program does include the optional categorically needy, it must provide these individuals with the same Medicaid benefits as those provided to people in the mandatory categories (Oberg and Polich, 1988).

Medically Needy Groups

At their option, state Medicaid programs may elect to cover a group known as the "medically needy." These individuals include people who would be eligible for Medicaid under one of the mandated or optional groups, except for the fact that their income and/or assets are higher than allowed by the state. Such individuals become Medicaid-eligible under the medically needy provision if their medical expenses reduce their "net" income to the Medicaid eligibility threshold or less. Thus the medically needy consist of families and children, or elderly, blind, or disabled individuals, who "spend down" to Medicaid eligibility by incurring high out-of-pocket medical expenses (Medicare and Medicaid Statistical Supplement, 1995). This spending-down process is especially important for granting Medicaid eligibility to institutionalized persons who incur extremely large medical expenses (Medicare and Medicaid Statistical Supplement, 1992).

Thirty-four states and the District of Columbia cover medically eligible persons in their Medicaid programs (Centers for Medicare and Medicaid Services, 2005c). When a state chooses to have a program for the medically needy, certain groups of people must be covered. These include certain children younger than age 18 and pregnant women who would be eligible for Medicaid if they met the income and asset requirements (Centers for Medicare and Medicaid Services, 2003b). States may include other groups and may offer different benefits to different groups under the medically needy option (Medicare and Medicaid Statistical Supplement, 1992).

FINANCING AND ADMINISTRATION

Because Medicaid is funded by both federal and state governments, these entities share responsibility for administering this program. Through the CMS, the federal government establishes broad guidelines under which states must design and operate their individual programs. At the state level, a single agency must be designated as responsible for the Medicaid program. Within the federal guidelines, states have responsibility for establishing eligibility criteria, determining the type and scope of services to be covered, setting rates of payment for services, and administering their programs. Because states differ in exactly how they carry out these responsibilities, Medicaid programs vary considerably from state to state. A person who is Medicaid-eligible in one state may not be eligible in nearby states, and the services provided may differ considerably between states (Centers for Medicare and Medicaid Services, 2002a; Medicare and Medicaid Statistical Supplement, 1995). Thus, while one may speak of Medicare as a program that is essentially uniform across the entire United States, there are actually 56 different Medicaid programs (one for each state, territory, and the District of Columbia).

Medicaid is entirely optional in the sense that the federal government does not require any state to have a Medicaid program. All 50 states do have Medicaid programs, of course, but they do so at their own discretion. Medicaid does not provide health care services for all poor Americans. Even in states with the broadest eligibility provisions, as illustrated by the case scenario, Medicaid is unlikely to provide care for poor individuals unless they are children, pregnant, elderly, blind, or disabled. As a consequence, it is important to recall that low income is only one criterion determining Medicaid eligibility (Centers for Medicare and Medicaid Services, 2003b). In 2002, for example, only 37% of Americans younger than age 65 who were living in poverty were covered by Medicaid (Kaiser Commission on Medicaid and the Uninsured, 2003b).

The portion of Medicaid program costs that is paid by the federal government for provider services is known as the Federal Medical Assistance Percentage (FMAP). Each state's FMAP is determined annually through the use of a formula that compares a given state's average per capita income to the national average. By law, the FMAP can be no greater than

83% and no less than 50% for any given state. States that are wealthier in terms of average per capita income have a smaller share of their Medicaid costs paid by the federal government than do relatively poorer states. In 2006, the FMAP ranged from a high of 76% in Mississippi to 50% in 12 states. There are some exceptions to the FMAP rules. Most administrative costs, for example, are matched at 50%, while higher than normal matching rates are allowed for some specific services and types of patients.

The total amount of money that the federal government spends on Medicaid has no set limit. It must match state government spending at the percentages established by law (Centers for Medicare and Medicaid Services, 2002b, 2005b). Thus, as state spending on Medicaid has escalated over time, so has the amount of money that the federal government contributes to the program.

State programs make payments directly to participating health care providers for services delivered to Medicaid patients. These providers must accept the amount of Medicaid reimbursement as payment in full; they may not bill patients for any difference between actual charges and Medicaid's approved charges (balance billing). Payment levels are subject to federally mandated conditions to which states must adhere. For example, payments must be high enough to attract sufficient numbers of providers so that services will be available to Medicaid recipients to the same extent that those services are available to the general population in a given geographic area. As another example of the conditions that must be met, Medicaid payments for institutional services may not exceed the amounts that would be paid by Medicare (Medicare and Medicaid Statistical Supplement, 1995).

MEDICAID SERVICES AND COST SHARING

Services Covered

To receive federal matching funds, state Medicaid programs are required to offer a specified list of services to the mandatory and optional categorically needy groups. These required services include the following:

- Inpatient hospital services
- Outpatient hospital services
- Physician services
- Rural health clinic services (provided in facilities located in rural areas determined to have shortages of health services or primary medical care providers)
- Federally qualified health center services (such as services provided in migrant health centers or community health centers)

- Laboratory and X-ray services
- Nursing facility services for individuals age 21 or older
- Early and periodic screening, diagnosis, and treatment (EPSDT) services for individuals younger than 21 years of age (includes physical examinations, immunizations, vision and hearing services, health education, and a variety of other diagnostic and treatment services)
- Family planning services and supplies
- Home health services for persons eligible for skilled nursing services
- Nurse-midwife services
- Certified pediatric nurse practitioner and certified family nurse practitioner services
- Prenatal care (Centers for Medicare and Medicaid Services, 2002b)

States also may receive federal funding for provision of a variety of optional services to the mandatory and optional categorically needy groups. States are under no obligation to cover any of these additional services, and the number of optional services provided by Medicaid programs varies widely. Outpatient prescription drugs are an optional service, although they are covered by Medicaid programs in all 50 states. The following are examples of optional services that may be available:

- Outpatient prescription drugs and prosthetic devices
- Physical and rehabilitative therapy
- Optometrist services and eyeglasses
- Services in an intermediate care facility for the mentally retarded
- Transportation services
- Home and community-based care for certain persons with chronic impairments (Centers for Medicare and Medicaid Services, 2002a)

If a state chooses to cover medically needy persons in its Medicaid program, it must at least provide prenatal and delivery services for pregnant women, ambulatory services to individuals younger than age 18 and to persons entitled to institutional services, and home health services for individuals entitled to nursing facility services. Additional requirements exist for states that cover services in institutions for mental diseases or intermediate care facilities for the mentally retarded (Centers for Medicare and Medicaid Services, 2002b).

Cost Sharing

States have broad discretion in determining reimbursement methodologies and payment rates within federal guidelines. Many states require Medicaid recipients to contribute to the cost of their health care in the form of deductibles, co-payments, or co-insurance (Centers for Medicare and Medicaid Services, 2002a). However, the magnitude of this cost sharing cannot be so great that it would present a serious barrier to receiving needed services. For example, in 2004, more than 80% of states imposed co-payments on outpatient Medicaid prescriptions, but most ranged between $0.50 and $3.00 (Kaiser Commission on Medicaid and the Uninsured, 2004). Likewise, nursing home patients are expected to contribute most of their income to help pay for their care. There are certain services, however, for which cost sharing cannot be required (for example, emergency care, family planning services, pregnancy-related services, and services provided to children younger than age 18) (Centers for Medicare and Medicaid Services, 2002a).

EXPENDITURES

Growth in Medicaid Enrollment and Spending

In terms of both the number of beneficiaries and total expenditures, Medicaid has experienced tremendous growth since its inception. In 1972, Medicaid covered 17.6 million poor Americans, about 8.5% of the U.S. population, with total expenditures of less than $10 billion (National Center for Health Statistics, 1993). By 2004, the Medicaid program covered about 50 million persons, some 18% of the U.S. population, and expended more than $300 billion annually (Henry J. Kaiser Family Foundation, 2004).

Spending by Eligibility Group

There are considerable differences between the proportion of beneficiaries and the proportion of expenditures accounted for by the major enrollment groups. Although 51% of all Medicaid beneficiaries in 2002 were children, only 17% of Medicaid spending went to provide care for children. By comparison, the elderly represented only 10% of Medicaid beneficiaries, but accounted for 27% of total spending. Similarly, blind and disabled persons made up just 17% of recipients, but they were responsible for 44% of expenditures (Kaiser Commission on Medicaid and the Uninsured, 2003a). Thus Medicaid is a program in which relatively small segments of the recipient population account for the vast majority of total spending.

Spending by Type of Service

Medicaid spending also varies by type of health care service. Substantial portions of Medicaid payments are associated with inpatient hospitals, nursing homes, and prescribed drugs, with each segment accounting for more than 10% of total payments in 2001 (see **Figure 17-2**). These proportions have changed considerably for some services since the mid-1970s. Inpatient services (i.e., those delivered in inpatient hospitals, nursing homes, intermediate care facilities for the mentally retarded) accounted

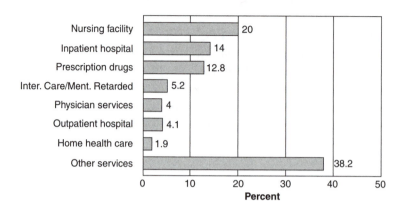

Figure 17-2 Distribution of Medicaid Payments by Type of Service, 2001. *Source:* Data from Center for Medicare and Medicaid Services.

___

for 66% of all Medicaid payments in 1975, but only 39.2% in 2001. Similarly, payments for physician services declined from 10% to 4% over the same period. Conversely, payments for prescription drugs increased from 6.7% to 12.8% between 1975 and 2001. The greatest change was in the "other services" category, which grew from 13.8% to 38.2%; this category includes managed care, which was essentially nonexistent in Medicaid in 1975 (Centers for Medicare and Medicaid Services, 2003a).

STATE FLEXIBILITY

General Requirements for Medicaid Programs

State Medicaid programs must operate within broad guidelines established by the federal government. In addition to meeting the eligibility and services restrictions already described, states must adhere to three other general requirements:

- *Statewideness.* A state's Medicaid plan must be in effect across the entire state; the services covered in one part of a state generally cannot differ from those covered in another part of the state.
- *Freedom of choice.* Medicaid recipients must be allowed to obtain covered services from any qualified participating provider.
- *Comparability of services.* The amount, duration, and scope of services must be equal for all persons in the mandatory and optional eligibility categories (Medicare and Medicaid Statistical Supplement, 1992).

Section 1115 and 1915b Waivers

Under the SSA, CMS is given the power to grant two types of waivers of these requirements: Section 1115 and Section 1915b waivers. These waivers have been extremely important in allowing states to experiment with managed care options for their Medicaid beneficiaries (Muirhead, 1996).

The Section 1115 waiver is intended to encourage state testing of innovative ideas that could be implemented nationwide (Medicare and Medicaid Statistical Supplement, 1995). These 5-year demonstration waivers, which are research-oriented and subject to rigorous evaluation, must be "budget neutral"—that is, they must not increase Medicaid costs and must enable more people to receive Medicaid benefits or provide new benefits to those individuals already covered by Medicaid. At least 80 Section 1115 waivers have been granted since 1965. In the 1970s, these waivers allowed states to implement new methods of providing home or community-based services and to facilitate implementation of EPSDT programs. Most of the recent Section 1115 demonstration waivers have involved implementation of Medicaid managed care programs (Henry J. Kaiser Family Foundation, 1999b; Muirhead, 1996; Vladeck, 1995).

Section 1915b waivers are more limited in scope than Section 1115 waivers. They target only current Medicaid recipients and do not seek to expand coverage to other uninsured individuals. Section 1915b waivers allow states to implement a variety of managed care practices. One example is a primary-care case management system in which primary-care physicians are paid fixed fees to manage the care of Medicaid patients who may be seeing multiple physicians (i.e., specialists). Other practices implemented under Section 1915b waivers include utilization of restricted provider networks and enrollment of Medicaid beneficiaries in MCOs (Muirhead, 1996). Over the years, at least 40 states have used 1915b waivers to implement mandatory managed care for some or all of their Medicaid beneficiaries (Henry J. Kaiser Family Foundation, 1999b). The Balanced Budget Act of 1997 eliminated the need for states to request a waiver to implement mandatory Medicaid managed care, except for a few special groups including children with special needs and Native Americans (Iglehart, 1999).

Managed Care

As evidenced by these waiver programs, many of the efforts aimed at reforming Medicaid have involved greater utilization of managed care organizations for delivery of health care services. As a result of a number of factors, including the need for cost containment in light of Medicaid's cost explosion, the proliferation of managed care in the private sector, and changes in federal policy that have promoted the expansion of Medicaid managed care through the waiver process, there has been tremendous growth in the number of Medicaid beneficiaries who are enrolled in managed care programs (Kaiser Commission on the Future of Medicaid, 1995). Between 1994 and 2004, the proportion of Medicaid beneficiaries enrolled in some form of managed care increased from 23% to 61% (Centers for Medicare and Medicaid Services, 2005a).

Medicaid's venture into managed care has been more successful than that of Medicare, possibly because the poor are easier to "force" into managed than are the elderly. While the expansion of states' Medicaid managed care programs have not been completely trouble-free, they have been able to install "midcourse corrections" designed to expand access to quality health care while slowing spending (Brown and Sparer, 2003).

COMPARISON OF MEDICARE AND MEDICAID

Medicare and Medicaid are similar in the sense that both are health insurance programs financed and administered by government entities, and that both are roughly equivalent in terms of the number of beneficiaries and total expenditures. In many ways, however, Medicare and Medicaid are very different. Philosophically, Medicare is a social insurance policy for which beneficiaries have paid through taxes; Medicaid is based on a welfare concept of redistributing wealth among citizens of the United States. There also are differences between the two programs with respect to financing, administration, eligibility, and benefits. Thus these two government programs actually represent two very different mechanisms for delivering health care benefits to selected segments of American society, thereby providing a vital "safety net" for many of the nation's most vulnerable citizens.

QUESTIONS FOR FURTHER DISCUSSION

1. If Medicare did not exist today, do you believe such a program would be enacted by Congress? Why or why not?
2. If you were speaking to a group of senior citizens, how would you explain the importance of Medicare supplemental insurance?
3. What do you see as the advantages and disadvantages of delivering services to Medicare beneficiaries through managed care plans?
4. What do you believe are the primary strengths and weaknesses of the Part D prescription drug coverage?
5. Should Medicaid be expanded to cover more low-income people? Why or why not?
6. Do you believe Medicaid eligibility criteria should be uniform from state to state? Why or why not?
7. In the long term, do you believe that managed care will have a positive or negative effect on Medicaid and its recipients? Why?
8. How would you restructure Medicaid to ensure that it best meets the needs of low-income Americans at a reasonable cost?

KEY TOPICS AND TERMS

Assignment
Benefit period
Centers for Medicare and Medicaid Services
Cost sharing
Federal Medical Assistance Percentage
Managed care
Mandated categorically needy
Medicaid
Medically needy
Medicare
Medicare Advantage
Medicare participating
Medicare supplement (Medigap) insurance
Medicare Part A
Medicare Part B
Medicare Part C
Medicare Part D
Optionally categorically needy
Qualified Disabled and Working Individuals
Qualified Medicare Beneficiaries
Specified Low-Income Medicare Beneficiaries
Supplemental Security Income
Temporary Assistance for Needy Families
Waivers

REFERENCES

AARP. (2003). *What does the new Medicare drug benefit mean for you?* Retrieved from http://www.aarp.org/bulletin/prescription/Articles/a2003-11-26-foryou.html

Ball, R. M. (1995). What Medicare's architects had in mind. *Health Affairs, 14*(4), 62–72.

Brown, L. D., & Sparer, M. S. (2003). Poor program's progress: The unanticipated politics of Medicaid policy. *Health Affairs, 22*(1), 31–44.

Center for the Study of Services. (1995). *Consumers' guide to health plans.* Washington, DC: Center for the Study of Services.

Centers for Medicare and Medicaid Services. (2002a). *Medicaid: A brief summary.* Retrieved from http://www.cms.hhs.gov/publications/overview-medicare-medicaid/default4.asp

Centers for Medicare and Medicaid Services. (2002b). *Medicaid services.* Retrieved from http://www.cms.hhs.gov/medicaid/mservice.asp

Centers for Medicare and Medicaid Services. (2003a). *Health Care Financing Review, Medicare and Medicaid supplement, 2003.* Retrieved from http://www.cms.hhs.gov/apps/review/supp/2003

Centers for Medicare and Medicaid Services. (2003b). *Medicaid eligibility.* Retrieved from http://www.cms.hhs.gov/medicaid/eligibility/criteria.asp

Centers for Medicare and Medicaid Services. (2003c). *Medicare and you.* Baltimore, MD: U.S. Department of Health and Human Services.

Centers for Medicare and Medicaid Services. (2003d). *Your Medicare benefits.* Baltimore, MD: U.S. Department of Health and Human Services.

Centers for Medicare and Medicaid Services. (2004). *Medicare enrollment—all beneficiaries.* Retrieved July, 2004 from http://www.cms.hhs.gov/Medicaid EnRpts/Downloads/04All.pdf

Centers for Medicare and Medicaid Services. (2005a). *Brief summaries of Medicare and Medicaid.* Retrieved from http://www.cms.hhs.gov/MedicareProgram RatesStats/downloads/MedicareMedicaidSummaries2005.pdf

Centers for Medicare and Medicaid Services. (2005b). *Medicaid at-a-glance 2005.* Baltimore, MD: U.S. Department of Health and Human Services.

Centers for Medicare and Medicaid Services. (2005c). *Medicare enrollment: National trends 1966–2005.* Retrieved from http://www.cms.hhs.gov/Medicare EnRpts/Downloads/HISMI05.pdf

Centers for Medicare and Medicaid Services. (2006). *Medicare premiums and deductibles for 2006.* Retrieved from http://www.cms.hhs.gov/apps/media/ press/release.asp?Counter=1557

Coleman, T. S. (1990). *Legal aspects of Medicare & Medicaid reimbursement: Payment for hospital and physician services.* Washington, DC: National Health Lawyers Association.

Davis, M. H., & Burner, S. T. (1995). Three decades of Medicare: What the numbers tell us. *Health Affairs, 14*(4), 231–243.

FamiliesUSA. (2000). *Welfare–Medicaid links: What every welfare advocate should know about Medicaid.* Retrieved from http://www.familiesusa.org/whatwelf .htm

Fein, R. (1989). *Medical care, medical costs* (2nd ed.). Cambridge, MA: Harvard University Press.

Friedman, E. (1987). Medicaid's overload sparks a crisis. *Hospitals, 61*(2), 50–54.

Friedman, E. (1990). Medicare and Medicaid at 25. *Hospitals, 64*(15), 38, 42, 46, 48, 50, 52, 54.

Ginsburg, P. B. (1988). Public insurance programs: Medicare and Medicaid. In H. E. Frech III (Ed.), *Health care in America* (pp. 179–218). San Francisco, CA: Pacific Research Institute for Public Policy.

Health Care Financing Administration. (1996). *Your Medicare handbook, 1996.* Baltimore, MD: U.S. Department of Health and Human Services.

Health Care Financing Administration. (1998). *A profile of Medicare chart book.* Baltimore, MD: U.S. Department of Health and Human Services.

Health Care Financing Administration. (2000a). *Link between Medicaid and Temporary Assistance for Needy Families (TANF).* Retrieved from http://www.hcfa. gov/medicaid/wrfs1.htm

Health Care Financing Administration. (2000b). *Medicaid: A brief summary.* Retrieved from http://www.hcfa.gov/pubforms/actuary/ormedmed/DEFAULT4. htm

Health Care Financing Administration. (2000c). *Medicare: A brief summary.* Retrieved from http://www.hcfa.gov/pubforms/actuary/ormedmed/DEFAULT3. htm

Hellman, S., & Hellman, L. H. (1991). *Medicare and Medigaps: A guide to retirement health insurance.* Newbury Park, CA: Sage.

Henry J. Kaiser Family Foundation. (1999a). *Analysis of benefits offered by Medicare HMOs, 1999: Complexities and implications.* Menlo Park, CA: Henry J. Kaiser Family Foundation.

Henry J. Kaiser Family Foundation. (1999b). *Medicaid and managed care.* Menlo Park, CA: Henry J. Kaiser Family Foundation.

Henry J. Kaiser Family Foundation. (2003). *Medicare+Choice.* Menlo Park, CA: Henry J. Kaiser Family Foundation.

Henry J. Kaiser Family Foundation. (2004). *Key Medicare and Medicaid statistics.* Retrieved from http://www.kff.org/medicaid/upload/KeyMedicareand MedicaidStatistics.pdf

Henry J. Kaiser Family Foundation. (2005a). *Medicare at a glance.* Menlo Park, CA: Henry J. Kaiser Family Foundation.

Henry J. Kaiser Family Foundation. (2005b). *Medicare chart book 2005.* Menlo Park, CA: Henry J. Kaiser Family Foundation.

Henry J. Kaiser Family Foundation. (2005c). *The Medicare prescription drug benefit.* Menlo Park, CA: Henry J. Kaiser Family Foundation.

Henry J. Kaiser Family Foundation. (2006a). *Medicare beneficiaries with creditable prescription drug coverage by type.* Retrieved April 18, 2006 from http://www. statehealthfacts.org/cgi-bin/healthfacts.cgi?actoin=compare&category=Medicare +Drug+Benefit&topic=Medicare+Rx+Drug+Coverage

Henry J. Kaiser Family Foundation. (2006b). *State Medicaid fact sheet.* Retrieved from http://www.kff.org/mfs/pdfs/mfs_highlow.pdf

Iglehart, J. K. (1999). The American health care system—Medicaid. *New England Journal of Medicine, 340*(5), 403–408.

Kaiser Commission on the Future of Medicaid. (1995). *Medicaid and managed care: Lessons from the literature.* Washington, DC: Henry J. Kaiser Family Foundation.

Kaiser Commission on Medicaid and the Uninsured. (2003a). *The Medicaid program at a glance.* Washington, DC: Henry J. Kaiser Family Foundation.

Kaiser Commission on Medicaid and the Uninsured. (2003b). *The uninsured and their access to health care.* Washington, DC: Henry J. Kaiser Family Foundation.

Kaiser Commission on Medicaid and the Uninsured. (2004). *Medicaid benefits: Online database.* Retrieved from http://www.kff.org/medicaid/benefits/service. jsp?gr=off&nt=on&so=0&tg=0&yr=2&cat=5&sv=32

Longest, B. B., Jr. (1994). *Health policymaking in the United States.* Ann Arbor, MI: Association of University Programs in Health Administration Press/Health Administration Press.

Medicare and Medicaid Statistical Supplement. (1992). *Health Care Financing Review, 14*(suppl).

Medicare and Medicaid Statistical Supplement. (1995). *Health Care Financing Review, 16*(suppl).

Medicare and Medicaid Statistical Supplement. (2001). *Health Care Financing Review, 21*(suppl).

Muirhead, G. (1996). More Medicaid programs turning to managed care. *Drug Topics, 140*(8), 50–51.

National Center for Health Statistics. (1993). *Health, United States, 1992.* Hyattsville, MD: Public Health Service, U.S. Department of Health and Human Services.

Oberg, C. N., & Polich, C. L. (1988). Medicaid: Entering the third decade. *Health Affairs, 7*(4), 83–96.

Pharmacy Times. (2006). *Medicare offers seniors advice for dealing with Part D glitches.* Retrieved from http://www.pharmacytimes.com/article.cfm?ID=3327

Social Security Administration. (2003). *Update 2003.* Retrieved from http://www.ssa.gov/pubs/10003.html

Social Security Administration. (2006). *Update 2006.* Retrieved from http://www.ssa.gov/pubs/10003.html

Ukens, C. (2006). *Medicare Part D off to rocky start.* Retrieved from http://www.drugtopics.com/drugtopics/article/articleDetail.jsp?id=283609

Vladeck, B. C. (1995). Medicaid 1115 demonstrations: Progress through partnership. *Health Affairs, 14*(1), 217–220.

Zarabozo, C., Taylor, C., & Hicks, J. (1996). Medicare managed care: Numbers and trends. *Health Care Financing Review, 17*(3), 243–261.

Pharmacoeconomics

Emily R. Cox and Kenneth W. Schafermeyer

Case Scenario

Bob is director of pharmacy for a large managed care organization, Gulf Coast Health. He manages all aspects of the health plan's pharmacy budget. The health plan has more than 300,000 members, located primarily in the southeastern United States, and last year it spent more than $78 million for pharmaceuticals. This spending was 20% higher than the expenditures for the previous year, which caused concern among Gulf Coast executives.

Bob has been asked to take a more active role in managing the pharmacy benefit. He is to begin by conducting a complete evaluation of new products that enter the market and comparing their value to existing products used to treat similar conditions. A new sulfonylurea has been approved by the Food and Drug Administration. The product is similar to products on the market and will be approved for the treatment of Type 2 diabetes. It does appear to have a more favorable side-effect profile than products currently on the market but is priced 20% higher per dose than the current therapies. As part of the formulary review process, Bob has asked his staff to conduct a pharmacoeconomic evaluation of this new product, comparing its costs and efficacy to those of the existing sulfonylureas.

LEARNING OBJECTIVES _____

Upon completion of this chapter, the student shall be able to:

- Define pharmacoeconomics and explain how it is used.
- Explain how perspective can affect a pharmacoeconomic study.
- Define and differentiate among CMA, CEA, CBA, and CUA (when should each be used, how they differ with regard to measuring costs and outcomes, and so on). Given a case study or a scenario, be able to calculate each value and use them to decide among alternatives.
- Define, differentiate, and give examples of inputs, outputs, and outcomes.
- Compare and contrast efficiency and effectiveness.
- Define, differentiate, and give examples of the four types of costs used in pharmacoeconomic analyses.
- Differentiate between a clinical endpoint and an outcome.
- Critically appraise a pharmacoeconomic study.

CHAPTER QUESTIONS

Begin formulating in your mind how Bob might begin to evaluate this new product.

1. Should Bob recommend that this product be covered?
2. Upon what criteria should he base his decision?
3. What alternative therapies would be compared with the new product?

INTRODUCTION

From 1997 through 2003, spending for pharmaceuticals experienced double-digit growth rates (Centers for Medicare and Medicaid Services, 2006). Those most alarmed by rising pharmaceutical costs are, of course, those responsible for paying for and managing these costs. Payers of pharmaceuticals include employers, managed care organizations (MCOs), and a myriad of health care institutions such as inpatient hospitals and the Veterans Administration. Those responsible for managing these costs are the individuals within these institutions who, through their own expertise and with the help of outside management organizations such as pharmacy benefit management (PBM) companies, attempt to constrain pharmacy costs in the face of limited budgets.

Decision makers charged with managing pharmacy costs have historically focused on the ingredient cost of the product along with its clinical profile in assessing a product's value. This is often referred to as the "silo" approach to evaluating pharmaceuticals. However, this approach does not consider how pharmaceuticals affect other health care costs, such as hospitalizations, physician visits, or laboratory services. All of these are important aspects to consider so as to capture the true value of pharmaceuticals.

"Pharmacoeconomics" is a term used to describe a compilation of methods that evaluate the economic, clinical, and humanistic dimensions of pharmaceutical products and services. More formally, pharmacoeconomics identifies, measures, and compares the costs and consequences of the use of pharmaceutical products and services (Bootman, Townsend, and McGhan, 1996). In its most simplistic form, a pharmacoeconomic evaluation compares the economic resources consumed (inputs) to produce the health and economic consequences of products or services (outcomes). This relationship is presented graphically in **Figure 18-1.**

The economic evaluation of health care began to take shape in the late 1970s with the writings of Weinstein and Stason (1977). The techniques used were taken from the field of public economics, particularly methods related to cost-benefit analysis. The application of economic evaluation to pharmacy began around the same time. These early writings and studies on the subject did not evaluate pharmaceuticals but rather pharmacy services (Bootman, McGhan, and Schondelmeyer, 1982; Bootman, Wertheimer, Zaske, and Rowland, 1979). The focus shifted to evaluation of products after the term "pharmacoeconomics" appeared in the literature in 1986 (Townsend, 1986). A tremendous growth in the number of pharmacoeconomic studies appearing in the literature has occurred since that time.

Pharmacoeconomic evaluations have been used as a tool in selecting formulary products, developing treatment guidelines, conducting disease management programs, establishing prior authorization policies, implementing step-therapy programs, and designing prescription drug benefit programs (Motheral, Grizzle, Armstrong, Cox, and Fairman, 2000). Together with information on a product's clinical efficacy and safety, pharmacoeconomic information assists decision makers in optimizing the use of prescription therapy.

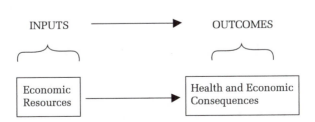

Figure 18-1 Economic Evaluation of Health Care

The economic evaluation of pharmaceuticals and pharmacy services grew out of the need to establish value or to respond to the question of value. Statements of product or service value center on two attributes: cost and benefit. From the consumer's perspective, the price paid should reflect the benefit gained from use of the product or service. Several factors have created the need to monitor the value of pharmaceuticals more closely: increased cost and thus growing concern on the part of payers, increased number of alternatives available to treat illness and disease, growing demand for pharmaceuticals, and the introduction of high-cost biotechnology products.

To conduct pharmacoeconomic evaluations, four methodological approaches are used: cost-minimization analysis (CMA), cost-benefit analysis (CBA), cost-effectiveness analysis (CEA), and cost-utility analysis (CUA). More recently, a fifth approach, cost-consequence analysis (CCA), has gained acceptance within the literature. This chapter covers each of these methods, including its advantages and disadvantages and its application to pharmaceutical products and services.

First, however, it is important to distinguish between several terms that are often confused with one another: efficiency, efficacy, and effectiveness. Efficiency can refer to a number of economic goals, such as properly allocating resources or increasing production. In our context, efficiency refers to the lowest cost per unit of output. It should be noted that an output is not the same as an outcome. For example, reducing the cost of prescriptions (outputs) may be efficient but it does not necessarily improve health outcomes.

Efficacy and effectiveness address outcomes. Efficacy answers the question, Does the product work? This question is answered through the clinical trial process, where it is determined whether the product does more good than harm. Effectiveness, however, seeks to determine whether the product works in real-world practice settings. Effectiveness answers the question, Does the product work in those individuals it was designed to treat?

COMPARING PHARMACOECONOMIC METHODOLOGIES

As shown in **Table 18-1,** each pharmacoeconomic method measures costs in monetary units (e.g., U.S. dollars). The methods differ from each other, however, in how consequences are measured.

In both CMA and CEA, the consequences or outcomes of the intervention being evaluated are measured in natural units of effectiveness. Natural units of effectiveness are typically clinical measures of a product's effectiveness, such as mm Hg or blood glucose levels. Natural units of effectiveness also include years of life saved, judgments of clinical success, or cases averted because of an intervention.

Table 18-1 Measurement of Costs and Consequences under Different Pharmacoeconomic Methodologies

Methodology	Cost	Consequences
Cost-minimization	Dollars	Natural units
Cost-effectiveness	Dollars	Natural units
Cost-benefit	Dollars	Dollars
Cost-utility	Dollars	Quality-adjusted life years (QALYs)
Cost-consequence analysis	Dollars	Natural units
		Dollars or QALYs

CBA measures the consequences of the intervention in dollars, whereas CUA measures the consequences of therapy in quality-adjusted life-years (QALYs). CCA also measures costs in dollars, but is different from the other methods in that multiple outcome measures are presented to the decision maker. Each of these methods will be covered in greater detail later in the chapter.

The remainder of this chapter will not only familiarize readers with the terminology and concepts of pharmacoeconomics, but also present some of the basic guidelines for conducting pharmacoeconomic studies and equip students and practitioners for critical appraisal of the literature.

STEPS FOR CONDUCTING A PHARMACOECONOMIC EVALUATION

Before the specifics of each method are presented, some important points need to be considered. When conducting a pharmacoeconomic evaluation, it is important to (1) define the problem and state the objective; (2) identify the perspective and the alternative interventions to be compared; (3) identify and measure the outcomes of each alternative; and (4) identify, measure, and value the costs of all alternatives. Other important aspects of pharmacoeconomic evaluations to be discussed are discounting and performing sensitivity analysis.

Define the Problem and State the Objective

All pharmacoeconomic evaluations should begin with a clear and concise statement of the problem or question to be addressed. In the chapter-opening case scenario, Bob could evaluate the alternative drug therapies for a specific indication or patient population, or he could compare the new therapy to a diet and exercise regimen for a specific study population such as newly diagnosed patients. Examples of problem statements include "Is the new sulfonylurea cost effective for the treatment of Type 2 diabetes?" and, more broadly, "What is the most cost-effective regimen for the treatment of Type 2 diabetes?"

Identify the Perspective

Establishing the perspective of a study is an important step in pharmaco-economic evaluation. Pharmacoeconomic evaluations can be conducted from several different perspectives, including those of the employer, the patient, the health insurance plan, society, and the government. For example, the perspective of the case scenario could be that of either the health plan or Gulf Coast Health's major employer group. The study perspective is an important factor in determining the costs considered relevant, the choice of outcomes measured, and the time period over which the product or service will be evaluated.

An example from the literature highlights the importance of perspective and how it can influence the results of the study. A cost-benefit analysis of a routine varicella (chickenpox) vaccination program for healthy children was conducted from two perspectives: that of society and that of the payer of health services (e.g., a health plan) (Lieu et al., 1994). The study found that from a payer's perspective, the vaccine had a benefit-to-cost ratio that was less than 1 (i.e., the benefits were less than the costs). However, when conducted from a societal perspective, the benefit-to-cost ratio was greater than 1, suggesting that the program should be implemented. The difference in findings derived from which costs were considered relevant from the different perspectives. From society's perspective, costs related to lost workdays avoided because of the vaccine were relevant and, therefore, were included. From a payer's perspective, these costs were not considered relevant and, therefore, were not included in the analysis.

Identify Alternative Interventions

The decision as to which alternatives should be compared in pharma-coeconomic evaluations is important. A simple question to ask when considering which alternatives to compare is, Have all relevant treatment alternatives been considered in addressing the research question? In many studies, the alternatives involve drug-to-drug comparisons; in other situations, drug therapy is compared to diet and exercise or surgical procedures.

Alternatives are compared only when one of the alternatives is both more costly and more effective than the other options. In **Table 18-2,** for example, nine scenarios exist in the comparison of alternatives A and B. Alternative A is either more costly than B, as costly as B, or less costly than B. The same relationship applies to the degree of effectiveness. In our case scenario, it is believed that the new sulfonylurea coming onto the market is more effective but also more costly. If alternative A represents existing products on the market and alternative B is the new sulfonylurea, this scenario would fall in the lower-right cell of Table 18-2. The researcher would then analyze the differences in costs and effects between these

Table 18-2 Cost and Effectiveness Comparison Grid

Cost	Effectiveness		
	A>B	A=B	A<B
A>B	Analyze	B dominates	B dominates
A=B	A dominates	Indifferent	B dominates
A<B	A dominates	A dominates	Analyze

two alternatives. The question becomes, Is the additional gain in benefit or effectiveness worth the additional cost? In those scenarios where one alternative dominates the other, such as in the upper-right cell, where A is more costly and less effective than B, no analysis is necessary because it is clear that B dominates A.

Identify and Measure Outcomes of Each Alternative Intervention

When a clinician thinks about evaluating pharmaceutical products, the products' clinical effects immediately come to mind. In general terms, treatment could result in one of several outcomes (listed in order from most desirable to least desirable):

- A cure (health is restored)
- Improved quality of life
- Decreased incidence of morbidity
- Extended life
- Relief or reduction in symptoms
- No effect
- Increased morbidity (e.g., drug interactions or adverse drug reactions)
- Death

Some of these outcomes are easier to measure than others. Death, for example, is easy to measure and quantify. In contrast, measures such as decreased risk of morbidity and improved quality of life are less exact. Outcomes may be difficult to measure because of the long follow-up required to determine whether the outcome has been achieved. For example, the desirable outcome for treatment of hypertension would be prevention of strokes or heart attacks (i.e., decreased incidence of morbidity). Achieving a normal blood pressure reading (e.g., diastolic reading < 90 mm Hg) is not, in itself, the desired outcome; it is merely an intermediate measure or clinical indicator.

Although we would prefer to measure final outcomes, this process can require years, even decades. However, given that normal blood pressure is correlated with fewer heart attacks and strokes, we often accept intermediate measures as surrogate indicators of outcomes. For diabetes, for example, the desirable outcomes are prevention of complications (e.g., retinopathy, neuropathy, nephropathy). Because these outcomes also occur over the long term, we use intermediate measures such as blood glucose and glycosylated hemoglobin (HbA_{1c}) levels as predictors of risk for complications of diabetes. For patients with asthma, we might desire an outcome of fewer complications (e.g., respiratory infections) or fewer emergency department visits or hospitalizations; the clinical indicators correlated with these outcome measures are peak-flow meter readings.

The outcomes discussed in the preceding paragraph were described in clinical terms. In fact, outcomes can also be described in humanistic terms (e.g., patient quality of life or patient satisfaction) or in economic terms such as cost per day, cost per course of therapy, or cost per member per month (PMPM). For a patient with asthma, for example, we could measure outcomes not only as the clinical endpoint "peak-flow rate" but also in terms of the patient's quality of life or the cost of treatment over a given period of time. Using economic measurement assumes that a patient is achieving the desired outcomes will need less intervention and treatment, such as physician visits, antibiotics, emergency department visits, or hospital admissions.

Identify, Measure, and Value Costs

As stated previously, pharmacoeconomics identifies, measures, and compares the costs and consequences of the use of pharmaceutical products and services. From a measurement aspect, two components exist: costs and consequences. Some of the issues related to identifying and measuring consequences or outcomes of therapy have been covered already. Our focus now shifts to three considerations that affect the cost side of the equation: identifying, measuring, and placing a value on resources or costs.

Identifying Relevant Costs

The first step in measuring costs is identifying all relevant resources consumed in association with the product or service under evaluation. To determine whether a cost is relevant, consider this question: Would this cost have been incurred had the program not been implemented?

As a method of identification, costs are often categorized as direct medical, direct nonmedical, indirect, or intangible costs.

Direct medical costs are resources consumed for medical services or products that are directly related to the product or service being evaluated. They include physician services, emergency department visits, laboratory services, prescribed medications, and hospitalizations. These costs are typically services covered by third-party payers, such as insurance companies, MCOs, or the government.

Direct nonmedical costs are those nonmedical resources consumed as the result of providing the product or service. They include transportation to treatment facilities and additional housing expenses incurred by the patients and their family when traveling to health care facilities outside their hometown. Other examples are special diets and exercise equipment required as a component of treatment or rehabilitation. These costs are not typically covered by third-party payers and are usually the responsibility of the patient.

Intangible costs are costs associated with pain and suffering resulting from treatment or the illness itself. Whereas these "costs" are important aspects of the product or service being evaluated, they can be very difficult to measure or quantify. Nevertheless, from the patient's perspective, these are real costs that the individual must bear.

Indirect costs are those costs "indirectly" associated with the product or service under evaluation. Illness and disease have an impact on resources outside the medical sector. For example, people who are sick may be unable to work or be less productive. This loss of productivity is an important cost that should be captured in an evaluation. The inclusion of indirect costs is controversial in the literature, primarily because of the difficulty in measuring lost productivity and establishing causal links between illness and lost productivity. Nevertheless, many pharmacoeconomic studies attempt to measure the impact of morbidity or the ill effects of the treatment or health condition on worker productivity. These costs are often borne by patients, caregivers, employers, the government, and society.

Different types of costs are borne by different parties and, consequently, the responsibility for payment of health care expenditures is fragmented. Managed care organizations, for example, determine what they will pay for in their statement of benefits; the patient then pays the remaining costs. In some cases, either patients or payers may try to shift costs to each other. When reviewing a pharmacoeconomic study, one should be aware of whether true cost savings have occurred or just cost shifting.

Measuring Costs

Once costs have been identified, the next step is to measure them. Depending on the type of cost, measurement often involves counts of units of resources consumed. These units can be amount of time or occurrence of certain events, such as hospitalizations or physician visits. For example, the number of office visits, hospitalizations, or laboratory services would be counted per patient over the time period of the evaluation. Measuring the cost of personnel services, whether it is nursing or pharmacist time, involves counts in units of time. However, some would argue that personnel time is a fixed cost and would be incurred whether the program was implemented or not. The inclusion of this cost is warranted if the time spent on the program detracts from other required responsibilities.

Valuing Costs

Once costs have been measured, the final step involves placing a dollar value on the resource or service. In a perfectly competitive market, the value of the resource would be based on the market price of the commodity or service. Of course, the price does not reflect the true opportunity cost for many health care products or services. Opportunity cost—an important concept in the valuation of resources—is defined as the value of a resource in its next best use.

To illustrate the idea of opportunity cost, consider a pharmacist who owns and operates his own independent pharmacy. The pharmacist has decided to expand the pharmaceutical care services he provides by providing flu vaccines to local senior citizens. As part of the proposal he has developed, he needs to estimate the additional hours he will spend on this service and place a value on these hours. The value of his time would not be based on the wages the pharmacist pays himself (which often vary based on the profitability of the business), but rather would be based on wages he would earn if he were employed elsewhere. In other words, his time should be valued based on the market price he could obtain if he were employed as a pharmacist at another local community pharmacy.

A critical component in the valuation of resources goes back to the issue of perspective. Perspective is important in health care, as in other sectors of the economy, because of the many ways in which the price of a commodity can vary by consumer. Consider the difference in price paid by a teaching hospital and the price paid by an independent pharmacy for the same pharmaceutical product. As discussed earlier, the resource should be valued based on its opportunity costs. However, because opportunity costs are often difficult to infer, researchers often use reference prices or reimbursement rates.

Reference prices are published list prices that serve as a reference for providers of those services or products. For example, a reference price for pharmaceuticals is the average wholesale price (AWP) assigned to products by the manufacturer. Many reference price lists are publicly available for a myriad of health care products and services (Else, Armstrong, and Cox, 1997).

Another method of valuing resources is by identifying actual reimbursement rates for services. Actual reimbursement rates are difficult to obtain because they are considered proprietary and thus are not publicly available.

What is controversial about using reference price lists or reimbursement rates as a proxy for actual cost is that these costs do not reflect the opportunity costs of using that resource elsewhere. Thus cost data should be adjusted when they are known to be very different from market prices. This adjustment ensures that costs are a true reflection of the opportunity cost of using those resources. Many methodological issues exist regarding valuation of costs, and readers should be aware of these controversies in conducting any economic evaluation (Copley-Merriman and Lair, 1994).

Sensitivity Analysis

Sensitivity analysis involves testing key outcome or cost assumptions of an analysis to determine how sensitive the results are to variation or uncertainty in these estimates. In many pharmacoeconomic evaluations, the accuracy with which costs can be identified, measured, or valued will vary. Variation around the measurement of outcomes also exists.

Numerous methods are available to test the impact of uncertainty within pharmacoeconomic evaluations (Briggs, Sculpher, and Buxton, 1994). As an example, suppose that the average per-patient direct medical costs were estimated to be $200, which varied around the mean by $100. To determine whether the results of the analysis would hold true if actual costs varied, the investigator could vary direct medical costs from a low of $100 ($200 − $100) to a high of $300 ($200 + $100). If the results of the analyses are the same when using different cost assumptions, then the researcher can more easily defend his or her conclusions. In critiquing studies, it is important to determine the key areas of uncertainty within a study and note whether researchers addressed areas of uncertainty through sensitivity analysis.

Discounting

The final step in calculating costs relates to the issue of discounting. In those instances where the program or service being evaluated extends beyond one year, adjustment should be made for differences in timing that may occur between alternatives. The purpose of discounting is to determine the present value of all costs and to incorporate society's time preference for money. We all have a preference for when we would like to receive money. Most, if not all, of us would rather receive $10 today rather than $10 one year from now. Because money can generate interest income, $10 received today is worth more than $10 received one year from now. In most, if not all, cases, people prefer to incur costs later and reap benefits earlier. This same time preference applies to health care costs. Thus costs or benefits of alternatives realized at different times should be discounted to a present value to make valid comparisons.

The effects that discounting, or failure to discount, can have on study results are presented in **Table 18-3.** In this example, the total costs of two competing programs A and B are the same ($85,000), but the costs occur at different time periods. Assuming that money received today is worth 4% more than money received one year later (a 4% discount rate), the

Table 18-3 Discounted versus Undiscounted Costs

Program	Year					Undiscounted	Discounted at 4%
	0	1	2	5	10		
A	$25,000	$15,000	$15,000	$10,000	$20,000	$85,000	$75,022
B	$40,000	$20,000	$15,000	$10,000		$85,000	$81,318

present value of costs are $75,022 for program A and $81,318 for program B, a difference of more than $6,000.

The choice of a discount rate is important, as it can significantly affect the results of the evaluation. The U.S. Public Health Service Panel on Cost-Effectiveness in Health and Medicine recommends using a discount rate of 3% (Gold, Siegel, Russell, and Weinstein, 1996). Drummond and colleagues suggest several other factors to consider when discounting (Drummond, O'Brien, Stoddart, and Torrance, 1998). These factors include the following:

- Presenting results in their undiscounted form so that the reader can evaluate the impact of discounting
- Using sensitivity analysis to vary the discount rate over a range of values
- When discounting affects the results, being clear with readers so that they are aware of its influence on the study's findings

PHARMACOECONOMIC METHODOLOGIES

Cost-Minimization Analysis

Cost-minimization analysis (CMA) compares the costs and consequences of two or more therapeutic interventions that are equivalent in terms of their outcomes or consequences. Thus the purpose of CMA is to choose the least costly alternative among interventions with equivalent outcomes. CMA is often confused with cost analysis, in which only the costs of therapy are evaluated. However, consequences are also evaluated in CMA to show or "prove" equivalency.

The requirement of equivalent outcomes limits the application of CMA to those situations where equivalency has been established. They include, but are not limited to, comparisons between branded and generic products, comparisons of different routes of administration of the same drug, and comparison of different settings for the administration of the same drug therapy—for example, inpatient versus home therapy. In all of these instances, the evidence supporting equivalent outcomes should be clearly stated and, where appropriate, statistically confirmed.

Because the consequences of alternatives being compared are shown to be equivalent, CMA focuses on cost differences. These differences in cost can be presented as average cost per patient or average total cost of care if the number of patients is the same under each alternative.

Cost-Effectiveness Analysis

Cost-effectiveness analysis (CEA) is the most commonly used pharmacoeconomic method. Its popularity is attributable in part to the way in which outcomes or consequences are measured (i.e., natural units of effectiveness). CEA is restricted to those situations in which the outcomes of the alternatives are all measured on the same scale, such as mm Hg or serum cholesterol levels. The purpose of CEA is to compare the costs and consequences of two or more alternatives to determine which alternative can achieve the best outcome at the lowest cost.

The term "cost-effective" is often misused in the literature. The judgment of whether a product is cost-effective is relative and often subjective. It is relative in the sense that when a product or service is deemed cost-effective, this distinction is made in comparison to the costs and outcomes of other alternatives. It is subjective in the sense that the decision maker determines whether the additional cost is worth the additional gain in effectiveness. Some guidelines exist to determine under what range of values a product would be considered cost-effective (for example, cost per QALY gained). In many other situations, it is left to the decision maker to determine what qualifies as cost-effective.

Results of a CEA take the form of an incremental ratio of costs to outcomes. **Table 18-4** presents the average total costs per patient and the average outcome per patient for three therapies used to treat a common toenail fungus. Also shown in the table are the average cost-effectiveness ratios and the incremental ratios. The outcome is measured simply as number of successful cases. When determining whether an alternative is cost-effective, one has to ask, Are you willing to pay $122, $155, or $187 per successfully treated patient? The investigator might be willing to pay all three prices, but certainly $122 per successful treatment appears to be the more efficient treatment regimen when compared to doing nothing. Of course, comparing an alternative to doing nothing is not a realistic approach.

Incremental cost-effectiveness ratios are a more appropriate way to compare product alternatives in cost-effective analysis. What additional amount must be paid to obtain the additional successfully treated cases? Comparing alternatives A and B (because B is both more costly and more effective), we see the additional cost of $65 would provide an additional gain in the rate of successfully treated cases of 0.25. The cost per additional successfully treated case is $260 ($65 ÷ 0.25). Comparing alternatives A and C, the incremental ratio is $43 per additional successfully

Table 18-4 Average and Incremental Cost-Effectiveness Ratios

Alternative	Average Cost Per Patient	Outcome (Success Rate)	Average Cost-Effectiveness Ratio	Incremental Cost-Effectiveness Ratio
A	$ 85	0.55	$155/successful case	
B	$150	0.80	$187/successful case	$260/additional successful case treated
C	$ 95	0.78	$122/successful case	$43/additional successful case treated

treated case. Based on this information, alternative C appears to be the most cost-effective alternative, given that the additional successfully treated cases cost less, on average, than the average cost of treatment under alternative A ($155 per successful case).

No established guidelines exist to determine whether an alternative is cost-effective in this example of antifungal therapies. In this scenario, decision makers may have been willing to pay $155 or even $187 per successfully treated case because the idea of cost-effectiveness is value for money. They may have been willing to pay these costs to obtain the benefit of successful treatment. In comparing all three alternatives, however, they discovered that alternative C is the most efficient (i.e., least costly for a given level of output) and most cost-effective option.

Cost-Benefit Analysis

Cost-benefit analysis (CBA) was first defined as "a way of assessing the desirability of projects, where it is important to take a long view (in the sense of looking at repercussions in the future) and a wide view (in the sense of allowing for side effects of many kinds on many persons, industries, regions, etc.), i.e., it implies the numeration and evaluation of all relevant costs and benefits" (Prest and Turvey, 1965, p. 721). The two aspects of CBA—taking a long and wide view—have made it most applicable to decisions with a broad societal impact, such as whether to fund immunization programs or whether to implement child safety seat legislation. In evaluating each of these programs, researchers would take a long view (estimating the value of the lives lost in terms of future productivity on the community) and the wide view (estimating not only the direct benefits but also the indirect benefits to the community from reduced risk of illness to those not immunized).

In measuring outcomes in dollars, CBA enjoys an advantage over other economic evaluations: It can compare alternatives that are not measured using the same natural unit of effectiveness. For example, CBA could compare an immunization program to child safety seat regulations to determine which program would yield the highest net benefit (benefits minus costs).

One of the methodologically challenging aspects of CBA is measuring and valuing benefits in dollars. Two broad categories of direct benefits can be measured in CBA: personal health benefits and medical resource benefits. The measurement and valuation of medical resource benefits have already been discussed. The measurement of personal health benefits is more challenging. Personal health benefits include the alternative's effects on morbidity or mortality. Changes in morbidity are reflected in two ways: changes in medical resource consumption for treatment of illness, and intangible benefits such as reduction in pain and suffering. The impact on mortality is captured as number of lives saved. Two methods are commonly used to value lives saved: the human capital approach and the willingness-to-pay (WTP) approach.

The human capital approach measures the value of a life saved in terms of the income that the person could have earned over his or her remaining productive years. The criticism of the human capital approach of valuing human life is that it focuses on the productivity of the individual and not his or her value to family and friends. Also, because of imperfections in the labor market, this method tends to undervalue women and minorities.

Willingness-to-pay values both the intervention's impact on lives saved and intangible benefits. In measuring WTP values, individuals are presented with a hypothetical statement describing the illness or disease and asked to express their willingness to pay to reduce the risk of death, pain, or suffering (Gafni, 1991). The advantage of WTP is that, in theory, it measures the full range of benefits, including productivity and intangible benefits. The disadvantage is that the WTP approach is a difficult method to apply and relies on individuals' abilities to comprehend and respond to hypothetical statements regarding small changes in health risks.

Presentation of Results

Two methods are most commonly used to present results in CBA: net benefit and cost-to-benefit or benefit-to-cost ratios.

Net Benefit. The formula for calculating net benefits (NB) when costs (C) and benefits (B) do not extend beyond one year is presented in Equation 1 following. The formula for calculating the net benefit when either costs and/or benefits extend beyond one year, also known as net present value (NPV), is presented in Equation 2. If the project lifetime extends beyond one year, the net benefits should be adjusted using an appropriate discount rate (r).

1. $NB = \sum_{i=1}^{x} B_i - \sum_{i=1}^{y} C_i$

2. $NPV_i = \sum_{t=0}^{n} \dfrac{B_t - C_t}{(1 + r)^t}$

where:

NPV_i = present value of net benefit received from project i

B_t = benefits received from the project in year t

C_t = costs of the project in year t

$1/(1 + r)$ = discount factor at rate of interest r

n = lifetime of the project

Equation 1 calculates the net benefit (NB) as the sum of all benefits (B), minus the sum of all costs (C). Equation 2 discounts costs and benefits to their net present value using the appropriate discount rate.

Unlike CEA where the decision rule for determining cost-effectiveness can be subjective, the decision rules in CBA are definite. The decision criteria when results are presented as net benefit, assuming a limited budget, would be to choose the project that provides the greatest net benefit or—if funds allow—to choose those projects that provide a positive net benefit.

Ratio Analysis. The formulas used in calculating benefit-to-cost ratios when costs and benefits are measured within a one-year period and when they extend beyond one year, are presented in Equations 3 and 4, respectively.

3. BC ratio $= \sum_{i=1}^{x} B_i \div \sum_{i=1}^{y} C_i$

4. BC ratio $= \sum_{t=0}^{n} \dfrac{B_t}{(1 + r)^t} \div \sum_{t=0}^{n} \dfrac{C_t}{(1 + r')^t}$

where:

B_t = benefits received from the project in year t

C_t = costs of the project in year t

$1/(1 + r)$ = discount factor at rate of interest r

n = lifetime of the project

The decision rule for choosing among projects when results are presented as ratios would be to choose those projects with a benefit-to-cost ratio greater than 1, or inversely where the cost-to-benefit ratio is less than 1. Assuming limited resources, the task would then be to select the project or projects with the highest benefit-to-cost ratio or lowest cost-to-benefit ratio.

How results are presented (net benefit versus ratios) can influence the decision. As an example, **Table 18-5** presents four hypothetical program options with their costs and benefits. Results are calculated both as net benefit and benefit-to-cost ratios.

Based on the information in Table 18-5 and assuming unlimited resources, the free oral contraceptives, the statewide drug abuse program, and the smoking cessation programs would be considered because their benefits are greater than their costs and the benefit-to-cost ratios are all greater than 1. Under conditions of limited resources, if one were to choose the project with the greatest net benefit, the choice would be the drug abuse treatment program. If the decision were based on benefit-to-cost ratio, however, the choice would be the free oral contraception program.

It is generally agreed that presenting results in terms of the net benefit provides decision makers with more information. For example, presenting results as a ratio does not provide information on the magnitude of both costs and benefits. Although the drug abuse treatment program included in Table 18–5 provides the greatest net benefit, it also requires an outlay by the state of $2 million.

Summary. Cost-benefit analysis remains a unique method of assessing the costs and benefits of programs and therapy interventions. However, it is applicable only when outcomes are easily converted to dollars and is most appropriate in situations where the objectives are broad in scope.

Table 18-5 Presentation of Results in Hypothetical Cost-Benefit Analysis

Option	Benefits ($)	Costs ($)	Net Benefit	Benefit-to-Cost Ratio
Free oral contraceptives at County Health Department	$45,000	$20,000	$25,000	2.25
Statewide drug abuse treatment program	$2 million	$1.5 million	$500,000	1.33
Additional police protection in high-crime neighborhoods	$85,000	$90,000	−$5,000	0.94
Smoking cessation program	$200,000	$100,000	$100,000	2.00

Cost-Utility Analysis

Cost-utility analysis (CUA) is often considered an extension of CEA in which outcomes are measured as lives saved. Most people would agree, however, that the alternative that provides more additional years of life is not always the preferred choice. The quality of the life-years gained should also be considered. For example, suppose a patient with cancer expects a modest gain in life expectancy with chemotherapy. However, during her treatment she experiences a great deal of discomfort and her physical strength is weakened to the extent that she cannot carry out activities of daily living, such as bathing or dressing. When the quality of those additional years of life is considered, the preference for those extended years of life may be diminished. CUA measures both the quantity and quality aspects of gains in life-years; in other words, it adjusts the gains in life-years for quality, measured as QALYs.

In CUA, life-years are converted to QALYs by applying a utility value. Utility is often perceived as preference, and it is measured on a scale of 0.0 to 1.0, where 0 represents death and 1 represents perfect health. Most health states fall somewhere between these extremes. Therefore, 1 life-year with a utility of 1.0 equals 1.0 QALY, as do 2 life-years with a utility of 0.5. For example, if a patient survives on dialysis for 4 years and is determined to have a utility value of 0.6, then he or she has 2.4 QALYs.

As in CEA, both average and incremental cost-utility ratios are calculated. The additional cost of a given treatment is divided by the additional effectiveness. The only difference is that effectiveness is measured as a QALY rather than in life-years alone. For example, if patients with lung cancer can have either surgery alone or both surgery and chemotherapy, the analysis compares the cost utility of these alternatives. Assume that surgery adds 3 years of life at a cost of $14,000. Surgery and chemotherapy together result in an average of 5 years of life but cost $27,000. Assume further that surgery has a utility value of 0.80 and chemotherapy and surgery together have a utility value of 0.60. Which is the better alternative? The answer varies depending on whether a CEA or a CUA is conducted.

If effectiveness were measured as additional life-years, the incremental cost-effectiveness ratio would be

$$\text{Incremental CE ratio} = \text{Additional cost of chemotherapy} \div \text{additional life-years}$$

$$= (\$27,000 - \$14,000) \div (5 \text{ years} - 3 \text{ years})$$

$$= \$13,000 \div 2 \text{ years}$$

$$= \$6,500 \text{ per additional life-year}$$

If effectiveness as QALYs were measured, the incremental cost utility ratio would be

Incremental CU ratio = Additional cost of chemotherapy ÷ additional QALYs

= ($27,000 − $14,000) ÷ [(5 years × 0.6 utility)
− (3 years × 0.8 utility)]

= $13,000 ÷ (3.0 QALY − 2.4 QALY)

= $13,000 ÷ 0.6 QALY

= $21,667 per additional QALY

The $21,667 per additional QALY considers the patient's preference for each outcome, and as a result the alternative of chemotherapy plus surgery does not appear as attractive as surgery alone.

Cost-Consequence Analysis

Cost-consequence analysis (CCA) has been defined as an analysis that presents all costs and effects in a disaggregated format (Mauskopf, Paul, Grant, and Stergachis, 1998). Costs are listed in table format by type of costs (i.e., direct medical, direct nonmedical, indirect costs, and intangible costs) as are outcomes (i.e., clinical intermediaries, dollars, and QALYs). Decision makers can then choose among the costs and outcomes that best fit their perspective. The advantage of CCA lies in its comprehensiveness and transparency for decision makers. The disadvantage of CCA is that the researcher must identify, collect, and value costs and outcomes salient to a variety of perspectives. This burden of analysis, however, far outweighs the potential gain for decision makers.

Table 18-6 provides a framework for how costs and consequences would be presented in a CCA. All costs and consequences are identified and measured in units, and a cost is assigned to each unit. Based on this information, decision makers can choose the costs and consequences that are relevant for their purposes. They can then calculate average and incremental ratios for each alternative.

APPROACHES TO CONDUCTING PHARMACOECONOMIC STUDIES

Pharmacoeconomic evaluations can be conducted using several approaches, including randomized controlled trials, naturalistic designs, decision analysis, and retrospective analysis.

Randomized Controlled Trials

Randomized controlled trials involve randomly assigning patients to the alternative therapies being considered. A standard protocol is established, and patients are followed over a specified time period. Patients and investigators are blinded as to which alternative they receive. The advantage of this design is that it has strong internal validity—that is, the results are attributable to the intervention and not to other extrane-

Table 18-6 Presentation of Costs and Consequences in Cost-Consequence Analysis

	Drug A		Drug B	
	Units	Costs	Units	Costs
Costs (per patient)				
Direct medical	—	—	—	—
Drug therapy	—	—	—	—
Physician costs	—	—	—	—
Hospitalizations	—	—	—	—
Direct nonmedical				
Transportation	—	—	—	—
Caregiver time	—	—	—	—
Indirect				
Productivity (lost days/episode)	—	—	—	—
Consequences				
Clinical				
Cases successfully treated	—	—	—	—
Quality-of-life (QALY)	—	—	—	—

ous factors. The disadvantage is that randomized controlled trials can be costly, and the strict adherence to treatment protocols is not reflective of real-world practice settings.

Naturalistic Designs

Naturalistic designs are similar to clinical trials in that patients are randomly assigned to treatment groups, but the patients recruited and the follow-up care delivered would be representative of routine clinical care (Simon, Wagner, and Vonkorff, 1995). Whereas this type of study design does have its advantages, it can be expensive.

Decision Analysis

Decision analysis is a systematic approach to decision making under conditions of uncertainty. Rather than conducting the study prospectively or collecting data on individual patients, decision analysis synthesizes clinical data from the literature with data on resource use to simulate or model the question or problem. Two modeling types are often used to represent the decision process: decision analysis and Markov models. Decision analysis is employed when direct observation is not feasible or when time or money constraints prohibit collecting data prospectively. The advantage of decision analysis as compared to clinical or naturalistic trial study designs is that results can be obtained in a timely and cost-efficient manner.

The use of decision analytic models (also known as decision trees) is becoming increasingly popular in the literature. **Figure 18-2** depicts a simplified decision tree for the decision of whether to treat a particular disease with drug therapy. The decision node, represented by the square (□), designates the point at which the decision to treat or not to treat is made. If the decision is to treat, the process follows the branch of the tree for drug therapy. The branch then comes upon a chance or probability node, represented by a circle (○), at which point a probability exists of experiencing a side effect (pSE). Patients must either experience a side effect or not experience a side effect, so the probability of no side effect is therefore 1 minus the probability of a side effect or (1 − pSE). The terminal branch for each alternative (drug or no drug) is the chance of a bad outcome (pBOrx) or a good outcome (1 − pBOrx). The probabilities used in the model are derived from the published literature or expert opinion, and resource utilization is inferred from either accepted practice standards or expert opinion.

As an example, assume three antiepileptic medications could be used: Drug A costs $120 per month, Drug B costs $160 per month, and Drug C costs $230 per month. Assume also that Drug A is 60% effective, Drug B is 80% effective, and Drug C is more than 90% effective. The managed care organization has already decided that Drug C should be used only in those cases in which either Drug A or Drug B has been tried unsuccessfully. An unsuccessful trial of either Drug A or B will result in an additional physician office visit costing $30 plus the cost of Drug C. Which drug, A or B, would be more cost-effective?

One way to answer this question is to use a decision tree like the one depicted in **Figure 18-3.** For Drug A, the cost of effective treatment is multiplied by the probability of effectiveness (pE), whereas the cost of unsuccessful treatment ($120 for Drug A, plus $30 for the additional

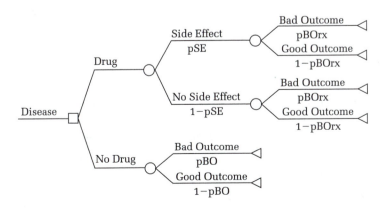

Figure 18-2 Decision Analysis Decision Tree

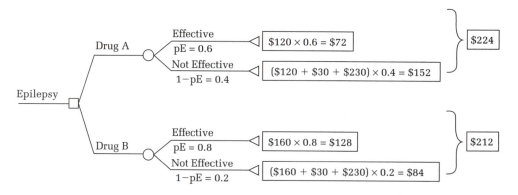

Figure 18-3 Hypothetical Decision Tree for First Line Epilepsy Treatment

office visit, plus $230 for the new Drug C) is multiplied by the probability that Drug A is not effective (1 − pE). The sum of these costs is compared to the sum of the same costs for Drug B. The results show that although Drug B costs more than Drug A, it is actually more cost-effective. Therefore, based on this information, Drug B would be preferred. As presented, the assumption is made that the products do not differ substantially in any other aspect, such as their side-effect profiles.

Decision trees are difficult to use for modeling chronic disease states in which patients may experience intermittent relapses and remissions. A convenient solution to this problem is to use Markov models. Markov models offer advantages when a problem involves risk that is continuous, when the timing of events is important, and when important events may happen more than once (Sonnenberg and Beck, 1993). The Markov model frames the decision in terms of health states and follows patients as they transition from one state to another.

Figure 18-4 illustrates a three-state Markov model in which the health states are Well, Ill, and Dead. When patients are well, there is a probability that they will become ill, stay symptom free, or die. When they experience symptoms, there is a probability that they could go into remission, stay symptomatic, or die. Of course, when they die, patients cannot change to other health states. In this way, Markov models simulate the natural progression of chronic diseases (Elliott and Payne, 2005).

The probabilities of moving from one state to the other are usually included in Markov models based on data published in the literature. (For example, a researcher could determine from the literature the probability that a patient with multiple sclerosis will either experience an asymptomatic period or die.) More sophisticated analyses may recognize that the probability of illness and death increases according to the duration of the disease, the age of the patient, and other variables. To the extent possible, these factors could also be included to determine probabilities of events. While pharmacoeconomics calculations using Markov

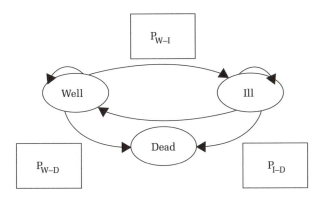

Figure 18-4 Three-State Markov Model. *Source:* Sonnenberg, F. A., and Beck, J. R. (1993). Markov models in medical decision making: A practical guide. In *Medical decision making, Vol. 13,* pp. 322–338. Philadelphia, PA: Hanley & Belfus.

models are beyond the scope of a single-chapter overview of pharmaco-economics, it is useful for students to know that Markov models are a better choice than decision trees for analysis of certain chronic diseases such as multiple sclerosis, osteoporosis, and arthritis.

Retrospective Analysis

Retrospective analysis of claims data (also known as observational data) can also be used to evaluate the costs and consequences of drug therapy. The advantages of using claims data are that they reflect routine clinical care, are comprehensive, and provide a large sample of patients to evaluate. Additionally, the evaluations can often involve less time and lower costs than randomized controlled trials or naturalistic designs. However, claims data were developed for billing and reimbursement purposes rather than to monitor and track health care costs and outcomes. As a consequence, several limitations apply to their use in pharmacoeco-nomic research—namely, the lack of information regarding clinical indicators, incompleteness of data, and inaccuracies in coding of diagnoses and procedures.

No particular study design is inherently superior to another. Each design approach has its advantages and disadvantages, and the final choice will depend on many factors. In critiquing a study with respect to study design, it is important to determine whether the disadvantage of a particular method affects the results.

CRITICAL APPRAISAL OF A PHARMACOECONOMIC STUDY

Many articles in the literature claim to study the cost-effectiveness or cost-benefit of alternative treatments. Readers should be cautioned, however, that many of these articles are flawed because they do not adequately identify, measure, or value costs and consequences. A number of guidelines have been published to assist researchers in conducting evaluations or evaluating the pharmacoeconomic literature (Dao, 1985; Jolicoeur, Jones-Grizzle, and Boyer, 1992; Task Force on Principles for Economic Analysis of Health Care Technology, 1995). Following is a list of questions that readers should ask when appraising a pharmacoeconomic study:

1. *What is the perspective of the study?* Is it the patient, the physician, an institutional provider, a managed care organization, or society? Results can vary widely depending on the perspective, so the author should make this clear.

2. *What type of study is it?* Is it a CMA, CEA, CBA, or CUA study, and does that methodology provide the best answer to the problem being posed?

3. *Were the competing treatment alternatives described and compared?*

4. *Were the relevant costs and consequences for each alternative properly identified?* This should include all relevant direct medical and nonmedical costs as well as indirect and intangible costs.

5. *Were the relevant costs and consequences for each alternative properly measured?* If a clinical indicator was used, then the relevance of this measurement should be documented. If a cost-minimization analysis was conducted, the author should have documented that the expected outcomes are identical.

6. *Were the relevant costs and consequences properly valued?* For example, the article should define how the costs were measured (e.g., standard costs or claims data) and whether any relevant opportunity costs were included.

7. *Were the instruments used to measure patient preferences or quality of life validated?* The article should explain how the instruments have been used in the past and whether experts in the field consider them valid.

8. *What are the assumptions and limitations of the study?* All assumptions and limitations should be clearly stated.

9. *Were costs and consequences adjusted for different time periods?* Articles that look at long-term consequences should recognize that dollars today will have a different value in later years. Therefore, the present and future values of money should be equated through a clearly defined discounting procedure.

10. *Was a sensitivity analysis performed?* If the analysis is built on certain assumptions, then the robustness of these assumptions should be tested by changing the assumptions to see whether the results are the same. For example, if an investigator assumes a discount rate of 3% and finds that the results of the analysis are the same even when a discount rate of 0% or 5% is used, he or she can have more confidence in the study results.

11. *Are the generalizations appropriate?* The study should not draw conclusions beyond the question that was studied. For example, the finding that a product is cost-effective in a managed care setting cannot be generalized to society.

CONCLUSIONS

As a larger number of students of pharmacy and practitioners become familiar with the concepts of pharmacoeconomics, the application of these tools in everyday practice will grow. The potential exists for pharmacoeconomic information to aid greatly in decision making in the ever more cost-conscious field of health care.

QUESTIONS FOR FURTHER DISCUSSION

1. Clinicians tend to focus their efforts on the measurement of outcomes of clinical therapy, including measures of clinical effectiveness or side effects. Discuss the importance of measuring the "inputs" of clinical therapy.
2. Discuss the reasons why a pharmaceutical company might use one methodological approach over another (e.g., decision analysis, naturalistic design, or retrospective analysis) in conducting a pharmacoeconomics evaluation for its product. How might this differ based upon where the product is in its life cycle (e.g., products at market maturity or products yet to be launched)?
3. Discuss how pharmacists in various practice settings (i.e., retail, hospital or managed care) might apply pharmacoeconomic principles.
4. Discuss why various decision makers might be more inclined to select one pharmacoeconomic method over another. Various decision makers could include: managed care organizations, public health officials, PBMs, physicians, hospital pharmacists, or members of a pharmacy and therapeutics committee.

KEY TOPICS AND TERMS

Benefit-to-cost ratio
Cost-benefit analysis
Cost-effectiveness analysis
Cost-consequence analysis
Cost-minimization analysis
Decision analysis
Decision tree
Direct medical costs
Direct nonmedical costs

Discounting
Effectiveness
Efficacy
Efficiency
Human capital approach
Incremental cost-effectiveness ratio
Indirect costs
Inputs
Intangible costs
Markov models
Net benefit
Net present value
Opportunity cost
Outcomes
Perspective
Pharmacoeconomics
Quality-adjusted life-years
Randomized controlled trials
Retrospective claims analysis
Sensitivity analysis
Willingness-to-pay approach

REFERENCES

Bootman, J. L., McGhan, W. F., & Schondelmeyer, S. W. (1982). Application of cost-benefit and cost-effectiveness analysis to clinical practice. *Drug Intelligence and Clinical Pharmacy, 16,* 235–243.

Bootman, J. L., Townsend, R. J., & McGhan, W. F. (1996). *Principles of pharmacoeconomics* (2nd ed.). Cincinnati, OH: Harvey Whitney Books.

Bootman, J. L., Wertheimer, A., Zaske, D., & Rowland, C. (1979). Individualizing gentamicin dosage regimens on burn patients with gram negative septicemia: A cost-benefit analysis. *Journal of Pharmacy Science, 68,* 267–272.

Briggs, A., Sculpher, M., & Buxton, M. (1994). Uncertainty in the economic evaluation of health care technologies: The role of sensitivity analysis. *Health Economics, 3,* 95–104.

Centers for Medicare and Medicaid Services, Office of the Actuary. (2006). *National health expenditure amounts, and annual percent change by type of expenditure: Selected calendar years 1960–2004.* Retrieved July 20, 2006 from http://www.cms.hhs.gov/NationalHealthExpendData/downloads/tables.pdf

Copley-Merriman, C., & Lair, T. J. (1994). Valuation of medical resource units collected in health economic studies. *Clinical Therapy, 16*(3), 553–567.

Dao, T. D. (1985). Cost-benefit and cost-effectiveness analysis of drug therapy. *American Journal of Hospital Pharmacy, 42,* 791–802.

Drummond, M. F., O'Brien, B. J., Stoddart, G. L., & Torrance, G. W. (1998). *Methods for the economic evaluation of health care programmes* (2nd ed.). New York: Oxford University Press.

Elliott, R., & Payne, K. (2005). *Essentials of economic evaluation in healthcare.* London: Pharmaceutical Products Press.

Else, B. A., Armstrong, E. P., & Cox, E. R. (1997). Data sources for pharmacoeconomic and health services research. *American Journal of Health-Systems Pharmacy, 54,* 2601–2608.

Gafni, A. (1991). Willingness-to-pay as a measure of benefits: Relevant questions in the context of public decisionmaking about health care programs. *Medical Care, 29*(12), 1246–1252.

Gold, M. R., Siegel, J. E., Russell, L. B., & Weinstein, M .C. (Eds.). (1996). *Cost-effectiveness in health and medicine.* New York: Oxford University Press.

Jolicoeur, L. M., Jones-Grizzle, A .J., & Boyer, J. G. (1992). Guidelines for performing a pharmacoeconomic analysis. *American Journal of Hospital Pharmacy, 49,* 1741–1747.

Lieu, T. A., Cochi, S. L., Black, S. B., Halloran, M. E., Shinefield, H. R., Holmes, S. J., Wharton, M., & Washington, A. E. (1994). Cost effectiveness of a routine varicella vaccination program for US children. *Journal of the American Medical Association, 271,* 375–381.

Mauskopf, J. A., Paul, J. E., Grant, D. M., & Stergachis, A. (1998). The role of cost-consequence analysis in healthcare decisionmaking. *Pharmacoeconomics, 13*(3), 277–288.

Motheral, B. R., Grizzle, A. J., Armstrong, E. P., Cox, E., & Fairman, K. (2000). Role of pharmacoeconomics in drug benefit decision-making: Results of a survey. *Formulary, 35,* 412–421.

Prest, A. R., & Turvey, R. (1965). Cost-benefit analysis: A survey. *Economics Journal, 75*(12), 683–735.

Simon, G. Wagner, E. & Vonkorff, M. (1995). Cost-effectiveness comparisons using "real world" randomized trials: The case of new antidepressant drugs. *Journal of Clinical Epidemiology, 48*(3), 363–373.

Sonnenberg, F. A. & Beck, J. R. (1993). Markov models in medical decision making: A practical guide. *Medical Decision Making, 13*(4), 322–338.

Task Force on Principles for Economic Analysis of Health Care Technology. (1995). Economic analysis of health care technology: A report on principles. *Annals of Internal Medicine, 122,* 61–70.

Townsend, R. J. (1986). Post marketing drug research and development: An industry clinical pharmacist's perspective. *American Journal of Pharmacy Education, 50,* 480–482.

Weinstein, M. C., & Stason, B. (1977). Foundations and cost-effectiveness analysis for health and medical practitioners. *New England Journal of Medicine, 296,* 716–721.

CHAPTER 19

International Health Care Services

Ana C. Quiñones and Linda E. Barry Dunn

Case Scenario

Jane has recently accepted a position as a health policy analyst and is investigating ways in which universal health care can be provided in the United States at a reasonable cost. Among other things, she is contemplating which types of health care services should be covered and how this coverage should be financed. As a first step, Jane decides to look at the health care systems of other countries. What data would Jane need to gather? How would this information be helpful?

Background

A health policy analyst who wants to determine how other countries have provided universal access to health care services at a reasonable cost might start by looking at the World Health Organization's (WHO) *World Health Report 2000, Health Systems: Improving Performance,* which compares health care systems around the world (World Health Organization, 2000a). The comparative analysis of health systems helps policy makers (and policy analysts like Jane) know how health systems perform and what they can do to improve those systems. The report asserts that much of the widening gap in death rates between the rich and poor, both within and among countries around the world, is explained by the differing degrees of efficiency with which health systems organize and finance themselves and react to the needs of their populations. This may explain, for instance, why countries with similar income levels and health expenditures vary greatly with regard to health outcomes. The WHO report finds that inequalities in life expectancy persist and are strongly associated with socioeconomic class, even in countries that enjoy good health.

To compare health systems, an analyst would review basic data such as per capita expenditures on health, immunization rates, infant mortality rates, mortality rates, or health care expenditures as a percentage of gross domestic product (GDP). The rankings contained in WHO's *World Health Report 2000* measure health systems' ability to achieve their goals (World Health Organization, 2000a). Achievement of these goals is based on the following measurements: (1) overall level of health or life expectancy; (2) responsiveness of how well people rated performance of their health care system; (3) fairness in responsiveness among different groups in the same country; and (4) fairness of financing among different groups, which looks at what proportion of income is devoted to health care (Hilts, 2000).

Based on this ranking system, the *World Health Report 2000* indicates that overall most European health systems perform the best. Among the highest-ranking countries are France, Italy, Singapore, Spain, Austria, and Japan (World Health Organization, 2000b). The United States outspends all other countries and ranks near the top on average health measures, but fails to deliver good health care to a large proportion of its population and distributes the cost relatively unfairly, leaving it ranked 37th on the WHO list (World Health Organization, 2000b).

Jane decides to start by researching four countries, each with a different type of health care delivery system. Three of those countries—Canada, Germany, and the United Kingdom—represent developed nations that fared better than the United States in the *World Health Report 2000* rankings. The fourth country, Cuba, received a health systems performance score of 39 but is worthy of examination because of its extraordinary health outcomes despite its developing nation status.

In her analysis, Jane would want to answer the following questions:

1. Is a ranking of a country's health care system based on how equitably resources are distributed a fair measurement of how a health care system performs?
2. Which factors, other than the amount of money spent on health care, could affect the overall health of a particular country?
3. Which aspects of various health care systems could be effectively applied in the United States?

LEARNING OBJECTIVES

Upon completion of this chapter, the student shall be able to:

- Describe the differences between the following health care models: socialized insurance program, decentralized national health program, and socialized medicine.
- Compare and contrast the health care delivery systems of a developing country and a developed country.
- Describe several factors that affect the health of a country's population.
- Describe the main characteristics of the health care plans of Canada, Germany, the United Kingdom, and Cuba.
- Describe some of the health care delivery strategies employed by other countries that might be useful to the United States.

CHAPTER QUESTIONS

1. What are the general features of the health care systems of
   a. Canada?
   b. Germany?
   c. The United Kingdom?
   d. Cuba?
2. How does the health care delivery system of a developing country differ from that of a developed country?
3. Describe several factors that affect the health of a country's population.
4. Describe some of the health care delivery strategies employed by other countries that might be useful to the United States.

INTRODUCTION

The failure of the U.S. health care system to provide universal access to health care services at a reasonable cost has prompted many observers to examine the health care systems of other countries for possible solutions. This chapter, therefore, highlights different methods of structuring and financing health care services. It provides an overview of the unique features of the health care systems of several countries and discusses the characteristics of and issues faced by health care systems in both developed and developing countries.

The chapter analyzes the major features of four health care systems that illustrate the variety of models of health care delivery available—namely, the health care systems of Canada, the United Kingdom, Germany, and Cuba. The discussion of each of these systems includes a brief description of the history of each country's health care system, the system's main features, the health status of the population, the structure of the health care system (i.e., health care facilities and workforce, with a focus on hospitals, physicians, and pharmaceuticals), health care financing (i.e., how the system is funded and what contributions are rendered by the government, citizens, and employers), and issues that appear to present concerns for each system. **Table 19-1** summarizes the key aspects of these systems, comparing them to the features of the U.S. health care system.

The health care systems discussed in this chapter can be classified as belonging to three broad models: (1) socialized insurance program (Canada); (2) decentralized national health program (Germany); and (3) socialized medicine (United Kingdom and Cuba). *Socialized* means that the government participates in or enforces participation in the country's health care scheme. Canada has socialized health insurance; the government administers health insurance. The United Kingdom and Cuba,

Table 19-1 Summary of Key Aspects of Health Care Delivery Systems

	United States	Canada	Germany	United Kingdom	Cuba
Total population, 2003	294,043,000	31,510,000	82,476,000	59,251,000	11,300,000
% of GDP devoted to health, 2002	14.6%	9.6%	10.9%	7.7%	7.5%
Total health care expenditure per capita, 2002	$5,274	$2,931	$2,817	$2,160	$2,360
Life expectancy at birth (years), 2003	Males: 75.0 Females: 80.0	Males: 78.0 Females: 82.0	Males: 76.0 Females: 82.0	Males: 76.0 Females: 81.0	Males: 75.0 Females: 79.0
Infant mortality rate (per 1,000), 2003	Males: 9 Females: 7	Males: 6 Females: 5	Males: 5 Females: 4	Males: 7 Females: 5	Males: 8 Females: 6
Universal coverage?	No	Yes	Yes	Yes	Yes
Hospital beds (per 10,000)	34 (2002)	44 (2002)	89 (2002)	42 (1997)	49 (2003)
Physicians (per 10,000)	28 (1999)	19 (2002)	34 (2003)	21 (2001)	60 (2003)
Pharmacists (per 10,000)	7.7 (2004)	2.9 (2005)	6.5 (2004)	7.8 (2004)	1.4 (2003)

	United States	Canada	Germany	United Kingdom	Cuba
Public health expenditure as % of health spending, 2002	55.1%	69.9%	78.5%	83.4%	86.5%
Hospital payment	Contracted-prospective DRGs; per diem; and discounted fee-for-services	Global budget	Cost-per-case; prospective budget; and DRGs	Annual block contracts; HRGs	National budget
Physician payment	Mix of fee-for-service and capitation	Fee-for-service; fee schedule	Capitation and service complex payments; DRGs; negotiated fee	Mix of fee-for-service and capitation	Salary
Drugs	Coverage by Medicare, Medicaid, and most private insurance; high cost-sharing requirements	Limited coverage—varies by province; some employer coverage	Coverage through sickness funds (co-payments required)	Through NHS	Full coverage

Sources: This table was compiled from various sources included in the references. Most statistics are available at the countries page of the World Health Organization Web site (http://www.who.int/countries/en/) and the Global Pharmacy Workforce and Migration Report (http://www.fip.org/hr/).

however, have socialized health care programs; the government employs health care practitioners, owns health care facilities, and administers the health care system. A decentralized national health program involves schemes in which the administration of health care delivery is divided among various groups.

DEVELOPED AND DEVELOPING COUNTRIES

Based on per capita income, the world can be divided into developed and developing countries. Developed nations (i.e., mostly capitalistic and social democratic societies in industrialized countries) have per capita incomes of more than $8,260 (Boyes and Melvin, 1999) and tend to have strong health infrastructures and positive health care outcomes. Developing countries account for 84% of the world's population but only 11% of global health expenditures.

The income and health expenditures gap between developing and developed countries underscores the enormous difference in terms of capacities and types of health services that can be provided. This translates into large differences in the health infrastructure and the health outcomes of populations in developing countries. A limiting factor for developing countries is the large portion of their budgets required to finance the most basic of primary health care services. If a basic package of health care services is estimated to cost approximately $15 to $20 per person, then a low-income country would be required to devote one quarter to one third of its government budget to the health sector just for these basic services (Schieber and Maeda, 1999).

Lack of resources, poor administrative capacity, and the competing needs for other social and economic programs have a profound effect on the burden of disease in developing countries (Schieber and Maeda, 1999). Worldwide, one death in every three is attributable to largely preventable communicable diseases such as infectious disease, maternal and perinatal conditions, and nutritional deficiencies. Communicable diseases that are mainly preventable remain the leading causes of death in developing countries; indeed, almost all deaths from communicable diseases occur in developing countries (Harvard School of Public Health, 2000). In developing countries, mortality for individuals younger than age 5 (i.e., the probability of a child dying before reaching his or her fifth year) is almost 10 times the level found in developed countries (Schieber and Maeda, 1999). Approximately one in every 500 women in developing countries dies from complications related to pregnancy and childbirth, compared with only one in 27,000 women in the established market economies (UNICEF, 1995).

In the next 30 years, important demographic and epidemiological changes are expected to occur in developing countries that will alter the demand for health services and increase the pressure to make new investments in their health care systems (Harvard School of Public Health, 2000; Schieber and Maeda, 1999). Life expectancy at birth is expected to increase for women in all regions. Men are not expected to do as well on the longevity front, partly because of the effects of tobacco use on their life expectancy (Harvard School of Public Health, 2000).

Although overall deaths from communicable diseases are expected to decline, a steep increase is expected in the number of deaths resulting from noncommunicable diseases (e.g., heart disease, stroke, cancer, diabetes) as well as the number of deaths from injuries. In part, the projected reduction in deaths from communicable diseases reflects increased income, education, and technological progress in the development of antimicrobials and vaccines. The expected increase in deaths from noncommunicable diseases and injury is largely driven by aging of the population as well as exposure to tobacco. By 2020, the burden of disease attributed to tobacco is expected to outweigh that caused by any single disease (Harvard School of Public Health, 2000). In the future, health systems in developing countries will need to change their health systems to focus on treatment and prevention of noncommunicable diseases instead of the more cost-effective and lower-cost interventions targeted toward communicable diseases—a trend that will further strain these already fragile health systems (Schieber and Maeda, 1999).

The health of a population or country is also influenced by a number of socioeconomic variables, such as the distribution of resources within a country, income per capita, the number of years of schooling in adults, and—to some extent—the ability to adopt new health technologies. Studies have also found the educational level and status of women to be indicators of the health outcomes in a household. Women are often the primary caregivers for the health and nutritional needs of other family members. As a consequence, greater educational attainment in women can contribute to improved understanding of disease prevention and better nutritional health within a household. When girls are offered educational opportunities, their value within the household increases. Thus the allocation of resources such as food and medicine within a household tends to be more equitable when parents place equal value on their children regardless of their gender.

A strong inverse relationship exists between per capita income and child mortality under 5 years of age. That is, as per capita income increases, infant mortality rates tend to decrease. However, variability exists among countries, indicating that social and cultural factors strongly influence these mortality rates, as do differences in the use of maternal and child health programs and the extent to which they achieve equity and efficiency in the delivery of health services (Schieber and Maeda, 1999). The distribution of limited health resources is also affected by whether services are administered through a public or private system. A strong direct relationship exists between an economy's health spending and its per capita gross domestic product (GDP—a measure of the value of the final goods and services produced in a given country). On a worldwide basis, for every 10% increase in per capita GDP, health spending increases by 13% (Schieber and Maeda, 1999).

Public health expenditures tend to be more responsive to income differences than private health expenditures. Thus, as countries' incomes increase, a larger share of total health spending tends to come from public sources. Public health expenditures account for 47% of health spending in low-income countries, 57% in middle-income countries, and 67% in high-income countries. These differing rates may be attributable to the relatively greater ability to tax and generate revenue in higher-income countries as well as governments' decisions to address health sector and health insurance market failures through public rather than private financing. The fact that such a large portion of health expenditures is privately financed in developing countries has important implications for both equity and efficiency in health care, because governments need to focus on efficient allocation of combined public and private resources (Schieber and Maeda, 1999). Typically, those countries with a higher proportion of publicly financed health care systems have also achieved better and more equitable health outcomes primarily through a more equitable distribution of scarce health resources. For this reason, certain socialist economic systems, even in developing countries, have achieved health outcomes that are comparable to those found in many industrialized countries.

Other factors—for example, public health improvements in drinking water, access to prenatal and perinatal care, population planning, immunizations, and the allocation of food supplies—also directly affect the health of a population. Rational and efficient investments in primary health care services could afford most developing countries a cost-effective package of basic primary care and emergency services, although data reveal that a disproportionate share of limited public health spending is allocated to tertiary care instead of primary care (Schieber and Maeda, 1999). In most developing countries, individuals in the highest income brackets can still enjoy access to health services (either within their country or by traveling outside the country) that is comparable to the best health care services available in higher-income countries. Nevertheless, the majority of people living in developing countries lack access to even basic primary health care services.

HEALTH CARE DELIVERY SYSTEMS IN SELECTED NATIONS

Canada's Health Care System

The origins of Canada's current health care system date back to the 1940s, when the first government-financed insurance was established for hospital services in Saskatchewan (Organization for Economic Cooperation and Development, 1994). In 1957, the Hospital Insurance and Diagnostic Service Act (HIDS) established public insurance that provided inpatient hospital care coverage for all Canadians. In 1966, the Medical Care Act established the main principles of Canada's current health care system:

1. Portability of benefits: Coverage is kept, even when the individual is absent from the province.
2. Comprehensiveness: All necessary physician and hospital services are covered.
3. Universality: All citizens of a province are entitled to the same services.
4. Accessibility: Reasonable access to services is assured.
5 Public administration: A nonprofit, public organization accountable to the provincial government runs the plan (Rozek and Mulhern, 1994).

This legislation was implemented on a province-by-province basis. By 1972, Canada's 10 provinces and two territories had implemented medical insurance measures, realizing the goal of national health insurance for the country. In 1984, the Canada Health Act aggregated the provisions of the Medical Care Act and HIDS into one updated piece of legislation.

As a consequence of these measures, Canada has 12 different health insurance plans. These plans are kept consistent through adherence to the five main principles of portability, comprehensiveness, universality, accessibility, and public administration. Failure to ensure that these principles are maintained would prevent a province from qualifying for federal subsidies (Rozek and Mulhern, 1994).

The Canadian system has been successful in providing universal access to care regardless of patients' ability to pay, and the services covered are extensive. As a result, the health status of the Canadian population is good. In 2004, life expectancy at birth was 78 years for men and 83 years for women. That same year infant mortality was 5 deaths per 1,000 births—compared to the rate of 6 deaths per 1,000 births in the United States (World Health Organization, 2006). Canada's success in providing universal access and caring for the less fortunate has been a great source of pride for its citizens, who view it as presenting a striking contrast to the U.S. system that leaves 45 million people uninsured. However, recent polls indicate that public confidence in the system is eroding as waiting lists increase and availability of physicians and services becomes more limited.

Structure: Health Care Facilities and Workforce

Although Canada has socialized health insurance, health care delivery systems in the country are mostly private. Hospitals are primarily nonprofit community and teaching hospitals, although 4% of hospitals belong to the federal government. Provinces set the standards for hospital facilities and staffing.

The Canada Medical Care Act explicitly prohibited private hospitals or insurance companies from providing or financing core medical services provided by the Canada Medical Care Act. However, a recent Canadian Supreme Court ruling struck down a Quebec law banning private medical insurance and private medical clinics. The court ruled that waiting lists at publicly financed hospitals had become so long that "the prohibition on obtaining private health insurance is not constitutional where the public system fails to deliver reasonable services" (Krauss, 2005). Supporters of the publicly financed system fear that the introduction of privately financed services will encourage physicians and private clinics to leave the publicly financed system for higher reimbursement—a system that favors better access to treatments for individuals with higher incomes (Canadian-healthcare, 2006).

The national health insurance program, called Medicare, covers physician care and the following hospital services: room and meals, nursing services, diagnostic procedures, and medications prescribed for inpatient use. Private insurance is available only as a supplement to the national health insurance. Until the recent court decision regarding private insurance, private policies provided coverage only for private or semiprivate rooms in a hospital and other services not covered through Medicare, such as cosmetic surgery, dental services, and outpatient medications for those not covered under the Canadian law (Rozek and Mulhern, 1994). Delivery systems other than hospitals are available to Canadians, but these options vary from province to province. These systems, which include community health centers and long-term care, aim to provide preventive care and other services for which an acute care hospital setting is not necessary (Rozek and Mulhern, 1994).

Under the Canada Health Act, primary-care doctors, specialists, and dental surgery are all covered by provincial policies. Approximately half of all Canadian physicians are general practitioners (GPs) or family physicians. Primary-care physicians function as gatekeepers, serving as the initial point of contact for patients at the forefront of Canadian health care. Approximately 30,000 primary-care doctors practice in Canada (Canadian-healthcare, 2006). Patients have free choice of physicians. Typically patients are referred to specialists by their primary-care physicians. Approximately 28,000 specialist doctors currently work in Canada.

The distribution of physicians across Canada is not homogeneous, and there is an undersupply in rural areas. A decrease in the supply of physicians is one of the latest concerns to arise regarding the country's health care resources (Iglehart, 2000). The government statistical agency estimates that more than 15% of the population does not have a primary-care physician (Krauss, 2004). This compares to an estimated 20% of U.S. residents who do not have a primary-care physician (Krauss, 2004).

Canada's physicians are paid lower salaries than their U.S. counterparts, with the average salary for a Canadian physician being about one-third less than that for a U.S. physician. Even so, physicians are the highest-paid professionals in Canada. Their salaries are higher than those of British and Japanese physicians and similar to those of German physicians. In 2002, there were approximately 2.1 physicians for every 1,000 residents in Canada, compared to 2.4 physicians per 1,000 residents in the United States (Anderson, Hussey, Krogner, and Waters, 2005).

Medicare covers outpatient prescription drugs for senior citizens, individuals with low incomes, and patients with specific disease states. Four provinces have implemented universal prescription plans called Pharmacare (Naylor, 1999). Most of the population relies on private insurance for outpatient prescription drug coverage, but subscribing to such supplemental coverage is often dependent on income.

Financing

The Canadian system is not one centralized plan, but rather 12 separate systems that are controlled by the provinces and territories. The universal insurance is paid for by personal and corporate taxes and distributed to each province according to budgets established on both national and provincial levels. Provinces may obtain additional funds from other sources such as lottery proceeds and sales taxes. The provinces of Alberta, British Columbia, and Ontario also charge health premiums to supplement health spending (Canadian-healthcare, 2006).

The provincial governments carefully plan how to allocate resources within their budgets. Because the government is the only insurer, administrative overhead is tightly controlled in Canada. In 1999, health administrative costs were $307 per capita in Canada compared with $1,059 per capita in the United States (Woolhandler, Campbell, and Himmelstein, 2003). The additional administrative costs in the U.S. system can be attributed to the nature of a pluralistic insurance system that has complex billing and reimbursement procedures that vary considerably among payers.

Costs are controlled through set fees for medical services. Every year, the government publishes a list of the fees that physicians are permitted to charge the government for treating patients. Physicians are then paid directly by the provincial government on a fee-for-service basis. Hospitals in Canada work on a budget that cannot be exceeded, which not surprisingly results in some strain in the system. Many hospitals have closed or merged, causing a "shrinking hospital sector" (Naylor, 1999). Because most hospitals are run at capacity in Canada, waiting lists are commonplace. For example, the waiting period for a coronary bypass in Canada can range from 3 to 6 months, compared with one day to a week in the United States.

While all inpatient prescription expenses are covered under the Canada Health Act, each province may offer varying levels of coverage for drugs prescribed on an outpatient basis. The publicly funded drug programs are generally established based on patients' age, income, and medical condition (Health Canada, 2006). Only those medications listed on the Medicare formularies are covered. In recent years, drug spending has been increasing and has become the second largest category of health care-related expenditures in Canada, after hospital services.

Although drug prices are set at the federal level, purchasing takes place at the provincial level. Provinces, therefore, face the responsibility of controlling increasing drug expenditures without having direct control over pricing (Anis, 2000).

Current Status

In recent years, Canada has struggled'with increased waiting times for diagnostic tests, hip and knee replacements, cancer treatments, and elective surgeries, among other things. In addition to the difficulties attributable to the maldistribution of physicians and long waiting lists for certain services, the federal government has decreased its contribution to provincial plans significantly, increasing the pressure on provincial governments. Coverage for services varies among the provinces, which can make it difficult for patients to receive care in other provinces than their own (Chidley, 1996). Moreover, the single-payer structure prevents the system from rapidly responding to local changes in the health care environment.

Dissatisfaction with the current waiting lists for services and the shortage of primary-care physicians in some areas has grown sharply as well. With the recent ruling by the Canadian Supreme Court that allows residents to purchase health services privately, some predict the creation of a two-tired health care system—where one branch is privately financed for those who can afford it and the other branch remains publicly financed. However, the current system has generally been strongly supported by most of the public, and most Canadian citizens identify with it as part of the Canadian national character (Krauss, 2005).

In 2003, the First Ministers' Accord on Health Care Renewal was adopted. This accord consisted of an agreement on a vision, principles, and action plan for renewal of the Canadian health system (Government of Canada, 2006). It incorporated an agreement on the value of a publicly funded health system, the need for reform, and the priorities for reform. The priorities established included additional investments in primary health care, home care, and catastrophic drug coverage to create a long-term, sustainable public health care system in Canada (Government of Canada, 2006). The federal government agreed to establish a health reform fund by 2004 for use by the provinces and territories to achieve the reform objectives. The health reform funding will eventually be integrated into the general health funding provided to each province (Government of Canada, 2006). It remains to be seen whether Canada's reform efforts will enable it to continue to achieve the health outcomes it has experienced in the past, but so far it continues to surpass the United States in terms of its national health coverage.

Germany's Health Care System

Germany's current health care system has its roots in the statutory health insurance system (sickness funds) for manual industrial workers instituted by Chancellor Bismarck in 1883 (Beske, 1988). This law, in conjunction with the accident insurance law of 1884 and the disability and old-age pension insurance law of 1889, remains the backbone of Germany's social security system. Although sickness funds started as coverage for certain occupations, they evolved to accept all qualified persons whose place of work fell within the geographical boundaries covered by the fund. During the 1990s, occupational and geographical limits on most of the sickness funds were lifted (Jackson, 1997). Today, only funds for small farmers, miners, and sailors remain closed (Busse, 2004). Moreover, potential enrollees cannot be discriminated against based on their age, gender, or other risk factors.

Thus Germany has no comprehensive national health plan. Instead, German citizens are covered by either the health insurance system (Krankenkasse, or "sickness funds") or the social welfare program for the unemployed. The sickness funds are considered "private corporations under public law" (Hoffmeyer, 1994), so the statutory system is decentralized. In 2003, 319 self-governing sickness funds were in charge of the health care insurance of the individuals they covered (Busse, 2004). Although insured individuals are allowed to change sickness funds at any time, they have to stay with their new fund for the next 18 months unless the new fund increases its contribution rate. This rule has recently been adopted because evidence has shown that healthier Germans consistently switched to funds with lower than average contribution rates.

Sickness funds can be classified in four main types. Most are company-based funds; the rest are either guild funds, general regional funds, or substitute funds (which originally covered white-collar groups) (Busse, 2004). Of those persons covered by sickness funds, 7% also carry supplemental private insurance for ambulatory and dental care (Beske, 1988).

By 1990, approximately 90% of the German population was covered through this statutory health insurance system, which provides a guaranteed health care package of comprehensive services (Hoffmeyer, 1994). Since 1994, this package has included long-term care, nursing home care, and home health care (Evans, Cuellar, and Wiener, 2000). The remaining 10% of the population had either private insurance (8%) or received free medical services (2%). The police, members of the armed forces, and welfare recipients all qualify for free medical care (Beske, 1988). Germans who earn more than a certain level of income have a choice of private insurance or voluntary membership in the sickness funds. Approximately 14% of the population covered through sickness funds joined voluntarily on this basis (Busse, 2004). Persons who elect to purchase private insurance, however, cannot switch back to a sickness fund (Jackson, 1997).

Three main values underlie the German health care system:

1. Self-governance: The system is administered by a self-managing organization (for example, the sickness funds).
2. Social partnership: Both the employer and the employee have a share in the system.
3. Social solidarity: Ensuring equality in health care through some members of society subsidizing other members' health care costs (Hoffmeyer, 1994).

A strong commitment to social solidarity exists in Germany (Jackson, 1997).

Germany's decentralized system appears to be successful in keeping its population healthy. The country's infant mortality rate was 4.5 deaths per 1,000 live births in 2003 (World Health Organization, 2006). Moreover, the percentage of infants with a low birth weight is smaller than that in the rest of Europe or the United States. In 2003, life expectancy was 76 years for men and 82 years for women in Germany (World Health Organization, 2006). These and other health status indicators are similar to those associated with other industrialized countries but significantly better than the indicators for the United States.

Structure: Health Care Facilities and Workforce

In 1990, Germany had a ratio of 10.8 hospital beds per 1,000 persons (Hoffmeyer, 1994). This ratio is high (almost twice that of the United

Kingdom and 60% higher than that of Canada) and has resulted in a surplus of hospital beds and consequent high operating costs for some hospitals (Beske, 1988). In recent years, the number of hospitals has been decreasing but it is still high. Government or nonprofit organizations own the majority of German hospitals.

There were approximately 34 physicians for every 10,000 people in Germany in 2003 (World Health Organization, 2006). This ratio indicates that there may currently be an oversupply of physicians that could eventually lead to increased health care costs. Physicians working in office-based practices act as gatekeepers for institutionalized care. If they wish to be reimbursed by sickness funds, physicians have to qualify and apply for accreditation with a regional association of physicians. Germans have freedom of choice of physicians. If a patient wants to switch physicians, however, he or she has to wait 3 months before selecting another office-based physician.

Germany has a well-developed pharmaceutical industry, with significant drug development occurring in the country (Spivey, Wertheimer, and Rucker, 1992). In 1995, Germany was the world's fourth largest producer of pharmaceuticals (Jacobzone, 2000). Medications are covered through the sickness funds and are available from both hospital and retail pharmacies. Retail pharmacies in Germany have to be owned by pharmacists, and each pharmacist can own only one pharmacy (Ulrich, 1999).

Financing

The statutory health system is financed primarily through payroll taxes; employers and employees make equal contributions to this system. The contributions represent a percentage of the employees' income up to a certain threshold. Sickness funds are financed to a lesser extent by pension funds, local unemployment offices, and welfare organizations (Hoffmeyer, 1994). Sickness funds with a high share of chronically ill participants receive a high-risk pool supplement, aimed at compensating them for 40% of their expenses for specific types of patients, over a certain limit (Busse, 2004).

Hospitals and most physicians negotiate their fees with the sickness funds. Physicians working in hospitals, however, are salaried employees. Payment for office-based physicians follows a fee-for-service point system; that is, each service is assigned a number of points and a conversion factor translates these points into German marks (Hoffmeyer, 1994). Each state has a union of physicians that provides services to the sickness funds that are in charge of negotiating budgets (Jost, 1998). Hospitals' payments have shifted from per diem rates to prospective cost-per-case payments. Patients are charged a co-payment for some benefits, but the majority of services are free at the point of delivery.

Sickness funds also provide reimbursement for approved medications. Reference pricing was introduced in 1989, whereby drugs with similar properties would be reimbursed at the same level. When a more expensive pharmaceutical is prescribed, the patient pays the difference. Prices for medications across the country are uniform because regulation determines the markup allowed to wholesalers and retailers. Patients pay co-payments reflecting the package size for the particular prescription drug (Ulrich, 1999).

Current Status

The 1993 Health Care Act introduced reforms to Germany's health care system, some of which are still being implemented. Among the short-term measures included in the reform package were ceilings on expenditures for office-based physicians and hospital services and on budgets for medicines prescribed by office-based physicians (Hoffmeyer, 1994). These measures were aimed at controlling two of the health care system's biggest problems: overutilization of health services and increased spending on drugs. Germany has also recently implemented a diagnosis-related group (DRG) payment system for hospital services and medical devices (Wood, personal communication, June 19, 2003).

Perhaps the biggest problem with Germany's health system relates to the country's high unemployment levels over the past decade. The slow-down in the German economy has created revenue problems for the sickness funds because their financing is based on wage-based premiums (Jost, 1998). Despite the pressures brought by reunification of East and West Germany, high unemployment rates, and the large percentage of elderly citizens (who account for approximately 16% of the population), the country has been successful in managing its health care system (Reinhardt, 1999).

In recent years, it has become apparent that some reform of the sickness funds will be necessary, and two different strategies have been proposed: citizen insurance and flat-rate premiums (Saltman and Dubois, 2005). Citizen insurance would require all Germans to buy a standard benefit package regardless of whether they participate in a sickness fund or a private insurance plan. The flat-rate premium would entail the implementation of a modest premium for all adults. Experts believe that citizen insurance would help perpetuate the existing system, whereas the flat-rate premium might erode the solidarity concept upon which the German health care system was developed.

The United Kingdom's Health Care System

The movement toward the United Kingdom's current health care system started after World War I (Harrison, 1988). In 1939, only half of the nation's population had insurance coverage (Allen, 1984), and people were concerned about creating a more rational and comprehensive health service. Planning for a comprehensive health care delivery system continued during World War II, although major disagreement existed between different players regarding the system administration, funding, and physicians' roles in the system.

The National Health Service Act was finally passed in 1946 (Harrison, 1988). The National Health Service (NHS) presented three innovations: (1) universal comprehensive service, (2) financing through general taxation with little or no charge at point of service. and (3) nationalization of the country's hospitals (Allen, 1984). This system can be defined as socialized medicine whereby most of the services are provided by practitioners who work for the government.

Since the implementation of the NHS, the United Kingdom has experienced longer life expectancy rates and concomitant changes in disease patterns. In 2004, life expectancy was 76 years for men and 81 years for women (World Health Organization, 2006). Infant mortality was 5 deaths per 1,000 live births in the same year (World Health Organization, 2006).

Structure: Health Care Facilities and Workforce

The United Kingdom's health care system includes three major components: hospitals, community services, and primary medical and dental care (Harrison, 1988). All of these services are available to the entire population, and only hospital care requires referral from a primary-care physician. Primary care is delivered by a wide range of health professionals, including family practitioners, nurses, dentists, pharmacists, and opticians (National Health Service, 2006).

Physicians work mainly in two settings: government hospitals and office practices. Physicians who work in NHS hospitals are salaried employees. Senior medical staff members, however, are allowed to hold contracts for private practice that account for as much as 10% of their gross income (Booer, 1994). GPs are in charge of primary care and act as the gatekeepers for hospital and specialty care. Patients have to register with a GP practice, but are allowed to change GPs whenever they like. The government controls the establishment of primary-care practices.

Secondary and tertiary care is provided by hospitals. Secondary care includes maternity care, pathology, radiology, and emergency care. Tertiary care deals with highly specialized services such as organ transplants and treatments for rare diseases.

As of 2002, physicians were organized into approximately 300 primary-care trusts (PCTs) (Bindman and Weiner, 2000; National Health Service, 2006). These groups include about 50 GPs each and are in charge of managing primary health services budgets for their patients (Enthoven, 2000).

PCTs control 80% of the total NHS budget. Given that providers are paid based on quality incentives rather than the quantity of care provided, physicians in PCTs have incentives to work as part of a primary-care team along with other health care providers, including nurses, midwives, and pharmacists. Pharmacists, for example, are currently being trained to prescribe some medications and/or approve patient refills and other primary care roles. Community trusts are in charge of those community services not provided by GPs, such as specialized mental health services.

Patients are not charged for their visits to health providers who work as part of the NHS system (National Health Service, 2006). Patients can also choose to receive care from private providers, but these services are not reimbursed by the NHS. Generally, private providers allow patients to receive services more quickly, but they do not appear to deliver higher-quality care (Keeler, 2006).

All drugs available through the NHS are reviewed by the National Institute for Clinical Excellence (NICE), which confirms the drugs' clinical efficacy and cost-effectiveness. (Morgan et al., 2006). The NHS creates a negative formulary that lists drugs that are excluded from coverage and then determines which drugs it will provide on a subsidized basis to the regional populations in its trusts (Morgan et al., 2006). Almost 70% of the medications prescribed in the United Kingdom are generics (Jacobzone, 2000). Prices for pharmaceutical products are negotiated by NHS and drug manufacturers (Jacobzone, 2000). Drug development in the United Kingdom is significant, and the U.K. drug industry continues to be one of the largest producers of pharmaceutical products worldwide (Spivey et al., 1992).

Financing

All health care through the NHS is free at the point of delivery to anyone who is a U.K. resident. All taxpayers, employees, and employers contribute to the system. Approximately 82% of the cost of health services is covered by general taxes. Employers and employees pay an additional 14.2%, and another 3.3% of expenditures is financed through small cost-sharing requirements for drugs and land sales taxes (British Studies Web pages, 2006).

Hospitals have to provide care within their annual contract constraints. Most contracts are specified as an annual block payment or budgeted amount. Hospitals are then paid a lump sum that covers a specific range of services and facilities that PCTs contract for. This reimbursement amount includes services such as inpatient hospital care, dialysis treatments, and day surgeries.

Primary-care funding is provided through an annual budget assigned by the Department of Health to each PCT. GPs have independent contracts with the PCTs they work for. Their payment is based on a complex equation involving a mix of capitation (60% of financing) and fee-for-service payments, with additional fees being mandated for special situations (such as working in deprived areas, night visits, and minor surgeries). Generally, physicians in the United Kingdom earn half of the amount earned by U.S. physicians (Keeler, 2006).

Additional trusts have been established to provide specialized or specific services. For example, mental health trusts serve people with mental health problems, care trusts combine social care and health care services, and ambulance trusts respond to life-threatening emergencies. All trusts operate within an annual budget allocated by the federal budget and based on the region and the size of the population they serve.

Current Status

The NHS is facing severe budget constraints, and it is feared that the program will prove inadequate to respond to increased technological advances and the aging of the U.K. population. Although a guaranteed health care package exists, it is not properly codified, and differences remain in various parts of the country (Booer, 1994). Because of these financial difficulties, treatments commonly available to patients in the United States, such as dialysis for individuals older than age 65, intensive care, and aggressive cancer treatments for terminal patients, are generally unavailable in the United Kingdom. Lack of facilities in some areas has resulted in waiting lists for certain hospital services, albeit not for emergency cases, pregnancy, or planned treatments such as chemotherapy (NHS A to Z HelpDirect, 2000). Some recent reforms aimed at improving the NHS include the creation of national clinical standards and external performance monitoring of NHS hospitals and PCTs.

In 2000, the NHS released *The NHS Plan*, a 10-year plan intended to increase the efficiencies of its services. This plan's publication was followed by a white paper titled the *NHS Improvement Plan and Creating a Patient-Led NHS*, which outlined the goals of giving patients more choice about their providers and health and increasing the country's health spending. The greater expenditures are expected to triple the investment made in the NHS from 1995 to 2008 (National Health Service, 2006). Other goals include increasing preventive care, expanding patient education for chronic conditions, creating new urgent care strategies, making health care services more convenient, and improving coordination of social and health care services (National Health Service, 2006). Other reforms will include the establishment of NHS Direct, a free nursing phone line, and future online appointment services through NHS Net, a computer-based network linking NHS organizations (Dobson, 1999). The United Kingdom has also stressed the removal of waiting lists by imposing its own form of DRG payments, called Healthcare Resource Groups (HRGs).

Although there is general dissatisfaction with waiting lists and restricted access to certain services, the United Kingdom has been able to achieve health outcomes that exceed those found in the United States and at a cost that is 60% less than the costs incurred by the U.S. system (Keeler, 2005). However, when faced long waiting lists in their own country, many British individuals travel to foreign countries such as India and other parts of Europe to seek treatment if they can afford to do so (Rai, 2005). Overall health spending is set by the British Parliament, which has defined efficient use of resources as a policy goal.

A 2002 survey of sicker adults in five health systems (the United States, the United Kingdom, Canada, New Zealand, and Australia) found that sicker British adults reported problems with waiting time and other non-financial barriers to care but were the most satisfied with their health system. (Blendon, Schoen, DesRosches, Osborn, and Zapert, 2003). In the same survey, sicker U.S. adults were most likely to be concerned about costs and coverage and to report access barriers due to costs; consequently, they were more likely to forgo medical care or not get recommended follow-up treatment, including skipping medications (Blendon et al., 2003). The government's current financial commitments to the existing U.K. system may mean that the country will continue to achieve high health outcomes at a fraction of what the United States spends on health care.

Cuba's Health Care System

Cuba's current health care system is the product of the socialist transformations that have occurred in this island-nation since the revolution of 1959. This system can be classified as socialized medicine. Cuba's health care system is ruled by five basic principles:

1. Health care is a right.
2. Health care is the responsibility of the state.
3. Preventive and curative services are integrated.
4. Everyone participates in the function of the health care system.
5. Health care activities are integrated with economic and social development (Santana, 1987).

Two main programs have been instrumental in achieving Cuba's basic health care principles: the Medicine in the Community Program (1975) and the Family Physician Program (1985) (Santana, 1987).

By the end of the 1960s, Cuba's health care resources had been aggregated into a single system. The Cuban Ministry of Public Health was established in conjunction with polyclinics (discussed in detail in the next section) that provided primary-care services at the local level. The Medicine in the Community Program was proposed in 1975 to promote, maintain, and improve individual and community health through individuals' participation in the functioning, organizing, and use of the system. The polyclinics were restructured to become responsible for the total health services of a geographical area and population, as well as teaching and research activities. However, the polyclinics' staffs were not able to integrate fully with the communities they served. Moreover, the number of persons assigned to a community team was sometimes too high, and continuity of care was not easy to achieve (Santana, 1987).

The Family Physician Program of 1985 changed the way primary care was delivered by increasing the number of family physicians and changing the role of the polyclinic. Under this program, a physician–nurse team works in a small office in charge of "the preventive, curative, and environmental health of a city block or rural area" consisting of roughly 600 to 800 persons. In 1990, 50% of the population was covered by the Family Physician Program (Roemer, 1993). By 2000, the program was expected to have enough family physicians to cover almost every city block (Cuba is mostly urban) (Santana, 1987). This goal proved difficult to reach, however, given Cuba's economic crisis, which continues to this day.

The restructuring of Cuba's health care system after the Cuban revolution of 1959 clearly improved the health of the nation's population. Cuba's health indicators are better than those of all other countries except those with industrial capitalist economies (Nayeri, 1995). Life expectancy is now 75 years for men and 79 years for women in Cuba (World Health Organization, 2006). Since the 1980s, in the Western Hemisphere, only the United States and Canada have ranked better than Cuba in terms of infant and child mortality indicators (Susser, 1993). The health profile of the majority of Cubans resembles that of their counterparts in developed societies; the leading health problems are chronic and degenerative diseases, including heart disease, cancer, and diabetes (Santana, 1987).

Structure: Health Care Facilities and Workforce

The Family Physician Program (Médico de Familia) currently constitutes the backbone of Cuba's health care delivery system. Family physicians and nurses are assigned to an office-consultation room (consultorio) in a given community. Living quarters either in the same building or nearby are provided for these caregivers (Ramers, 2001). Family physicians hold office hours during the mornings. In the afternoons, they follow patients in the hospital, make visits, and inspect community facilities such as food stores, pharmacies, and day care centers (Santana, 1987). Thus the family physician is in charge of the complete well-being of the whole community rather than just the health of a given number of patients.

Patients in need of additional services are referred to a polyclinic (policlínico). The polyclinic has evolved into an ancillary facility that provides laboratory and emergency services as well as specialty consultations. In addition, it serves as a setting for physician residency training. Each policlinic serves 30 to 40 consultorios (Dresang, Brebrick, Murray, Shallue, and Sullivan-Vedder, 2005). Hospital services are also available, but they focus on tertiary care. In 1995, there were 400 polyclinics and 263 hospitals in Cuba (Veeken, 1995).

Cuba prides itself on the advances it has achieved in medically related scientific endeavors. Resources have been allocated to training for primary care and to improving research into and knowledge of new diagnostic and treatment techniques (Santana, 1987). For example, computed tomography scans, organ transplants, and other high-technology facilities are all available in Cuba (Nayeri, 1995).

The health care workforce in Cuba has grown dramatically to fulfill the goals of the Family Physician Program. According to Cuban government statistics, Cuba had 71,000 physicians by November 2005 (Rios, 2005). This represents the highest family physician per capita ratio in the world (Dresang et al., 2005). A physician trained through the Family Physician Program spends 6 years learning medicine with a preventive, prophylactic, and epidemiological view. The majority of family physicians and medical students in Cuba are women. Also, the proportion of male nurses has increased, reflecting a change in traditional gender roles in the medical professions. Physicians' salaries remain modest, however (Santana, 1987).

A unique feature of Cuba's health care workforce is its internationalist focus. A number of Cuban physicians participate in a program that sends them abroad for 2 years of service to another country in Latin America, the Caribbean, Africa, the Middle East, or Asia (Nayeri, 1995). Cuba is also involved with the education of foreign doctors. The Escuela Latinoamerciana de Medicina (Latin American School of Medicine), which is sponsored by the Cuba government, was originally established to train doctors of poor origins from Latin American countries affected by Hurricanes George and Mitch in 1998. It currently has 7,200 students from 24 countries, including 4 African nations and the United States (Escuela Latinoamericana de Medicina, 2006). U.S. students in the program are exempted from the U.S. government's ban on travel to Cuba (Mullan, 2004).

Financing

The government controls health care in Cuba, so financing for health care is entirely public. Even providers' medical education is paid for by the state, which provides additional financial aid to students with dependents (Nayeri, 1995). National budgets established for health care services are an important part of the country's expenditures.

Current Status

Cuba is facing an economic crisis that is driven by two external factors: the fall of the Soviet bloc and the U.S. economic embargo (Nayeri, 1995). Before the Cuban revolution, most of the country's pharmaceutical products were imported; more than 80% came from the United States. Importation of goods, including drugs, shifted to the Soviet Union and Soviet bloc nations before the dissolution of this Soviet alliance in 1991. With the downfall of the Soviet bloc, Cuba lost the main supplier of its basic needs. Approximately 85% of its international trade ended with the collapse of the Soviet bloc, and the Cuban economy has been shrinking ever since. Cuba's unemployment rates, inflation rates, and budget deficit are high (Nayeri, 1995).

Cuba's situation is unique, in that a trade embargo imposed by the United States has influenced Cuba's health care system by affecting the flow of medical supplies and related materials to Cuba. This embargo has been in place since the 1960s and is one of the world's few sanctions that explicitly includes both food and medical supplies (Williams, 1997). The embargo was strengthened in the United States by passage of the Cuban Democracy Act of 1992, which prohibited foreign subsidiaries of U.S. companies from trading with Cuba (Barry, 2000). This measure effectively banned Cuba from purchasing half of the new world-class drugs available on the market (Barry, 2000; Williams, 1997). The lack of medical supplies and equipment has also reduced surgical rates in Cuba as well as the country's use of laboratory and radiological services such as mammography and other diagnostic tools (Williams, 1997).

Water supply and treatment is a serious problem in Cuba. Waterborne disease rates have doubled in recent years, and diarrhea is the second most common reason for a medical visit (Williams, 1997). Cuba cannot produce enough chlorine to disinfect its water supply, and the water delivery system is in disrepair because of the lack of pipes and equipment needed from the United States.

The Cuban government has tried to preserve both education and health care services, despite the ongoing economic crisis. For example, the use of alternative medicine (called "traditional medicine" in Cuba) has increased (Quick, 1997; Dresang et al., 2005). The Family Physician Program has not appeared to be affected by the economic pressures so far (Nayeri, 1995). Some health problems may be related to the scarcity of food supplies. Nevertheless, the infant mortality rate has remained low, at 7 deaths per 1,000 live births in 2003 (World Health Organization, 2006). Restrictions relating to U.S. embargo on Cuba were tightened in 2004, however (Garfield, 2004). Despite the Cuban population's satisfaction with the gains in health care delivered by the socialist regime, the future success of this nation's health care system remains uncertain.

INTERNATIONAL HEALTH CARE SYSTEMS: IMPLICATIONS FOR THE UNITED STATES

The United States has a fragmented, multiple-payer health care system that makes it difficult to reduce inefficiencies and inappropriate spending (Keeler, 2006). The failure of the U.S. health care system to provide universal access to health care services at a reasonable cost has prompted the examination of foreign health care systems for possible solutions.

After discussing the health-related issues of developed and developing nations and the major features of four health care systems representing a variety of models of health care delivery, Jane (introduced in the case scenario at the beginning of this chapter) has been able to extract several lessons. The same pattern is evident in each of the countries examined—namely, a cycle of unsustainable spending growth, followed by implementation of numerous cost-containment strategies (Anderson et al., 2005).

Policy makers continue to try to determine whether prices, technology, aging, waste, inefficiency, the legal system, new disease patterns, corporate consolidation, or too many consumers and providers are to blame for rising costs (Anderson et al., 2005). In the United States, recent cost-containment strategies have focused on increased cost-sharing requirements in an effort to decrease demand for services, albeit so far with negligible results. In comparison, both the United Kingdom and Canada have sought to limit the supply of services, resulting in waiting lists for elective procedures.

In 2002, the United States spent $5,267 per capita on health expenditures, whereas Germany spent $2,817 per capita, Canada spent $2,931 per capita, and the United Kingdom spent $2160 per capita for health care (Anderson et al., 2005). The United States continues to pay more per capita for health care than any other country. While part of this difference can be explained by higher U.S. incomes and cost of living, U.S. health spending is still $2,037 higher than the predicted value, after adjusting for each country's per capita GDP (Anderson et al., 2005). In 2002, the United States also spent $1,821 more per capita on health care than Switzerland, the country that had the second highest spending on health care on a per capita basis (Anderson et al., 2005).

Some important lessons can be learned by comparing how health services are structured in the various countries. Both Canada and the United Kingdom set annual budgets that restrict reimbursement and tend to limit supply of certain services, especially elective procedures. By contrast, both the United States and Germany have a plentiful supply of physicians, technology, and health resources. While this ready supply has been cited as a cost driver for these systems, it has also meant that many U.S. residents cannot afford basic medical services. In the United

States, resources are distributed in a decidedly non-egalitarian fashion. People who have the ability to pay for services, either through income or insurance, can enjoy the best possible health care in the world. An increasing number of individuals, however, lack access to even the most basic primary-care services. This system stands in contrast to the U.K. system, where approximately 80% of the annual health care budget is spent on primary-care services but spending on heroic end-of-life technology is limited.

Another interesting component in the comparisons of systems is the role played by government in financing the systems of care. In this regard, the United States is unique in its reliance on private systems and funding for health care. Generally, as most countries achieve a high per capita income, the government assumes a greater role in financing health care services through public expenditures. In the United States, expenditures on health care represent 45% of total public spending, compared with 86% of total public expenditures in the United Kingdom, 70% of total public expenditures in Canada, and 73% of total public expenditures in Germany. These contrasts in public funding reflect a strong ethos in the United States that emphasizes the private sector's role and responsibility in the health care delivery system. This preference also leads to a pluralistic, fragmented delivery system with unique opportunities to shift costs between public and private payers.

While a high per capita income is generally associated with improved health outcomes, both the United States and Cuba, in their own ways, demonstrate that increased expenditures alone cannot improve health outcomes. In Cuba, which has a low per capita income, health outcomes are comparable to those achieved in many developed countries. In contrast, in the United States, having a high per capita income and health care expenditures that exceed those in all other countries has not improved health outcomes considerably. Clearly, how fairly and equitably health resources are distributed is an important consideration when comparing health systems.

CONCLUSIONS

Although health care systems may differ from nation to nation, they enable us to compare and contrast those characteristics that move a system toward the goals of providing affordable, accessible, and equitable health care for all populations. As pointed out by the case scenario at the beginning of the chapter, lessons can be learned from both industrialized and developing countries. Health care systems constantly evolve and change. Many factors—including consumer activism, political change, and public and private financing efforts—influence these complex processes. The distribution of health care resources both globally and within a particular country has a profound impact on how health care services will be delivered and used.

The need for health personnel in a health care system, in terms of both the number of providers and the mix of skills, is directed by policy decisions within a particular country. If policies direct greater involvement of pharmacists or other allied health professionals, then significant resource planning must be undertaken to ensure the availability of appropriately trained personnel. Appropriately trained personnel may be one of many constraints that planners face when developing health care policies. The disparities in the distribution of health care resources will continue to strain all health care systems, but particularly those in developing countries where competing social and economic programs are equally justified for funding.

QUESTIONS FOR FURTHER DISCUSSION

1. Are there components or features of the health care delivery systems discussed in this chapter that should be adopted to improve health care delivery in the United States?
2. Are there components or features of the pharmaceutical sector of the countries discussed in this chapter that should be adopted to improve health care delivery in the United States?
3. Should a national drug policy be developed and adopted in the United States? If so, what should its goal be and how should it be structured?

KEY TOPICS AND TERMS

Comprehensive care
Decentralized national health program
Developed nation
Developing nation
Gross domestic product (GDP)
Infant mortality rate
Life expectancy
Portability
Sickness funds
Socialized health insurance
Socialized medicine
Social partnership
Social solidarity
Universality

REFERENCES

Allen, D. (1984). Health services in England. In M. W. Raffel (Ed.), *Comparative health systems* (pp. 197–257). University Park, PA: Pennsylvania State University Press.

Anderson, G., Hussey, P., Krogner, B., & Waters, H. (2005). Health spending in the United States and the rest of the industrialized world. *Health Affairs, 24*(4), 903–914.

Anis, A. H. (2000). Pharmaceutical policies in Canada: Another example of federal–provincial discord. *Canadian Medical Association Journal, 162*(4), 523–526.

Barry, M. (2000). Effect of the U.S. embargo and economic decline on health in Cuba. *Annals of Internal Medicine, 132*(2), 151–154.

Beske, F. (1988). Federal Republic of Germany. In R. B. Saltman (Ed.), *The international handbook of health-care systems* (pp. 93–106). Westport, CT: Greenwood Press.

Bindman, A. B., & Weiner, J. P. (2000). The modern NHS: An underfunded model of efficiency and integration. *Health Affairs, 19*(30), 120–122.

Blendon, R., Schoen, C., DesRosches, C., Osborn, R., & Zapert, K. (2003). Common concerns amid diverse systems: Health care experiences in five countries. *Health Affairs, 27*(3), 106–121.

Booer, T. (1994). The health care systems in the United Kingdom. In U. K. Hoffmeyer & T. R. McCarthy (Eds.), *Financing health care* (pp. 1071–1145). Dordrecht, Netherlands: Kluwer.

Busse, R. (2004). Disease management programs in Germany's statutory health insurance system. *Health Affairs, 23*(3), 56–67.

Boyes, W., & Melvin, M. (1999). *Fundamentals of economics.* Boston, MA: Houghton Mifflin.

British Studies Web Pages. (2006). *The British health and welfare system.* Retrieved May 18, 2006 from http:/≠elt.britcoun.org.pl/elt/h_what.htm

Canadian-healthcare. (2006). *Canadian health care.* Retrieved May 24, 2006 from http://www.canadian-healthcare.org

Chidley, J. (1996). Radical surgery: Cuts in public funding imperil Medicare's future. *Maclean's, 109*(49), 44–48.

Dobson, F. (1999). Modernizing Britain's national health services. *Health Affairs, 18*(3), 40–41.

Dresang, L. T., Brebrick, L., Murray, D., Shallue, A., & Sullivan-Vedder, L. (2005). Family medicine in Cuba: Community-oriented primary care and complementary and alternative medicine. *Journal of the American Board of Family Practice, 18,* 297–303.

Enthoven, A. C. (2000). In pursuit of an improving national health service. *Health Affairs, 19*(3), 102–119.

Escuela Latinoamericana de Medicina (ELAM). (2006). *Informaciones generales sobre el Proyecto ELAM.* Retrieved May 18, 2006 http://www.elacm.sld.cu/infogen.htm

Evans-Cuellar, A., & Wiener, J. M. (2000). Can social insurance for long-term care work? The experience of Germany. *Health Affairs, 19*(3), 8–25.

Garfield, R. (2004). Health care in Cuba and the manipulation of humanitarian imperatives. *Lancet, 364,*1007.

Harrison, S. (1988). Great Britain. In R. B. Saltman (Ed.), *The international handbook of health-care systems* (pp. 123–143). Westport, CT: Greenwood Press.

Harvard School of Public Health. (2000). *Burden of disease unit.* Retrieved August 29, 2000 from http://www.hsph.harvard.edu/organizations/bdu/index/htm

Health Canada. (2006). *Health care system delivery.* Retrieved May 24, 2006 from http://www.hc-sc.gc.ca

Hilts, P. J. (2000, June 21). Europeans perform highest in ranking of world health. *The New York Times,* p. 9.

Hoffmeyer, U. (1994). The health care system in Germany. In U. K. Hoffmeyer & T. R. McCarthy (Eds.), *Financing health care* (pp. 419–512). Dordrecht, Netherlands: Kluwer.

Iglehart, J. K. (2000). Revisiting the Canadian health care system. *New England Journal of Medicine, 342*(26), 2007–2012.

Jackson, J. (1997). The German health system: Lessons for reform in the United States. *Archives of Internal Medicine, 157*(2), 155–161.

Jacobzone, S. (2000). *Pharmaceutical policies in OECD countries: Reconciling social and industrial goals* (Vol. 40, pp. 1–98). Paris, France: Organization for Economic Cooperation and Development.

Jost, T. (1998). German health care reform: The next steps. *Journal of Health Politics, Policy and Law, 23*(4), 697–711.

Keeler, E. (2006). Can we say no? The challenge of rationing health care. *The New England Journal of Medicine.* 354 (12), 1327-1328.

Krauss, C. (2004, September 12). *Canada looks for ways to fix its health care system.* Retrieved May 10, 2006 from http://www.nytimes.com/2004/09/12

Krauss, C. (2005, June 10). *In blow to Canada's health system, Quebec law is voided.* Retrieved May 10, 2006 from http://www.nytimes.com/2005/06/10

Morgan, S., McMahon, M., Mitton, C., Roughead, E., Kirk, R., Kanavos, P., & Menon, D. Centralized drug review processes in Australia, Canada, New Zealand, and the United Kingdom. *Health Affairs,* 25(2), 337–348.

Mullan, F. (2004). Affirmative action, Cuban style. *New England Journal of Medicine, 351*(26), 2680–2682.

National Health Service (NHS). (2006). *About the NHS—how the NHS works.* Retrieved May 18, 2006, from http://www.nhs.uk/england/AboutTheNhs/Defalut.cmsx

Nayeri, K. (1995). The Cuban health care system and factors currently undermining it. *Journal of Community Health, 20*(4), 321–334.

Naylor, C. D. (1999). Health care in Canada: Incrementalism under fiscal duress. *Health Affairs, 18*(3), 9–26.

NHS A to Z HelpDirect. (2000). Retrieved September, 2000 from http://www.nhsatoz.org.

Organization for Economic Cooperation and Development. (1994). *The reform of health care systems.* Paris, France: Organization for Economic Cooperation and Development.

Quick, R. (1997). A health care revolution. *Nursing Times, 93*(29), 17.

Rai, S. (2005, April 7). *Low costs lure foreigners to India for medical care.* Retrieved May 10, 2006 from http://www.nytimes.com/2005/04/07

Ramers, C. (2001). Medicina Cubana: A fresh perspective. *The Western Journal of Medicine,* 175(2), 129.

Reinhardt, U. (1999). Mangled competition and managed whatever. *Health Affairs,* 18(3), 92–94.

Rios, A. (2005). 40 years after the first graduation on Pico Turquino, Cuba now has 71,000 doctors. *Granma International Online Edition.* Retrieved May 18, 2006 from http://www.granma.cu/ingles/2005/noviembre/juev17/47turquino.html

Roemer, M. I. (1993). Primary health care and hospitalization: California and Cuba. *American Journal of Public Health, 83*(3), 317–318.

Rozek, R., & Mulhern, C. (1994). The health care system in Canada. In U. K. Hoffmeyer & T. R. McCarthy (Eds.), *Financing health care* (pp. 255–344). Dordrecht, Netherlands: Kluwer.

Saltman, R. B., & Dubois, H. F. W. (2005). Current reform proposals in social health insurance countries. *Eurohealth, 11*(1), 10–14.

Santana, S. M. (1987). The Cuban health care system: Responsiveness to changing population needs and demands. *World Development, 15*(1), 113–125.

Schieber, G., & Maeda, A. (1999). Health care financing and delivery in developing countries. *Health Affairs, 18,* 193–205.

Spivey, R. N., Wertheimer, A. I., & Rucker, T. D. (1992). *International pharmaceutical services: Drug industry and pharmacy practice in 23 major countries of the world.* New York: Haworth Press.

Susser, M. (1993). Health as a human right: An epidemiologist's perspective on the public health. *American Journal of Public Health, 83*(3), 418–426.

Ulrich, V. (1999). Health care in Germany: Structure, expenditure, and prospects. In W. McArthur, C. Ramsay, and M. Walker (Eds.), *Healthy incentives: Canadian health reform in an international context.* Vancouver, Canada: The Fraser Institute. Retrieved March 2, 2007 from http://www.fraserinstitute.ca/admin/books/files/Healthy%20Incentives%20(all).pdf

UNICEF. (1995). *The Bamako initiative: Rebuilding health systems.* New York: UNICEF.

Veeken, H. (1995). Cuba: Plenty of care, few condoms, no corruption. *British Medical Journal, 311*(7010), 935–937.

Williams, R. (1997). In the shadow of plenty: Cuba copes with a crippled health care system. *Canadian Medical Association, 157*(3), 291–293.

Woolhandler, S., Campbell, T., & Himmelstein, D. (2003). Costs of health care administration in the United States and Canada. *New England Journal of Medicine, 349,* 768–775.

World Health Organization. (2000a). *The world health report 2000, health systems: Improving performance.* Geneva, Switzerland: WHO.

World Health Organization. (2000b). France, Italy provide best healthcare. *Reuters,* 21 June 2000.

World Health Organization. (2006). *Countries page.* Retrieved May 5, 2006 from http://www.who.int/countries/en/

CHAPTER

20

Health Care Reform

Catherine N. Otto and Craig A. Pedersen

LEARNING OBJECTIVES _____

Upon completion of this chapter, the student shall be able to:

- Describe the effects of lack of access to health care in the United States
- Compare and contrast demand and need with respect to health care delivery
- Identify potential outcomes of proposals addressing the insolvency of the Medicare program
- Discuss the federal government's provisions to support health care as a right: Kerr-Mills Act, Medicare, and Medicaid
- Summarize the key components of federally proposed cost-containment methods for health care
- Explain the key concepts of uncompensated care pools, employer mandates, and Medicaid waivers
- Compare and contrast Hawaii's Prepaid Health Care Act, the Oregon Health Plan, and TennCare
- Define employer and employee mandates, sin taxes, health savings accounts, and portability of health insurance coverage
- Discuss methods to increase access to health insurance in Massachusetts and Vermont

INTRODUCTION

An in-depth discussion of the topics covered in this chapter could fill an entire book. In many ways, Chapter 20 integrates material from other chapters of this text as well as information on history, politics, financing, and the structure of the U.S. health care system. It discusses the problems of the U.S. health care system, the politics of health care reform, past landmark efforts to reform the U.S. health care system, current reform efforts, and pharmacy's role in reform efforts. This chapter can serve as an introductory guide to this textbook or as a capstone to the information provided elsewhere in this text.

This chapter does not endorse any particular side on any of the controversial issues. Nor does it hold the answers to the complex problems the United States faces today regarding health care for its citizens. Instead, this chapter seeks to outline the issues, suggest questions for debate, and stimulate readers to look deep within themselves and their core values to come to a reasonable and rational opinion on these issues. Finally, it suggests that pharmacists have the opportunity and responsibility to work proactively to ensure that the profession of pharmacy plays an integral part in the future of health care in the United States.

IDENTIFICATION OF THE PROBLEM

The people and the government of the United States are unique in their approach to health and health care. The United States is the only developed country that does not ensure access to health care through guaranteed coverage. This structural uniqueness of the U.S. health care system fragments the financing system and makes it difficult for the poor and the sick to seek preventive care. Thus expensive safety nets are required that drive up costs and aggravate the problem of cost shifting.

As discussed in Chapter 19, which covered international health care systems, the United States spends more of its gross domestic product

(GDP) on health care and has higher per capita expenditures on health care than any other industrialized nation (Anderson and Poullier, 1999; *OECD Health Data 2006,* 2006). The cost of health care in the United States has been increasing since the early 1960s. This rise can be attributed to multiple factors, including an aging population, patient demand for the "best" care available, technological advancements, increasing therapeutic options, and general and health care inflation.

Yet, although the U.S. levels of spending exceed those of other industrialized nations and cost increases outstrip the growth of other components of the U.S. economy, researchers report that Americans are generally dissatisfied with the health care system (Donelan, Blendon, Schoen, Davis, and Binns, 1999; Smith, Altman, Leitman, Moloney, and Taylor, 1992). This dissatisfaction is rooted in the high cost of health care, lack of universal access, and lack of any demonstrated gains in life expectancy. Life expectancy at birth for female Americans was 80.1 years in 2003. The United States ranked below the OECD median of 80.3 years for women, and behind Japan (85.3 years), France (82.9 years), Sweden (82.5 years), Germany (81.4 years), and Canada (82.4 years). Men have considerably shorter life expectancies at birth of 74.8 years in the United States, compared with the OECD median of 75.9 years (*OECD Health Data 2006*). Meanwhile, the United States has spent a considerably larger percentage of its GDP on health care than these other countries. Clearly, the United States has not gained in life expectancy from the additional money spent. Therefore, a crisis appears to exist in U.S. health care.

AN ISSUE OF ACCESS

In the United States, access to health care is determined by age, economic status, and race/ethnicity. The enactment of Medicare and Medicaid in 1965 addressed some of the access issues for the elderly and the indigent. Even so, the number of uninsured Americans has increased from 27 million in 1977 to 45.5 million in 2004. Eighteen states have uninsured rates exceeding 18% for their residents younger than age 65 (Kaiser Commission on Medicaid and the Uninsured, 2005).

Nine million of the 45.5 million uninsured people in the United States are children. Half of families with incomes less than 100% of the federal poverty level have access to health insurance through their employer, yet 81% of uninsured adults are employed (Kaiser Commission on Medicaid and the Uninsured, 2005). Non-white Americans are more likely to be uninsured—Latino (34.6%), African American (20.1%), American Indian/Alaska Native (26.8%), Asian/Pacific Islander (18.9%)—compared to white Americans (11.4%) (Lillie-Blanton, Rushing, and Ruiz, 2003.)

Lack of access to health care in the United States has become a high-profile issue for several reasons. First, health insurance coverage is an important determinant of access to care. Second, lack of adequate health coverage puts individuals at risk for high medical expenses. Third, everyone ends up paying for costs shifted because of uncompensated care (Brown and Wyn, 1996).

THE BEST HEALTH CARE?

Does the United States have the best health care system in the world? Many say yes—we are the leaders. We have the latest and best treatment available anywhere in the world. Fuchs (1992) agrees that the United States is the leader in technological advances related to medicine. Physicians come from around the world to receive the most advanced training. Very wealthy patients come from around the world to receive care in the United States. At the same time, Fuchs suggests other dimensions in which the United States may not be the best: public health, service, efficiency, and distribution equity.

The United States ranks below average among developed countries in most public health measures. Frequently, access to providers is limited, and many providers lack the caring nature that patients desire. If the U.S. health care system were efficient, it seems that we should be able to spend amounts comparable to those spent by other countries to achieve the same level of public health. Also, the distribution of health care in the United States is clearly not equal. The large number of uninsured and underinsured Americans is evidence of this fact. Thus, Fuchs suggests, for the United States to claim to have the best health care system, improvements in efficiency (controlling the high cost of care), distributional equity (providing universal coverage), service, and public health are necessary (Fuchs, 1992).

The United States clearly has made judgments about the nature of access to its health care system. Structurally, health care is a privilege in the United States and not a right. Nevertheless, many have begun to question the wisdom of not providing universal health coverage for all Americans.

DEMAND VERSUS NEED

In the late 1960s, economists began analyzing demand versus need—an important component to understanding access to medical care in the United States. Needs are normative judgments concerning the quantity of medical services that ought to be consumed (Jeffers, Bognanno, and Bartlett, 1971). Frequently, needs are fixed by policy makers. An example is the need for prenatal care. Society and policy makers believe that every pregnant woman needs prenatal care. It is difficult to object to this position because, without such care, the health of the unborn infant is at risk.

Need is often criticized by economists as being too mechanical, as denying the individuality and autonomy of the patient, and as characterizing the human body as a machine that needs fuel in the form of food and repairs in the form of medication or spare parts from the surgeon. Demand, by comparison, implies patient autonomy, choice, and tailoring inputs to individual preferences (Boulding, 1996). Demand, therefore, is the quantity of medical services that patients think they ought to consume based on their perceptions of their health care needs (Jeffers et al., 1971). Individual tastes and preferences determine utilization (see Chapter 12 for further discussion of demand).

GOVERNMENT TRUST FUNDS

Medicare and Social Security trust funds are frequently cited in discussions about health care reform. The concern over these trust funds stems from widespread confusion about their function and about the organization and purpose of the Medicare and Social Security programs.

Only recently has the disposition of trust fund moneys become a concern. When Social Security was created in 1935, the Roosevelt administration was aware that the amount of money collected would exceed expenditures for many years. The solution was to create a trust fund to account for the receipt and disposition of these funds.

The first source of confusion centers on the money in these trust funds. By law, the Social Security Administration is required to "invest" the surplus funds in special U.S. Treasury bonds (Peterson, 1996). Therefore, the taxes collected flow into the U.S. Treasury, just like all other tax collections. And like most taxes collected, these revenues become part of the general fund, available for any use (e.g., roads, infrastructure, defense). No special savings account exists that surplus funds are deposited into and thus saved for future obligations. In essence, the trust funds are a bookkeeping device.

Of recent concern is the question of what happens when the Social Security trust fund is exhausted—an event projected to occur in 2040. Tax revenues are predicted to fall below program costs beginning in 2017 (Medicare Trustees, 2006).

Perhaps the greatest source of confusion related to Social Security is the common belief that the Social Security Administration functions like a private pension fund, when, in fact, it does not. In a private pension fund, funds are collected and invested to provide retirement income to participants when the time comes for them to retire. Social Security does not work that way. Taxes collected from an individual for Social Security benefits are not designated for that individual upon retirement. Instead, these taxes are paid to current beneficiaries. Thus the Social Security system allows for an intergenerational transfer of funds between the working population and those eligible for Social Security benefits.

The Medicare trust fund operates in a similar manner. Congress has frequently appropriated unspent funds collected under the Medicare tax for other purposes. Total expenditures from Medicare's two trust funds—Hospital Insurance and Supplementary Medical Insurance—are projected to amount to 3.2% of GDP in 2006 and to 7.3% of GDP in 2035 due to the increases in medical costs, utilization, the addition of Medicare Part D, and the aging of the baby-boom generation (Medicare Trustees, 2006).

Maintaining these trust funds will be a major challenge when the baby-boom generation reaches retirement age beginning in 2011. Currently, four workers contribute to the program per beneficiary; by the middle of the 21st century, only two workers will contribute to the program per beneficiary (O'Sullivan, 1996). Although U.S. citizens expect to use Medicare and Social Security when they retire, they are concerned that these programs will be difficult to maintain because of underfinancing and changing demographics. Substantial reforms will be required to ensure long-term solvency of the programs.

The year that the Hospital Insurance trust fund (Medicare Part A) has been projected to become insolvent has fluctuated over the past 25 years. For example, in 1982 the trust fund was forecast to become insolvent in 1987—only 5 years later. From 1987 to 1995, the projected year of insolvency ranged from 1999 to 2005 (O'Sullivan, 1996). Thus the potential insolvency of this trust fund is not a new issue. Nevertheless, Congress and the President must address the long-term financial solvency of Medicare.

A number of approaches have been suggested to reform the Medicare program, such as lower provider fee schedules, use of co-payments and increasing beneficiary premiums, eligibility changes, and health savings accounts.

HEALTH CARE REFORM EFFORTS BY THE FEDERAL GOVERNMENT

In an effort to eliminate some of the economic barriers to medical care for the elderly and medically indigent, the federal government has addressed the notion of health care as a right and not a privilege, at least for some people in the United States. Enactment of the Kerr-Mills Act and establishment of the Medicare and Medicaid programs in the 1960s paved the way for health care to be perceived as a basic human right.

Kerr-Mills Act

Amendments to the Social Security Act in 1960 provided health care coverage to elderly indigent individuals. This landmark legislation, known as the Kerr-Mills Act, was the first to provide health care to elderly or indigent persons on a broad scale. Many critics were concerned that the states would not implement this legislation in a timely manner. These predictions were confirmed. Many states had failed to adopt Kerr-Mills by 1963, when 90% of the funds were received by the five largest industrialized states (Starr, 1982).

Kerr-Mills did not provide health care coverage to the nonindigent elderly or the indigent nonelderly. These groups were not covered until amendments to the Social Security Act in 1965 established Medicare coverage for elderly persons (regardless of income) and Medicaid coverage for the poor.

Medicare and Medicaid

Medicare and Medicaid were significant health care reform programs (see Chapter 17). Before 1960, many elderly people in the United States lacked any kind of health insurance coverage. The Kerr-Mills Act and its successor, Medicare, addressed this need. Medicare Part A covers hospitalization, and Medicare Part B covers outpatient and physician bills. The third layer of reform was Medicaid, which covers indigent persons.

These programs reflected contrasting traditions. Medicare had popular support, and Social Security had made it acceptable for the elderly to receive government retirement benefits. Medicaid, however, was burdened by the stigma of public assistance (Starr, 1982). Medicare had uniform national criteria for eligibility, whereas Medicaid allowed states to determine the breadth of their programs. These differences persist today.

The Cost-Containment Era

By the early 1970s, Americans understood that their health care system was in a financial crisis. One survey in 1970 found that approximately three fourths of heads of households agreed with the statement, "There is a crisis in health care in the United States" (Starr, 1982). Terms used to describe costs included "skyrocketing" and "runaway inflation." Medical care had become very expensive, and costs were exceeding inflation at an alarming rate. Coupled with worries about high prices for medical care were concerns about access, such as the diminishing number of primary-care practitioners and patients' inability to obtain care from a physician on the weekends or in the evenings (Starr, 1982).

During this era, cost containment became a primary concern. Several strategies were implemented to control rising costs: voluntary hospital planning, wage and price freezes, changes in the amounts and methods of reimbursement for services, development of more cost-effective health care delivery systems, and regulatory programs such as utilization review and controls on hospital capital expenditures. Ultimately, most of those strategies proved unsuccessful in controlling costs.

Another significant health care reform effort was the 1972 amendments to the Social Security Act, which established professional standards review organizations (PSROs). PSROs were a national network of utilization review programs that had dual responsibility for medical cost containment and quality assurance. This program did not work, however, and it was replaced in 1983 by peer review organizations with a local focus.

Yet another cost-containment program was Section 1122 of the 1972 amendments to the Social Security Act, which required states to review proposed capital improvement expenditures of health care organizations and to provide authorization through a "certificate of need" at the state level. The certificate-of-need program was intended to reduce unnecessary duplication of services but was unsuccessful in meeting this goal. Some states have since eliminated the certificate-of-need requirements for capital improvements.

In 1973, President Richard Nixon signed the Health Maintenance Organization (HMO) Act. The HMO Act encouraged the use of these lower-cost health care delivery systems and provided financial assistance for development of nonprofit HMOs. This act constituted the federal government's first effort to develop an alternative to fee-for-service medicine (Iglehart, 1982). Health care reimbursement would be forever changed by this act.

Diagnosis-Related Groups

These cost-containment efforts did not appreciably restrain the growth of health care costs in the United States. By contrast, the 1983 implementation of diagnosis-related groups (DRGs), also referred to as the prospective payment system (PPS), was a landmark effort to control hospital reimbursement under Medicare. Medicare established a fixed schedule of fees to be paid to hospitals, where the fee varied for each diagnosis. If the actual cost to the hospital is less than the set fee, the hospital keeps the difference; if the service costs more than the set fee, the hospital absorbs the loss.

The objective of DRGs is to promote rational use of health care dollars and to stimulate competition among hospitals. Under this system, hospitals are reimbursed on an episode-of-care rather than a fee-for service basis, placing the hospital at risk for inpatient health care costs.

DRGs have substantially slowed the growth of hospital expenditures, but physician expenditures, which are not subject to the PPS, continue to grow. Concern also exists about hospitals "dumping" patients and discharging patients early (Epstein, Bogen, Dreyer, and Thorpe, 1991). Use of these mechanisms has the potential to hurt quality of care. (For further reading, see Chapter 6.)

Medicare Catastrophic Coverage Act of 1988

The Medicare Catastrophic Coverage Act (MCCA) was enacted in 1988 in response to rising Medicare costs. MCCA was one of the most controversial attempts to change Medicare (Greenberg, 1988). It extended days of hospital coverage by eliminating the annual 90-day allowance and the lifetime 60-day reserve. In addition, the act expanded Medicare Part B to increase home care benefits and provide outpatient prescription drug coverage. Preventive care was also included in the package. The prescription drug benefit was of particular interest because, for the first time, older persons were offered the opportunity to receive outpatient prescription drugs at a nominal cost.

So why was MCCA repealed? Congress selected the concept of self-funding to provide for the increased cost of the program. This new sensitivity about not passing costs along to the next generation or tapping general revenues was unique—and it eventually killed the program. The elderly—especially the wealthy elderly, who would have paid for a larger portion of the cuts—objected to paying for the increased benefits.

MCCA included components that were eventually incorporated into the Omnibus Budget Reconciliation Act of 1990. This act required pharmacists to keep patient profiles, conduct prospective drug utilization review, and provide counseling on prescriptions dispensed to Medicaid patients. For the first time, federal legislation mandated that pharmacists offer to counsel Medicaid patients.

Health Security Act

The Health Security Act was proposed by President Bill Clinton in 1993 during his first year in office. This legislation sought to create an employer mandate and provide universal health care coverage for Americans (Angell, 1993; Brock and Daniels, 1994). The primary innovation of this act was a concept known as "managed competition," which created networks of providers operating under competing managed care organizations (MCOs). The Health Security Act would have set limits for yearly expansion in health care premiums and established out-of-pocket caps, thereby limiting a family's financial exposure. Total spending was capped in the plan. The plan created a uniform package that included a standardized claim form, as well as standard billing and coding procedures. The proposal died before it reached Congress, however, with its failure being attributable to a lack of public understanding and support and strong opposition from the health insurance industry (Yankelovich, 1995).

Portability of Coverage

The Health Insurance Portability and Accountability Act of 1996 (HIPAA) addressed three issues in the health care reform debate: (1) preexisting condition exclusions, (2) elimination of health discrimination applications to eligibility rules, and (3) guaranteed renewability for plans that cover more than one employee. Later, HIPAA was expanded to address patient confidentiality issues.

Under HIPAA, individuals cannot be denied coverage because they have a preexisting medical condition if they agree to an exclusionary period for that condition, which cannot exceed more than one year. After one year, the policyholder can no longer be denied coverage for the preexisting condition. As long as the policyholder remains continuously enrolled in a plan, with breaks no longer than 63 days, the exclusion period cannot be re-imposed. In short, HIPAA guarantees that policies and benefits available to a specific group cannot be withheld if an exclusionary period has already been met.

The second part of the act addresses the discriminatory practice of eliminating individuals and groups from the insurance market based on risk, preexisting conditions, or utilization history. In the past, the practice of "cherry-picking," or selecting the healthiest groups, was commonplace in the insurance industry. Now, however, insurance companies are required to sell coverage to small employer groups and individuals who lose coverage without regard to their health history. This issue is especially important to employers with fewer than 50 employees. Previously, one employee with a high risk factor could jeopardize the coverage of all members of the small group (Cantor, Long, and Marquis, 1995). A significant component missing here is controls on insurance prices for these small groups and individuals.

The third component of HIPAA is that insurers must renew policies they sell to groups and individuals. Previously, insurance companies were allowed to eliminate costly individuals or groups from their policies by denying renewal of coverage.

Health Savings Accounts

The Medicare Prescription Drug, Improvement, and Modernization Act (MMA) of 2003 included a provision creating health savings accounts (HSA) (Remler and Giled, 2006). HSAs are a type of medical savings account (MSA)—a pilot project Congress created in 1996 for self-employed and employers with fewer than 50 employees as a method of paying for medical care expenses. Under MMA, an employer of any size may offer an HSA as a health insurance option to its employees (Minicozzi, 2006). Like MSAs, HSAs are tax-free savings accounts that are used for the out-of-pocket medical expenses for those individuals who select a high-deductible health insurance plan (e.g., $1,000 to $5,000 per individual or $2,000 to $10,000 per family). Contributions from pretax income are limited to the amount of the deductible ($2,600 for an individual or $5,100 for a family) and may be made by either the employer or the employee. Total out-of-pocket spending is capped at $5,000 for an individual and $10,000 for a family; after this point, the health insurance will cover all health care expenses. Balances in HSAs do not expire, but rather accumulate over time, even if the employee is no longer covered by a high-deductible health insurance plan (Remler and Giled, 2006).

MSAs and HSAs are designed to create price sensitivity among health care consumers. Patients with traditional health insurance coverage are largely unaware of the cost of medical care services. Economists suggest that this lack of knowledge is one of the reasons why health care costs have risen so dramatically over the years (American College of Physicians, 1996). Unlike most health insurance plans, MSAs and HSAs do not shield the consumer from the cost of medical care. The consumer becomes directly responsible for dollars spent on health care and thus becomes more price sensitive. Consumers are at partial risk for expenditures, because money comes from their MSAs or HSAs to pay for care. As a consequence, they have an incentive to avoid medical care that is not worth the cost (Goodman and Pauly, 1995). Proponents of MSAs and HSAs have suggested that these accounts will reduce wasteful utilization of resources and hold down health care cost inflation rates (Hsiao, 1995).

Critics of MSAs and HSAs remain concerned about the prospect of adverse selection with these accounts. As discussed in Chapter 14, adverse selection occurs when insured individuals can accurately predict their future need for health insurance coverage (Folland, Goodman, and Stano, 1997). Consumers know more about their health than the insurance company, so sick people might enroll in a health plan in higher proportions than other plans. With these types of plans, the fear is that healthy individuals would drop their low-deductible health insurance in favor of MSAs combined with high-deductible plans. Premiums in the low-deductible plan would then skyrocket because only the sick would participate in the plan (Gardner, 1995).

Although access to health care in the United States may not be significantly altered by either MSAs or HSAs, the growth of health care spending may be slowed by their adoption. However, consumers may be unwilling or unable to determine the appropriateness, quality, and cost of health care services given the specialized nature of health care delivery, and thus do little to decrease spending. Also, consumers who have limited resources may forego necessary care, potentially resulting in increased spending to compensate for their delays in seeking treatment.

HSAs represent a radical change in health care reform—moving away from the concept of collective responsibility and toward the notion of individual accountability (Robinson, 2005). Their consequences—intended and unintended—to health care delivery systems, employer health insurance costs, and individual health outcomes are unknown.

HEALTH CARE REFORM EFFORTS BY THE STATES

Reforms at the state level have primarily consisted of adjustments to the financing of health care delivery. A number of states, however, have developed unique approaches intend to expand access to health care for their citizens. These approaches include uncompensated care pools subsidized by taxes on acute care services, employer mandates to provide health insurance for employees, and a federal waiver allowing states to expand access to the Medicaid program.

Uncompensated Care Pools

The American Hospital Association estimates that U.S. hospitals provide more than $16 billion of uncompensated care each year (Weissman, 1996). States have set up uncompensated care pools, also referred to as "free care pools," to reimburse hospitals for a portion of these uncompensated services delivered to uninsured and underinsured individuals who meet some means test, usually based on level of income. Uncompensated care pools are primarily financed by placing a tax on the hospital bills of individuals who have health insurance, but they may also be supported by funds from general tax revenues. Hospitals apply to the pool for reimbursement for those patients who are unable to pay for their hospital care.

Uncompensated care pools do not increase access to health care services, unlike the expansion of Medicaid programs. These programs simply finance acute care received in a hospital setting. However, the existence of an uncompensated care pool creates an incentive for hospitals to offer charitable care. In the current competitive market, without the availability of an uncompensated care pool, many public hospitals would close or reduce the care offered to indigent individuals (Weissman, 1996). An uncompensated care pool is only one aspect of financing health care for a state's citizens. It is most effective when used in conjunction with other state programs that increase access to primary care services.

Employer Mandates

In 1974, long before there was a national debate about universal access to health care, Hawaii passed the Prepaid Health Care Act, a type of legislation referred to as an employer mandate (Budde, Patrick, and Budde, 1995; Lewin and Sybinsky, 1993). The Prepaid Health Care Act requires all employers to provide a standard, state-established health insurance package for their employees who work 20 or more hours per week. The program requires both employer and employee to share in the cost of the health insurance package. The employer pays at least 50% of the cost of the insurance. Employees pay up to 1.5% of their monthly salaries toward the monthly health insurance premium (Lewin and Sybinsky, 1993). The act does not require employers to provide health insurance coverage for their employees' dependents; however, given the competition for employees, most employers offer this benefit.

The Prepaid Health Care Act does not mandate a specific type of health insurance—just a minimum set of basic services. These minimum services include hospitalization, emergency treatment, surgical services, physician office visits, laboratory tests, radiology services, and maternity services (Lewin and Sybinsky, 1993). Within the state, the options for health insurance include fee-for-service and managed care plans.

Health insurance in Hawaii is less expensive than it is in the states on the mainland. Considering that the cost of living in Hawaii is significantly higher than in most of the United States, one might expect that the cost of health insurance would also be higher. There are two explanations for this phenomenon (Lewin and Sybinsky, 1993). First, because the employer mandate requires all employers to provide health insurance, there is less need to subsidize health care for uninsured individuals; this allows health insurance companies to use community rating rather than experience rating, which is frequently used when insuring small businesses. Thus small businesses and large employers are offered similar rates. Second, because Hawaii has experienced a lower rate of hospitalization and a subsequent higher rate of outpatient physician visits than the rest of the country, health insurance premiums can be reduced.

Health outcomes for Hawaiian citizens have been better than those for the rest of the U.S. population with respect to extended longevity, low infant mortality, and low premature morbidity and mortality for cancer, cardiovascular disease, and pulmonary disease (Lewin and Sybinsky, 1993). One might think that the environment—the sunshine—and perhaps a healthy lifestyle cause these outcomes. In reality, these factors do not appear to affect health outcomes in Hawaii significantly. Although Hawaiians exhibit health risk behaviors common to all Americans, their commitment to outpatient care and prevention—instead of hospitalization—has improved health outcomes and decreased costs. Hawaiians visit their physicians twice as often and are hospitalized half as often as the national average (Lewin and Sybinsky, 1993). With less costly outpatient care and the use of preventive measures, expensive hospitalizations are used less frequently; this allows health insurance to remain at a lower rate than in other states.

From Hawaii's experience, it appears that an employer mandate could eliminate the largest percentage of uninsured individuals in the United States. However, since Hawaii's Prepaid Health Care Act was passed in 1974, several other states have passed employer mandate ("play-or-pay") legislation. These states have been unable to implement their laws because of the Employee Retirement Income Security Act (ERISA), which restricts the types of mandates that states can impose on the benefits that employers offer their employees. Because Hawaii's Prepaid Health Care

Act was enacted before ERISA was passed in 1974, it was not initially affected by ERISA. Yet, since ERISA has been enacted, no amendments have been made to Hawaii's Prepaid Health Care Act. Changes that might improve Hawaii's program, such as requiring coverage of dependents or adjusting the employer and employee contributions to the health insurance premiums, cannot be implemented because they would violate ERISA.

The intent of ERISA is to protect employees' retirement plans. Under ERISA, the federal government is solely responsible for regulating employee benefit plans, with its authority superseding any state laws (Gostin and Widiss, 1993). ERISA does not apply to the regulation of insurance. However, one half to two thirds of employers provide health care benefits for their employees with self-insurance. Self-insurance, also referred to as self-funded arrangements, involves setting aside money specifically to pay for employees' medical expenses rather than purchasing an insurance policy to protect them against financial loss. Employers that use self-insurance for their employees' health benefits are exempt from state employer mandates under ERISA.

Although ERISA has provided protection for employees in terms of retirement benefit programs, its enactment has halted state employer mandates, such as Hawaii's, that would have improved individuals' access to health care. ERISA is the roadblock to the full implementation of the employer mandate legislation passed by a number of states in the late 1980s, such as that included in the Oregon Basic Health Services Act of 1989.

Employer Versus Employee Mandates

Frequently, discussion about federal health care reform turns into a debate over employer versus employee mandates. Employer mandates place the burden for financing on the employer. Employee mandates place the burden on the employee.

Economists argue that benefits are a component of reimbursement. Direct payments and benefits are both considered employee compensation. For example, the Medicare contribution for employees and employers is set at 1.45% each. If the employer did not have to pay this Medicare tax, he or she could afford to provide a higher wage to the employee. Either way, the employee "pays" the tax—whether directly through taxes or indirectly through lower compensation.

Thus the distinction between employer and employee mandates matters in the sense of the wage a worker receives, although total compensation remains constant. When the employee is forced to participate through payroll deduction, he or she is more likely to realize the true cost of the mandate. However, employer mandates shield the employee from the true cost. This price sensitivity is at the core of theory behind cost sharing. For this reason, increasing patient cost sharing is always a component of health care reform.

Medicaid and State Requests for Waiver

Medicaid program costs have increased annually since the program went into effect in 1966. They are now the fastest-growing state expenditures, often limiting the ability of states to support higher education and other social programs. The increasing proportion of state budgets—as much as 20%—devoted to Medicaid has prompted states to look at methods to limit the growth of this spending (Holahan, Coughlin, Ku, Lipson, and Rajan, 1995). The federal government allows states to enroll Medicaid patients into managed care plans and to experiment with other cost-containment programs through a Medicaid waiver procedure. (See Chapter 17 for a full discussion of the Medicaid waiver procedure.) Examples from two states, Oregon and Tennessee, that received Medicaid waivers and used managed care to expand access to Medicaid are presented next.

Oregon Health Plan

Oregon's Basic Health Services Act of 1989 consisted of three bills to provide health insurance to the then 450,000 uninsured Oregonians. Senate Bill 27 expanded Medicaid to 120,000 uninsured low-income persons. Instead of determining who will be covered, the Oregon Health Plan (OHP) assumed that everyone will receive coverage and addressed what will be covered based on values assessed in town meetings, ratings for health states, subjective judgments about treatment effectiveness, and reprioritization based on commissioner judgment (Kaplan, 1994). Using this information, a prioritized list of diagnoses and treatments was created. Once the budget was determined, a line was drawn on that list of diagnoses; the diagnoses above the line were funded, and those below the line were not covered. The other two bills include Senate Bill 534, which established a high-risk pool for health insurance coverage for individuals previously uninsurable because of preexisting conditions, and Senate Bill 1076, a play-or-pay approach for small businesses to provide health insurance for their employees (Bussman, 1993).

To obtain its Medicaid waiver from the Centers for Medicare and Medicaid Services (CMS) the Oregon Health Services Commission had to revise this plan by eliminating the quality-of-life component and resubmitting its waiver application to CMS. The revised proposal is considered to be more subjective than the original proposal and to lack its most scientifically justifiable and reproducible portion (Kaplan, 1994). The loss of the scientific basis of the OHP experiment means that analysts will have difficulty assessing the outcomes and subsequently making recommendations for future programs that allocate health care dollars in this manner.

A key component of the OHP, in addition to its ranking protocol for funding care for only a specific number of conditions from the prioritized list of disease processes, is its use of managed care as a delivery and financing system to control costs. The success of the OHP, in terms of its ability to enroll more individuals, was linked to the availability of numerous MCOs throughout Oregon. At the time of the plan's implementation, one third of the Oregon population was already in HMOs, and 31% of Medicaid recipients were already in capitated health plans (Gold, Chu, and Lyons, 1995).

Although two of the three bills from the Oregon Basic Health Services Act of 1989 are in effect, the play-or-pay mandate for all employers was not implemented because Oregon was unable to obtain a congressional waiver from ERISA (Leichter, 1999).

Although there was considerable debate about the explicit rationing program proposed in the OHP, the plan has functioned more as a mechanism for defining the benefits package rather than as a rationing instrument. The OHP has been funded through an increase in state funding and a cigarette tax—frequently referred to as a "sin tax"—and by moving recipients into managed care plans rather than by rationing care from the list of approved services. These changes in funding were manageable because of Oregon's growing economy and because Medicaid expenditures were already low before the program started. When the OHP began, Oregon ranked 46th in Medicaid spending as a proportion of the state budget (Jacobs, Marmor, and Oberlander, 1999).

The list of OHP noncovered services has not been strictly enforced by providers. For example, procedures to diagnose the noncovered conditions are allowed, and individuals with noncovered conditions often have comorbidities that allow for treatment (Jacobs et al., 1999). Because managed care companies receive capitated payments for a specified number of enrollees, noncovered services are often delivered. In addition, OHP recipients may appeal decisions for denial of those services that are listed below the funding line. To date, there have been 40 to 80 appeals per year, out of 362,000 patient encounters (Leichter, 1999). Although the Oregon state legislature has the authority to identify the number of services provided from the list each biennium, CMS must approve any changes to the list of funded services. CMS appears to be reluctant to make further reductions in the number of procedures covered by the OHP (Leichter, 1999).

The OHP was successful in extending health care to an additional 130,000 low-income individuals. An estimated 4,000 individuals were assisted under the high-risk pool that provides health insurance for individuals with preexisting conditions. The percentage of uninsured Oregonians fell from 17% to 11% in 1996, and the percentage of children without health insurance fell from 21% to 8%, each less than the national averages of 15% (Jacobs et al., 1999).

Although the OHP is considered a success at improving access to health care, its record has been marred by a recession and Oregon's high unemployment rate, which combined to produce the state's budget deficit in 2003. Increases to premiums and co-payments, reductions to provider reimbursements, and limits on provided services were instituted midyear to the approximately 100,000 people who qualify for the expansion portion of the OHP (Colburn, 2003c). Given continued reductions in state income tax receipts, the Oregon legislature was faced with the prospect of instituting cuts to enrollment (Steves, 2003). Changes to the OHP resulted in hospitals incurring large budget deficits due to reductions in reimbursements (Rojas-Burke, 2003), hospitals filing a lawsuit to block payment reductions (Colburn, 2003b), and pharmacies losing revenue because they could not require co-payments before filling prescriptions (Colburn, 2003a).

TennCare

In 1993, Tennessee, motivated by problems similar to those in Oregon (an increasing portion of the state budget allocated to Medicaid and an increasing proportion of the population being uninsured), expanded its Medicaid program to include previously uninsurable and uninsured individuals through a program called TennCare. The foundation of the TennCare program was the enrollment of recipients in managed care plans.

Like other states that were expanding access to their Medicaid programs, Tennessee based its program on using managed care as the key component to improve access and contain costs. However, only two of the state's nine established HMOs and 20 preferred provider organizations (PPOs) chose to participate in the TennCare program. Ten new MCOs were then created specifically for TennCare participants (Mirvis, Chang, Hall, Zaar, and Applegate, 1995).

Cost sharing was a key element of the TennCare program. It required premiums, co-payments, and deductibles using a sliding scale based on income (Mirvis et al., 1995). Cost sharing was not required for individuals who qualified for Medicaid; it was required only for individuals who were enrolled in the expanded portion of the Medicaid program. Initially, TennCare expanded both the number of recipients eligible for health care services and the quantity of services recipients could obtain (Mirvis et al., 1995).

In May 2000, TennCare had an enrollment of 1.3 million, of which 800,000 persons were Medicaid eligible and 500,000 persons were from the uninsured and uninsurable categories (Bureau of TennCare, 2000). Although TennCare appeared successful—it resulted in a decrease in the uninsured population and a reduction in costs for treatment of diabetes and pediatric asthma (Fox and Lyons, 1998; External Quality Review

Organization, 1997)—there have been severe reductions to the program since its introduction (Hurley, 2006).

Throughout its history, TennCare has experienced numerous problems. The inception, development, and implementation of the TennCare plan were extraordinarily fast paced. The new MCOs created specifically to serve the program recipients had little time to organize their delivery systems. Potential TennCare participants did not know which providers were associated with which MCO or even which MCOs were participants in TennCare (Mirvis et al., 1995).

The program has also periodically closed enrollment to new enrollees in the uninsured and uninsurable categories. In November 1999, facing a state budget deficit and rising costs, TennCare was closed to any new uninsurables and uninsured until a future date. Benefits were altered to match those offered by private health insurance, and the program imposed a limit of seven prescriptions or refills per month for adults. Cost sharing was changed by eliminating deductibles and using co-payments instead (Fortune, 1999). The pharmacy component of the services was carved out of the MCO program to reduce risk to the MCOs and to take advantage of the federal drug rebate program. A single statewide preferred drug formulary was later implemented in July 2003; only those drugs listed were covered for TennCare recipients (Bureau of TennCare, 2003).

Since the program's implementation, more than 200,000 people have lost their health care coverage through TennCare—the largest reduction in U.S. history (Hurley, 2006). TennCare's lack of long-term success can be attributed to both the imposition of a managed care model in a state with limited experience in this delivery system and state budget deficits.

Other State Initiatives to Increase Access to Health Insurance

Legislation to provide universal access had not been attempted since the late 1980s, but two states—Massachusetts and Vermont—passed sweeping legislation intended to increase access to health insurance in 2006. Both accomplished this feat with bipartisan support from Republican governors and Democrat-controlled legislatures. The primary focus of these reforms is a requirement that individuals purchase health insurance policies. Both states also require employers to pay an assessment to help finance the programs.

Massachusetts passed an individual health insurance mandate in April 2006, requiring all residents 18 years and older to purchase a minimum level of health insurance by July 1, 2007 (Steinbrook, 2006). Failure to comply with the law will result in a fine of 50% of the cost of an affordable insurance premium. Although this program is not an employer mandate, it does have an employer financing component, requiring businesses with 11 or more full-time employees that do not provide or contribute to health insurance to pay a fee of $295 per employee per year. The state will subsidize the premium payments for families who earn less than 300% of the federal poverty level. The law also expands Medicaid to include the children of families who earn up to 300% of the federal poverty level (Steinbrook, 2006).

Other key features of the Massachusetts program include the creation of the Commonwealth Health Insurance Connector to administer the insurance components of the laws. This organization will also serve as a clearinghouse to link individuals and businesses with fewer than 50 employees with insurance products. Health insurance will be portable for individuals who purchase health insurance through the Connector (Steinbrook, 2006).

In May 2006, Vermont passed the 2006 Health Care Affordability Act, which created Catamount Health. This health insurance program is offered by Blue Cross/Blue Shield of Vermont and is available to anyone who has been uninsured for previous 12 months effective October 1, 2007 (Blue Cross/Blue Shield of Vermont, 2006). Premiums will be subsidized based on income for persons with incomes at or below 300% of the federal poverty level, both for those who enroll in Catamount Health and for those who are employed with comparable employer-sponsored health insurance (VPIRG, 2006). Employers will be assessed a fee—$365 per year per full-time equivalent—for each uninsured employee. Exemptions for 8 employees will be allowed in 2007 and 2008, for 6 employees for 2009, and for 4 employees in 2010 and thereafter (Vermont State Legislature, 2006).

Vermont's Health Care Affordability Act also creates a chronic disease management plan called Blueprint for Health, which will incorporate early disease screening, promote patient self-management tools, and financially reward health care providers for using proactive chronic care management tools (VPIRG, 2006).

OTHER HEALTH CARE REFORM INITIATIVES

Although it was not created with state or federal legislation, the Drug Effectiveness Review Project (DERP), designed by researchers at Oregon Health and Science University to evaluate drugs for the Oregon Medicaid program in 2003, has created an information clearing house for clinical effectiveness for drugs for public policy (Drug Effectiveness Review Project, 2006a). As of 2006, 15 states and 2 nonprofit organizations participated in DERP (Drug Effectiveness Review Project, 2006b). Three Agency for Healthcare Research and Quality-Designated Evidence-Based Practice Centers are responsible for conducting the analyses—at Oregon Health and Science University, RAND, and University of North Carolina at Chapel Hill. Participating organizations provide input regarding the questions to study, maintain the freedom to interpret the final reports, develop their own preferred drug lists for their Medicaid programs, and negotiate their own prices with pharmaceutical companies (Neumann, 2006). Recently, the Consumer Union and *Consumer Reports* have begun using information from DERP reports to create a consumer drug report (Findlay, 2006).

Criticisms of the DERP include a need for more openness in the process—a request to include other stakeholders in the process, such as consumer advocates and pharmaceutical company representatives; too much reliance on published randomized control trials rather than on observational studies; and the lack of cost-effectiveness analyses performed simultaneously with analyses of the clinical value of therapeutic drug classes (Neumann, 2006). Recommendations for peer reviewers are requested from advocacy organizations to critique DERP reports. Results of randomized control trials are given priority—as the gold standard for clinical research studies, when they are available. DERP has chosen to leave the cost component of cost-effectiveness analysis to the user; however, the reports provide a baseline to perform a cost-effectiveness analysis (Gibson and Santa, 2006).

DERP is a unique collaboration of states and organizations using scientific methodologies to evaluate the effectiveness and safety of drugs. Its effect on public policy and health outcomes has yet to be determined.

THE PHARMACY PROFESSION AND HEALTH CARE REFORM: A CALL FOR ACTION

The pharmacy profession is in a unique position to influence health care reform efforts. Pharmacists have more contact with the general public than do other health care professionals. Community pharmacists have ample opportunities to interact with patients who receive a prescription or who are visiting the pharmacy to pick up an over-the-counter drug product or other products stocked on pharmacy shelves. Whether dispensing a prescription to a patient or helping a customer in the store, pharmacists have direct and frequent contact with the public.

Private insurance plans implement cost-sharing mechanisms including co-payments, co-insurance, deductibles, and maximum limit caps. Most plans use electronic claims submission from the pharmacy; a few require patients to file their own claims and be reimbursed. Pharmacists who deal with these issues on a daily basis are familiar with the major issues of debate and the sources of frustration.

Drug expenditures are frequently perceived to be a problem that drives much of the debate over prescription drug coverage. Much of this focus stems from the public's concern with insurance plans that cover less than 100% of prescription costs. Coverage for prescriptions has historically been lower than physician or hospital coverage. As recently as the Kefauver hearings (in 1959), little or no drug coverage existed, and in 1986, patients paid for more than 75% of their prescription medications (Health Insurance Institute of America, 1989).

Although insurance coverage for prescription drugs has broadened in recent years, it still lags behind coverage for other components of medical care. Consumers are less sheltered from the burden of paying for prescription medications than from the burden of paying for other medical care services because of the higher utilization of prescription services coupled with the higher percentages of cost sharing they are forced to bear. Pharmacists are in the position to understand the patient's perspective, and they also have the opportunity to manage reimbursement from the third-party payer's perspective.

Pharmaceutical care offers members of the pharmacy profession an opportunity to move from providing a product to providing true service. It gives pharmacists the chance to secure a place we define in the future of the changing health care marketplace. A pharmacist who becomes a disease state manager will be better able to influence public policy and health care system change. Pharmacists should get involved in their professional associations, in community groups, and in insurance plans. They should understand the perspectives of different players so that they can address the concerns of others as well as promote the pharmacist's perspective.

Health care system reform should not frighten pharmacists. It should provide a challenge and an opportunity to carve out a niche in tomorrow's health care system.

CONCLUSIONS

At the core of health care reform is people's willingness to pay for changes to the health care system. Financing is the key to reform, but the current political climate remains difficult to read. Some suggest that politicians are unwilling to risk reelection to make bold, sweeping changes to the system. Others see health care reform as inevitable. Both groups may be partially correct.

As health care costs grow and the proportion of uninsured individuals rises, state and federal governments will continue to develop programs to address these issues. At the state level, other states may model their programs after the Massachusetts plan. As the use of managed care increases and providers fear exclusion from access to patient populations, more legislation (such as any-willing-provider laws) is likely to be introduced. States will continue to play a significant role in addressing the escalation of health care costs and the increase of uninsured individuals unless major reform occurs at the federal level.

This chapter has highlighted the rapid changes occurring in the health care system. Of course, the issues discussed here are merely the tip of the iceberg. The challenge is to follow the evolution of and items of discussion concerning health care reform. Successful pharmacists will diligently meet this challenge.

QUESTIONS FOR FURTHER DISCUSSION

1. Which health care reform solutions are most viable?
2. What should be done to save Medicare?
3. Should the United States move toward a basic health benefit for all?
4. Should the Oregon Health Plan pay for treatment of diseases that consistently get better with self-treatment (such as colds)?
5. Should states impose a fee on employers that do not offer their employees health insurance? Why? Why not? What are the intended and unintended consequences of this type of financing mechanism?

KEY TOPICS AND TERMS

Cost containment
Diagnosis-related groups
Employee mandate
Employee Retirement Income Security Act
Employer mandate
Health savings account
Health Insurance Portability and Accountability Act
Health Security Act
Kerr-Mills Act
Managed care
Managed competition
Medicaid
Medicaid waiver
Medicare
Medicare Catastrophic Coverage Act
Oregon Health Plan
Sin tax
Social Security
TennCare
Trust fund
Uncompensated care pool

REFERENCES

American College of Physicians. (1996). Position paper: Medical savings accounts. *Annals of Internal Medicine, 125,* 333–340.

Angell, M. (1993). The beginning of health care reform: The Clinton plan. *New England Journal of Medicine, 329,* 1569–1570.

Anderson, G. F., & Poullier, J. P. (1999). Health spending, access, and outcomes: Trends in industrialized countries. *Health Affairs, 18,* 178-192.

Blue Cross/Blue Shield of Vermont. (2006). *The Health Care Affordability for Vermonters Act.* Retrieved from http://www.bcbsvt.com/pages/PDFs/Catamount-brochure.pdf

Boulding, K. E. (1996, October). The concept of need for health services. *Milbank Memorial Fund Quarterly, 44,* 202–223.

Brock, D. W., & Daniels, N. (1994). Ethical foundations of the Clinton administration's proposed health care system. *Journal of the American Medical Association, 271,* 1189–1196.

Brown, E. R., & Wyn, R. (1996). Public policies to extend health care coverage. In R. J. Anderson, T. H. Rice, & G. F. Kominski (Eds.), *Changing the U.S. health care system: Key issues in health services, policy, and management* (pp. 41–61). San Francisco, CA: Jossey-Bass.

Budde, J. C., Patrick, W. K., & Budde, M. T. (1995). Hawaii HealthQUEST: A managed care demonstration project. *Hawaii Medical Journal, 54,* 720–722.

Bureau of TennCare. (2000). *About TennCare.* Retrieved from http://www.state.tn.us/tenncare/about/htm

Bureau of TennCare. (2003). *Important TennCare pharmacy changes.* Retrieved from http://www.state.tn.us/tenncare/carveout.coverltr.pdf

Bussman, J. W. (1993). The Oregon Health Plan: A rational approach to care for the underserved. *Journal of Health Care for the Poor and Underserved, 4,* 203–209.

Cantor, J. C., Long, S. H., & Marquis, M. S. (1995). Private employment-based health insurance in ten states. *Health Affairs, 14,* 199–234.

Colburn, D. (2003a, January 8). Oregon pharmacies plan co-pay suits. *The Oregonian,* p. B2.

Colburn, D. (2003b, March 18). Oregon hospitals sue state over cutting low-income health plan payments. *The Oregonian,* p. B7.

Colburn, D. (2003c, April 30). 10,000 low-income Oregonians will be cut from state health plan. *The Oregonian,* pp. B1, B4.

Donelan, K., Blendon, R. J., Schoen, C., Davis, K., & Binns, K. (1999). The cost of health system change: Public discontent in five nations. *Health Affairs, 18,* 206–216.

Drug Effectiveness Review Project. (2006a). *Drug Effectiveness Review Project. OHSU.* Retrieved from http://www.ohsu.edu/drugeffectiveness.index.htm

Drug Effectiveness Review Project. (2006b). *Drug Effectiveness Review Project description.* Retrieved from http://www.ohsu.edudrugeffectiveness/description/index.htm

Epstein, A. Z. M., Bogen, J., Dreyer, P., & Thorpe, K. E. (1991). Trends in lengths of stay and rates of readmission in Massachusetts: Implications for monitoring quality of care. *Inquiry, 28,* 19–28.

External Quality Review Organization. First Mental Health, Inc. (1997). *TennCare, inpatient admissions due to diabetes: A report of regional and managed care organization variation.* Retrieved from www.//www.state.tn.us/governor/Nov1999/tenncare.htm

Findlay S. D. (2006, June 6). Bringing the DERP to consumers: "*Consumer Reports* best buy drugs." *Health Affairs, 25,* w283–w286. 10.1377/hlthaff.25.w283

Folland, S., Goodman, A. C., & Stano, M. (1997). *The economics of health and health care* (2nd ed.). Englewood Cliffs, NJ: Prentice-Hall.

Fortune, B. (1999). *Governor proposes major changes to TennCare.* News release. Office of Governor Don Sundquist. Retrieved from http://www.state.tn.us/governor/Nov1999/tenncare.htm

Fox, W. F., & Lyons, W. (1998). *The impact of TennCare: A survey of recipients.* Center for Business and Economic Research, University of Tennessee, Knoxville. Retrieved from http://www.state.tn.us/tenncare/reports

Fuchs, V. R. (1992). The best health care system in the world? *Journal of the American Medical Association, 268,* 916–917.

Gardner, J. (1995). Medical savings accounts make waves. *Modern Healthcare, 25*(9), 57.

Gibson, M., & Santa, J. (2006, June 6). The Drug Effectiveness Review Project: An important step forward. *Health Affairs, 25,* w272–w275. 10.1377/hlthaff.25.w2720

Gold, M., Chu, K., & Lyons, B. (1995). *Managed care and low-income populations: A case study of managed care in Oregon.* Washington, DC: Mathematica Policy Research, Inc.

Goodman, J. C., & Pauly, M. V. (1995). Tax credits for health insurance and medical savings accounts. *Health Affairs, 14,* 126–139.

Gostin, L. O., & Widiss, A. I. (1993). What's wrong with the ERISA vacuum? *Journal of the American Medical Association, 269,* 2527–2532.

Greenberg, R. B. (1988). Medicare Catastrophic Coverage Act of 1988. *American Journal of Hospital Pharmacy, 45,* 2518–2525.

Health Insurance Institute of America. (1989). *Source book of health insurance data. 1989.* Washington, DC: Health Insurance Association of America.

Holahan, J., Coughlin, T., Ku, L., Lipson, D. J., & Rajan, S. (1995). Insuring the poor through Section 1115 waivers. *Health Affairs, 14*(1), 199–216.

Hsiao, W. C. (1995). Medical savings accounts: Lessons from Singapore. *Health Affairs, 14,* 260–266.

Hurley, R. E. (2006, April 25). TennCare—a failure of politics, not policy: A conversation with Gordon Bonnyman. *Health Affairs, 25,* w217–w225. 10.1377/hlthaff.25.w217

Iglehart, J. K. (1982). The future of HMOs. *New England Journal of Medicine, 307,* 451–456.

Jacobs, L., Marmor, T., & Oberlander, J. (1999). The Oregon health plan and the political paradox of rationing: What advocates and critics have claimed and what Oregon did. *Journal of Health Politics, Policy and Law, 24*(1), 161–180.

Jeffers, J. R., Bognanno, M. E., & Bartlett, J. C. (1971). On the demand versus need for medical services and the concept of "shortage." *American Journal of Public Health, 61,* 46–63.

Kaiser Commission on Medicaid and the Uninsured. (2005). *The uninsured and their access to health care.* Retrieved from http://www.kff.org/uninsured/1420-07.cfm

Kaplan, R. M. (1994). Value judgment in the Oregon Medicaid experiment. *Medical Care, 32,* 975–988.

Leichter, H. M. (1999). Oregon's bold experiment: Whatever happened to rationing? *Journal of Health Politics, Policy and Law, 24*(1), 147–160.

Lewin, J. C., & Sybinsky, P. A. (1993). Hawaii's employer mandate and its contribution to universal access. *Journal of the American Medical Association, 269,* 2538–2543.

Lillie-Blanton, M., Rushing, O. E., & Ruiz, S. (2003). *Key facts, race, ethnicity and medical care.* Menlo Park, California: Henry J. Kaiser Family Foundation.

Medicare Trustees. (2006, May). *2006 Annual report of the boards of trustees of the federal hospital insurance and federal supplementary medical insurance trust funds.* Washington, DC: U.S. Government Printing Office.

Minicozzi, A. (2006). Medical savings accounts: What do the data tell? *Health Affairs, 25,* 256–267.

Mirvis, D. M., Chang, C. F., Hall, C. J., Zaar, G. T., & Applegate, W. B. (1995). TennCare—health system reform for Tennessee. *Journal of the American Medical Association, 274,* 1235–1241.

Neumann, P. J. (2006, June 6). Emerging lessons from the Drug Effectiveness Review Project. *Health Affairs, 25,* w262–w271. 10.1377/hlthaff.25.w262

OECD health data 2006: A comparative analysis of 30 countries. Paris, France: Organisation for Economic Cooperation and Development.

O'Sullivan, J. (1996). *Medicare: Financing the Part A Hospital Insurance program* (95–650 EPW). Washington, DC: CRS Report for Congress, Congressional Research Service, Library of Congress.

Peterson, W. C. (1996). Those Social Security trust funds. *Omaha World Herald,* p. 15B.

Remler, D. K., & Giled, S. A. (2006). How much more cost sharing will health savings accounts bring? *Health Affairs, 25*(4), 1070–1078.

Robinson, J. C. (2005). Health savings accounts—the ownership society in health care. *New England Journal of Medicine, 353*(12), 1199–1201.

Rojas-Burke, J. (2003, January 28). Spending cuts, recession puts state's hospitals under pressure. *The Oregonian,* pp. C1, C3.

Smith, M. D., Altman, D. E., Leitman, R., Moloney, T. W. & Taylor, H. (1992). Taking the public's pulse on health system reform. *Health Affairs,* 11, 125-133.

Starr, P. (1982). *The social transformation of American medicine.* New York: Basic Books.

Steinbrook, R. (2006). Health care reform in Massachusetts: A work in progress. *New England Journal of Medicine, 354*(20), 2095–2098.

Steves, D. (2003, July 11). New figures may force cuts in Oregon health plan. *The Register Guard,* pp. A1, A9.

Vermont State Legislature. (2006). *2006 health care reform initiatives, quick overview. State of Vermont.* Retrieved from http://www.leg.state.vt.us/Health-Care/2006_HC_Affordability_Act_Leddy_Summary.htm

VPIRG. (2006). *The 2006 Vermont Health Care Affordability Act—frequently asked questions.* Retrieved from http://www.vpirg.org/campaigns/healthCare/documents/06.06.27_FINAL.CatamountQA.pdf

Weissman, J. (1996). Uncompensated hospital care: Will it be there if we need it? *Journal of the American Medical Association, 276,* 823–828.

Yankelovich, D. (1995). The debate that wasn't: The public and the Clinton health care plan. *Brookings Review, 13,* 36–41.

Glossary

Academic detailing: a tool used by managed care organizations (MCOs) in which a health plan representative (or the contracting pharmacy benefit manager [PBM]) visits targeted physicians to provide information regarding the most cost-effective use of selected drugs and to encourage physicians to prescribe in ways that will reduce overall costs while maintaining program quality. The targeted physicians are usually identified by the practice profiling program as ones with higher than average costs or unusual prescribing patterns.

Accreditation: the formal review process that institutions, such as schools and colleges of pharmacy and hospitals, periodically undergo to ensure that they are meeting predetermined quality and standards.

Accrediting agencies: independent organizations that develop standards for entities such as hospitals, home care providers, and colleges and universities, among others. Accrediting organizations are not federal or state agencies.

Activities of daily living (ADLs): activities that are performed during the course of a normal day, such as bathing, toileting, dressing, and eating.

Activity–passivity model of care: as described by Szasz and Hollender, practitioner–patient communication in which the patient is passive. This interaction can be compared to a parent–infant relationship.

Actual acquisition cost (AAC): the price that pharmacies pay for drug products after subtracting all discounts.

Actuary: an insurance company employee who conducts a statistical analysis of an insured population to estimate the income (premiums) that must be earned to cover the estimated expenses, usually expressed as cost per member per month (PMPM).

Adjudication: the process of reviewing or screening claims to determine payment.

Adulterated: made impure by adding extraneous, improper, or inferior ingredients.

Adverse drug reaction: an undesirable or harmful reaction to a drug that occurs at doses normally used for the treatment, prevention, or diagnosis of a disease.

Adverse selection: a situation in which individuals or companies purchase insurance only when they expect a loss.

Alternative health therapy: nontraditional sources of health care, such as use of herbal and nutritional supplements, acupuncture, support groups, meditation, and massage therapy, among others.

Ambulatory care: health care services provided to a patient who is not an inpatient in a health care institution (e.g., a nursing home or hospital) and can walk or move about to obtain these services.

American Hospital Association (AHA): a national organization composed hospitals, health care organizations, and individual members. It provides education to the public and its members, and advocates for and represents its membership in legislative and regulatory issues.

Ambulatory patient groups (APGs): a type of prospective payment for outpatient services that is based on diagnosis.

Asepsis: a practice introduced in the late 19th century that consists of washing hands and using sterilized instruments for surgery in an effort to stop the spread of infectious diseases.

Average manufacturer's price (AMP): a proposed method for estimating pharmacy acquisition costs that is based on actual costs charged by manufacturers rather than the wholesale list price.

Average wholesale price (AWP): the list price established by the manufacturer. AWP is higher than the actual acquisition cost (AAC) that pharmacies pay for drug products and is discounted by the payer to arrive at the estimated acquisition cost (EAC).

Balanced Budget Act of 1997: law that required the implementation of a prospective payment system (PPS) for home health services, reductions in reimbursement rates for home medical equipment, and implementation of competitive bidding processes. Under a PPS, a home health agency is paid a flat rate to care for a Medicare recipient.

Benefit-to-cost ratio: a method of representing outcomes in a cost-benefit analysis whereby total benefits are divided by total costs.

Biopsychosocial model of care: a model of care in which the social, emotional, and psychological aspects of the patient are taken into account, as well as the patient's physical status, in understanding his or her health or illness.

Blue Cross and Blue Shield: originally a nonprofit health insurance established in 1929 offering comprehensive plans. Most Blue Cross and Blue Shield plans switched to for-profit status in the 1990s.

Brand-name drug product: the original product first developed, marketed, and made available by a pharmaceutical company; contrast this with a *generic drug product*.

Bricks-and-mortar: a term for the situation in which an establishment's (usually a business establishment's) operations are conducted in a physical space, as opposed to online. Many establishments have both online and bricks-and-mortar presences.

Capitation: a type of prospective payment in which providers are paid a fixed amount each month for each enrolled patient, regardless of the amount of health care services actually provided.

Catastrophic hazard: a situation in which an insurance company incurs excessive losses due to widespread and catastrophic events such as hurricanes, acts of war, and earthquakes. Companies that provide casualty insurance limit their exposure for catastrophic events by trying to avoid insuring large numbers of policyholders in the same geographic area.

Centralized pharmacy services: pharmacy services that are provided from a single location from within the hospital.

Certification: process by which a non-regulatory agency recognizes an individual who has met certain qualifications, such as successfully completing an examination following an intensive course of self-study.

Certified pharmacy technician (CPhT): an individual designated and recognized for completing the certification requirements administered by The Institute for the Certification of Pharmacy Technicians (ICPT) or the Pharmacy Technician Certification Board (PTCB).

Changes in demand: a shift in an entire demand curve such that the quantity demanded changes even though price remains constant. An increase in demand is represented by a rightward shift of the demand curve; a decrease in demand is illustrated by a leftward shift of the demand curve.

Changes in quantity demanded: a movement along a given demand curve caused by a change in price. The demand schedule shows that as the price charged increases, the quantity demanded decreases.

Therefore, a change in quantity demanded is caused solely by a change in the price charged to customers.

Changes in quantity supplied: a movement along a given supply curve caused by a change in price. The supply schedule shows that, as the price that customers are willing to pay increases, the quantity supplied increases. Therefore, a change in quantity supplied is caused solely by a change in the price charged to customers.

Changes in supply: a shift in an entire supply curve such that that the quantity supplied changes even though price customers are willing to pay remains constant. An increase in supply is represented by a rightward shift of the supply curve; a decrease in supply is illustrated by a leftward shift of the supply curve.

Charitable hospitals: Medical care facilities in the 19th century that housed impoverished patients who had no friends or relatives to care for them. These institutions provided patients with only the bare necessities. The public generally perceived these institutions as places to die; professionals saw them as places to develop clinical experience.

Children's Health Insurance Program (1997): a program that expanded health insurance to at least half of the 11 million U.S. children lacking health insurance.

Chronic diseases: illnesses that last a long time, affecting patients either continuously or episodically. Chronic illnesses such as heart disease and cancer began to appear with greater frequency in the early 20th century.

Clinical testing of new drugs: the phase of testing required by the FDA in which the drug entity is first used in human subjects to determine its safety and efficacy.

Co-insurance: a form of patient cost sharing that requires patients to pay a specified percentage (usually 20%) of the cost of covered services; the plan pays the remainder.

Community chain pharmacy: a retail pharmacy that serves the general public and that is owned by a larger corporation (e.g., Walgreens, CVS, Rite-Aid).

Community health centers (CHCs): federally supported health centers that provide primary-care services (e.g., physicians, physician extenders, laboratory services, dental services, social services, and pharmaceutical services) to underserved areas in urban and rural areas of the United States.

Community independent pharmacy: a retail pharmacy that serves the general public and that is independently owned, usually by a pharmacist.

Community pharmacy: any independent, chain, or supermarket-based pharmacy that provides pharmaceutical products and services to ambulatory patients.

Community rating: a method of setting insurance premiums based on the insurance company's overall expenses for a specific geographic area during the previous year.

Complements: products that tend to influence the purchase of other related products, such that an increase in the price of one good can cause a decrease in the demand for another good.

Comprehensive: characteristic whereby essential health care benefits are covered.

Comprehensive health reform: extensive reform legislation that would broadly and fundamentally change the health care system in reference to financing and delivery.

Consumer drug use: the act of using medications by the general public.

Consumer model of care: a practitioner–patient model of care in which patients have a greater autonomy in decision making and are somewhat skeptical "buyers" of medical care.

Continuing care retirement community: a retirement community that provides a continuum of independent living, assisted living, and skilled nursing care on a single campus.

Coordination of benefits: a provision in insurance contracts that is designed to prevent duplicate payments by more than one insurance plan for the same medical care by limiting total reimbursement from all insurance plans for the same event to the amount of the actual loss. Health insurance policies usually pay after automobile, homeowners', or workers' compensation insurance policies have paid their portion.

Co-payment: a form of patient cost sharing that requires patients to pay a specified dollar amount every time a service is received (e.g., $50 per hospital admission or $5 per prescription).

Cost-benefit analysis: a method used to evaluate two or more alternatives where the input and outcomes are measured in dollars.

Cost-consequence analysis: a method used to evaluate two or more alternatives where the inputs are measured in dollars and the outcome is measured using a variety of methods, including natural units of effectiveness, quality-adjusted life-years (QALYs), or dollars.

Cost containment: concept considered to either decrease health care spending or restrain the growth of health care spending. It has become the focus of much of health care reform since the 1970s.

Cost-effectiveness analysis: a method used to evaluate two or more alternatives where the inputs are measured in dollars and the outcome is measured in natural units of effectiveness.

Cost-minimization analysis: a method used to evaluate two or more alternatives where the inputs are measured in dollars and the consequences or outcomes of the alternatives are identical.

Cost sharing: a provision in managed care plans requiring patients to share in the cost of services received. Cost sharing attempts to optimize utilization of health services by making patients more cost-conscious. It can take many forms, including co-payments, co-insurance, deductibles, out-of-pocket limits, or maximum benefits.

Cost-utility analysis: a method used to evaluate two or more alternatives where the input is measured in dollars and the outcome is measured as life-years saved or patient-preference weighted outcome.

Counterdetailing: see *academic detailing.*

Counterfeiting: creating fraudulent medical products and passing them off as the real thing.

Cyberpharmacy: see *Internet pharmacy.*

Decentralized national health program: a type of health care system where the administration of health care delivery is divided among various groups.

Decentralized pharmacy services: pharmacy services that are provided from satellite locations in patient care areas, or specialized areas, such as the operating room or emergency department.

Decision analysis: a systematic approach to decision making under conditions of uncertainty. This approach uses existing data and models the outcomes based on the best available data.

Decision tree: a type of decision analysis whereby all possible consequences of a decision are mapped in a branching or tree shape.

Deductible: a form of patient cost sharing that requires patients to pay their own health care expenses until a specified dollar amount has been paid out-of-pocket during a given period of time, usually a year.

Demand: the ability and willingness of a consumer to pay for a good or service.

Demand curve: a graphic representation of a demand schedule.

Demand schedule: a table or chart that shows the amounts of a commodity consumers are willing and able to purchase at each specific price charged in a set of possible prices during some specified period of time.

Two variables exist: (1) the price charged by the supplier (independent variable) and (2) the quantity demanded by the consumer at each given price (dependent variable). It is assumed, for the sake of simplicity, that all other variables are held constant.

Developed nation: any country with a high standard of living that is characterized by high per capita incomes, strong health infrastructures, and positive health care outcomes. Also known as an industrialized country.

Developing nation: any country with a low standard of living that is characterized by low per capita incomes, weak health infrastructures, and poor health care outcomes.

Diagnosis-related group (DRG): a categorization of diseases of conditions created initially by the federal government as a means to reimburse hospitals prospectively for services provided to patients.

Direct medical costs: the medical inputs or resources consumed that are directly related to the product or service being evaluated.

Direct nonmedical costs: those nonmedical resources consumed that are directly related to the product or service being evaluated.

Direct-to-consumer advertising (DTCA): the act of advertising prescription medications to the general public through a variety of media.

Discounted fee-for-service: a retrospective reimbursement rate in which health care providers are paid a negotiated fee each time a service is provided. The agreed-upon rate is lower than the providers' usual and customary charges to cash-paying patients.

Discounting: the process of converting dollars, either paid out or received over time periods of more than one year, to their present value. The purpose is to incorporate the time preference for money into the analysis.

Disease management: a system of coordinated health care interventions and communications for populations with conditions in which patient self-care efforts are a significant component of care.

Dispensary: separate, freestanding institutions in urban neighborhoods designed to provide medical care for the poor, usually employing a physician and/or pharmacist.

Dispense as written (DAW): a provision in the participating pharmacy agreement that allows full reimbursement for the higher-cost multiple-source drug product if the pharmacy indicates on the prescription claim that the prescriber demanded a brand-name product instead of its generic equivalent.

Dispenser: points of distribution for medications through the pharmaceutical supply chain (e.g., manufacturer, wholesaler, pharmacy).

Drug therapy monitoring: verifying drug, dose, and route of administration and monitoring for medication-related problems to optimize drug therapy.

Drug use control: the system of knowledge, understanding, judgments, procedures, skills, controls, and ethics that assures optimal safety in the distribution and use of medications.

Drug use evaluation (DUE): an evaluation of the use of one or more drugs prescribed for one or more diseases or conditions within the context of quality assurance and risk management procedures.

Drug utilization evaluation: see *drug use evaluation.*

Drug utilization review (DUR): the review of physician prescribing, pharmacist dispensing, and patient use of drugs with the goal of ensuring that drugs are used appropriately, safely, and effectively. A DUR may be conducted prospectively or retrospectively.

Drug wholesaler: a company that buys pharmaceuticals directly from manufacturers and then resells those drugs to individual pharmacies.

Duration of treatment: a measure of how long patients continue receiving treatment. For hospitals, this means length of stay; for physicians, the episode of care; and for pharmacies, the number of prescription refills.

Earned discount: the difference between the average wholesale price and the pharmacy's actual acquisition cost.

Economic resources: (1) land, including all natural resources, (2) labor, and (3) capital, including physical resources produced by labor. Economists refer to these three basic economic resources as factors of production because they are used to produce those things that people desire (commodities).

Economics: the study of how individuals and societies allocate their limited resources in attempts to satisfy their unlimited wants.

Effectiveness: the ability of a product to produce an effect in real-world practice, typically outside of the well-controlled setting of clinical trials.

Efficacy: the ability of a product to produce an effect, typically demonstrated in randomized controlled clinical trials.

Efficiency: a term used to describe the goal of producing the greatest output for the lowest net cost.

Elastic demand: a situation in which consumers are relatively sensitive to price changes, such that an increase in price will result in a decrease in total revenue.

Elasticity: economic concept that measures the responsiveness of consumer demands to a change in price.

Electronic data interchange (EDI): the transfer of data between organizations using networks or the Internet.

Elimination period: a restriction found in group insurance policies that is aimed at reducing adverse selection by restricting coverage for preexisting health problems until after the policyholder has been covered for a given period of time. Expenses related to pregnancy and childbirth, for example, may not be covered for the first 9 months of a new policy. Elimination periods are often waived when new employees are hired and during open enrollment periods.

Emergency services: a wide range of "emergent and urgent" services provided in hospital emergency rooms to emergency medical services (e.g., 9-1-1, emergency medical vans, paramedics, trauma centers, and emergicenters).

Employee mandate: a requirement usually set by a state law requiring all employees to purchase health insurance.

Employee Retirement Income Security Act (ERISA): a federal law designed to protect employees' benefits, including health insurance and retirement plans. Self-insured plans are exempt from state employer mandates under ERISA.

Employer mandate: a proposal that would require employers to provide health insurance for all their workers or pay a tax that would create an insurance pool for the uninsured.

Equilibrium price: the price corresponding to the point where the demand curve and the supply curve intersect; the price where the market can rest without a natural tendency to increase or decrease price.

Equilibrium quantity: the quantity corresponding to the point where the demand curve and the supply curve intersect; the quantity where the market can rest without a natural tendency to increase or decrease the quantity supplied or demanded.

Estimated acquisition cost (EAC): the amount paid by a pharmacy benefit manager (PBM) for drug ingredient costs, calculated as a percentage of the average wholesale price.

Exclusive provider organization (EPO): a form of PPO in which no coverage is provided for care received outside the provider network.

Experience rating: a method of setting insurance premiums based on the insurance company's overall expenses for a specific subset of insured individuals—usually an employer group—based on the group's experience for the previous year.

Factors explaining changes in mortality rates and life expectancy: improvements in public health measures (e.g., garbage collection, pure water, clean air, sewerage disposal), improvements in lifestyle (e.g., domestic sanitary practices, diet), and therapeutic interventions (e.g., anesthetics, antibiotics, surgical procedures).

Fee-for-service (FFS): reimbursement in which a fee is paid to a provider for each service performed. FFS was the predominant reimbursement mechanism before managed care; some MCO contracts still allow a discounted FFS. FFS provides incentives to increase the quantity of services provided.

First dollar coverage: a reimbursement mechanism in which there is no provision for patient cost sharing.

Fiscal intermediary: an organization that facilitates exchanges between health care payers and health care providers by underwriting and/or administering health care benefit programs.

Flat of the curve: a point where additional health care expenditures produce relatively little incremental benefit to the patient.

Flexner Report: a report on the state of medical education in the United States sponsored by Carnegie Foundation and prepared by Abraham Flexner in 1910. The report examined such factors as entrance requirements, teaching, labs, financing, and clinical status. Recommendations of the report resulted in closure of inadequate medical schools and new emphasis on scientific, lab-based medical education.

Floor-stock distribution: a drug distribution system that involves supplying the nursing staff units with a predetermined number of dosage forms, which are stored in a separate drug room on each patient care area. Nurses dispense the medications to any number of patients from this supply, and then they reorder from the pharmacy as needed.

Formal care or caregiving: care that is provided by health care workers in an institution or offered by other organizations.

Formulary: a list of medications compiled by a hospital or pharmacy benefit manager (PBM) that contain either those drugs approved for use within the hospital or for reimbursement by the PBM. Medications are included based on the relative clinical benefit and cost of the medication as compared to other agents within a similar therapeutic class.

Full-time equivalent (FTE): a unit of labor supply equal to one person working full-time, approximately 40 hours per week.

Gatekeeper: a central component of most HMOs in which primary-care physicians must coordinate and authorize all medical services, including laboratory services, specialty referrals, and hospitalizations. In many gatekeeper systems, a patient must receive a referral from his or her primary-care physician to receive coverage for a specialist's care. The rationale underlying this approach is that it avoids unnecessary and often expensive referrals to specialists. The gatekeeper may be financially at risk—not only for the services that he or she provides, but also for the medical services provided by specialists to whom a patient is referred.

Generic drug product: a drug product manufactured by a company other than the one that originally developed the product, after the original product's patent has expired.

Gross domestic product (GDP): the market value of all final goods and services produced within a country within a given period of time.

Gross margin (GM): the difference between the selling price and the cost to the pharmacy for the product that was sold.

Group-model HMO: a type of HMO characterized by contracts with large, multispecialty medical groups offering services exclusively to the HMO on a capitated basis.

Group policies: insurance plans sponsored by employer groups for employees and their dependents. Group policies are usually less expensive than individual policies because they are less subject to adverse selection and because they are less expensive to sell and administer.

Guidance cooperation model of care: as described by Szasz and Hollender; practitioner–patient communication in which the patient is active in the interaction, but defers to medical expertise. This interaction can be compared to a parent–adolescent relationship.

Health belief model: a health behavior theory that describes the likelihood an individual will take action to change a behavior. Components of this theory include susceptibility and severity of disease, perceived benefits and barriers, cues to action, self-efficacy, and demographic, sociopsychological, and structural variables.

Health department: a public health agency at the federal, state, or local level that is established to identify and manage health problems that affect individuals and population groups (e.g., environmental sanitation, communicable diseases, chronic diseases, immunizations, maternal and child health clinics, and prevention services).

Health insurance: a situation in which individuals or employers "buy" a plan from a company to assist them in paying for health care costs incurred. Insurance coverage varies, but often includes physician visits, hospitalizations, laboratory tests, and other medical expenses.

Health Insurance Portability and Accountability Act of 1996 (HIPAA): a law enacted by Congress that limits the amount of time a preexisting condition may be excluded from coverage to one year, requires insurance companies to sell health insurance policies to small employers and individuals who lose coverage without regard to their health history, requires insurance companies to renew policies they sell to groups and individuals, and outlines standards for patient confidentiality.

Health maintenance organization (HMO): a type of managed care organization that shares risk with a network of health care providers by requiring that the providers assume some risk, either directly or indirectly, and that generally does not provide coverage for medical care that is received outside the network. The risk arrangement can take many forms, such as capitation or risk pools. The gatekeeper is a central component of most HMOs. The four basic types of HMO models are staff models, group models, network models, and independent practice associations.

Health Maintenance Organization Act of 1973: a federal law that set standards and provided start-up funds for health maintenance organizations—specialized insurance plans that involve restrictive provider networks and primary-care gatekeepers that are responsible for referrals to other health care services and risk sharing with providers. This act also required employers with more than 25 employees to offer a HMO plan.

Health Plan Employer Data and Information Set (HEDIS): a group of performance measures developed by NCQA, which gives plan sponsors objective information that they can use to evaluate MCOs.

Health savings account (HSA): a provision of the Medicare Prescription Drug Improvement and Modernization Act that established tax-free savings accounts to be used for out-of-pocket medical expenses for those individuals who select a high-deductible health insurance plan.

Health Security Act: a Clinton administration proposal that would have imposed an employer mandate and established managed competition in which health providers would compete for patients based on cost and value.

Heroic medical therapy: an aggressive type of patient care that used depletive and strengthening measures to return the patient's diseased body to equilibrium. Methods used included leeches, tonics, medical instruments, and medicines to bleed, purge, puke, or sweat patients.

Home care: provision of heath care services in a patient's home that are intended to restore and maintain the patient's optimal level of well-being in a familiar environment.

Home care standards for pharmacists: standards established by the American Society of Health-System Pharmacists that apply to activities pertaining to home care pharmacy practice. These standards establish a minimum level of pharmacy services within this component of pharmacy practice.

Home health services: services usually associated with nursing care provided through a home health agency. They may also include speech and physical therapy or other types of rehabilitation therapies, homemaker services, social services, and hospice care.

Home infusion therapy: the parenteral administration of drugs, solutions, and nutrition to patients in their homes.

Horizontal integration: integration of two or more hospitals—frequently a large, urban, tertiary care hospital and a small community hospital—to provide a larger number of services and increase the hospitals' managerial efficiency.

Hospice: care provided for individuals who are terminally ill or close to death.

Hospital clinics: ambulatory care clinics in hospitals that range from family practice and internal medicine (e.g., general medicine, cardiology, dermatology) to surgical clinics (e.g., general surgery, urology, orthopedics, plastic surgery).

Hospital Survey and Construction Act of 1946 (Hill-Burton Act): a federal law that established hospitals in rural, town, and city areas that were previously underserved and provided renovations and extensions to already-existing hospitals. This act contributed to the growth of major medical centers, which are now widespread in the United States.

Hospitals at the turn of the 20th century: orthodox physicians and trustees sought private paying patients from the middle and upper classes. These institutions implemented the germ theory of disease and introduced new aseptic and antiseptic techniques and new technology such as X-rays. The architectural design focused on private and semiprivate rooms rather than the ward arrangement prevalent in charitable hospitals.

Human capital approach: a method used to value lives saved in terms of the income that the person could have earned the remaining productive years of his or her life.

Humoralism: Galen's second-century concept that saw the human body as interrelated and in natural balance. Health equaled a human body in balance; disease meant the body's system was in disequilibrium.

Incremental cost-effectiveness ratio: a ratio comparing the additional cost incurred to the additional benefit provided by one alternative relative to another option.

Incremental health reform: step-by-step, slow passage of individual pieces of health legislation.

Indemnity: a form of insurance that traditionally required patients to submit claims for reimbursement. Today the term is often used to refer to any health insurance plan with fee-for-service reimbursement and few cost controls.

Independent practice association (IPA)-model HMO: a type of HMO in which physicians form a separate legal entity, usually a corporation or partnership, that then contracts with the MCO. The IPA usually shares risk with the MCO and individual providers are paid by the IPA for services provided to enrolled patients for a negotiated fee. The IPA may reimburse physicians on a discounted FFS basis or may share some risk with them. These physicians typically have their own private practices and are allowed to provide services to patients enrolled in other MCOs.

Indian Health Service (IHS): managed by the U.S. Public Health Service, the system of hospitals and ambulatory care centers that provides health care and pharmacy services to nearly 1.5 million American Indians and Alaska natives living on or near reservations.

Indirect costs: those costs "indirectly" associated with the product or service under evaluation. Examples of indirect costs include the cost of lost productivity associated with an illness and the costs borne by caregivers.

Induced demand: the increased demand for health care services that is created by the availability of insurance payment. Health care providers, especially physicians, can increase utilization of health services by creating more demand for the services they provide.

Inelastic demand: a situation in which consumers are relatively insensitive to price changes, such that an increase in price will not result in a decrease in demand.

Infant mortality rate: the number of children younger than one year of age who die during a particular year divided by the number of live births during the same year.

Infectious diseases: communicable, contagious diseases that historically killed large numbers of people. These diseases are always present (endemic) or appear occasionally with great intensity (epidemic). They include pneumonia, gastritis, measles, smallpox, and scarlet fever.

Informal care or caregiving: care provided by family or friends to an individual.

Inpatient prospective payment system (IPPS): the reimbursement or payment mechanism used for Medicare beneficiaries receiving hospital care. Payment is based on the patient's diagnosis and is determined prior to the patient receiving care. Also referred to as the DRG payment method.

Inputs: as related to pharmaceuticals, all resources—including but not limited to human capital and supplies—that are needed to produce optimal outcomes.

Institutional pharmacy: the practice of pharmacy usually found in hospitals and larger health care systems and organizations.

Instrumental activities of daily living (IADLs): activities that are required for independent living, but are not necessarily performed on a daily basis, such as meal preparation, housework, balancing a checkbook, driving, and using a telephone.

Insurable hazard: a type of pure risk that can lead to specific, measurable, and substantial losses that are unanticipated for an individual, but that are anticipated and relatively predictable for the group as a whole.

Insurable interest: a situation in which the individual who will receive payment for an insurance claim actually experiences a loss when an insurable hazard occurs.

Intangible costs: those costs that cannot be measured or tracked easily or are not associated with a medical or nonmedical resource. Intangible costs are often associated with the pain and suffering due to illness or disease.

Intensity of services: a measure of the types and numbers of services provided. It includes the service mix (types of services), the quantity (per capita use), and the quality of services.

Interdisciplinary: those professionals who work together for the patient's good and who also communicate effectively among themselves and with the patient.

Internet pharmacy: a retail entity in which consumers can purchase pharmaceuticals via an Internet Web site. Also known as a cyberpharmacy.

Investigational new drug (IND): a chemical entity that shows promise as a potential new drug and has been approved by the FDA for clinical testing.

Joint Commission on Accreditation of Healthcare Organizations (JCAHO): a nonprofit organization that sets standards of practice for, evaluates, and accredits more than 15,000 health care organizations and programs in the United States.

Kerr-Mills Act of 1960: an amendment to the Social Security Act that provided health care coverage to poor elderly individuals.

Law of demand: an economic principle that states that, as the price charged for a product or service falls, the corresponding quantity demanded rises; alternatively, as the price charged increases, the corresponding quantity demanded falls. In short, an inverse relationship exists between the price charged and the quantity demanded.

Law of diminishing marginal utility: an economic principle states that the value of any additional goods declines as one consumes more of it. In other words, the more we have of a good, the less we desire it.

Law of large numbers: an insurance principle that states that the larger the number of insured persons, the more accurate the predictions regarding losses. With losses being more predictable, the risk of this loss actually decreases.

Law of supply: an economic principle that states that, as the price customers are willing to pay falls, the corresponding quantity supplied falls; alternatively, as the price customers are willing to pay increases, the corresponding quantity supplied increases. In short, a direct relationship exists between the price customers are willing to pay and the quantity supplied.

Legend drug: a term used to describe a class of drugs created by the Durham-Humphrey Amendments in 1952 that were required to bear the legend, "Caution: Federal law prohibits dispensing without a prescription."

Length of stay (LOS): the amount of time a patient stays in the hospital, calculated from admission to discharge.

Licensure: permission granted by a regulatory body to an individual meeting predetermined qualifications, allowing him or her to practice in a particular occupation or profession.

Life expectancy: average number of years remaining for a person of a given age to live.

Locus of control: a health behavior theory that refers to whether an individual feels the attainment of a particular outcome is within his or her control (e.g., internal locus of control) or outside of it (e.g., external locus of control).

Long-term care services: a set of services—whether health, personal, or social—that is provided over a period of time to individuals who have lost some aspect of functioning.

Mail-order pharmacy: the practice of pharmacy in which consumers mail in their prescriptions to a pharmacy to be filled and mailed back.

Major medical insurance: a type of insurance policy designed to help offset expenses incurred by catastrophic illness or injury. These policies usually have high deductibles and are not designed to cover minor expenses.

Managed behavioral health care: specialty managed care organizations that attempt to reduce the costs of health care by carving out mental health services and using mental health practitioners at discounted fees thus reducing the length of mental health treatment, decreasing the use of hospital treatment, and increasing the use of ambulatory mental health care treatment.

Managed care: the application of cost and quality controls to health care by controlling patient demand and provider supply. The defining feature of managed care is the use of provider networks through a contractual arrangement specifying the types of services to be provided and the reimbursement to be received in return.

Managed care organization (MCO): an organization designed to manage the cost and quality of a health insurance program. The differentiating feature of managed care plans versus fee-for-service plans is the use of a provider network. MCOs are categorized according to their degrees of (1) risk sharing, (2) provider exclusivity, (3) out-of-network coverage, and (4) physician autonomy and organization.

Managed competition: a provision of the Health Security Act that would have organized health care providers into health alliances that would compete with one another for patients based on cost and value.

Manufacturing and distribution: the production of prescription drugs that meet FDA standards for best manufacturing practices. Prescription drugs are sold and distributed by the drug manufacturer to the pharmacy via a direct or wholesale route. In the pharmacy, the drugs are dispensed by the pharmacist for the patient, via the prescription, and are ultimately taken or consumed by the patient.

Marginal utility: the additional utility received from consuming one additional unit of a particular good or service.

Market structure: the categorization of firms based on attributes such as the numbers of buyers and sellers, product differentiation, pricing behavior, and so on. The four types of market structures are perfect competition, monopolistic competition, monopoly, and oligopoly.

Markov model: a type of decision analysis suited to those situations in which the patient may transition from one state to another. The simplest example of a Markov model features a three-state transition—from well to ill to dead.

Maximum allowable cost (MAC): the amount paid by a pharmacy benefit manager (PBM) for the drug ingredient cost for a multiple-source drug. The MAC is usually set at the price of a low-cost generic product without regard as to whether a brand-name or generic product was actually dispensed.

Means testing: a requirement that participants in a program have less than a specified level of income or assets before enrollment or benefits would be granted. Such a requirement may also mandate using a sliding-scale payment mechanism for participation in a program, such that individuals with higher incomes would pay a larger amount than persons with lower incomes.

Medicaid: Title XIX of the Social Security Act; a joint program between the federal and state governments that pays for medical care for individuals who receive case assistance through the Supplemental Security Income (SSI) program and certain low-income pregnant women, children, and other vulnerable groups.

Medicaid waiver: a provision established by the Omnibus Budget Reconciliation Act (OBRA) of 1981 that allows states to apply for exceptions to federal Medicaid guidelines for the purpose of either establishing Medicaid managed care plans or creating new initiatives to curb costs or improve delivery of Medicaid services.

Medicalization: redefining or relabeling of a personal or social problem as a medical condition, thus necessitating treatment for it in the health care system.

Medicare: Title XVIII of the Social Security Act; a federal social health insurance program for individuals 65 years of age and older, individuals who receive disability benefits from Social Security or the Railroad Retirement Board, or individuals with end-stage renal disease requiring dialysis or kidney transplantation.

Medicare Catastrophic Coverage Act: a 1988 proposal to expand Medicare Part B coverage to include outpatient prescription drug coverage.

Medicare Part D: a provision that created a new voluntary outpatient prescription drug benefit for Medicare recipients; it became available in 2006.

Medication adherence: successfully following a specified medication treatment regimen.

Medication assistance programs (MAPs): programs that provide lower-income patients with access to brand-name prescription products from pharmaceutical companies at little or no cost to patients.

Medication delivery: a delivery system for prescription drugs in community and institutional settings that ensures medications are used safely and effectively.

Medication therapy management services (MTMS): a broad range of activities within the scope of practice of pharmacists and other qualified health care providers intended to ensure that patients with multiple diseases and on many medications get the greatest benefit possible from their medication regimen.

Medication-utilization evaluation (MUE): an objective evaluation of selected drug use in the hospital, which is compared to specific criteria established for these medications.

Mental health: functioning at a satisfactory level of physical, mental, and social well-being; a harmonious balance between the individual, his or her social group, and the larger environment context.

Monopolistic competition: a market structure similar to perfect competition except that it does not have standardized and interchangeable products.

Monopoly: a market structure that has only one seller of a product that has no close substitutes.

Monopsony: a market structure that has only one buyer, but several competing suppliers.

Moral hazard: a situation in which patients, with insurance coverage, overconsume health care services to the extent that the additional health benefits achieved from consuming additional health services are not really worth their full costs. Nevertheless, because the enrollees are paying only a fraction of the costs, they still want to use the services. Overconsumption of health services owing to moral hazard increases total health expenditures and insurance premiums.

Mutual participation model of care: as described by Szasz and Hollender, a practitioner–patient communication in which the patient assumes an active role and is equally powerful to the practitioner. This model is most commonly seen with patients who have chronic diseases and can be compared to a parent–adult child relationship.

National Committee for Quality Assurance (NCQA): an independent, nongovernment agency that promotes performance standards, quality assurance, review standards, and accreditation for HMOs.

Net benefit: a method used to represent outcomes in a cost-benefit analysis where the time frame of the analysis is less than or equal to one year.

Net present value: a method used to represent outcomes in a cost-benefit analysis where the time frame of the analysis goes beyond one year.

Network: a defined group of providers, typically linked through contractual arrangements, who supply a full range of primary and acute health care services. Managed care enrollees who use providers outside the network may receive reduced coverage or even no coverage.

Network-model HMO: a type of HMO characterized by nonexclusive contracts with large medical groups. While networks typically bear risk, the nonexclusivity of the arrangement reduces the influence of the risk on the physician's behavior.

New drug application (NDA): the application submitted by a pharmaceutical manufacturer to the FDA for approval of a drug product that has completed the FDA's clinical testing requirements.

New technologies: "advances in communications and networking technologies . . . [including] telemedicine" (National Library of Medicine, 2001).

Nonprescription (over-the-counter [OTC], nonlegend) products: pharmaceutical products that can be purchased without a prescription.

North American Pharmacy Licensure Examination (NAPLEX): an examination created by the National Associated of Boards of Pharmacy (NABP) and used to determine, along with a state's jurisprudence examination, an individual's eligibility to acquire licensure to practice pharmacy.

Off-label drug use: use of drugs for an indication for which they do not have formal approval from the FDA.

Oligopoly: a market structure that consists of a few sellers and many buyers. Firms in oligopolies are often interdependent, and a dominant firm can exert influence through price leadership.

Oligopsony: a market structure that consists of only a few buyers, but several competing suppliers.

Open enrollment period: a short period of time when employees are allowed to join the employer's health insurance plan. Open enrollment, without restrictions for preexisting conditions, is usually available to new employees immediately upon being hired and to incumbent employees during a short period of time (i.e., approximately two weeks) each year.

Opportunity cost: a term used in economics for valuing a resource based on its highest-valued alternative use or market value.

Oregon Health Plan: The Oregon Basic Health Services Act of 1989 expanded the state's Medicaid program to include previously uninsured citizens. To determine what was covered, the program evaluated treatment options based on their effectiveness and their cost.

Orthodox (allopathic, regular, or mainstream) physicians: physicians who possessed some didactic medical education and underwent apprenticeship to develop their clinical skills. They practiced heroic medicine.

Outcome: the impact or effect of drug therapy.

Participating pharmacy agreement: a contract between a pharmacy and a pharmacy benefit manager (PBM) that specifies the rights and duties of each party with regard to prescription drug coverage.

Patent medicines: cheap concoctions in tonic or pill form that were widely advertised in newspapers and popular magazines and sold in pharmacies or by traveling tradesmen.

Patent registration: the period of time during which a manufacturer has exclusive rights to develop, market, and produce a product without competition from other manufacturers.

Patient-centered model of care: a model in which the focus of the practitioner shifts from disease orientation (the body) to the person as a whole. Practitioners are encouraged to view the illness from the patient's eyes.

Patient cost sharing: a provision in health insurance plans that provides financial incentives for patients to avoid using unnecessary health care services by making them pay a portion of the cost of the service. Patient cost-sharing methods include co-payments, co-insurance, deductibles, out-of-pocket limits, and maximum benefit limits.

Patient-induced demand: an increase in the quantity of services demanded resulting from insurance coverage that lowers patients' out-of-pocket expenses. By isolating patients from the true cost of health care services, health insurance has encouraged patients to consume more health care services than they would if they were bearing the full cost of the product or service themselves.

Per diem: a type of prospective reimbursement in which hospitals are paid a flat rate for each day of hospital care provided to covered individuals without regard to the actual costs incurred.

Perfect competition: a market structure characterized by (1) many buyers and sellers, (2) freedom of entry and exit, (3) standardized products, (4) full and free information, and (5) no collusion.

Perspective: the point of reference (typically the decision maker) from which the pharmacoeconomic analysis will be conducted.

Pharmaceutical care: the responsible provision of drug therapy for achieving specific outcomes that improve a patient's quality of life; a term used to define a pharmacy's mission in taking responsibility for patients' medication-related outcomes.

Pharmaceutical manufacturer: a company that participates in the manufacturing of drug products.

Pharmaceutical marketing: techniques used to publicize pharmaceutical products to prescribers and users of those products.

Pharmaceutical research and development (R&D): the process through which a pharmaceutical company discovers and develops new drug entities.

Pharmaceutical Research and Manufacturers of America (PhRMA): a U.S.-based organization that represents the interests of research-based pharmaceutical companies.

Pharmacoeconomics: the evaluation of the inputs and outcomes associated with pharmaceuticals or pharmacy services.

Pharmacoinformatics: the field of informatics that focuses on the creative use of computers and other technologies in support of pharmaceutical services, including patient care, education, and research.

Pharmacotherapy: the use of drugs to treat illness.

Pharmacy benefit manager (PBM): a specialized company that adjudicates prescription drug claims and manages the prescription drug coverage for a third-party payer by containing costs and influencing the quality of services provided.

Pharmacy education: the education that a pharmacist receives in the United States that leads to a doctor of pharmacy degree (PharmD). The PharmD replaced the baccalaureate degree as the entry-level required degree in 2004.

Pharmacy information services: provision of drug and health information by using textbooks, library, and Web-based sources to answer questions and provide information to patients and health professionals.

Pharmacy practice: practice settings where a pharmacist may work, including community pharmacy (e.g., independent, chain, supermarket, and megastore pharmacy), institutional (e.g., hospital, nursing facility, home care, and community health center), education, government, and pharmaceutical industry.

Pharmacy practice residency: an organized, directed, postgraduate training program designed to develop competencies in a defined area of pharmacy practice. These programs may be one or two years.

Pharmacy technician: an assistant to a pharmacist whose roles and functions include medication preparation, customer service, and other activities as deemed appropriate by the employer within the context of state law.

Pharmakon: the Greek term for "drug," meaning remedy, poison, or magical charm.

Physician profiling: a tool used by managed care organizations to analyze the practice patterns of physicians on cost and quality dimensions. Measures are generally expressed as a rate over a specific period of time within the physician's patient population (e.g., the average dollars spent per patient per month).

Point of service plan (POS): a type of managed care organization that is a hybrid of a health maintenance organization and a preferred provider organization. As with a PPO, when care is received from a provider outside the network, partial coverage is provided. As with an HMO, physicians may be at risk or contract exclusively with the plan.

Population effects: a measure of the number of patients and the mix of various demographic factors within the group (e.g., gender, age, socioeconomic status, and other factors) that affect utilization. For hospitals, this means the number of hospital admissions; for physicians, the number of new patients; and for pharmacies, the number of new prescriptions.

Portability: a characteristic whereby health care benefits are readily transportable when individuals change their jobs or place of residence.

Postmarketing surveillance: the act of collecting information about a drug's use after it has been on the market for some time and is used more widely in the population.

Preferred provider organization (PPO): a type of managed care organization that creates a network of providers who agree to discount their charges for services delivered to enrolled beneficiaries. Beneficiaries are free to see any provider they choose, but have a financial incentive (i.e., lower out-of-pocket expenses) to receive care from providers in the preferred network.

Prescriber: a health care professional who is licensed to prescribe medications.

Prescription: an order written by a prescriber for a patient that describes therapy that a patient should receive.

Preventive health care: performance of activities or behaviors for the purpose of avoiding or deterring disease and maintaining health.

Primary care: ambulatory services for common ailments provided by primary-care (first-order or gatekeeper) providers, who include physicians (e.g., family practice, internal medicine, pediatrics, obstetrics, and gynecology), nurse practitioners, and physician assistants.

Professional: a person who possesses specialized technical knowledge, is licensed to practice, and is motivated by a desire to be of service to others.

Prospective drug utilization review (DUR): see *drug utilization review*.

Psychopharmacology: the treatment of mental disorders with the use of prescription drugs.

Psychotherapy: a variety of treatment modalities for treating and evaluating individuals with mental and/or emotional disorders.

Public policy: health or drug policy (e.g., a political position, statement, or viewpoint) that affects the public (community or population). Public policy is often determined at the community, state, and/or federal government level.

Pure risk: a type of risk in which there is a possibility of a loss but no possibility of a gain. This type of risk is insurable.

Quackery: pretending to have medical knowledge or credentials so as to defraud the public; manufacturing or selling nontherapeutic nostrums or medical devices that generally cause harm.

Quality: originally applied to manufacturing, meaning the state of zero defects and reliable engineering processes. It now applies to health care, meaning the reduction of preventable errors and reduced variability in evidence-based best practices (Kerzner, 1995). Quality is considered one of three major facets of the "iron triangle" of health care—cost, access, and quality.

Quality-adjusted life-years (QALYs): an outcome measured as life-years gained adjusted for patient preference or another means of weighting/adjusted gains in life-years.

Quality assurance: quality of care considerations that typically include both assessment of care and a feedback loop to the health care organization that recommends either a continuation or a change in care.

Randomized controlled trials: a research design model in which the unit of analysis (typically a patient) is randomized to one of multiple study arms (typically treatment and control or placebo).

Rebate: payment received by a pharmacy benefit manager (PBM) from a pharmaceutical manufacturer in return for putting a specific drug on the PBM's formulary or giving the drug preferred status. The amount of a rebate may be based on performance (i.e., a certain level of prescribing) or market share (i.e., the percentage of all prescriptions within a given therapeutic class that are dispensed for the company's product).

Regulatory agencies: federal and state agencies that regulate components of the health care industry, such as the Department of Public Health (DPH), the Drug Enforcement Administration (DEA), and the Food and Drug Administration (FDA).

Reinsurance: a type of insurance that protects insurance companies from extraordinary, unexpected losses. Insurance companies are willing to accept some risk of having claims exceed income, but obtain reinsurance to protect them from catastrophic losses. The reinsurance company pools the risks faced by many insurance companies together.

Report card: a periodic report sent by a managed care organization (MCO) to inform providers about how their general performance and compliance with plan guidelines compared with the same characteristics for their colleagues or to the MCO's standards. Typical information on report cards includes cost per patient per month, number of prescriptions per patient per month, percentage of brand-name versus generic prescriptions, compliance with formulary guidelines, and prescribing patterns for selected prescription drugs.

Retrospective claims analysis: analysis that relies on paid administrative pharmacy or medical claims data. It is retrospective in the sense that researchers are typically evaluating events or measuring associations that have occurred in the past.

Retrospective drug utilization review (DUR): see *drug utilization review.*

Risk-bearing: the amount of risk borne by the providers, which can range from full risk to no risk. Physicians typically accept risk in the form of capitation and risk pools; hospitals accept capitation as well as per diem and DRG reimbursement.

Risk pool: an arrangement in which an HMO places a portion of payments in a pool as a source for any subsequent claims that exceed projections, with the provider and the HMO sharing in the surplus (or loss) from the risk pool at the end of the year.

Roemer's law: "A built bed is a filled bed." This statement reflects the historical tendency for health care providers to increase hospital admissions and the use of health care technology when excess capacity exists.

Sectarians (irregular physicians): rivals to orthodox physicians who sought education or training outside the orthodox medical educational system. They represented various beliefs, therapies, or medical systems that competed with the orthodox practice of medicine and included homeopaths and eclectics.

Self-care: the act of consumers selecting and using products or processes to treat health ailments without the supervision of a health care professional.

Self-dosing: do-it-yourself medicine. It uses traditional practices, family recipes, and folk and herbal medicines to treat oneself and one's family.

Sensitivity analysis: a methodological approach whereby assumptions made in modeling are tested to determine how sensitive the results are to changes in key assumptions within the model.

Service benefit: a form of health insurance plan in which health care providers submit claims and are paid directly by the insurance plan.

Shortage: a situation that occurs when the market price is below the equilibrium price, resulting in a quantity supplied that is less than the quantity demanded.

Sickness funds: the common name for the quasi-public, third-party payers characterizing Germany's health care system.

Sin tax: a tax applied to nonessential items, such as alcohol and tobacco products.

Single-payer plan: a plan in which the government is the primary financer in one, all-inclusive health care system.

Skilled nursing facility (SNF): a facility that provides basic medical and nursing care, as well as additional services or therapies, that can include restorative, physical, and occupational therapies.

Social cognitive theory: a health behavior theory that describes an individual's expectations in relation to changing behavior. The model includes two main components: (1) outcome expectations, or the individual's belief that a behavior leads to a specific outcome, and (2) efficacy expectations, or the individual's belief that he or she has the ability to perform this behavior.

Social healers: usually female healers who treated friends and neighbors in rural and small-town communities in the 18th and 19th centuries. Patients sought simple medicines and treatments for boils or wounds as well as advice. Social healers were often also midwives.

Socialized health insurance: a type of health care system where the government provides health insurance to all citizens.

Socialized medicine: a type of health care system where the government participates in or enforces participation in the country's health care system, employs health care practitioners, owns health care facilities, and administers the health care system.

Social partnership: characteristic whereby both the employer and the employee contribute funds to the health care system.

Social Security: a program created by the Social Security Act of 1935 that provides a minimum level of income for qualified individuals who are 65 years of age or older or who are disabled.

Social solidarity: a characteristic whereby some members of a country subsidize other members' health care costs.

Speculative risk: a type of risk in which there is the possibility of either a gain or a loss. Business ventures and gambling are examples of activities in which there is speculative risk. This type of risk is not insurable.

Staff-model HMO: a type of HMO characterized by direct ownership of health care facilities and direct employment physicians. Physicians in a staff-model HMO typically bear no direct risk, but the HMO can influence the physician through utilization review (the review of the necessity and efficiency of patients' utilization patterns).

Subrogation: the process in which an insurance company enforces a coordination of benefits provision by determining which insurance company is required to pay first if a particular patient has duplicate coverage.

Substance abuse disorders: disorders related to the use and abuse of various substances, both legal and illegal. Also referred to as addictive disorders and chemical disorders.

Substitutes: related products that may be interchanged by consumers. When the price of one good increases, the quantity demanded for that good decreases and the demand for its substitute increases.

Supplier-induced demand: an increase in demand created by the service provider. Physicians may induce demand for their own services by ordering follow-up care or referring patients to physician-owned laboratory, pharmacy, radiology, or other diagnostic or treatment services.

Supply: the ability and willingness of a supplier to provide a good or service.

Supply curve: a graphic representation of a supply schedule.

Supply schedule: a table or chart that shows the amount of a commodity suppliers are willing and able to supply at each specific price that customers are willing to pay in a set of possible prices during a specified period of time.

Surplus: a situation in which the market price exceeds the equilibrium price, resulting in a quantity supplied that is greater than the quantity demanded.

Taxonomy: the classification of objects or phenomena into an ordered system that indicates natural relationships.

Technology: the technical means that a person uses to improve his or her surroundings by extending user capabilities and performing repetitive tasks.

Telehealth: providing health care, at a distance, through the use of technologies, including medical, pharmacy, and public health.

Telepharmacy: using technologies to support and deliver pharmaceutical services at a distance, most often in rural areas.

TennCare: Tennessee's program to extend Medicaid coverage to include previously uninsured citizens in managed care plans.

Theory of planned behavior (TPB): a health behavior theory that is an extension of the theory of reasoned action. It includes an additional component relating to the degree an individual has control over the behavior, such as knowledge, time, money, and opportunity.

Theory of reasoned action (TRA): a health behavior theory that hypothesizes an individual's behavior is related to his or her behavioral intention or the likelihood that the person will perform a behavior. According to the model, two main factors contribute to this intention: (1) attitude toward performing the behavior (beliefs and outcome), and (2) the subjective norm (what "important" individuals think of the behavior and the motivation to comply) associated with the behavior.

Tiered co-payments: a type of patient cost sharing that specifies multiple co-payment levels that are designed to encourage the use of preferred drug products, such as generics and lower-cost brand-name drugs.

Total revenue: the average price charged per unit multiplied by the quantity demanded ($TR = P \times Q$).

Transtheoretical model: often referred to as stages of change or readiness to change model. This health behavior theory theorizes that a patient progresses through five stages before a change in behavior occurs: (1) pre-contemplation, (2) contemplation, (3) preparation, (4) action, and (5) maintenance.

Trust fund: a fund that accounts for the moneys collected as Social Security and Medicare taxes.

Uncompensated care pool: an account financed by a tax on hospital bills or general tax revenue that establishes a pool of money used to reimburse hospitals for a portion of the cost of providing medical care to underinsured and uninsured patients.

Underwriting: the process of insuring. Underwriters attempt to calculate the amount of financial risk that they assume for insurable events, estimate losses and administrative expenses (with the aid of actuaries), and set the level of premiums needed to cover expenditures and provide for a reasonable profit.

Unit-dose distribution: a drug distribution system in which each dose of medication is separately packaged and labeled with the drug name, strength, lot number, and expiration date in a ready-to-administer form.

Universality: characteristic whereby all health care benefits are provided for all citizens of a given country.

U.S. drug approval process: the process identified by the FDA, and which pharmaceutical manufacturers must abide by, for products to be approved for use in the United States.

U.S. Federal Trade Commission (FTC): the federal agency that governs unfair business practices.

U.S. Food and Drug Administration (FDA): the federal agency that is responsible for assuring the safety and effectiveness of many food and drug products.

U.S. Pharmacopeia (USP): a nongovernmental, national, public agency responsible for setting standards for all prescription and over-the-counter medicines, dietary supplements, and other health care products manufactured and sold in the United States.

Utility: economic term for the satisfaction obtained from purchasing a particular good or service.

Utilization review: a tool used by managed care organizations (MCOs) to review the necessity and efficiency of health care services, with the aim of decreasing costs and enhancing the safety and quality of services. See also *drug utilization review.*

Vertical integration: the provision of a continuum of health care services. For hospitals, it entails expanding health care services beyond traditional acute medical care to include nursing home care, home health care, and outpatient and rehabilitation services.

Web-based pharmacy: see *Internet pharmacy.*

Willingness-to-pay approach: a method used to value lives saved and/or the intangible benefits and health risks associated with a product or service, whereby individuals express their willingness to pay to reduce a health risk.

Index

page numbers followed by t denote tables; those followed by f denote figures; those followed by ex denote exhibits